THE WASHINGTON MANUAL™

Endocrinology **Subspecialty Consult**

Third Edition

Editors

Janet B. McGill, MD, MA, FACE
Professor of Medicine
Division of Endocrinology, Metabolism,
    and Lipid Research
Washington University School of Medicine
St. Louis, Missouri

Thomas J. Baranski, MD, PhD
Associate Professor of Medicine
Division of Endocrinology, Metabolism,
    and Lipid Research
Washington University School of Medicine
St. Louis, Missouri

William E. Clutter, MD
Associate Professor of Medicine
Division of Endocrinology, Metabolism,
    and Lipid Research
Washington University School of Medicine
St. Louis, Missouri

Series Editors

Katherine E. Henderson, MD
Assistant Professor of Clinical Medicine
Division of Medical Education
Washington University School of
    Medicine
Barnes-Jewish Hospital
St. Louis, Missouri

Thomas M. De Fer, MD
Professor of Medicine
Division of Medical Education
Washington University School of
    Medicine
St. Louis, Missouri

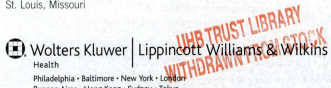

Wolters Kluwer | Lippincott Williams & Wilkins
Health
Philadelphia • Baltimore • New York • London
Buenos Aires • Hong Kong • Sydney • Tokyo

Senior Acquisitions Editor: Sonya Seigafuse
Senior Product Manager: Kerry Barrett
Vendor Manager: Bridgett Dougherty
Senior Marketing Manager: Kimberly Schonberger
Manufacturing Manager: Ben Rivera
Design Coordinator: Stephen Druding
Editorial Coordinator: Katie Sharp
Production Service: Aptara, Inc.

© 2013 by Department of Medicine, Washington University School of Medicine

Printed in China

Library of Congress Cataloging-in-Publication Data

The Washington manual endocrinology subspecialty consult. – 3rd ed. / editors,
Thomas J. Baranski, William E. Clutter, Janet B. McGill.
    p. ; cm. – (Washington manual subspecialty consult series)
Includes bibliographical references and index.
  ISBN 978-1-4511-1407-2 (alk. paper)
  I. Baranski, Thomas J. II. Clutter, William E. III. McGill, Janet B.
  IV. Washington University (Saint Louis, Mo.). School of Medicine.
  V. Title: Endocrinology subspecialty consult. VI. Series: Washington
manual subspecialty consult series.
  [DNLM: 1. Endocrine System Diseases–Handbooks. 2. Metabolic
Diseases–Handbooks. WK 39]
  616.4′8--dc23

                                                    2012020563

The Washington Manual™ is an intent-to-use mark belonging to Washington University in St. Louis to which international legal protection applies. The mark is used in this publication by LWW under license from Washington University.

Care has been taken to confirm the accuracy of the information presented and to describe generally accepted practices. However, the authors, editors, and publisher are not responsible for errors or omissions or for any consequences from application of the information in this book and make no warranty, expressed or implied, with respect to the currency, completeness, or accuracy of the contents of the publication. Application of the information in a particular situation remains the professional responsibility of the practitioner.

The authors, editors, and publisher have exerted every effort to ensure that drug selection and dosage set forth in this text are in accordance with current recommendations and practice at the time of publication. However, in view of ongoing research, changes in government regulations, and the constant flow of information relating to drug therapy and drug reactions, the reader is urged to check the package insert for each drug for any change in indications and dosage and for added warnings and precautions. This is particularly important when the recommended agent is a new or infrequently employed drug.

Some drugs and medical devices presented in the publication have Food and Drug Administration (FDA) clearance for limited use in restricted research settings. It is the responsibility of the health care provider to ascertain the FDA status of each drug or device planned for use in their clinical practice.

To purchase additional copies of this book, call our customer service department at (800) 638-3030 or fax orders to (301) 223-2320. International customers should call (301) 223-2300.

Visit Lippincott Williams & Wilkins on the Internet: at LWW.com. Lippincott Williams & Wilkins customer service representatives are available from 8:30 am to 6 pm, EST.

10 9 8 7 6 5 4 3 2 1

CCS0712

Contributing Authors

Ana Maria Arbelaez, MD
Assistant Professor of Pediatrics
Division of Pediatric Endocrinology
  and Diabetes
Washington University School of Medicine
St. Louis, Missouri

Shunzhong Bao, MD
Fellow
Division of Endocrinology, Metabolism, and
  Lipid Research
Washington University School of Medicine
St. Louis, Missouri

Thomas J. Baranski, MD, PhD
Associate Professor of Medicine
Division of Endocrinology, Metabolism, and
  Lipid Research
Washington University School of Medicine
St. Louis, Missouri

Carlos Bernal-Mizrachi, MD
Assistant Professor of Medicine
Division of Endocrinology, Metabolism, and
  Lipid Research
Washington University School of Medicine
St. Louis, Missouri

Kim Carmichael, MD
Associate Professor of Medicine
Division of Endocrinology, Metabolism, and
  Lipid Research
Washington University School of Medicine
St. Louis, Missouri

Sara Chowdhury, MD
Clinical Fellow
Division of Endocrinology, Metabolism, and
  Lipid Research
Washington University School of Medicine
St. Louis, Missouri

Roberto Civitelli, MD
*Sydney M. and Stella H. Schoenberg
  Professor of Medicine*
*Professor of Orthopaedic Surgery and of
  Cell Biology and Physiology*
Director, Bone and Mineral Diseases
Division of Endocrinology, Metabolism, and
  Lipid Research
Washington University School of Medicine
St. Louis, Missouri

William E. Clutter, MD
Associate Professor of Medicine
Division of Endocrinology, Metabolism,
  and Lipid Research
Washington University School of Medicine
St. Louis, Missouri

Philip E. Cryer, MD
*Irene E. and Michael M. Karl Professor of
  Endocrinology and Metabolism in Medicine*
Division of Endocrinology, Metabolism,
  and Lipid Research
Washington University School of Medicine
St. Louis, Missouri

Kathryn Diemer, MD
Assistant Professor of Medicine
Division of Bone and Mineral Diseases
Washington University School of Medicine
St. Louis, Missouri

Judit Dunai, MD
Clinical Fellow
Division of Endocrinology, Metabolism,
  and Lipid Research
Washington University School of Medicine
St. Louis, Missouri

Simon J. Fisher, MD, PhD
Associate Professor of Medicine, Cell Biology, and Physiology
Division of Endocrinology, Metabolism, and Lipid Research
Washington University School of Medicine
St. Louis, Missouri

Stephen J. Giddings, MD, PhD
Associate Professor of Medicine
St. Louis VA Medical Center
Washington University School of Medicine
St. Louis, Missouri

Anne C. Goldberg, MD, FACP, FAHA
Associate Professor of Medicine
Division of Endocrinology, Metabolism, and Lipid Research
Washington University School of Medicine
St. Louis, Missouri

Scott Goodwin, MD
Clinical Fellow
Division of Endocrinology, Metabolism, and Lipid Research
Washington University School of Medicine
St. Louis, Missouri

Paul Hruz, MD, PhD
Associate Professor of Pediatrics
Division of Pediatric Endocrinology and Diabetes
Washington University School of Medicine
St. Louis, Missouri

Mariko Johnson, MD
Clinical Fellow
Division of Endocrinology, Metabolism, and Lipid Research
Washington University School of Medicine
St. Louis, Missouri

Prajesh M. Joshi, MD
Clinical Fellow
Division of Endocrinology, Metabolism, and Lipid Research
Washington University School of Medicine
St. Louis, Missouri

Kavita Juneja, MD
Clinical Fellow
Division of Endocrinology, Metabolism, and Lipid Research
Washington University School of Medicine
St. Louis, Missouri

Nadia Khoury, MD
Clinical Fellow
Division of Endocrinology, Metabolism, and Lipid Research
Washington University School of Medicine
St. Louis, Missouri

Janet B. McGill, MD, MA, FACE
Professor of Medicine
Division of Endocrinology, Metabolism, and Lipid Research
Washington University School of Medicine
St. Louis, Missouri

Dominic N. Reeds, MD
Associate Professor of Medicine
Division of Geriatrics and Nutritional Science
Washington University School of Medicine
St. Louis, Missouri

Amy E. Riek, MD
Instructor in Medicine
Division of Endocrinology, Metabolism, and Lipid Research
Washington University School of Medicine
St. Louis, Missouri

David A. Rometo, MD
Clinical Fellow
Division of Endocrinology, Metabolism, and Lipid Research
Washington University School of Medicine
St. Louis, Missouri

Julie Silverstein, MD
Instructor in Medicine
Division of Endocrinology, Metabolism, and Lipid Research
Washington University School of Medicine
St. Louis, Missouri

Richard I. Stein, PhD
Research Assistant Professor, Center for
  Human Nutrition
Behavioral Director, Weight Management
  Program
Washington University School of Medicine
St. Louis, Missouri

Garry Tobin, MD
Associate Professor of Medicine
Division of Endocrinology, Metabolism,
  and Lipid Research
Washington University School of Medicine
St. Louis, Missouri

Dwight A. Towler, MD, PhD
Lang Professor of Medicine
Division of Endocrinology, Metabolism,
  and Lipid Research
Washington University School of Medicine
St. Louis, Missouri

Zhiyu Wang, MD, PhD
Clinical Fellow
Division of Endocrinology, Metabolism,
  and Lipid Research
Washington University School of Medicine
St. Louis, Missouri

Michael P. Whyte, MD
*Professor of Medicine, Pediatrics,
  and Genetics*
Division of Bone and Mineral Diseases
Washington University School of Medicine
Medical-Scientific Director, Center
  for Metabolic Bone Disease and
  Molecular Research, Shriners
  Hospitals for Children, St. Louis
St. Louis, Missouri

Kevin Yarasheski, PhD
*Professor of Medicine, Cell Biology,
  and Physiology, and Physical Therapy*
Division of Endocrinology, Metabolism,
  and Lipid Research
Washington University School of Medicine
St. Louis, Missouri

Chairman's Note

I t is a pleasure to present the new edition of *The Washington Manual*™ Subspecialty Consult Series: *Endocrinology Subspecialty Consult*. This pocket-size book continues to be a primary reference for medical students, interns, residents, and other practitioners who need ready access to practical clinical information to diagnose and treat patients with a wide variety of disorders. Medical knowledge continues to increase at an astounding rate, which creates a challenge for physicians to keep up with the biomedical discoveries, genetic and genomic information, and novel therapeutics that can positively impact patient outcomes. The *Washington Manual* Subspecialty Series addresses this challenge by concisely and practically providing current scientific information for clinicians to aid them in the diagnosis, investigation, and treatment of common medical conditions.

I want to personally thank the authors, which include house officers, fellows, and attendings at Washington University School of Medicine and Barnes Jewish Hospital. Their commitment to patient care and education is unsurpassed, and their efforts and skill in compiling this manual are evident in the quality of the final product. In particular, I would like to acknowledge our editors, Drs. Thomas J. Baranski, William E. Clutter, and Janet B. McGill, and the series editors, Drs. Katherine Henderson and Tom De Fer, who have worked tirelessly to produce another outstanding edition of this manual. I would also like to thank Dr. Melvin Blanchard, Chief of the Division of Medical Education in the Department at of Medicine at Washington University School of Medicine, for his advice and guidance. I believe this Subspecialty Manual will meet its desired goal of providing practical knowledge that can be directly applied at the bedside and in outpatient settings to improve patient care.

Victoria J. Fraser, MD
Dr. J. William Campbell Professor
Interim Chairman of Medicine
Co-Director of the Infectious Disease Division
Washington University School of Medicine

Preface

T his third edition of *The Washington Manual™ Endocrinology Subspecialty Consult* was written by Washington University endocrine fellows and faculty members. The manual is designed to serve as a guide for students, house staff, and fellows involved in inpatient and outpatient endocrinology consults. It is not meant to serve as a comprehensive review of the field of endocrinology. Rather, it focuses on practical approaches to endocrine disorders commonly seen in consultation, with emphasis on key components of evaluation and treatment.

Several changes in content were made with the third edition. All chapters have been updated to provide the latest information on the pathophysiology and treatment of endocrine disorders. A new chapter has been added that covers Inpatient Management of Diabetes. Drug dosing information was reviewed and updated in each chapter. Clinical pearls are highlighted in boldfaced text within the chapters.

We are indebted to the remarkable efforts of the fellows and attending physicians who contributed to the current edition of this manual and worked enthusiastically to provide high-quality, contemporary, concise chapters.

TJB
WEC
JBM

Contents

PART I. HYPOTHALAMIC AND PITUITARY DISORDERS

PART II. THYROID DISORDERS

PART III. ADRENAL DISORDERS

PART IV. GONADAL DISORDERS

PART V. DISORDERS OF BONE AND MINERAL METABOLISM

Pituitary Adenomas

Zhiyu Wang and Julie Silverstein

GENERAL PRINCIPLES

- Pituitary adenomas are benign neoplasms arising in the adenohypophysial cells.
- Pituitary tumors constitute 10% of intracranial tumors.
- The most frequent primary pituitary tumors are pituitary adenomas.
- Pituitary adenomas occur in 10% to 15% of the general population[1] and are usually benign.
- Most pituitary adenomas are sporadic, but some arise as a component of genetic syndromes.
- Pituitary carcinomas are rare.[2]

Classification

According to the tumor size, pituitary adenomas are classified as **microadenomas** (<10 mm in greatest diameter) or **macroadenomas** (≥10 mm in greatest diameter). Depending on the cell of origin, they can be **hormone-producing,** or **functionally inactive** (Table 1-1).[3]

Etiology

Pituitary adenomas arise as a result of monoclonal pituitary cell proliferation. Several different mutations have been associated with pituitary adenomas.[4]

- Activating *gsp* mutations are present in 40% of GH-secreting adenomas. These are point mutations of the G protein alpha subunit (Gs alpha) gene, which activate Gs alpha protein and increase cyclic adenosine monophosphate (cAMP) levels, leading to GH hypersecretion and cell proliferation.
- H-ras gene mutations have been identified in metastatic pituitary carcinomas.
- Pituitary tumor transforming gene (PTTG) is abundant in all pituitary tumor types, especially prolactinomas.
- A truncated form of FGFR-4 is immunodetected in about a third of prolactinomas.
- Multiple endocrine neoplasia type 1 (MEN-1) is characterized by combined tumor formation or hyperfunction of pancreatic islets, anterior pituitary, and parathyroid glands.
- Carney's complex is characterized by pituitary adenomas, cardiac myxomas, schwannomas, and thyroid adenomas with spotty skin pigmentation.
- Hypothalamic factors may promote and maintain growth of transformed pituitary adenomatous cells. There is emerging data that dysregulation of cell-cycle control proteins, and loss of reticulin network play a role in pituitary tumor formation.[4]

TABLE 1-1	FUNCTIONAL CLASSIFICATION OF PITUITARY ADENOMAS		
Adenoma type	**Incidence (%)**	**Hormone overproduction**	**Clinical relevance**
Lactotroph	30	Prolactin (PRL)	Hyperprolactinemia, hypogonadism, and galactorrhea
Somatotroph	15	Growth hormone (GH)	Acromegaly or gigantism
Corticotroph	15	ACTH	Cushing's disease
Gonadotroph	10	FSH/LH, alpha subunit	Usually nonfunctioning
Thyrotroph	<1	TSH	Hyperthyroidism or silent when inactive TSH subunits are secreted
Plurihormonal adenomas	15	Multiple hormones, GH/PRL most common	Mixed syndromes
Null cell adenomas	20	None	No hormonal dysfunction
"Silent" adenomas	rare	Positive hormone(s) staining, but clinically silent	No hormonal dysfunction

DIAGNOSIS

Clinical Presentation

- The clinical presentation of pituitary adenomas depends on whether or not the tumor is hormonally functional or nonfunctional and on whether or not there is mass effect or hemorrhage.
- The diagnosis is sometimes made when a pituitary tumor is found incidentally on imaging studies performed for other reasons.[5]

Hormonal Hypersecretion

- **Prolactinomas** (see Chapter 2)
  Hyperprolactinemia causes hypogonadism in men and premenopausal women. Men present with decreased libido and impotence. Women often present with abnormal menses or infertility and galactorrhea.[6] There is often a delay in the diagnosis in postmenopausal women due to lack of clinical manifestations.
- **Somatotroph adenomas** (see Chapter 3)
  Acromegaly is growth hormone oversecretion occurring in the postpubertal phase of life. **Gigantism** is growth hormone excess that occurs before fusion of the epiphyseal

growth plates in children or adolescents. Acromegaly is characterized by skeletal overgrowth and soft tissue enlargement. Acromegalic patients have an increase in mortality related to associated cardiovascular, respiratory, gastrointestinal, and metabolic disorders.[7] The onset of acromegaly is insidious and often results in a delay in diagnosis.

- **Corticotroph adenomas** (see Chapter 14)
  ACTH–secreting tumors cause **Cushing's disease**.[8] The classic symptoms and signs of hypercortisolism are not always present and are often not specific. Obesity (predominantly central fat distribution), hypertension, glucose intolerance or diabetes, hirsutism, and gonadal dysfunction are common. Hypercortisolism produces skin thinning, easy bruising, abdominal striae, and proximal muscle weakness (inability to climb stairs or rise from a deep chair). Psychiatric abnormalities occur in 50% of patients (depression, lethargy, paranoia, and psychosis). Long-standing Cushing's disease can cause osteoporosis and aseptic necrosis of the femoral and humeral heads. Patients may present with poor wound healing and frequent superficial fungal infections.
- **Thyrotroph adenomas**
  Hyperthyroidism due to a TSH-secreting pituitary adenoma is very rare.[9] Thyrotroph adenomas usually present as large macroadenomas, and >60% are locally invasive.
- **Gonadotroph adenomas**
  Gonadotroph adenomas are usually macroadenomas and present with visual disturbances, symptoms of hypopituitarism or headache.[10] Most are clinically nonfunctioning.

Hormonal Hyposecretion (Hypopituitarism)

- Hypopituitarism can be a result of any hypothalamic or pituitary lesion.[11]
- Gonadotrophs are most commonly affected. Patients present with hypogonadism with low or inappropriately normal FSH and/or LH levels (secondary hypogonadism).
- Corticotrophs and thyrotrophs are most resistant to mass effects and the last to lose function. TSH or ACTH deficiency usually indicates panhypopituitarism. ACTH deficiency causes secondary adrenal insufficiency. TSH deficiency causes secondary hypothyroidism.
- GH deficiency is often present when two or more other hormones are deficient.
- Prolactin deficiency is rare and occurs when the anterior pituitary is completely destroyed, as in apoplexy.

Mass Effect

- Local effects are closely related to the size and location of the adenoma.
- Headaches are common and may not correlate with the size of the adenoma.
- Visual defects are also common.
  - Upward compression and pressure on the optic chiasm may result in bitemporal hemianopsia, loss of red perception, scotomas, and blindness.
  - Lateral invasion may impinge on the cavernous sinus, leading to lesions of the III, IV, VI, and V1 cranial nerves, causing diplopia, ptosis, ophthalmoplegia, and facial numbness.
- Direct hypothalamic involvement may cause several endocrine disorders such as:
  - Diabetes insipidus (see Chapter 4).
  - Appetite/behavioral disorders (obesity, hyperphagia, anorexia, adipsia, and compulsive drinking).
  - Sleep and temperature dysregulation.

- Cerebrospinal fluid rhinorrhea, caused by inferior extension of the adenoma, is a very rare presentation.
- Uncinate seizures, personality disorders, and anosmia can occur if temporal and frontal brain lobes are invaded by the expanding parasellar mass.

Pituitary Apoplexy
- Pituitary apoplexy is an endocrine emergency, often resulting from spontaneous hemorrhage and/or infarction of a rapidly growing or large pituitary adenoma.[12]
- Symptoms include severe headache, neck stiffness, progressive cranial nerve damage, bilateral visual disturbances, change in consciousness, cardiovascular collapse, and coma. Acute adrenal insufficiency may also occur. Patients may experience long-term pituitary insufficiency.
- Pituitary imaging reveals intraadenomal hemorrhage and stalk deviation.

Differential Diagnosis
- For a list of common sellar and parasellar masses, see Table 1-2.
- **Sellar/parasellar cysts**
  - **Craniopharyngiomas** are the most common and are calcified, cystic, suprasellar tumors arising from embryonic squamous cell rests of Rathke's cleft. Craniopharyngiomas have a bimodal peak of incidence, occurring predominantly in children between the ages of 5 and 10 years; a second peak occurs in late middle age.[13] Craniopharyngiomas are slow growing. Large craniopharyngiomas can obstruct CSF flow and cause increased intracranial pressure. Children present with headache, vomiting, visual field deficits, and growth failure. Adults may present with neurologic symptoms, anterior pituitary hormone deficits, and DI.
  - **Rathke's cleft cysts** are benign, noncalcified lesions that mimic hormonally inactive adenomas or craniopharyngiomas. They have a particularly low recurrence rate after partial excision.
- **Pituitary granulomas**
  - **Sarcoidosis** of the hypothalamic-pituitary region occurs in most patients with CNS involvement and can cause hypopituitarism with or without symptoms of an intrasellar mass. Sarcoidosis has a predilection for the hypothalamus, posterior pituitary, and cranial nerves.[14] The most common hormonal abnormalities are hypogonadotropic hypogonadism, mild hyperprolactinemia, and DI.
  - **Langerhans' cell histiocytosis (LCH)**
    - Langerhans' histiocytosis is characterized by infiltration of dendtritic cells (Langerhans' cells).[15] It can be unifocal or multifocal and affect multiple sites, such as bone, skin, lung, pituitary, hypothalamus, liver, and spleen.
    - LCH occurs more often in children and is almost always associated with diabetes insipidus. Anterior pituitary dysfunction occurs in 20% of patients.[16]
    - Hand–Schüller–Christian (HSC) disease includes the triad of DI, exophthalmos, and lytic bone disease. Other features of the disease include axillary skin rash and a history of recurrent pneumothorax. Children can present with growth retardation and anterior pituitary hormone deficits.
    - MRI may reveal a thickened pituitary stalk or a diminished posterior pituitary bright spot, and possibly bone lesions.
- **Hypophysitis** is characterized by either focal or diffuse infiltration of the pituitary by inflammatory cells.[17]
  - **Lymphocytic hypophysitis** affects mostly women in late pregnancy or during the postpartum period. Other autoimmune diseases (autoimmune thyroiditis)

TABLE 1-2 COMMON SELLAR AND PARASELLAR MASSES

Benign tumors
Pituitary adenoma
Craniopharyngioma
Meningioma

Primary malignant tumors
Germ cell tumor
Sarcoma
Chordoma
Pituitary carcinoma
Lymophoma

Metastatic malignant tumors
Lung cancer
Breast cancer
GI tract
GU tract

Cysts
Rathke's
Epidermoid
Dermoid
Arachnoid

Pituitary hyperplasia
Lactotroph hyperplasia during pregnancy
Thyrotroph hyperplasia due to longstanding primary hypothyroidism
Gonadotroph hyperplasia due to longstanding primary hypogoandism
Somatotroph hyperplasia due to ectopic GHRH

Miscellaneous lesions
Aneurysms
Hypophysitis
Infections
Giant cell granulomas
Sarcoidosis
Others

may also be present. The diagnosis is confirmed by histology or resolution of the mass over time. Partial recovery of pituitary function and resolution of the sellar mass can occur spontaneously or with use of corticosteroids and hormone replacement.

○ **Granulomatous hypophysitis** is not usually associated with pregnancy. Pituitary histology shows features of chronic inflammation and granulomas.
• **Pituitary hyperplasia** usually presents as generalized enlargement of the pituitary.[18] Pituitary hyperplasia may be caused by:
  ○ Lactotroph hyperplasia during pregnancy
  ○ Thyrotroph hyperplasia secondary to long-standing primary hypothyroidism
  ○ Gonadotroph hyperplasia in long-standing primary hypogonadism
  ○ Very rarely, somatotroph hyperplasia in ectopic secretion of growth hormone-releasing hormone (GHRH)

- **Pituitary metastases** most commonly arise from breast carcinomas (women) and lung carcinomas. A rapidly enlarging mass is highly suggestive of a metastatic lesion.[19]
- **Pituitary carcinomas** are rare.[19] They may produce GH, ACTH, or prolactin, or they may be clinically nonfunctioning. The diagnosis can only be established when the lesion metastasizes.

Diagnostic Testing

Laboratories

- **Hormonal hypersecretion**
  - ○ **Prolactinoma**
    - ▪ Serum prolactin levels are usually proportional to the tumor mass. Values are generally >250 ng/mL in macroprolactinomas.[6]
    - ▪ Hyperprolactinemia between 20 and 200 ng/mL can be due to microprolactinomas, stalk compression from a sellar masse, medication induced hyperprolactinemia, or due to the "hook effect" (see Chapter 2).
  - ○ **Acromegaly**
    - ▪ GH secretion in normal subjects is pulsatile, diurnal, and affected by a variety of factors.[7]
    - ▪ The initial laboratory tests to be ordered in a patient suspected of having acromegaly should be IGF-1 and GH levels. Current guidelines recommend an elevated IGF-1 and failure to suppress GH during an oral glucose tolerance test (OGTT) to confirm the diagnosis (see Chapter 3).
  - ○ **Cushing's disease**
    - ▪ Patients with clinical signs or symptoms of Cushing's syndrome should be screened for Cushing's disease with either a 24-hour urine free cortisol, a low-dose dexamethasone suppression test, or a late-night salivary cortisol.[8]
    - ▪ An elevated ACTH level in the setting of biochemically confirmed Cushing's syndrome suggests either a pituitary source (Cushing's disease) or ectopic ACTH syndrome. A high-dose dexamethasone suppression test and/or inferior petrosal sinus sampling (IPSS) can be used to differentiate between the two (see Chapter 14).
  - ○ **TSH-secreting adenomas**
    - ▪ Elevated thyroid hormone levels in the setting of an elevated or inappropriately normal TSH suggests the diagnosis.[9] An elevated pituitary glycoprotein hormone alpha-subunit (α-GSU) may be present.
    - ▪ Similar laboratory values may be seen in the presence of circulating antibodies against TSH. Therefore, a methodologic interference in the measurement of TSH must be ruled out. Dynamic testing, such as T3 suppression and TRH stimulation can be used to differentiate a TSH-secreting adenoma from thyroid hormone resistance syndromes.
  - ○ **Gonadotroph adenomas**
    - ▪ Most non-functioning pituitary adenomas arise from gonadotroph cells.
    - ▪ Although circulating LH and FSH levels may be elevated in a minority of patients, this is rarely clinically significant.
- **Hypopituitarism**
  - ○ **Corticotropin deficiency** (secondary adrenal insufficiency)
    - ▪ ACTH deficiency produces hypotension, shock, nausea, vomiting, fatigue, and hyponatremia (see Chapter 11).
    - ▪ Dynamic testing to evaluate the HPA axis can be done with a cosyntropin stimulation test or insulin-induced hypoglycemia.

- Cosyntropin stimulation test may be normal in recent-onset corticotropin deficiency, because it takes time for adrenals to atrophy after acute disruption of ACTH secretion.
  ○ **Thyrotropin deficiency** (secondary hypothyroidism)
    - A low serum free T4 in the setting of an inappropriately low/normal TSH suggests secondary hypothyroidism.[20]
    - A free T4 level should be used as the follow-up test for secondary hypothyroidism.
  ○ **GH deficiency**
    - Measurement of basal GH does not distinguish reliably between normal and subnormal GH secretion.
    - Patients with multiple pituitary hormone deficits (three or four) and a low IGF-1 are likely GH deficient.[21]
    - Low serum IGF-1 in a patient with pituitary disease may suggest the diagnosis of GH deficiency.
    - Stimulation tests include the GHRH-arginine stimulation test and the insulin tolerance test.
  ○ **Gonadotropin deficiency** (secondary hypogonadism)
    - May be secondary to hyperprolactinemia.
    - Normal menses in premenopausal women not on birth control suggests an intact pituitary-gonadal axis. In female patients with abnormal menses, serum LH/FSH, prolactin, and estradiol levels should be checked.
    - Low serum testosterone in the setting of an inappropriately low or normal LH in males suggests the diagnosis.
- **Pituitary incidentalomas**
  ○ Evaluation of pituitary incidentalomas should depend on the size of the lesion.
  ○ Macroadenomas should be screened for both hypersecretion (hyperprolactinemia, acromegaly, or Cushing's disease) and hypopituitarism. Visual field defects should also be evaluated if the tumor abuts the optic chiasm.
  ○ Microadenomas should be screened only for hypersecretion. Evaluation for hypopituitarism or visual abnormalities is not necessary unless the patient has related symptoms or signs.
  ○ Asymptomatic non-functioning incidentalomas may be followed up by periodic MRI for tumor growth. Tumor growth without treatment occurs in about 10% of microadenomas and 24% of macroadenomas.[5]

Imaging Studies
- **Pituitary MRI:** MRI with a focus on the pituitary (contiguous sections detect lesions of 1 to 3 mm) is the best imaging study to visualize pituitary tumors.[22] MRI detects tumor effects on soft tissue structures, cavernous sinus or optic chiasm, sphenoid sinus, and hypothalamus. T1-weighted sections in the coronal and sagittal plane distinguish most pituitary masses. Pituitary adenomas usually take up less gadolinium than the normal pituitary tissue but more than the CNS. T2-weighted images are important for diagnosing high-signal hemorrhage. Teenage girls exhibit increasing gland convexity during their menstrual cycle. During pregnancy, the gland should normally not exceed 12 mm. A thickened stalk may indicate the presence of hypophysitis, a granuloma, or an atypical chordoma.
- **Pituitary CT** allows better visualization of bony structures, including the sellar floor and clinoid bones. Calcifications associated with craniopharyngiomas, which may not be visible on MRI, can be seen on CT.

TREATMENT

The goals of pituitary adenoma therapy are to alleviate local compressive mass effects, to correct hormone hypersecretion, and preserve normal pituitary function.

Surgical Management

- General indications:
  - ○ Functioning GH-, TSH-, or ACTH-secreting adenomas, and nonfunctioning macroadenomas.
  - ○ Progressive compressive features including visual compromise, hypopituitarism, or other CNS dysfunctions.
  - ○ Hemorrhage especially with sudden visual field compromise.
  - ○ Patients who are intolerant or resistant to medical therapy.
- The transsphenoidal microsurgical approach is the procedure of choice for >90% of pituitary tumors. The adenoma is selectively removed. Normal pituitary tissue is identified and preserved if possible.
- Major complications:
  - ○ CSF leakage, DI, and SIADH are the most common transient complications
  - ○ Iatrogenic hypopituitarism, permanent DI, or SIADH
  - ○ Local damage

Radiotherapy

- Pituitary irradiation is usually reserved for large tumors with incomplete resection or for patients who have a contraindication for surgery.
- Gamma knife delivers high-dose radiation to the tumor while sparing surrounding tissue as compared to conventional radiation. They have similar long-term efficacy.
  - ○ Major complications include hypopituitarism (develops in up to 80% of patients after 10 years), optic nerve damage, and brain necrosis. It is unclear whether or not the risk of cancer is increased.

Medical Therapy

- **Dopamine agonists** are usually the first line therapy for prolactinomas of all sizes. They decrease hyperprolactinemia due to any cause and decrease the size and secretion of most prolactinomas.[6]
  - ○ Bromocriptine and cabergoline are both commonly used. Cabergoline is more potent, better tolerated, and longer-acting as compared to bromocriptine.
  - ○ Dopamine agonists can be added in combination with somatostatin analogs (SSAs) for acromegaly therapy.
- **SSAs,** including octreotide (Sandostatin) and lanreotide (Somatuline) bind to somatostatin receptor subtypes (SSTRs) and act as inhibitors to a number of endocrine cells.[23]
  - ○ SSAs are the mainstay of medical therapy for acromegaly and TSH-secreting pituitary adenomas.
- The growth hormone receptor antagonist (Pegvisomant) inhibits peripheral GH action. It is highly effective in reducing IGF-1 levels in acromegaly.
- Temozolomide is an oral chemotherapeutic agent that has been used in the treatment of aggressive pituitary tumors.[24]
- Ketoconazole and metyrapone may be used to inhibit cortisol synthesis in Cushing's disease.[8] Occasionally mitotane is used to achieve biochemical control.

MONITORING/FOLLOW-UP

- Postsurgical patients should be evaluated for complete tumor resection and hormone dysfunction in 4 to 6 weeks.
- Follow-up after pituitary irradiation is essential, because the response to therapy may be delayed and the incidence of hypopituitarism increases with time.
- Follow-up MRI may not be necessary in patients with normal posttherapy pituitary function, but should be done in patients with persistent or recurrent disease.

REFERENCES

1. Daly AF, Tichomirowa MA, Beckers A. The epidemiology and genetics of pituitary adenomas. *Best Pract Res Clin Endocrinol Metab* 2009;23(5):543–554.
2. Scheithauer BW, Gaffey TA, Lloyd RV, et al. Pathobiology of pituitary adenomas and carcinomas. *Neurosurgery* 2006;59(2):341–353.
3. Saeger W, Lüdecke DK, Buchfelder M, et al. Pathohistological classification of pituitary tumors: 10 years of experience with the German Pituitary Tumor Registry. *Eur J Endocrinol* 2007;156(2):203–216.
4. Dworakowska D, Grossman AB. The pathophysiology of pituitary adenomas. *Best Pract Res Clin Endocrinol Metab* 2009;23(5):525–541.
5. Molitch ME. Pituitary tumours: Pituitary incidentalomas. *Best Pract Res Clin Endocrinol Metab* 2009;23(5):667–675.
6. Klibanski A. Clinical practice. Prolactinomas. *N Engl J Med* 2010;362(13):1219–1226.
7. Molitch ME. Clinical manifestations of acromegaly. *Endocrinol Metab Clin North Am* 1992;21(3):597–614.
8. Nieman L, Biller B, Finding J, et al. The diagnosis of Cushing's syndrome: An endocrine society clinical practice guideline. *J Clin Endocrinol Metab* 2008;93:1526–1540.
9. Beck-Peccoz P, Persani L, Mannavola D, et al. Pituitary tumours: TSH-secreting adenomas. *Best Pract Res Clin Endocrinol Metab* 2009;23(5):597–606.
10. Greenman Y, Stern N. Non-functioning pituitary adenomas. *Best Pract Res Clin Endocrinol Metab* 2009;23(5):625–638.
11. Arafah BM. Reversible hypopituitarism in patients with large nonfunctioning pituitary adenomas. *J Clin Endocrinol Metab* 1986;62(6):1173–1179.
12. Turgut M, Ozsunar Y, Başak S, et al. Pituitary apoplexy: An overview of 186 cases published during the last century. *Acta Neurochir (Wien)* 2010;152(5):749–761.
13. Garnett MR, Puget S, Grill J, et al. Craniopharyngioma. *Orphanet J Rare Dis* 2007;2:18.
14. Bell NH. Endocrine complications of sarcoidosis. *Endocrinol Metab Clin North Am* 1991;20(3):645–654.
15. Kaltsas GA, Powles TB, Evanson J, et al. Hypothalamo-pituitary abnormalities in adult patients with langerhans cell histiocytosis: Clinical, endocrinological, and radiological features and response to treatment. *J Clin Endocrinol Metab* 2000;85(4):1370–1376.
16. Carpinteri R, Patelli I, Casanueva FF, et al. Pituitary tumours: Inflammatory and granulomatous expansive lesions of the pituitary. *Best Pract Res Clin Endocrinol Metab* 2009;23(5):639–650.
17. Honegger J, Fahlbusch R, Bornemann A, et al. Lymphocytic and granulomatous hypophysitis: Experience with nine cases. *Neurosurgery* 1997;40(4):713–722; discussion 722–723.
18. Melmed S. Mechanisms for pituitary tumorigenesis: The plastic pituitary. *J Clin Invest* 2003;112(11):1603–1618.
19. Kaltsas GA, Grossman AB. Malignant pituitary tumours. *Pituitary* 1998;1(1):69–81.
20. Lania A, Persani L, Beck-Peccoz P. Central hypothyroidism. *Pituitary* 2008;11(2):181–186.
21. Clemmons DR. The diagnosis and treatment of growth hormone deficiency in adults. *Curr Opin Endocrinol Diabetes Obes* 2010;17(4):377–383.

22. Melmed S, Kleinberg D. Anterior pituitary. In: Kronenberg HM, Melmed S, Polonsky KS, eds. *Williams Textbook of Endocrinology,* 11th ed. Philadelphia, PA: Saunders/Elsevier, 2008: 155–261.

23. Fleseriu M, Delashaw JB Jr, Cook DM. Acromegaly: A review of current medical therapy and new drugs on the horizon. *Neurosurg Focus* 2010;29(4):E15.

24. Raverot G, Sturm N, de Fraipont F, et al. Temozolomide treatment in aggressive pituitary tumors and pituitary carcinomas: A French multicenter experience. *J Clin Endocrinol Metab* 2010;95(10):4592–4599.

Prolactinoma

2

Mariko Johnson and Julie Silverstein

GENERAL PRINCIPLES

Definition
Prolactinomas are prolactin-secreting pituitary tumors.

Classification
- Based on size
  - **Microprolactinomas** are tumors <10 mm in greatest diameter.
  - **Macroprolactinomas** are tumors ≥10 mm in greatest diameter.
- Based on local invasion
  - Microprolactinomas by definition are confined to the pituitary.
  - Macroprolactinomas can invade local structures such as the cavernous and sphenoid sinuses and compress the optic chiasm.
- Based on metastatic spread
  - Most prolactinomas are benign and confined to the pituitary.
  - Malignant prolactinomas are extremely rare and are defined by the presence of metastases to the bone, lymph nodes, lung, liver, or spinal cord.

Epidemiology
- Prolactinomas are the most common secretory pituitary tumors with an estimated prevalence of 100 per million population.[1] Large autopsy series have found pituitary microadenomas in 10% of individuals.[2] Prolactinomas account for 40% of pituitary adenomas.[3]
- Microprolactinomas occur more often in women with a female:male ratio of 20:1.[4]
- Macroprolactinomas occur with similar frequency in men and women.[4]

Associated Conditions
- Prolactinoma is the most frequent pituitary tumor occurring in the multiple endocrine neoplasia syndrome.
- Prolactinomas may also secrete other hormones. The most frequent mixed tumors are growth hormone (GH)/prolactin-secreting adenomas.

DIAGNOSIS

Clinical Presentation
- Prolactinomas cause symptoms on the basis of hormonal secretion and mass effect.
  - Symptoms due to hyperprolactinemia can include galactorrhea and symptoms of hypogonadism. Galactorrhea occurs via direct action of prolactin on the estrogenized breast. Hypogonadism occurs due to inhibitory effects of prolactin on

gonadotropin secretion or via direct compression of gonadotrophs. Therefore, hypogonadism can occur with tumors of any size and may be reversible if prolactin levels are controlled.

- ○ Symptoms due to mass effect include headache and visual field defects. Ophthalmoplegia and rhinorrhea are signs of more advanced disease. Headaches are caused by the expanding tumor. Visual field defects are caused by compression of the optic chiasm. Ophthalmoplegia may occur when tumors expand laterally and invade the cavernous sinus. Rhinorrhea may occur if the tumor invades the sphenoid or ethmoid sinuses or after rapid drug-induced tumor shrinkage. Hypothyroidism and adrenal insufficiency occur via direct compression of thyrotrophs or corticotrophs by a macroprolactinoma. Unlike hypogonadism, if these hormonal deficiencies are present as a result of a macroprolactinoma, they are generally not reversible.

- The clinical presentation of prolactinomas can vary based on the gender and age of the patient.
  - ○ Premenopausal women may present with galactorrhea and/or hypogonadism (infertility, oligomenorrhea, or amenorrhea). Women who are amenorrheic for long periods are at risk for osteopenia and osteoporosis and are less likely to present with galactorrhea.
  - ○ Postmenopausal women rarely present early in the course of disease since menses are no longer present and galactorrhea is rarely present due to low estrogen levels. Hyperprolactinemia is often not recognized in postmenopausal patients until a prolactinoma has become sufficiently large to produce symptoms of mass effect such as headache or visual field defects.
  - ○ Men present with secondary hypogonadism and symptoms of decreased libido, impotence, infertility, loss of body hair, or gynecomastia. More subtle manifestations include decreased cognitive function and energy, and loss of muscle and bone mass. Men almost never have galactorrhea.
- The clinical presentation of prolactinomas can vary based on the size of the tumor.
  - ○ Symptoms of mass effect generally only occur in the presence of a macroadenoma.

History
The history should focus on symptoms of hormonal overproduction and mass effect. It should also seek to define possible alternate causes for hyperprolactinemia. Symptoms or history of hypothyroidism, adrenal insufficiency, renal disease, or cirrhosis should be sought. Current medications should be carefully reviewed. Any family history of pituitary tumors or syndromes of endocrine neoplasia should be noted.

Physical Examination
The physical examination should evaluate for bitemporal visual field defects, galactorrhea (in premenopausal females), as well as for signs of hypothyroidism or hypogonadism.

Diagnostic Criteria
- **The first requirement for a diagnosis of prolactinoma is a persistently elevated prolactin level.** The likelihood of prolactinoma can be roughly estimated based on the degree of elevation in the prolactin.[5]
  - ○ Levels above normal but <100 ng/mL: possible prolactinoma
  - ○ Levels 100 to 200 ng/mL: likely prolactinoma
  - ○ Levels >200 ng/mL: usually diagnostic of prolactinoma

TABLE 2-1	DIFFERENTIAL DIAGNOSIS OF HYPERPROLACTINEMIA: MNEMONIC HIGH PROLACTIN

Hypothyroidism
Idiopathic
Glucocorticoid insufficiency
Hyperplasia of lactotrophs
Physiologic (nipple stimulation or pregnancy)
Renal failure
Opiates/other drugs (estrogen, antipsychotics, antidepressants,
    antihypertensives, antiemetics)
Liver failure
Adenoma
Convulsion
Trauma (chest wall)
Irradiation
No abnormality (Macroprolactinemia)

- Alternate causes of mild to moderate prolactin elevations should be considered and if possible excluded (see Section on Differential Diagnosis).
- Once persistent hyperprolactinemia is established and alternate causes excluded, a pituitary protocol brain MRI should be performed to define tumor size and anatomy. Microprolactinomas may be too small to be seen on MRI.

Differential Diagnosis

- Many factors other than a prolactinoma can lead to hyperprolactinemia and a differential diagnosis can be remembered using the mnemonic HIGH PROLACTIN (Table 2-1).[14]
- **Medications**
  Many medications cause elevations in prolactin (Table 2-2). These include dopamine antagonists as well as others.
- **Physiologic causes**
  Physiologic causes of increased prolactin levels include pregnancy and nipple stimulation.
- **Lactotroph adenomas** (prolactinomas)
- **Lactotroph hyperplasia**
  Lactotroph cells are inhibited by dopamine. Compression of dopamine-secreting neurons, which are found in the hypothalamus and pituitary, releases this tonic inhibition and permits lactotroph hyperplasia. Compression can occur due to tumors of the hypothalamus, infiltrative diseases, disruption of the hypothalamic-pituitary stalk in head trauma, or non-functioning pituitary macroadenomas.
- **Hypothyroidism**
  Most patients with hypothyroidism have normal prolactin levels. Rarely, patients with hypothyroidism present with elevated prolactin values. Thyroid hormone replacement typically restores normal prolactin values.
- **Chest wall injury**
  Chest wall injuries, irritating lesions (e.g., herpes zoster), and spinal cord injuries can activate neural reflexes similar to nipple stimulation and increase prolactin levels.

TABLE 2-2 MEDICATIONS THAT MAY CAUSE HYPERPROLACTINEMIA

Antipsychotics
Typical antipsychotics
Certain atypical antipsychotics
   Risperidone
   Molindone
   Quetiapine
   Olanzapine

Antidepressants
Tricyclic antidepressants
Monoamine oxidase inhibitors
Fluoxetine (no other SSRIs)*

Antihypertensives
Verapamil
Reserpine
Methyldopa
Drugs of abuse
   Opiates
   Cocaine

Gastrointestinal medications
Metoclopramide
Domperidone
Prochlorperazine

Other
Estrogens
H2 blockers*

---
*Case reports exist but data are not well established.

- **Renal or hepatic failure**
  Elevations in prolactin levels may be seen in renal or hepatic failure due to decreased prolactin clearance.
- **Adrenal insufficiency**
  Glucocorticoids have a suppressive effect on prolactin gene transcription and release.
- **Idiopathic hyperprolactinemia**
  In some patients with prolactin concentrations between 20 and 100 ng/mL, no cause can be found. Some of these patients have undetectable lactotroph microadenomas. Long-term follow-up has revealed that in one-third of these patients prolactin levels return to normal, in 17% prolactin levels rise to 50% over baseline, and in the remaining 50% prolactin levels remain stable or decrease.[6]
- **Macroprolactinemia** ("Big Prolactin")
  Prolactin can circulate as a monomer or in aggregates (usually bound to IgG). Monomeric hyperprolactinemia leads to classical symptoms and signs such as menstrual disturbance and galactorrhea. In contrast, the presence of circulating prolactin aggregates (macroprolactinemia) is felt to be a benign variant.[7] In long-term

follow-up of such patients, few had initial symptoms and none had symptom progression.[7] Macroprolactinemia can be distinguished from monomeric hyperprolactinemia by polyethylene glycol precipitation. Some, but not all, laboratories routinely test for macroprolactinemia.

Diagnostic Testing

Laboratories
- Laboratory testing begins with a serum prolactin level.
- If the serum prolactin is elevated, a serum TSH, a comprehensive metabolic panel, and a pregnancy test (in premenopausal females) may be ordered to begin to rule out secondary causes.
- A prolactin with serial dilutions should be measured in all patients with a pituitary macroadenoma who have a mild to moderate prolactin elevation to exclude the Hook effect.
  - ○ Distinguishing a prolactinoma from a nonfunctioning pituitary macroadenoma is of utmost importance because prolactinomas are best treated medically, whereas nonfunctioning tumors require surgery.
  - ○ An immunoradiometric assay is frequently used for measurement of serum prolactin levels. Falsely low values can occur when a large amount of prolactin saturates the antibodies. This is known as the Hook effect.
  - ○ Mild to moderate prolactin elevations (<200 ng/mL) in the setting of a pituitary macroadenoma may be due to stalk compression but may also be due to the Hook effect. This artifact can be excluded by performing an additional prolactin determination on diluted serum. If the diluted specimen yields a value that is the same or higher, the diagnosis of macroprolactinoma can be made.
- Screening for hypopituitarism should be considered in all patients with macroprolactinomas.

Imaging
- **MRI with gadolinium** enhancement provides the best anatomic detail of the hypothalamic-pituitary area.
- **Visual field testing** should be obtained in patients with tumors that are adjacent to or compressing the optic chiasm.

TREATMENT

- **All macroprolactinomas require treatment** whether or not compressive symptoms are present.
- **Not all microprolactinomas require treatment** and should be treated only when symptoms caused by hyperprolactinemia or rapidly increasing prolactin levels indicative of an enlarging tumor are present. As such, microprolactinomas in postmenopausal women rarely require treatment.
- Prolactinomas are unique among pituitary tumors in that **first-line treatment is medical, not surgical.**
- **The mainstays of management for prolactinomas are the dopamine agonists bromocriptine and cabergoline.**
- Most patients will respond to therapy within weeks of initiation, as evidenced by symptoms and prolactin levels. The majority of patients will also have a >25% decrease in the size of the adenoma.[3]

- A normal prolactin level should be the target of therapy for macroprolactinomas.
- Restoration of gonadal function and relief from symptoms should be the goal of therapy for microprolactinomas, and achieving a normal prolactin level may not be necessary.

Medications

- **Bromocriptine**

Bromocriptine is an ergot derivative D2 receptor agonist. It can be administered orally once or twice a day at doses of 2.5 to 20 mg/day and produces reduction in prolactin levels to the normal range in 70% to 90% of cases.[1] Women resume regular ovulatory menses, and galactorrhea should resolve after 2 to 3 months of therapy. For macroprolactinomas, the reduction in tumor size is usually associated with improved visual fields, reduction of hyperprolactinemia, and improvement in other pituitary function (owing to reduced mass effect). Most series suggest that bromocriptine therapy has little or no effect on later surgical results for microadenomas; however, in patients with macroadenomas, bromocriptine treatment lasting >6 to 12 weeks has been associated with perivascular fibrosis of the tumor, which can complicate complete tumor resection.[8] The most common side effects of bromocriptine are nausea and vomiting. Orthostatic hypotension may occur when initiating therapy.

- **Cabergoline**

Cabergoline is a nonergot D2 receptor agonist with a long half-life, and can be given orally at 0.25 to 1 mg twice a week. A large comparator study of cabergoline and bromocriptine demonstrated the superiority of cabergoline over bromocriptine in both efficacy and tolerability.[9] Cabergoline leads to a greater reduction in prolactin secretion, decrease in tumor size, and improvement in gonadal function than bromocriptine. Side effects are much less frequent and less severe than with bromocriptine. Recent studies have shown that cabergoline can cause valvular fibrosis at the higher doses used for treatment of Parkinson's disease.[10] For hyperprolactinemic disorders, a considerably lower dose of cabergoline is used. At these lower doses, there appears to be minimal risk of valvular abnormalities though large randomized studies have not yet been performed and the true risk remains to be defined.[10]

- **Other dopamine agonists**

Quinagolide is not yet approved for use in the United States.

Surgical Management

Pituitary surgery is reserved for patients who are refractory to or intolerant of dopamine agonists, have persistent visual field deficits despite medical therapy, or have other neurologic signs in the context of a cystic macroadenoma or pituitary apoplexy.[3] Pituitary surgery aimed at debulking the tumor to reduce the risk of potential expansion is indicated for women with macroprolactinomas desiring pregnancy. Trans-sphenoidal surgery by an experienced neurosurgeon can be offered to patients with microadenomas who do not wish to receive lifelong medical therapy.

Radiotherapy

Radiotherapy is not a primary therapy for prolactinomas. Its use is limited to patients with macroprolactinomas that are refractory to medical treatment and surgery or in the rare case of a malignant prolactinoma.[3]

SPECIAL CONSIDERATIONS

Pregnancy

• During pregnancy, the normal pituitary increases in size, owing to marked lactotroph hyperplasia due to the effect of estrogen on prolactin synthesis. The risk of tumor expansion is small (<3%) for microprolactinomas but significant (30%) for macroprolactinomas.[11]

• Patients with prolactinomas wishing to become pregnant should be referred to specialists in high-risk obstetrics and endocrinology.

• No increase in adverse fetal events has been demonstrated with use of either bromocriptine or cabergoline.[12,13] However, experience with cabergoline in pregnancy is more limited than bromocriptine, making bromocriptine the drug of choice in pregnancy.

• In women with microprolactinomas desiring fertility, bromocriptine should be titrated to normalize prolactin levels and restore regular menses. Barrier contraception should be recommended until menstrual cycles become regular so that a pregnancy test can be performed immediately if a cycle is missed. Once pregnancy is confirmed, bromocriptine should be discontinued in order to limit fetal exposure to the drug.

• In women with macroprolactinomas, control of tumor size should ideally be attained prior to conception because of the growth potential of these tumors during pregnancy. These patients should be pretreated with bromocriptine for a sufficient period to cause substantial tumor shrinkage in addition to regular menses. Only then should contraception be discontinued. If the tumor does not shrink sufficiently in size, prepregnancy transsphenoidal surgical debulking can be considered. Once pregnancy is achieved, bromocriptine should be discontinued followed by close surveillance for symptoms of tumor enlargement.

• Monitoring prolactin levels in pregnant patients is of no benefit, as levels do not always rise during pregnancy and may not rise with tumor enlargement. Visual field testing and imaging is reserved for patients with symptoms of tumor enlargement. Reinstitution of bromocriptine therapy at the lowest effective dose during pregnancy is the treatment of choice for patients with symptomatic tumor enlargement. Transsphenoidal surgery or delivery (if pregnancy is far enough advanced) should be performed if there is no response to bromocriptine and vision is progressively worsening.

MONITORING/FOLLOW-UP

• Available guidelines suggest routine follow-up but do not specify an optimal interval for biochemical or radiologic assessment.[3]

• Our opinion is that once stable, prolactin levels should be followed on a yearly basis and MRI evaluation should be repeated only if either clinical signs of tumor growth appear or if prolactin levels rise significantly.

• Visual field testing and MRI evaluation should be repeated at regular intervals if a visual field defect was present at diagnosis.

• Several recent studies demonstrate that cabergoline or bromocriptine can be tapered safely in a subset of patients but the rate of remission has been variable between studies.[11]

• Tapering of dopamine agonists can be considered when the prolactin level has been normal for at least 3 years and the size of the tumor has decreased significantly.[3] These patients require close follow-up to monitor for recurrence of hyperprolactinemia and tumor growth.

REFERENCES

1. Colao A. Pituitary tumours: The prolactinoma. *Best Pract Res Clin Endocrinol Metab* 2009;23: 575–596.
2. Buurman H, Saeger W. Subclinical adenomas in postmortem pituitaries: Classification and correlations to clinical data. *Eur J Endocrinol* 2006;154:753–758.
3. Casanueva FF, Molitch ME, Schlechte JA, et al. Guidelines of the Pituitary Society for the diagnosis and management of prolactinomas. *Clin Endocrinol (Oxf)* 2006;65:265–273.
4. Ambrosi B, Faglia G. Epidemiology of pituitary tumors. In: Faglia G, Beck-Peccoz P, Ambrosi B, Travaglini P, Spada A, eds. *Pituitary Adenomas: New Trends in Basic and Clinical Research.* Amsterdam: Elsevier Science Publishers, 1991:159–168.
5. Aron D, Findling J, Tyrrell B. Hypothalamus & pituitary gland. In: Gardner D, Shoback D, eds. *Greenspan's Basic & Clinical Endocrinology,* 8th ed. New York, NY: McGraw-Hill, 2007:101–156.
6. Martin TL, Kim M, Malarkey WB. The natural history of idiopathic hyperprolactinemia. *J Clin Endocrinol Metab* 1985;60:855–858.
7. Wallace IR, Satti N, Courtney CH, et al. Ten-year clinical follow-up of a cohort of 51 patients with macroprolactinemia establishes it as a benign variant. *J Clin Endocrinol Metab* 2010;95:3268–3271.
8. Molitch ME. Medical Therapy of pituitary tumors. In: Thapar K, Kovacs K, Scheithauer B, Lloyd R, eds. *Diagnosis and Management of Pituitary Tumors.* Totowa, NJ: Humana Press Inc., 2001:247–268.
9. Webster J, Piscitelli G, Polli A, et al. A comparison of cabergoline and bromocriptine in the treatment of hyperprolactinemic amenorrhea. Cabergoline Comparative Study Group. *N Engl J Med* 1994;331:904–909.
10. Valassi E, Klibanski A, Biller BM. Clinical Review: Potential cardiac valve effects of dopamine agonists in hyperprolactinemia. *J Clin Endocrinol Metab* 2010;95:1025–1033.
11. Klibanski A. Clinical practice. Prolactinomas. *N Engl J Med* 2010;362:1219–1226.
12. Krupp P, Monka C. Bromocriptine in pregnancy: Safety aspects. *Klin Wochenschr* 1987;65: 823–827.
13. Colao A, Abs R, Barcena DG, et al. Pregnancy outcomes following cabergoline treatment: Extended results from a 12-year observational study. *Clin Endocrinol (Oxf)* 2008;68:66–71.
14. Molitch ME. Medication-induced hyperprolactinemia. *Mayo Clin Proc* 2005;80:1050–1057.

Acromegaly

3

Nadia Khoury and Julie Silverstein

GENERAL PRINCIPLES

- Acromegaly is a disorder characterized by overproduction of growth hormone (GH).
- Overproduction of GH results in progressive skeletal, skin, and organ growth that is associated with significant morbidity and premature mortality if left untreated.

Definition

- **Acromegaly** is growth hormone oversecretion occurring in the postpubertal phase of life.
- When GH oversecretion occurs before puberty, it may cause rapid growth and hypogonadism with failure of growth-plate closure, resulting in **gigantism**.

Epidemiology

- The incidence of acromegaly is low—about three cases per million people per year.
- Acromegaly is insidious, resulting in a lag time between disease onset and diagnosis. Older studies indicate this was almost 10 years but newer studies indicate this has decreased to 2 to 3 years.[1]

Pathophysiology

- Acromegaly is most commonly due to a pure somatroph pituitary adenoma (60%). Adenomas that secrete a combination of growth hormone and prolactin are also seen (25%). Adenomas that secrete GH and TSH are rare.[2]
- Molecular studies of the pathogenesis of somatotroph adenomas are ongoing. A mutation in the Gsα protein has been seen in up to 40% of somatotroph adenomas.[2]
- GH secretion, stimulated by GH-releasing hormone (GHRH) from the hypothalamus, causes increased IGF-1 secretion from the liver. Normally, GH secretion is inhibited by both somatostatin from the hypothalamus and insulin-like growth factor 1 (IGF-1) from peripheral tissue. IGF-1 causes growth of bone and cartilage, impaired glucose tolerance, and changes in protein and fat metabolism.

DIAGNOSIS

The diagnosis of acromegaly involves first recognizing the phenotype and then performing the appropriate hormonal work up. Lastly, imaging of the pituitary is performed.

Clinical Presentation

Patients with acromegaly present with **skeletal overgrowth and soft tissue enlargement.** Changes can be subtle over time and may best be recognized by comparing previous photographs of the patient. Symptoms related to hormonal deficiencies may arise as a result of compression of the remaining pituitary gland by the enlarging mass.

History
- Patients may complain of having to increase hat, ring, or shoe size.
- Headache is the second most common symptom, even when the adenoma is small.
- The voice tends to be deeper, related to sinus and laryngeal hypertrophy.
- Malodorous sweating, especially at night, may occur.
- Paresthesias related to carpal tunnel syndrome and other peripheral neuropathies occur, as do visual disturbances related to increased skeletal growth in the skull or to compression of the optic chiasm by the pituitary adenoma.
- Arthralgias and myalgais occur in 30% to 70% of patients with large joints affected more prominently. Spinal osteoarthritis with resulting backache, usually in the lumbar spine, also occurs. Rarely, spinal involvement leads to nerve compression leading to lumbar spinal stenosis or sciatica.[3]
- Dyspnea at rest or with exertion can happen with more advanced disease due to remodeling of myocardium.
- Endocrine symptoms related to compression of the remaining pituitary gland can be those of hypothyroidism (cold intolerance, fatigue, weight gain), hypogonadism (reduced libido, infertility, irregular menses), and hyperprolactinemia (irregular menses, galactorrhea).

Physical Examination
- Hypertension occurs in 20% to 50% of patients.[4]
- The extremities are broad with wide, thick, and stubby fingers.
- The nose is widened and thickened, the forehead and cheekbones are prominent, and facial lines are more visible. Mandibular overgrowth leads to prognathism, teeth separation, and jaw malocclusion.
- Skin can be sweaty and oily (70%), as well as coarse and thick. Skin tags occur more frequently and can grow in size.
- While arthropathy occurs, objective findings are less prominent. Decreased joint mobility may be seen in later disease. Joint effusions are rare.

Differential Diagnosis
- Other causes of increased growth hormone must be excluded. Exogenous use of GH should be considered in adolescent patients and body builders.
- Pituitary somatotroph carcinoma is exceptionally rare.
- Extra-pituitary GH oversecretion is rare but can occur with ectopic pituitary adenomas in the sphenoid sinus or nasopharyngeal cavity or, much more rarely, by a peripheral tumor such as a pancreatic neuroendocrine tumor. GHRH hypersecretion that causes pituitary somatotrophs to oversecrete GH has been seen with pancreatic and bronchial carcinoid tumors.
- Acromegaly is seen with the genetic syndromes of McCune–Albright and Carney complex. Acromegaly can be seen as part of the multiple endocrine neoplasia type 1 (MEN1) syndrome.

Diagnostic Testing
Laboratories
- The initial laboratory tests for a patient suspected of having acromegaly should be **IGF-1 and GH levels**. Current guidelines recommend an elevated IGF-1 and

failure to suppress GH during an oral glucose tolerance test (OGTT) to confirm the diagnosis. An OGTT may not be needed if GH and IGF-1 levels are elevated in a patient with clear signs and symptoms of acromegaly.[5]

- During an **OGTT**, blood is drawn at baseline for glucose and GH levels, 75 grams of oral glucose is administered, and then blood is drawn for GH and glucose every 30 minutes for 2 hours. Using ultrasensitive assays, if the GH level falls to <0.3 mcg/L during the OGTT, acromegaly is excluded.[4] False positives may occur in patients with diabetes, chronic hepatitis, renal failure, and anorexia. Patients with acromegaly can have suppressed GH levels (<0.3 mcg/L) during an OGTT.[6]
- TRH or GHRH stimulation tests should not be used because they yield discordant results.[7]
- Assessment of the remainder of pituitary hormones, including measurement of prolactin and free T4, should also take place. If indicated by symptoms, a cosyntropin stimulation test to diagnose adrenal insufficiency may be needed.

Imaging
- The initial imaging study should be magnetic resonance imaging (MRI) of the brain, with and without gadolinium contrast to evaluate for pituitary adenoma.
- Radiographs of the extremities and cranium will show abnormalities related to bone and cartilage overgrowth. Bone mineral density is not significantly decreased but there is a higher prevalence of vertebral fractures.
- Echocardiography can show hypertrophy of the interventricular septum and left ventricular posterior wall as well as diastolic, and less often systolic, dysfunction.

TREATMENT

- The goals of treatment include relief of symptoms, reduced tumor volume, and improvement of long-term morbidity and mortality. A GH level <1 mcg/L and an IGF-1 level in the normal range is the goal.[5]
- If left untreated, acromegalic patients live on average 10 years less than control patients. Death is most commonly due to cardiovascular disease.
- An algorithm presenting the three major treatment modalities is presented in Figure 3-1.

Medications
In general, all medical therapy for acromegaly should stop if a woman becomes pregnant, due to lack of available safety information.[8]

Somatostatin Analogs
- Somatostatin analogs, including **octreotide** (Sandostatin) and **lanreotide** (Somatuline), act as agonists on somatostatin receptors on the tumor to decrease GH secretion. These drugs are also available as monthly depot injections.
- They achieve adequate IGF-1 suppression in up to 50% of patients.[9]
- The use of these agents is most appropriate as first line therapy for tumors that have a low probability of surgical cure, as a temporizing measure before surgery to improve comorbidities, to control symptoms before radiation therapy achieves full effects, or after surgery when full biochemical control is not achieved.[8]
- The initial does of octreotide LAR is 10 mg IM q month. The dose is increased at 2 to 3 month intervals until plasma IGF-1 levels are normal or until a maximal dose of 40 mg IM q month is reached.

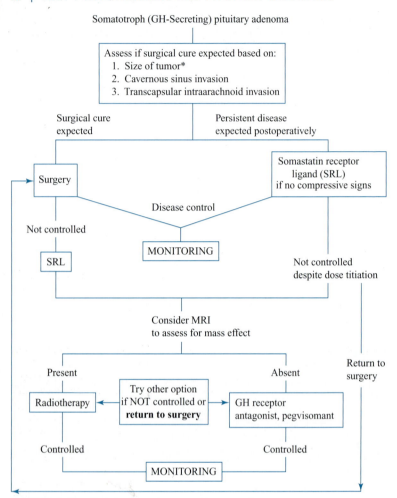

FIGURE 3-1 Algorithm for Management of Acromeagly.
*Influence of tumor size on surgical outcome is uncertain. As a rough guideline, tumor less than 2 cm has greater chance of surgical success.

- The initial dose of lanreotide is 60 mg via deep SC injection q month. The dose is increased as above until IGF-1 levels are normal or a maximal dose of 120 mg q month is reached.
- Side effects include abdominal bloating and cramping, which occur early and usually improve over the first few months of treatment. Gallstones occur more frequently but usually do not cause acute cholecystitis. Rarely, pancreatitis can occur.
- Patients should remain on the same dose for 3 months to assess adequacy of treatment.

GH Receptor Antagonist: Pegvisomant

- Pegvisomant (Somavert) blocks GH action in peripheral tissues by antagonizing the GH receptor. This agent can be used when adequate biochemical control is not achieved with other treatment modalities and possibly as monotherapy or in combination with a somatostatin analog.
- This results in normalization of IGF-1 levels in 89% of patients; however, a significant rise in GH levels is seen. It is unclear whether or not this increase in GH levels is associated with an increase in tumor size; however, two patients have required surgery for rapidly enlarging pituitary tumors while receiving pegvisomant.[10]
- The initial dose is 10 mg SC q day. The dose is increased in 5 mg increments at 4-week intervals until plasma IGF-1 is normal or a maximal dose of 30 mg is reached.
- 25% of patients have elevated liver enzymes so these should be followed every 6 months.

Dopamine Agonists

- The dopamine agonist **cabergoline** (Dostinex), inhibits secretion of GH by stimulating dopaminergic receptors on the adenoma, though only <10% achieve biochemical control with monotherapy.[11]
- The initial dosing of carbegoline is 0.25 mg twice per week.
- Side effects include nausea and orthostatic hypotension, so the medication should be started at low doses and gradually titrated up. With long-term therapy, there may be an increased risk of cardiac valvular abnormalities.

Radiation Therapy

- Radiation therapy should never be used as first-line therapy. It is usually employed after surgery fails to achieve hormonal control or decrease tumor growth.
- Both conventional fractionated radiotherapy and stereotactic radiotherapy (gamma-knife) have been used to treat somatotroph adenomas. Treatment with gamma-knife therapy appears to provide faster normalization of GH levels (though studies are flawed by selection bias), with less damage to surrounding brain tissue. Use of gamma-knife therapy is limited by tumor size and proximity to the optic nerves.[12]
- Full response to treatment with fractionated therapy may not be seen for up to 15 years.
- Up to 60% of patients develop hypopituitarism after radiotherapy, with this rate equal in conventional radiotherapy and gamma-knife therapy at 5 to 10 years. There may be an increased risk of secondary tumors and stroke over time with both forms of radiotherapy.[8]

Surgical Management

- Surgery results in the most rapid reduction in GH levels. However, its efficacy depends on the size of the adenoma and the experience of the surgeon.
- Control rates quoted in studies are best achieved with an experienced neurosurgeon, performing at least 50 pituitary operations per year.[13]
- Trans-sphenoidal surgery is appropriate for intrasellar microadenomas, noninvasive macroadenomas, and when the tumor is causing compressive symptoms. Craniotomy is rarely required. Control rates for macroadenomas are lower (~50%) than for microadenomas (90%). Tumors with cavernous sinus involvement or transcapsular intraarachnoid invasion have even lower cure rates.

COMPLICATIONS

- The standardized mortality ratio for patients with acromegaly is 1.72. Insulin resistance develops due to elevated IGF-1 levels. Patients must be screened for development of **type 2 diabetes mellitus**.
- **Pituitary dysfunction**, including hypothyroidism, hypogonadism, adrenal insufficiency, and hyperprolactinemia may occur due to local tumor effects and must be adequately screened for as described in Diagnostic Testing section.
- **Obstructive sleep apnea** occurs in 25% to 60% of patients with acromegaly. Though this may improve with treatment of acromegaly, some will continue to require nocturnal positive end-expiratory pressure.
- **Cardiovascular morbidity** is increased related to hypertension, left ventricular hypertrophy, diastolic and systolic dysfunction, and arrhythmias. Standard management of these complications is needed.
- Although it is controversial whether or not acromegalics have an increased risk of cancer, the rate of death is higher in patients with acromegaly who have colon cancer.[4] Current guidelines recommend at least one baseline colonoscopy and follow-up based on international guidelines for colonic polyps.[8]

MONITORING/FOLLOW-UP

- **Biochemical testing:**
  - In patients who have undergone surgery, IGF-1 and GH levels should be checked 3 months after surgery. An IGF-1 level in the normal range or random GH <1 mcg/L by ultrasensitive assay define control.[5]
  - An OGTT can also be used to assess outcome. Although many authors recommend using a nadir GH level <0.3 mcg/L to define control, current guidelines recommend a nadir GH level <0.4 mcg/L.[14]
  - Only IGF-1 levels are measured with GH receptor antagonist therapy and the OGTT should not be used in patients receiving somatostatin analogs. A full assessment of pituitary function should occur 3 months after surgery.
  - Ongoing assessment for pituitary dysfunction is needed after radiation therapy.
- **Tumor control by imaging**
  - Repeat MRI can be performed at 3 to 4 months after surgery to establish a baseline. Initial MRI after starting medical therapy should be at 3 to 6 months.[8]
  - The subsequent timing of MRI depends on disease control. If disease control is achieved by surgery, MRI may only be needed every 2 to 3 years. In patients who are not adequately controlled, MRI should likely be followed yearly.
  - With growth hormone receptor antagonist therapy, an MRI should be performed 6 months after initiation of therapy and then yearly because of the potential risk of tumor enlargement.

REFERENCES

1. Nachtigall L, Delgado A, Swearingen B, et al. Changing patterns in diagnosis and therapy of acromegaly over two decades. *J Clin Endocrinol Metab* 2008;93:2035–2041.
2. Melmed S. Acromegaly pathogenesis and treatment. *J Clin Invest* 2009;119:3189–3202.
3. Chanson P, Salenave S, Kamenicky P, et al. Acromegaly. *Best Pract Res Clin Endocrinol Metab* 2009;23:555–574.

4. Melmed S. Acromegaly. *N Engl J Med* 2006;355:2558–2573.
5. Guistina A, Chanson P, Bronstein D, et al. A consensus on criteria for cure of acromegaly. *J Clin Endocrinol Metab* 2010;95:3141–3148.
6. Ribeiro-Oliveira A, Faje A, Barkan A. Limited utility of oral glucose tolerance test in biochemically-active acromegaly. *Eur J Endocrinology;* 2010 OCT 6. [Epub ahead of print]
7. Cook DM, Ezzat S, Katznelson L, et al. AACE medical guidelines for clinical practice for the diagnosis and treatment of acromegaly. *Endocr Pract* 2004;10:213–225.
8. Melmed S, Colao A, Barkan A, et al. Guidelines for acromegaly management: An update. *J Clin Endocrinol Metab* 2009;94:1509–1517.
9. Newman CB, Melmed S, Snyder PJ, et al. Safety and efficacy of long-term octreotide therapy of acromegaly: Results of a multicenter trial in 103 patients—a clinical research center study. *J Clin Endocrinol Metab* 1995;80:2768–2775.
10. Trainer PJ, Drake WM, Katznelson L, et al. Treatment of acromegaly with the growth-hormone receptor antagonist pegvisomant. *N Engl J Med* 2000;342:1171–1177.
11. Abs R, Verhelst J, Maiter D, et al. Cabergoline in the treatment of acromegaly: A study in 64 patients. *J Clin Endocrinol Metab* 1998;83:374–378.
12. Landolt AM, Haller D, Lomax N, et al. Stereotactic radiosurgery for recurrent surgically treated acromegaly: Comparison with fractionated radiotherapy. *J Neurosurg* 1998;88:1002–1008.
13. Ahmed E, Stratton P, Adams W. Outcome of transphenoidal surgery for acromegaly and its relationship to surgical experience. *Clin Endocrinol (Oxf)* 1999;50:561–567.

Diabetes Insipidus

4

Prajesh M. Joshi and Julie Silverstein

GENERAL PRINCIPLES

Definition
- Diabetes insipidus (DI) is a disorder of water balance caused by the non-osmotic renal loss of water leading to the excretion of a large volume of dilute urine.
- Polyuria is defined by a 24-hour urine output >30 to 50 mL/kg in adults and >100 mL/kg in children.[1]

Classification
- **Central DI** is caused by either complete or partial deficiency of antidiuretic hormone (ADH) secretion from the posterior pituitary gland.
- **Nephrogenic DI** is caused by end-organ unresponsiveness of the kidneys to ADH. It can be complete or partial.
- **Dipsogenic DI** is caused by excessive and inappropriate fluid intake due to a defect in thirst mechanism.[1,2]

Epidemiology
- All forms of DI are rare with an estimated prevalence of central DI of 1/25,000.[3] No gender predilection has been seen. Most cases present in adulthood, although familial central DI and nephrogenic DI usually present during childhood.
- Overall incidence of transient DI after transsphenoidal surgery of the pituitary has been reported to be 18.3% to 31%, while only 0.5% to 2% of patients develop permanent dysfunction. Approximately 67.5% to 80% of patients with clinical evidence of postoperative DI need treatment with DDAVP (an ADH analog) at least once during the course of their management.[1]

Etiology
- See **Table 4-1** for a list of causes of diabetes insipidus.
- Central DI is caused by destruction of ADH-producing cells in the hypothalamus and posterior pituitary gland. The destruction can be traumatic, infectious, neoplastic, or infiltrative in origin resulting in complete or partial lack of ADH.
- Nephrogenic DI is caused by either congenital or acquired impaired renal responsiveness to ADH.

Pathophysiology
- ADH is synthesized in the supraoptic and paraventricular nuclei of the hypothalamus and transported to the posterior pituitary gland for storage and secretion. Osmoreceptors in the hypothalamus are very sensitive to changes in plasma osmolality, primarily determined by the sodium concentration.
- The release of ADH is inhibited until the osmolality rises above a threshold level, after which ADH secretion rises rapidly in proportion to the plasma osmolality. ADH is also secreted in response to volume depletion.

TABLE 4-1	CAUSES OF DIABETES INSIPIDUS
Central DI	Head trauma (may remit after 6 months)
	Postsurgical (develops 1–6 days after surgery and often disappears, recurs, or becomes chronic)
	Tumors—craniopharyngioma, pinealoma, meningioma, germinoma, glioma, benign cysts, leukemia, lymphoma, metastatic breast or lung
	Infections—TB, syphilis, mycoses, toxoplasmosis, encephalitis, meningitis
	Granulomatous disease—sarcoidosis, histiocytosis X, Wegener's granulomatosis
	Cerebrovascular disease—aneurysms, thrombosis, Sheehan's syndrome, cerebrovascular accident
	Idiopathic—sporadic or familial (rare autosomal dominant trait)
Nephrogenic DI	Congenital—rare inherited disorder caused by inherited mutations in the AVP receptor (X-linked recessive) or in the water channel of the renal tubule (autosomal recessive)
	Acquired—much more common and less severe
	Medications (lithium, amphotericin B, demeclocycline, cisplatin, aminoglycosides, rifampin, foscarnet, methoxyflurane, vincristine)
	Electrolyte disorders (hypercalcemia, hypokalemia)
	Chronic tubulointerstitial diseases (polycystic kidney disease, medullary sponge kidney, obstructive uropathy, papillary necrosis)
	Sickle cell disease and trait
	Multiple myeloma, amyloidosis
	Sarcoidosis

AVP, arginine vasopressin; DI, diabetes insipidus; TB, tuberculosis.
From Fried LF, Palevsky PM. Hyponatremia and hypernatremia. *Med Clin North Am* 1997;81: 585–609, with permission.

- ADH primarily acts on the distal tubules and collecting ducts of the kidneys to increase water reabsorption.
- The effects of ADH are mediated via a G protein-coupled V2 receptor that signals the translocation of aquaporin-2 channels into the apical membrane of the principal cells in the collecting duct. In conjunction with aquaporin-3 and aquaporin-4 channels on the basal–lateral surface of these cells, water is then allowed to flow freely down the osmotic gradient from the relatively dilute tubular fluid to the highly concentrated renal medulla. Therefore, decreased production or activity of ADH results in impaired water reabsorption in the nephron, leading to a dilute urine and loss of free water.
- An intact thirst mechanism is very effective in preventing hypernatremia (hypertonic dehydration). DI leads to a decrease in the absorption of free water which leads to an increase in basal plasma osmolality of as little as 1% to 2% which is sufficient to induce thirst. Once this threshold is reached, even a small increase in hypertonicity stimulates a very large increase in water intake, which prevents hypernatremia.

DIAGNOSIS

Patients with DI present with increased thirst and polyuria, with urine volume typically exceeding 3 L/day. Symptoms of hypernatremia (e.g., weakness, altered mental status, coma, or seizures) may develop with significant or rapid dehydration.

Clinical Presentation
History
- A thorough history including the patient's age, the rate of onset, duration and degree of polyuria, family history, history of head trauma/surgery, dietary habits, fluid intake, the presence/absence of thirst, the presence of headaches or vision changes, medication history, the presence of psychiatric illness, and a history of diabetes mellitus and/or renal failure is essential for diagnosis and to differentiate DI from other causes of polyuria.
- A history of nocturia is often present in DI.
- Patients with DI often crave cold liquids.

Physical Examination
Orthostatic hypotension and skin tenting may be signs of volume depletion.

Diagnostic Criteria
- Diagnosis of DI is made when polyuria is present in the setting of an inappropriately low urine osmolality (<300 mOsm/kg) for a given plasma osmolality. The urine specific gravity is usually <1.001 to 1.010.[1,2]
- Plasma sodium may be normal or elevated (i.e., in someone who does not have an intact thirst mechanism).

Differential Diagnosis
- Several conditions can present with polyuria. Simultaneous measurement of urine and plasma osmolality is essential to differentiate the various causes.
- **Hypotonic polyuria** (Uosm <300 mOsm/kg) can be either physiologic (due to an increase in free water intake leading to appropriate suppression of ADH, free water diuresis, and a normal serum osmolality) or pathologic (due to a decrease in the production or action of ADH).
- **A fully concentrated urine (urine osmolality 800 to 1200 mOsm/kg) in the setting of hypernatremia essentially rules out DI** and other causes should be considered (e.g., insensible water losses from skin, lungs, and GI tract and/or salt loading from feedings, medications, or intravenous fluids).
- **Non-hypotonic polyuria** (Uosm >300 mOsm/kg) is caused by **solute diuresis,** most commonly due to diuretics and hyperglycemia. Glucosuria in the setting of a urine specific gravity >1.010 is characteristic of polyuria due to hyperglycemia. If glucose is absent in the urine, other less common types of solute diuresis (such as relief from urinary obstruction, recovery from renal failure, or administration of large amounts of sodium, mannitol or radiocontrast dye) should be considered.
- If hyponatremia is present, polyuria is most likely due to **primary polydipsia**.
- **Chronic hypokalemia and hypercalcemia** can cause partial nephrogenic DI. On the other hand, hypokalemia can also be a consequence of DI, and hypercalcemia can be caused by volume depletion. Patients with chronic kidney disease may also develop partial DI as a consequence of defects in the renal concentrating capacity.

Diagnostic Testing

Water (Fluid) Deprivation Test

- This is the standard method for differentiating polyuria caused by primary polydipsia, central and nephrogenic DI.
- **This test is unnecessary, and could even be dangerous, in the setting of hypertonic hypernatremia**, in which primary polydipsia is not a consideration. Likewise, if the patient has hypotonic hyponatremia, DI is virtually ruled out. Therefore, a water deprivation test **should only be performed in a patient with hypotonic polyuria with a normal plasma sodium/osmolality.**
- Procedure
  - Drugs that influence ADH secretion or action should be discontinued if possible. Caffeine, alcohol, and tobacco should be avoided for at least 24 hours.
  - Patient's water intake is restricted starting after dinner unless the patient is producing >10 L of urine/day, in which case the deprivation test is only done during the day under close supervision. Body weight, plasma osmolality, serum sodium, urine osmolality, and urine volume should be followed hourly.
  - Fluids are withheld until,
    Body weight decreases by 5% and plasma sodium and osmolality reach the upper limits of normal (sodium >145 mEq/L and osmolality >295 mOsm/kg)
    OR
    A stable hourly urinary osmolality (variation of <5% over 3 hours) is established.
- Interpretation of the test
  - In healthy individuals, water deprivation increases plasma osmolality, which stimulates ADH secretion resulting in retention of water by the kidney (hence increasing urine osmolality).
  - In complete DI, with absent ADH or ineffective ADH, the urine osmolality remains less than plasma osmolality.
  - In partial DI and primary polydipsia, urine osmolality will be greater than plasma osmolality, but the urine will remain sub-maximally concentrated.
  - If a diagnosis of primary polydipsia has been excluded, ADH can be given to help differentiate between central and nephrogenic DI. DDAVP (desmopressin) 0.03 mcg/kg can be given subcutaneously and urine osmolality measured at 30, 60, and 120 minutes. If the urine osmolality increases >50% from the level achieved during dehydration, the diagnosis of central DI is established.
  - Plasma vasopressin should be measured before and after water deprivation unless the results are unequivocal. The levels should be analyzed as a function of the concurrent plasma and urine osmolality.[5] Patients with central DI and primary polydipsia have basal levels of plasma ADH that are subnormal. Patients with nephrogenic DI have normal to elevated basal levels. During water deprivation, ADH levels rise in primary polydipsia and nephrogenic DI but remain subnormal in central DI.
- Pitfalls of water deprivation test
  - The diagnosis of partial DI may be difficult, since there may be enough ADH secretion to partially concentrate the urine.
  - ADH secretion or action should be normal in patients with primary polydipsia, but the associated chronic polyuria can lead to "washout" of the medullary interstitium, resulting in loss of the transtubular osmolar gradient that is required to maintain the maximum urinary concentrating ability of the kidneys, hence making it difficult to differentiate from partial DI.

Hypertonic Saline Test

- The hypertonic saline test may be used if the water restriction test is inconclusive or cannot be performed. It may be useful to diagnose partial central DI, partial nephrogenic DI, and primary polydipsia.[3]
- Hypertonic (3%) saline is infused at 0.05 to 0.1 mL/kg/minute for 1 to 2 hours, and plasma osmolality and sodium are measured every 30 minutes.
- ADH is measured once the serum sodium and osmolality are above the upper limits of normal (sodium >145 mEq/L and osmolality >295 mOsm/kg).
- Normograms have been established to distinguish between primary polydipsia, partial central DI, and partial nephrogenic DI. However, this test **may be contraindicated in patients at risk for complications of volume overload** (e.g., those underlying heart disease or congestive heart failure).

TREATMENT

Replacement of Water Deficit

- Water deficit should be calculated and replaced orally with water whenever possible. Hypotonic saline can be given intravenously in a patient who cannot tolerate oral intake.
- If hypernatremia has developed rapidly over a period of hours, the water deficit can be corrected to decrease the plasma sodium at 1 mEq/L/hour. If hypernatremia developed slowly, the rate should be no more than 0.5 mEq/L/hour, up to a maximum of 8 to 10 mEq/L/day, using the smallest volume of fluid possible to avoid cerebral edema.[4]
- The water deficit can be calculated from the serum sodium using the following formula:

$$\text{Water deficit (L)} = \text{Total Body Water}^* \times ([Na+]serum - 140) \div 140$$

  For example, if a 70 kg man has serum sodium of 150 mEq/L, the calculated water deficit is 3 L [$\{0.6 \times 70 \times (150 - 140)\} \div 140$]. To decrease the sodium at a rate of 0.5 mEq/L/hour, 3 L of D5W can be administered over 20 hours [$(150-140 \text{ mEq/L}) \div 0.5 \text{ mEq/L/hour}$] at a rate of 150 mL/hour (3 L $\div$ 20 hours)

- Alternatively, the change in serum sodium for each liter of fluid given can be approximated from the following equation:

$$\text{Change in serum Na+} = ([Na+]infusate - [Na+]serum) \div (\text{Total Body Water}^* + 1)$$

  For the same person, the calculated decrease in sodium per liter of D5W would be $(0 - 150) \div (0.6 \times 70 + 1) = -3.5$ mEq/L. To decrease the sodium at an initial rate of 0.5 mEq/L/hour, D5W should be infused at approximately 143 mL/hour (0.5 mEq/L/hour $\div$ 3.5 mEq/L $\times$ 1000 mL). This formula is particularly useful when choosing a hypotonic fluid other than D5W.

  Total body water = Total body weight in kg $\times$ 0.6 in men/0.5 in women

- It should be noted that both of these strategies offer only approximations of the expected change in sodium and the rate of infusion needs to be adjusted to account for other ongoing free water losses.
- The fluid infusion rate may need to be decreased if DDAVP is used to treat DI, and plasma sodium and volume status should be assessed frequently (every 2 to 4 hours).

Treating the Underlying Defect

Central DI

- **DDAVP (desmopressin)** is an ADH-analog, which is a potent antidiuretic with no vasopressor activity and a longer duration of action than ADH. It is the most common agent used to treat central DI. It is available in parenteral, oral, and intranasal preparations.

- DDAVP given intravenously or subcutaneously has a rapid onset of action and is usually given at a dose of 1 to 2 mcg once or twice daily.
- Intranasal DDAVP also has a rapid onset of action and can be given at a dose of 1 to 4 sprays/day (1 spray = 10 mcg) in 1 to 3 divided doses/day.
- Oral DDAVP has an onset of action of 30 to 60 minutes and can be given at a dose of 0.1 to 0.4 mg one to four times a day with a maximum dose of 1.2 mg/day.
- Use of oral DDAVP has been shown to be very effective, but may be limited in some patients owing to variable gut absorption and reduced bioavailability.
- Conversion from intranasal to parenteral preparation is easily accomplished by reducing the dose by a factor of ten; conversion from intranasal to oral requires that the dose be titrated due to the variable bioavailability with oral preparations.

Acute Postsurgical Central DI

- Patients who are awake and alert and have an intact thirst mechanism should be able to maintain adequate fluid intake to prevent hypernatremia. Although these patients may not need drug therapy, they need to be closely monitored and drug therapy should be considered in patients who develop bothersome nocturia.
- If DDAVP is indicated, a simple and safe method of dosing a patient who has an intact thirst mechanism and who is tolerating oral intake is to start with 0.05 to 0.1 mg of oral DDAVP and assess for response (decreased urine output, increased urine osmolality, and decreased thirst). If the response is not appropriate within a few hours, the dose should be increased by 0.1 mg every few hours until an appropriate response (urine output <300 mL/hour) is achieved. The patient should continue to receive DDAVP on an as needed (PRN) basis until a stable regimen is found.
- Throughout the dose titration, patients should be given free access to water and told to drink only when thirsty to avoid water intoxication and hyponatremia.
- If oral intake is inadequate, intravenous administration of hypotonic fluid (D5W, 45% NaCl or 0.2% NaCl) should be used. Normal saline should be avoided in patients with DI unless needed for initial volume resuscitation/hypovolemia (solute load to kidneys worsens renal water loss).

Chronic Central DI

- Chronic DI in patients with an intact thirst mechanism should be treated with a fixed dosing regimen of DDAVP. The lowest possible dose (based on patient's symptoms) should be used to minimize the risk of hyponatremia. Patients are usually able to correct their free water losses by increasing their fluid intake (directed by their thirst mechanism).
- Bedtime dosing of DDAVP helps some patients to reduce disabling nocturia.
- Management is extremely difficult in adipsic patients with DI. In general, they are managed with a fixed dose of DDAVP and adequate hydration. They are instructed to adjust their fluid intake based on indirect indicators of water balance (e.g., daily weight measurements) or serum sodium when feasible.

Nephrogenic DI

- In acquired nephrogenic DI, correction of associated electrolyte disorders or discontinuation of offending drugs usually improves diabetes insipidus.
- A low sodium diet and a thiazide diuretic (e.g., hydrochlorothiazide 25 mg once or twice daily) can be used to control nephrogenic DI.

- Thiazides cause an overall reduction in electrolyte-free water excretion by stimulating proximal tubular sodium and water reabsorption, hence diminishing sodium/water delivery to the ADH-sensitive sites in the collecting tubules.
- Amiloride, which is a potassium sparing diuretic, may enhance the effect of thiazide diuretics by increasing sodium excretion and the resulting antipolyuric response to volume depletion. It can be used in lithium-induced DI because it acts by blocking sodium channels in the collecting ducts through which lithium enters and interferes with the tubular response to ADH.
- NSAIDs can also be a useful adjunct to treatment because they may decrease glomerular filtration as well as decrease the synthesis of prostaglandins that normally antagonize the action of ADH.
- DDAVP may be effective in patients with partial nephrogenic DI.

SPECIAL CONSIDERATIONS

Diabetes Insipidus After Pituitary Surgery

- Transient DI usually develops on postoperative days 1 to 3 and generally lasts 1 to 7 days.[5]
- Although rare, DI after transsphenoidal surgery can be associated with a triphasic pattern characterized by early DI, followed by normal urine output (or SIADH) due to release of stored hormone (lasts 24 hours to several days), followed by permanent DI (occurs once the hormone stores are depleted).[4]
- Microadenoma (secondary to stalk manipulation and exploration), intraoperative CSF leak, non-pituitary sellar lesions (i.e., craniopharyngiomas or rathke's cleft cysts), young age, male sex, suprasellar extension, and Cushing's disease have been shown to be predictors for DI after pituitary surgery.[6]
- Postoperative pituitary patients require close monitoring of their fluid intake and output, electrolytes, and urine specific gravity.
- Treatment is the same as in acute postsurgical central DI (see Treatment section).

COMPLICATIONS

- Overtreatment and undertreatment can result in hyponatremia and hypernatremia, respectively. Therefore, frequent monitoring is recommended.
- It is essential for a patient with DI to have access to water. A patient, who loses access to water, as may occur during a medical emergency or surgery, is at high risk for dehydration and hypernatremia. Under these circumstances, urine output and serum sodium concentration should be followed closely and hypotonic fluid and DDAVP (on a PRN basis) should be administered.

MONITORING/FOLLOW-UP

- Patients with central DI treated with DDAVP on a fixed dosing schedule should be monitored for the development of hyponatremia.
- Weight monitoring at home can be used for estimation of water loss/retention in adipsic patients.
- Occasional withdrawal of DDAVP is reasonable to confirm recurrence of polyuria.

PATIENT EDUCATION

- All patients with DI should be educated to wear or carry a medical alert tag or card.
- All patients with DI (and their family members) should be educated about the signs and symptoms of hyper/hyponatremia.

REFERENCES

1. Roberson GL. Differential diagnosis of polyuria. *Annu Rev Med* 1988;39:425–442.
2. Ball SG. Diabetes insipidus. *Medicine* 2005;33:18–19.
3. Zerbe RL, Robertson GL. A comparison of plasma vasopressin measurements with a standard indirect test in the differential diagnosis of polyuria. *N Engl J Med* 1981;305: 1539–1546.
4. Adrogue HJ, Madias NE. Hypernatremia. *N Engl J Med* 2000;342:1493–1499.
5. Ausiello JC, Bruce JN, Freda PU. Postoperative assessment of the patient after transsphenoidal pituitary surgery. *Pituitary* 2008;11:391–401.
6. Nemergut EC, Zuo Z, Jane JA, et al. Predictors of diabetes insipidus after transsphenoidal surgery: A review of 881 patients. *J Neurosurg* 2005;103:448–454.

Syndrome of Inappropriate Antidiuretic Hormone

Scott Goodwin and Thomas J. Baranski

GENERAL PRINCIPLES

Definitions

The syndrome of inappropriate secretion of antidiuretic hormone (SIADH) is a disorder in which water excretion is impaired by the unregulated secretion of ADH leading to free water retention and varying degrees of dilutional hyponatremia.[1]

Epidemiology

Hyponatremia is the most common electrolyte abnormality in hospitalized patients, with a prevalence estimated to be as high as 30% in some series.[2]

Etiology

- The causes of SIADH are summarized in Table 5-1.
- Prognosis is dependent on the underlying etiology as well as the severity of the hyponatremia and associated symptoms. SIADH usually resolves with therapy for the underlying etiology.

Pathophysiology

- Antidiuretic hormone (ADH), also known as vasopressin, is a key component of the homeostatic mechanisms that regulate water balance.
- In normal individuals, ADH is released from cells in the neurohypophysis in response to increased serum osmolality or decreased intravascular volume. ADH exerts its activity in the kidneys via the vasopressin V2 receptor to increase water permeability at the distal tubule and collecting duct of the nephron, enhancing water reabsorption at these sites.[3]
- With excess ADH, dilutional hyponatremia develops because water cannot be excreted normally. Therefore, the hallmark of SIADH is an inappropriately elevated urine osmolality in the setting of a low plasma osmolality.[3]

DIAGNOSIS

Clinical Presentation

- As with other causes of hyponatremia, symptoms are dependent on the degree of hyponatremia and the rapidity at which it develops.
- It is rare to have symptoms with serum sodium levels of ≥125 mEq/L, but with acute hyponatremia (<48 hours) patients may complain of malaise and nausea.[4]
- At serum sodium levels of <125 mEq/L, patients may present with neuropsychiatric signs and symptoms, ranging from muscular weakness, headache, lethargy, ataxia, and psychosis to cerebral edema, increased intracranial pressure (ICP), seizures, and coma.[4]

TABLE 5-1	CAUSES OF THE SYNDROME OF INAPPROPRIATE ANTIDIURETIC HORMONE

CNS (excess ADH release)
Acute intermittent porphyria
Bleeding (hematoma/hemorrhage)
CVA
Delirium tremens
Guillain–Barré syndrome
Head trauma
Hydrocephalus
Infections (meningitis/encephalitis/abscess)
Tumors

Medications
Bromocriptine mesylate (Bromocriptine)
Carbamazepine (Tegretol)
Chlorpropamide
Clofibrate
Cyclophosphamide
Desmopressin (DDAVP)
Ecstasy
Haloperidol (Haldol)
Nicotine
Opiates
Oxytocin
Phenothiazines
SSRIs
TCAs
Vinblastine
Vincristine

Miscellaneous
HIV
Nausea
Neuropsychiatric disorders (increased thirst, ADH release at lower osmolality, increased renal sensitivity to ADH)
Pain
Postoperative state (excessive amounts of electrolyte-free water)

Neoplasms (ectopic ADH secretion)
Duodenal carcinoma
Lymphoma
Mesothelioma
Olfactory neuroblastoma
Pancreatic carcinoma
Prostate carcinoma
Small cell carcinoma of lung
Thymoma
Pulmonary diseases
Bronchiectasis
COPD

(continued)

TABLE 5-1	CAUSES OF THE SYNDROME OF INAPPROPRIATE ANTIDIURETIC HORMONE (*Continued*)

Cystic fibrosis
Pneumonia (PCP, TB, aspergillosis)
Positive pressure ventilation

ADH, antidiuretic hormone; CNS, central nervous system; COPD, chronic obstructive pulmonary disease; CVA, cerebrovascular accident; SSRIs, selective serotonin reuptake inhibitors; TCAs, tricyclic antidepressants; PCP, *Pneumocystis carinii* pneumonia; TB, tuberculosis.

Adapted from Ellison DH, Berl T. The syndrome of inappropriate antidiuresis. *N Engl J Med* 2007;356:2064–2072.

- Signs of either volume depletion or overload are not consistent with SIADH and should prompt an evaluation for other causes of hyponatremia.[5]

Diagnostic Criteria

- SIADH is a diagnosis of exclusion, and therefore, other causes of hyponatremia must be ruled out.
- Essential diagnostic criteria include:[1–3]
  - **Low plasma osmolality:** a plasma osmolality <275 mOsm/kg is consistent with SIADH, and will rule out hypertonic causes of hyponatremia.
  - **Inappropriately elevated urine osmolality and urine sodium concentration:** a urine osmolality >100 mOsm/kg and urine sodium concentration >20 to 40 mEq/L are consistent with SIADH.
  - **Euvolemia:** volume depletion or overload should prompt an evaluation for an alternative diagnosis.
  - **Normal renal, adrenal, and thyroid function tests.**
  - **No recent use of diuretic agents.**
- Supplemental diagnostic criteria that are not needed to make a diagnosis of SIADH, but could be useful in situations of uncertainty, include:
  - **Abnormal water load test**, which is defined as the inability to excrete at least 80% of a water load (20 mL/kg water ingested in 10 to 20 minutes) after 4 hours and/or the failure to dilute urinary osmolality to <100 mOsm/kg. This test should be administered after the serum sodium level is >125 mEq/L through water restriction and/or saline administration.
  - No significant correction of plasma sodium with volume expansion, but improvement after fluid restriction.

Differential Diagnosis

- SIADH is a diagnosis of exclusion that should be differentiated from other known causes of euvolemic hypotonic hyponatremia. **Euvolemic hypotonic hyponatremia** is characterized by low to normal total body sodium and normal to elevated total body water.[1]
- The most common cause of euvolemic hypotonic hyponatremia is SIADH, but other causes of euvolemic hypotonic hyponatremia that must be excluded include:[2]
  - **Hypothyroidism** rarely causes hyponatremia, and the mechanisms by which this occurs are not entirely understood. Proposed mechanisms include dysregulation of ADH release or clearance, or both, as well as effects on vascular tone, cardiac output, and renal blood flow.

○ **Adrenal insufficiency** is also an unusual cause of hyponatremia. ADH is an adrenocorticotropic hormone (ACTH) secretagogue and is subject to negative feedback by glucocorticoids. Hyponatremia from adrenal insufficiency is thought to be caused by the loss of negative feedback on ADH secretion.

○ **Primary polydypsia** may lead to hyponatremia if free water intake exceeds the capacity of the kidneys to excrete free water.

○ **Potomania** was classically described in binge beer drinkers, but is now found more commonly in people with unusual dietary habits or eating disorders (e.g., anorexia nervosa). These patients develop hypotonic hyponatremia in the setting of dilute urine because of low solute intake and excretion. Free water clearance is dependent on solute excretion by the kidneys. If solute intake is decreased because of a restricted diet, solute excretion will also be decreased, and the kidneys will not be able to clear as much free water.

○ **Thiazide diuretics** typically cause hypotonic hyponatremia associated with hypovolemia, but patients can be euvolemic if free water intake is increased to compensate for thirst and volume depletion.

○ **Reset osmostat syndrome** is a variant of SIADH in which there is a shift in the set-point for ADH release to a lower plasma osmolality. Therefore, the patient may have inappropriately concentrated urine in the setting of hypotonic hyponatremia, but will be able to dilute urine normally in response to a water load and concentrate urine in response to dehydration.

○ **Nephrogenic syndrome of inappropriate antidiuresis** is a rare genetic syndrome in which all of the criteria for SIADH are met, but in which ADH levels are undetectable. It results from gain-of-function mutations in the renal vasopressin V2 receptor causing increased water resorption.[6]

TREATMENT

- SIADH is usually self-limited, and the primary management strategy is to correct the underlying etiology. However, immediate treatment strategies are based on the severity of the hyponatremia and any associated symptoms.
- Rate of correction:
  ○ Overly aggressive correction of hyponatremia may result in the development of **central pontine myelinolysis** (CPM), a potentially devastating neurologic condition; therefore, correction of hyponatremia should always be done with caution. If the rate of development of hyponatremia is rapid (<48 hours), an equally rapid rate of correction is felt to be safe. However, resolving the symptoms should be the primary goal, whereas correction to normonatremia should be performed more judiciously.[7] In cases where the acuity or chronicity of the hyponatremia is not known, the rate of correction should be limited to 1 to 2 mEq/L/hour for the first 3 to 4 hours, and by no more than 0.5 mEq/L/hour thereafter, for a maximum correction of 10 mEq/L per 24 hours.[7]
- With any chosen therapeutic strategy, plasma sodium, and volume status should be assessed frequently (initially every 2 hours, and reduced to every 4 hours when the correction rate is stable) to monitor and make adjustments to therapy.

Nonpharmacologic Therapies

- **Fluid restriction** is the mainstay of therapy for most patients with SIADH so that free water excretion in the urine exceeds dietary intake. In asymptomatic hyponatremia due to SIADH, an appropriate prescription for fluid restriction can be estimated by measuring plasma sodium and a spot urine sample for sodium. These values can then be used to determine the urine-to-plasma (U/P) electrolyte ratio:

$$\text{U/P ratio} = ([Na+]_{urine} + [K+]_{urine}) \div [Na+]_{plasma}$$

where $[Na+]_{urine}$ = mEq/L of sodium in the urine, $[K+]_{urine}$ = mEq/L of potassium in the urine, and $[Na+]_{plasma}$ = mEq/L of sodium in the plasma.

- If the U/P ratio is ≥1, free water should be maximally restricted. If the ratio is 0.5 to 1, free water should be restricted to ≤500 mL/day, and if the ratio is ≤0.5, free water should be restricted to ≤1000 mL/day.[8]

Medications

First Line

- **Intravenous saline** can improve SIADH-induced hyponatremia if the osmolality of the intravenous fluid is greater than the osmolality of the urine. This usually requires the use of hypertonic saline. *Hypertonic saline should be reserved ONLY for treatment of acute or symptomatic hyponatremia.*[8] Many strategies have been employed to calculate the initial rate of hypertonic saline. One simple formula to estimate the increase in plasma sodium for one liter of fluid:

$$\text{Change in } [Na+]_{plasma} = ([Na+]_{infusate} - [Na+]_{plasma}) \div (\text{total body water} + 1)$$

where $[Na+]_{infusate}$ = mEq/L of sodium in the infusate (e.g., 3% saline is 513 mEq/L), and total body water = body weight (kg) × (0.6 for men or 0.5 for women). For example, if a 70 kg man is having seizures and has a plasma sodium of 110 mEq/L, the calculated increase in sodium per liter of 3% saline would be (513 − 110) ÷ (0.6 × 71) = 9.4 mEq/L. To increase the sodium at an initial rate of 2 mEq/L/hour, 3% NaCl should be infused at 213 mL/hour (2 mEq/L/hour ÷ 9.4 mEq/L × 1000 mL). If one can estimate the expected change of sodium in 1 L of intravenous fluid, a rate can be calculated for that infusion to avert over-correcting too quickly.

- **Oral salt tablets** increase serum sodium by the same mechanism as hypertonc saline. Salt tablets are usually reserved for treatment of chronic or asymptomatic hyponatremia.[7]

Second Line

- **Loop diuretics** can enhance the effect of solute loading with oral salt or intravenous saline by increasing free water excretion and impairing the renal responsiveness to ADH.[7]
- **Demeclocycline** acts on the renal collecting tubules to diminish responsiveness to ADH, resulting in increased free water excretion. The typical dose of 300 to 600 mg twice daily is typically reserved for chronic or asymptomatic SIADH-induced hyponatremia.[7] The major side effect is nephrotoxicity, so renal function should be monitored closely.
- **Vasopressin receptor antagonists** exert their activity on renal V2 receptors resulting in a selective water diuresis without affecting sodium excretion.[7,9] Examples include intravenous conivaptan and oral tolvaptan. Multiple studies have shown these agents to effectively increase serum sodium level when compared to placebo. However, trials comparing vasopressin receptor antagonists versus traditional therapies (water restriction or salt administration) have not been performed.[10,11] Intravenous conivaptan can exert its effect in as little as 1 to 2 hours, permitting a more rapid initial elevation on serum sodium.[10] While this may be an initial benefit in patients who are symptomatic, careful monitoring must be maintained to avoid

overly rapid correction of hyponatremia. Thirst increases significantly with these agents and water restriction is needed to ensure the rise of serum sodium.[11] The financial expense also limits the use of these agents. Therefore, the vasopressin receptor antagonists are typically used in conjunction with traditional therapies in the rare patients who have severe hyponatremia (serum sodium <115 to 120) and neurologic symptoms.[9]

REFERENCES

1. Adrogue HJ, Madia NE. Hyponatremia. *N Engl J Med* 2000;342:1581–1589.
2. Robinson, AG. Posterior Pituitary. In: Gardner DG, Shoback D, eds. *Greenspan's Basic & Clinical Endocrinology,* 8th ed. New York, NY: McGraw-Hill Companies 2007:157–168.
3. Ball SG, Baylis PH. Vasopressin, diabetes insipidus, and syndrome of inappropriate antidiuresis. In: DeGroot LJ, Jameson JL, eds. *Endocrinology,* 5th ed. Philadelphia, PA: Elsevier; 2006:537–556.
4. Sterns RH, Nigwekar SU, Hix JK. The treatment of hyponatremia. *Semin Nephrol* 2009; 29:282–299.
5. Ellison DH, Berl T. The syndrome of inappropriate antidiuresis. *N Engl J Med* 2007;356: 2064–2072.
6. Decaux G, Vandergheynst F, Bouko Y, et al. Nephrogenic syndrome of inappropriate antidiuresis in adults: High phenotypic variability in men and women from a large pedigree. *J Am Soc Nephrol* 2007;18:606–612.
7. Verbalis JG, Goldsmith SR, Greenberg A, et al. Hyponatremia treatment guidelines 2007: Expert panel recommendations. *Am J Med* 2007;120:1–21.
8. Furst H, Hallows KR, Post J, et al. The urine/plasma electrolyte ratio: A predictive guide to water restriction. *Am J Med Sci* 2000;319:240–244.
9. Cawley MJ. Hyponatremia: Current treatment strategies and the role of vasopressin antagonists. *Ann Pharmacother* 2007;41:840–850.
10. Zeltser D, Rosansky S, Van Rensburg H, et al. Assessment of the efficacy and safety of intravenous conivaptan in euvolemic and hypervolemic hyponattremia. *Am J Nephrol* 2007; 27:447–457.
11. Schrier RW, Gross P, Gheorghiade M, et al. Tolvaptan, a selective oral vasopressin V2-receptor antagonist, for hyponatremia. *N Engl J Med* 2006;355:2099–2112.

Evaluation of Thyroid Function

6

William E. Clutter

GENERAL PRINCIPLES

- The major hormone secreted by the thyroid is **thyroxine** (T_4), which is converted by deiodinases in many tissues to the more potent **triiodothyronine** (T_3). Both are reversibly bound to plasma proteins, primarily **thyroxine-binding globulin (TBG)**, and also thyroxine-binding prealbumin (TBPA) and albumin. Only the free (unbound) fraction enters cells and produces biologic effects.
- T4 secretion is stimulated by **thyroid-stimulating hormone (TSH)**. In turn, pituitary TSH secretion is inhibited by thyroid hormones, forming a sensitive negative-feedback loop that keeps free T_4 levels within a narrow normal range. TSH secretion is stimulated by hypothalamic thyrotropin-releasing hormone (TRH).
- Diagnosis of thyroid disease is based on clinical findings, palpation of the thyroid, and measurement of plasma TSH and thyroid hormones.

DIAGNOSIS

Clinical Presentation

- **Thyroid palpation** determines the size and consistency of the thyroid, and the presence of nodules, tenderness, or a thrill. Auscultation may detect a bruit over the gland in severe hyperthyroidism.
- **Examination of the eyes** includes assessment for lid lag and proptosis in suspected hyperthyroidism and periorbital edema in suspected hypothyroidism. **Skin examination** may reveal warm, moist skin in hyperthyroidism and dry, cool skin or myxedema in hypothyroidism. **Neurologic signs** include brisk tendon reflex relaxation and fine tremor in hyperthyroidism and delayed reflex relaxation in hypothyroidism.

Diagnostic Testing

Laboratories[1]

- **Thyroid-stimulating hormone**
  - **Plasma TSH is the initial test of choice in most patients with suspected thyroid disease,** except when thyroid function is not in a steady state or TSH secretion by the pituitary may be abnormal (Table 6-1).
  - TSH levels are elevated in even very mild primary hypothyroidism and are suppressed to <0.1 μU/mL in even very mild hyperthyroidism. Therefore, **a normal plasma TSH level excludes hyperthyroidism and primary hypothyroidism**. Because even slight changes in thyroid hormone levels affect TSH secretion, **abnormal TSH levels are not specific for clinically important thyroid disease**. Changes in plasma TSH lag behind changes in plasma T_4, and TSH levels may be misleading when plasma T_4 levels are changing rapidly, as during treatment of hyperthyroidism, or in the first few weeks after changes in the dose of thyroxine.

TABLE 6-1	PLASMA TSH MEASUREMENT

Appropriate uses

Diagnosis of suspected hyperthyroidism or primary hypothyroidism

Monitoring and adjustment of therapy for primary hypothyroidism

Monitoring TSH suppression therapy for thyroid cancer

Inappropriate uses

Evaluation of suspected secondary hypothyroidism

Monitoring and adjustment of therapy for secondary hypothyroidism

Within several weeks of a change in thyroxine dose

During early stages of treatment of hyperthyroidism

○ **Plasma TSH is mildly elevated** (<20 μU/mL) in some euthyroid patients recovering from **nonthyroidal illnesses** and in **mild** (or **subclinical**) **hypothyroidism.**

○ TSH levels may be suppressed to <0.1 μU/mL in **severe nonthyroidal illness,** in **mild** (or **subclinical**) **hyperthyroidism,** and during treatment with dopamine or high doses of glucocorticoids (Table 6-2). Also, TSH levels remain <0.1 μU/mL for some time **after hyperthyroidism is corrected.** TSH levels decrease in the first trimester of **pregnancy** (owing to thyroid stimulation by chorionic gonadotropin) and may fall to <0.1 μU/mL.

○ TSH levels are usually within the reference range in secondary hypothyroidism due to pituitary or hypothalamic disease, and not useful for detection of this rare form of hypothyroidism.

• **Plasma free T_4**

Measurement of plasma free T_4 confirms the diagnosis and assesses the severity of **hyperthyroidism** when plasma TSH is <0.1 μU/mL (Table 6-3). It is also used to diagnose **secondary hypothyroidism** and adjust thyroxine therapy in patients with pituitary disease. Most laboratories measure free T_4 by one of several types of immunoassay.

• **Plasma free T_4 measured by equilibrium dialysis**

Plasma free T_4 by equilibrium dialysis (ED) is the most reliable measure of clinical thyroid status, but results are seldom rapidly available. ED is needed only in rare cases in which the diagnosis is not clear from measurement of plasma TSH and free T_4 by immunoassay.

• **Plasma total T_4**

Plasma total T_4 assays measure both bound and free hormone. Because altered levels of TBG cause abnormal total T_4 levels in euthyroid patients, total T_4 is less reliable than free T_4 and should not be used, except when free T_4 may be artifactually

TABLE 6-2	CAUSES OF A SUPPRESSED PLASMA TSH

Clinical hyperthyroidism

Subclinical hyperthyroidism

Recently resolved hyperthyroidism

First trimester of pregnancy

Nonthyroidal illness

Dopamine therapy

High-dose glucocorticoid therapy

TABLE 6-3	APPROPRIATE USES OF PLASMA FREE T$_4$

Confirmation of the diagnosis and severity of hyperthyroidism
Confirmation of the severity of primary hypothyroidism
Diagnosis of suspected secondary hypothyroidism
Monitoring and adjustment of therapy for secondary hypothyroidism

elevated by heparin treatment (see Effect of Drugs on Thyroid Function Tests in this chapter). Some common causes of increased TBG are estrogen treatment, including oral contraceptives, and pregnancy. Low TBG levels are common in cirrhosis, nephrotic syndrome, and many severe illnesses.

- **Plasma total T$_3$**
Although T$_3$ is the biologically active hormone, much of it is derived from deiodination of T$_4$ within target cells, making T$_4$ the major circulating thyroid hormone. Plasma T$_3$ level is affected by alterations in plasma TBG just as is plasma T$_4$. This test has very limited use in the evaluation of suspected thyroid disease, and **should only be measured in patients with suspected hyperthyroidism with suppressed plasma TSH but normal plasma free T$_4$.** Some of these patients have clinical hyperthyroidism with elevation of plasma T$_3$ alone (**T$_3$ toxicosis**). Plasma T$_3$ assays are not useful in the diagnosis of hypothyroidism. Many laboratories offer assays of plasma free T$_3$, but their reliability is unknown.

- **Plasma thyroglobulin**
  ○ Thyroglobulin (Tg), the precursor of thyroid hormones, is a glycoprotein synthesized only by thyroid follicular cells. Most thyroglobulin is broken down within the thyroid to release T$_4$ and T$_3$, but a small amount enters the circulation intact. Plasma thyroglobulin levels are increased in all thyroid diseases and are undetectable when all thyroid tissue has been removed. The only use of plasma thyroglobulin assays is **monitoring of patients with papillary or follicular thyroid carcinoma after total thyroidectomy** to detect persistent or recurrent disease.
  ○ An assay for **antithyroglobulin antibodies** should always be done in conjunction with the thyroglobulin assay, since the presence of such antibodies renders the thyroglobulin assay useless.

- **Antithyroid antibodies**
Patients with autoimmune thyroid diseases (Hashimoto's thyroiditis, painless thyroiditis, and Graves' disease) often have **autoantibodies against thyroid peroxidase, thyroglobulin,** or both. Measurement of these antibodies has a very limited role in thyroid diagnosis. They can be used to confirm that primary hypothyroidism or a euthyroid goiter is due to Hashimoto's thyroiditis, but this diagnosis can usually be made on clinical grounds.

- **Thyroid-stimulating immunoglobulins**
Thyroid-stimulating immunoglobulins (TSIs) are **autoantibodies to the TSH receptor** that mimic the stimulatory effect of TSH on thyroid growth and hormone production, and cause hyperthyroidism in **Graves' disease.** Measurement of these antibodies is seldom needed to make this diagnosis, which is usually obvious on clinical grounds. Its primary use is in **pregnant women with a history of Graves' disease treated by radioactive iodine or thyroidectomy.** These patients may still have high levels of TSI, which can no longer produce hyperthyroidism in the mother, but can cross the placenta and cause neonatal hyperthyroidism. Assay of TSI in the third trimester has some value in predicting this rare complication.

- **Plasma calcitonin**

  Calcitonin is the secretory product of thyroid parafollicular or C cells. Although it has no apparent physiologic role, it is a useful tumor marker for **medullary carcinoma of the thyroid** (MCT), which is derived from parafollicular cells. Mild elevations of plasma calcitonin are not specific for MCT.

- **Radioactive iodine uptake**

  Radioactive iodine uptake (RAIU) is the percentage of a small oral dose of iodine-131 (^{131}I) retained by the thyroid after 24 hours. It occasionally helps in **differential diagnosis of hyperthyroidism** (see Chapter 8), and is also used to calculate the dose for RAI therapy. Large doses of exogenous iodine in the form of x-ray contrast media or iodine-containing drugs suppress RAIU temporarily. The normal range of RAIU for dietary iodine intake in the United States is 10% to 30%. Note that RAIU is a number, not an image.

Imaging

Although thyroid imaging tests are widely used, they have very limited value in the assessment of patients with suspected thyroid disease, since clinically important abnormalities of thyroid anatomy are readily assessed by palpation.

- **Radioisotope thyroid scan**

  ○ Radioisotope thyroid scans use technetium-99m pertechnetate, which is taken up by the sodium-iodine symporter of thyroid cells. These scans can determine the functional activity of thyroid nodules: hypofunctioning ("cold"), isofunctioning ("warm"), or hyperfunctioning ("hot").

  ○ Almost all thyroid carcinomas are hypofunctioning, but unfortunately for the usefulness of this test, so are most benign nodules, resulting in a very low positive predictive value (PPV). This test has been supplanted in the evaluation of thyroid nodules by fine-needle aspiration cytology (FNAC).

  ○ The only indication for radioisotope thyroid scanning is the presence of **a single palpable thyroid nodule in a patient with hyperthyroidism**. If the nodule is hyperfunctioning and causing hyperthyroidism, it is assuredly benign and does not require biopsy. On the other hand, a hypofunctioning nodule in a gland affected by Graves' disease should be evaluated by FNAC.

- **Ultrasonography**

  ○ High-resolution ultrasonography (US) of the thyroid has become widely used, despite a lack of evidence that its use improves the clinical outcome in patients with thyroid disease. Its primary role is in the evaluation of thyroid nodules. It differentiates solid from cystic nodules and may be used to guide fine-needle biopsy, particularly of nonpalpable nodules.

  ○ The critical limitation of US is the **high prevalence of incidental thyroid nodules, which are found in 20% to 60% of the population.** Most of these nodules are of no clinical importance, and their detection leads only to unnecessary anxiety, further testing, and even unnecessary surgery. **US has no role in the evaluation of diffuse goiters, or of patients with hypo- or hyperthyroidism.**

Diagnostic Procedures

Fine-needle aspiration cytology

FNAC is the method of choice for evaluating thyroid nodules for the presence of malignancy. It is a safe and simple bedside procedure, and provides a definitive diagnosis in the great majority of patients. If the specimen obtained is inadequate for diagnosis, the procedure should be repeated. Complications are rare and consist mostly of transient painful swelling of the nodule due to bleeding within it.

SPECIAL CONSIDERATIONS

- **Effect of nonthyroidal illness on thyroid function tests**
  Many illnesses alter thyroid tests without causing true thyroid dysfunction (the nonthyroidal illness or euthyroid sick syndrome).[2] These changes must be recognized to avoid mistaken diagnosis and therapy.
  - **The low T_3 syndrome** occurs in many illnesses, during starvation, and after trauma or surgery. Conversion of T_4 to T_3 by type 1 deiodinase is decreased, and plasma T_3 levels are low. Plasma free T_4 and TSH levels are normal. This may be an adaptive response to illness, and thyroid hormone therapy is not beneficial.
  - **The low T_4 syndrome** occurs in severe illness. Plasma total T_4 levels fall due to decreased levels of TBG and perhaps due to inhibition of T_4 binding to TBG. **Plasma free T_4 measured by equilibrium dialysis usually remains normal.** However, when measured by commonly available immunoassays, free T_4 may be low. **TSH levels decrease early in severe illness,** sometimes to <0.1 μU/mL. **During recovery they rise, sometimes to levels higher than the normal range** (although rarely >20 μU/mL).
- **Effect of drugs on thyroid function tests**
  A number of drugs affect thyroid function tests (Table 6-4). Iodine-containing drugs (**amiodarone** and **radiographic contrast media**) may cause hyperthyroidism

TABLE 6-4	EFFECTS OF DRUGS ON THYROID FUNCTION TESTS
Effect	**Drug**
Decreased free and total T_4	
True hypothyroidism (TSH elevated)	Iodine (amiodarone, radiographic contrast)
	Others (see Chapter 9)
Inhibition of TSH secretion	Glucocorticoids
	Dopamine
Multiple mechanisms (TSH normal)	Phenytoin
Decreased total T_4 only	
Decreased TBG (TSH normal)	Androgens
Inhibition of T_4 binding to TBG (TSH normal)	Furosemide (high doses), salicylates
Increased free and total T_4	
True hyperthyroidism (TSH <0.1 μU/mL)	Iodine (amiodarone, radiographic contrast)
Inhibited T_4 to T_3 conversion (TSH normal)	Amiodarone
Increased free T_4 only	
Displacement of T4 from TBG in vitro (TSH normal)	Heparin, low-molecular-weight heparin
Increased total T_4 only	
Increased TBG (TSH normal)	Estrogens, tamoxifen, raloxifene

T_3, triiodothyronine; T_4, thyroxine; TBG, thyroxine-binding globulin; TSH, thyroid-stimulating hormone.

or hypothyroidism in susceptible patients. Other drugs alter thyroid function tests, especially plasma total T_4, without causing true thyroid dysfunction. In general, plasma TSH levels are reliable in determining whether true hyperthyroidism or hypothyroidism is present.

- **Evaluation of thyroid function in pregnancy**
  Thyroid hormone is critical for fetal brain development, and several changes occur in maternal thyroid function during pregnancy.[3] **TBG and total T_4 levels** rise early in pregnancy. **Chorionic gonadotropin** is homologous to TSH, and very high levels in the first trimester stimulate the TSH receptor, causing a transient **fall in TSH levels** by stimulating T_4 secretion. The mother usually remains euthyroid, but rarely she develops a transient clinical hyperthyroidism, often associated with hyperemesis gravidarum.

  ○ **The placenta contains high levels of type 3 deiodinase (D3), which inactivates T_4 and severely limits T_4 transfer from mother to fetus.** Nevertheless, some T_4 crosses the placenta and is important for early fetal brain development. **In mothers with preexisting hypothyroidism, increased T_4 metabolism by placental D3 means that their levothyroxine dose must usually be increased to maintain euthyroidism.** Urinary iodine excretion increases, and in areas of iodine deficiency, it becomes more difficult for the thyroid to maintain adequate hormone secretion, with development of a transient goiter. If the iodine deficiency is too severe, the fetus receives inadequate thyroid hormone, and endemic cretinism results.

  ○ Thyroid disorders and pregnancy often coincide (because of the frequency of thyroid disease in young women). Important interactions between the two include (a) the normal decrease in TSH in the first trimester, which may be mistaken for hyperthyroidism; (b) in hypothyroid women, the frequent need to increase levothyroxine dose in pregnancy; (c) the complexity of treating hyperthyroidism in pregnant women without adversely affecting the fetus; and (d) the occasional occurrence of a transient hyperthyroidism caused by painless thyroiditis in the months after delivery.

REFERENCES

1. Dufour DR. Laboratory tests of thyroid function: Uses and limitations. *Endocrinol Metab Clin North Am* 2007;36:579–594.
2. Adler SM, Wartofsky L. The nonthyroidal illness syndrome. *Endocrinol Metab Clin North Am* 2007;36:657–672.
3. Abalovich M, Amuino N, Barbour LA, et al. Management of thyroid dysfunction during pregnancy and postpartum: An Endocrine society clinical practice guideline. *J Clin Endocrinoll Metab* 2007;92:S1–S47.

Euthyroid Goiter and Thyroid Nodules

7

William E. Clutter

GENERAL PRINCIPLES

Definition
- Euthyroid goiter is defined as thyroid enlargement with normal thyroid function. There are three forms: **diffuse goiter, multinodular goiter (MNG)**, and a **solitary thyroid nodule.**
- **The diagnosis of euthyroid goiter is based on palpation of the thyroid and evaluation of thyroid function.** If the thyroid is enlarged, the examiner should determine whether the enlargement is diffuse or multinodular, or whether a single nodule is palpable.

Epidemiology
All three forms of euthyroid goiter are common, especially in women. Imaging studies, such as thyroid scans or ultrasonography, provide no useful additional information about goiters that are diffuse or multinodular by palpation and should not be performed in these patients. Furthermore, **20% to 60% of people have nonpalpable thyroid nodules that are detectable by ultrasound.** These nodules rarely have any clinical importance, but their incidental discovery may lead to unnecessary diagnostic testing and treatment.

EUTHYROID DIFFUSE GOITER

GENERAL PRINCIPLES

Almost all euthyroid diffuse goiters in iodine-sufficient regions such as the United States are caused by **chronic lymphocytic thyroiditis (Hashimoto's thyroiditis). Iodine deficiency** also causes diffuse colloid goiter in much of the world. Because Hashimoto's thyroiditis may also cause hypothyroidism, **plasma thyroid-stimulating hormone (TSH)** should be measured even in patients who are clinically euthyroid. The presence of antithyroid antibodies confirms the diagnosis of Hashimoto's disease, but this test is seldom needed. Thyroid imaging should not be performed.

DIAGNOSIS

- Diffuse goiter is diagnosed by thyroid palpation. Imaging is not needed and often detects incidental, clinically unimportant nodules.
- Small diffuse goiters usually are **asymptomatic,** and therapy is seldom required. Larger goiters may cause **compressive symptoms** such as **dysphagia, dyspnea,** or **neck fullness.**

TREATMENT

Patients should be followed annually with thyroid palpation and measurement of plasma TSH to monitor for the development of hypothyroidism. Most diffuse goiters do not progressively enlarge, but in a few, thyroidectomy may be needed to relieve compressive symptoms or for cosmetic reasons.

MULTINODULAR GOITER

GENERAL PRINCIPLES

MNG is caused by nodular hyperplasia of thyroid follicles. It occurs most commonly in iodine-deficient regions, but is also very common in iodine-sufficient areas such as the United States, primarily in **older patients and in women.**

DIAGNOSIS

- MNG is diagnosed by thyroid palpation. Most patients are asymptomatic and require no treatment. In a few patients, **hyperthyroidism (toxic MNG)** develops (see Chapter 8). In some patients, the goiter causes compressive symptoms, and treatment is required.
- The risk of malignancy in MNG is comparable to the frequency of incidental thyroid carcinoma in clinically normal glands. Evaluation for thyroid carcinoma with fine-needle aspiration cytology (FNAC) is warranted if there is a dominant nodule (a nodule that is disproportionately larger than the other nodules).
- Some centers have adopted a policy of performing thyroid ultrasonography (US) in all patients with MNG, and evaluating all nodules larger than 1 cm by FNAC. This policy dramatically increases the number of thyroid biopsies and the cost of managing this common condition. **There is no evidence that routine thyroid US improves clinical outcomes in patients with MNG, and it is not recommended.**[1]

TREATMENT

- Subtotal thyroidectomy is the treatment of choice for patients with compressive symptoms. If the patient is a poor candidate for surgery or refuses surgery, a high dose (about 50 mCi) of radioactive iodine (RAI) will reduce gland size and improve symptoms in most patients.[2]
- Thyroxine treatment has little if any effect on the size of MNGs and should not be used.

SINGLE THYROID NODULES

GENERAL PRINCIPLES

Single thyroid nodules are palpable in about 5% of women and 1% of men. They are usually due to benign nodular hyperplasia or thyroid adenomas, but about 5% are thyroid carcinomas, and the main diagnostic task is diagnosing or excluding carcinoma.

DIAGNOSIS

Clinical Presentation

- Most thyroid nodules present as a **painless lump in the neck** discovered by the patient or physician.
- **Clinical findings that increase the likelihood of carcinoma** include age <20 years, the presence of cervical lymphadenopathy, a history of radiation to the head or neck in childhood, and a family history of medullary thyroid carcinoma or multiple endocrine neoplasia (MEN) syndromes type 2A or 2B. A hard, fixed nodule; recent nodule growth; or hoarseness due to invasion of the recurrent laryngeal nerve also suggests malignancy. However, most patients with thyroid carcinomas have none of these risk factors, and their lesions cannot be distinguished clinically from benign nodules. Thus, **nearly all palpable single thyroid nodules should be evaluated with FNAC.**
- A few solitary thyroid nodules are **adenomas producing hyperthyroidism** (see Chapter 8). Some thyroid nodules present with the sudden onset of pain and tenderness, indicating hemorrhage into a preexisting, usually benign, nodule. Solitary nodules rarely cause compressive symptoms.

Diagnostic Testing

- **Plasma TSH** should be measured, since a nodule in a hyperthyroid patient is more likely to be benign. **If plasma TSH is suppressed**, a radioisotope thyroid scan should be performed. If the nodule is hyperfunctioning and causing hyperthyroidism, it is assuredly benign and does not require biopsy. On the other hand, a hypofunctioning nodule in a gland affected by Graves' disease should be evaluated by FNAC. **This is the only indication for radioisotope scanning in patients with a thyroid nodule.**
- **Plasma calcitonin** should be measured if there is a family history of medullary carcinoma or MEN 2A or 2B.
- **The key diagnostic evaluation is FNAC,** the results of which are classified into five major diagnostic categories[3] (Table 7-1):
  - ○ Nodules with **benign** cytology should be reevaluated periodically by palpation, since there is a low risk of false-negative cytology. Repeat biopsy should be considered if the nodule enlarges. Levothyroxine therapy has little or no effect on the size of single thyroid nodules, and is not indicated.
  - ○ If the specimen is **nondiagnostic or unsatisfactory,** the biopsy should be repeated.
  - ○ Nodules with **malignant** cytology or cytology suspicious for malignancy should be treated by total thyroidectomy followed by treatment described in the Thyroid Carcinoma section in this chapter.

TABLE 7-1	DIAGNOSTIC CATEGORIES OF FINE-NEEDLE ASPIRATION CYTOLOGY
Benign	
Nondiagnostic or unsatisfactory	
Malignant or suspicious for malignancy	
Atypical	
Follicular neoplasm	

○ About 5% to 15% of nodules with **atypical** cytology are malignant. These lesions are usually evaluated by repeat biospy. If the repeat biopsy does not provide a definitive diagnosis, a lobectomy is often performed, with completion thyroidectomy if carcinoma is confirmed.

○ Nodules that are **follicular neoplasms** are malignant 15% to 30% of the time. These patients should be treated with a lobectomy, with completion thyroidcdectomy if carcinoma is confirmed.

• Some centers have adopted a policy of performing thyroid US in all patients with a single palpable nodule, and performing FNAC on all nodules larger than 1 cm. Some ultrasonographic features of thyroid nodules are suggestive of malignancy, but they are neither sensitive nor specific enough to establish or exclude the diagnosis. There is no evidence that routine thyroid US improves clinical outcomes in these patients, and it is not recommended.

THYROID CARCINOMA

GENERAL PRINCIPLES

Most thyroid malignancies are differentiated carcinomas arising from follicular cells (**papillary or follicular carcinomas**) (Table 7-2).[4] These cancers retain many properties of normal thyroid cells: they **take up iodine** and **synthesize thyroglobulin**, although less efficiently than normal thyroid tissue. **Their growth and function is stimulated by TSH.** These three properties are used in treatment and follow-up of thyroid carcinoma.

Classification

• **The most common type of thyroid cancer is papillary carcinoma**, which is a slow growing tumor that may remain localized for years. It characteristically metastasizes first to cervical lymph nodes. Microscopic foci of papillary carcinoma are common at autopsy. Thus, a small papillary carcinoma found incidentally in a thyroid removed for other reasons, is usually not clinically important.

• **Follicular carcinoma** is more aggressive, and may metastasize early to lung and bone. Many thyroid cancers have mixed papillary and follicular morphology; these behave like papillary carcinoma.

• **Anaplastic** carcinoma is a rare, rapidly progressive thyroid cancer with a very poor prognosis.

TABLE 7-2	MAJOR TYPES OF THYROID CANCER
Type	**Frequency**
Follicular cell origin	
Papillary	80%
Follicular	15%
Anaplastic	Rare
C-cell (parafollicular cell) origin	
Medullary carcinoma	5%
Thyroid lymphoma	Rare

Hyperthyroidism

William E. Clutter

8

GENERAL PRINCIPLES

Hyperthyroidism is the syndrome caused by thyroid hormone excess. Thyrotoxicosis is a synonym. It affects about 2% of women and 0.2% of men.

Etiology

- **Graves' disease**[1] is the most common cause of hyperthyroidism, especially in young patients. This autoimmune disorder may also cause **proptosis** (exophthalmos) or **pretibial myxedema,** neither of which is found in other causes of hyperthyroidism (Table 8-1).
- **Toxic multinodular goiter** (MNG) is a common cause of hyperthyroidism in older patients.
- Unusual causes of hyperthyroidism include **iodine-induced hyperthyroidism** (usually precipitated by drugs such as **amiodarone** or radiographic contrast media), **thyroid adenomas, subacute thyroiditis** (a painful tender goiter with transient hyperthyroidism), **painless thyroiditis** (a nontender goiter with transient hyperthyroidism, most often seen in the postpartum period), and **factitious hyperthyroidism** (surreptitious ingestion of thyroid hormone). The other causes of hyperthyroidism are extremely rare.

Pathophysiology

- Graves' disease is an autoimmune disorder in which autoantibodies (**thyroid-stimulating immunoglobulins, TSIs**) bind to the thyroid-stimulating hormone (TSH) receptor and mimic the effects of TSH. Graves' disease is much more common in women. It occurs at any age, but is most common in young adults. A family history of Graves' disease or Hashimoto's disease is common. Patients have a **diffuse goiter,** which is soft and nontender. Increased blood flow sometimes causes a thyroid bruit or thrill. There is diffuse hyperplasia of follicular cells with a lymphocytic infiltrate. The natural history of Graves' disease may be marked by exacerbations and remissions of hyperthyroidism.

  Graves' disease and Hashimoto's disease are clearly related. Both are autoimmune in origin and cluster in the same families, and antithyroid antibodies are present in both. Sometimes, one evolves into the other (e.g., patients with Graves' disease may later become hypothyroid even if treated only with antithyroid drugs). Graves' disease includes two extrathyroidal signs caused by the underlying autoimmune disease, not by thyroid hormone excess. They are not seen with other causes of hyperthyroidism.
  - **Graves' ophthalmopathy,** characterized by inflammation and edema of retroorbital tissues (extraocular muscles and fat), causes forward protrusion of the globe (proptosis or exophthalmos).

TABLE 8-1	CAUSES OF HYPERTHYROIDISM

Graves' disease
Toxic multinodular goiter
Toxic adenoma
Iodine and iodine-containing drugs (e.g., amiodarone, iodinated contrast agents)
Painless thyroiditis
Subacute thyroiditis
Factitious hyperthyroidism
Ectopic thyroid tissue (struma ovarii)
Chorionic gonadotropin-induced (choriocarcinoma, hydatidiform mole)
TSH-secreting pituitary adenoma

TSH, thyroid-stimulating hormone.

- ○ **Pretibial myxedema,** a rare plaque-like thickening of the skin over the shins, is due to accumulation of glycosaminoglycans in the dermis.
- In **toxic multinodular goiter (MNG),** areas of autonomous function (i.e., not regulated by TSH) develop within a MNG and produce excess thyroid hormone. Patients are usually elderly and have a longstanding MNG.
- **Thyroid adenomas** occasionally cause hyperthyroidism. Thyroid carcinomas produce hormone very inefficiently and almost never cause hyperthyroidism, so a thyroid nodule in a hyperthyroid patient is usually benign.
- Certain forms of **thyroiditis** disrupt follicles, release stored hormone, and cause transient hyperthyroidism (lasting from a few weeks to a few months), often followed by a similar period of hypothyroidism.
  - ○ **Subacute thyroiditis** is a granulomatous inflammation that causes a painful, tender goiter.
  - ○ **Painless thyroiditis** is a form of lymphocytic thyroiditis that may cause hyperthyroidism, especially in the postpartum period (i.e., the first few months after delivery). Patients often have a small diffuse nontender goiter, and may be suspected of having Graves' disease. Although some authors refer to Hashimoto's thyroiditis as a rare cause of hyperthyroidism, these patients likely have coexisting Graves' disease.
- **Iodine-induced hyperthyroidism** (Jod-Basedow phenomenon; German for iodine plus German eponym for Graves' disease) usually occurs in patients with euthyroid goiters after large doses of iodine (e.g., **x-ray contrast medium** or **amiodarone**). Presumably, areas of autonomous function in these glands produce excess thyroid hormone only when high iodine levels permit. After iodine exposure ends, hyperthyroidism gradually resolves. Amiodarone also produces direct toxic effects on the thyroid which may contribute to hyperthyroidism.
- **Factitious use of thyroid hormone** is usually for the purpose of weight loss. Recently, hyperthyroidism due to thyroid hormone-containing "nutritional supplements" has been reported.
- Very high levels of chorionic gonadotropin (which weakly cross-reacts with the TSH receptor) secreted by trophoblastic tumors can cause hyperthyroidism.

TABLE 8-2 MANIFESTATIONS OF HYPERTHYROIDISM

Symptoms
Heat intolerance, increased sweating
Weight loss (often with increased appetite)
Anxiety, irritability
Palpitations
Oligomenorrhea
Increased stool frequency
Dyspnea
Fatigue, weakness

Signs
Brisk reflexes, fine tremor
Lid lag, stare
Sinus tachycardia
Atrial fibrillation
Warm, moist skin
Palmar erythema, onycholysis
Hair loss
Muscle weakness and wasting
Exacerbation of heart failure or coronary artery disease
Periodic paralysis (primarily in Asian men)

DIAGNOSIS

Clinical Presentation

- **Symptoms** include heat intolerance and weight loss (due to increased metabolic rate), weakness, palpitations, oligomenorrhea, and anxiety (Table 8-2). **Signs** include brisk tendon reflexes, fine tremor, proximal weakness, stare, and eyelid lag. Cardiac abnormalities may be prominent, including sinus tachycardia, atrial fibrillation, and exacerbation of coronary artery disease or heart failure. **In the elderly,** hyperthyroidism may present with only atrial fibrillation, heart failure, weakness, or weight loss, and a high index of suspicion is needed to make the diagnosis.
- Graves' disease may cause additional findings that are not due to hyperthyroidism (Table 8-3). Symptoms of ophthalmopathy include increased lacrimation, foreign

TABLE 8-3 MANIFESTATIONS OF GRAVES' DISEASE

Diffuse goiter
Ophthalmopathy
   Retrobulbar pressure or pain
   Periorbital edema, scleral injection
   Exophthalmos (proptosis)
   Extraocular muscle dysfunction
   Exposure keratitis
   Optic neuropathy (rare)
Pretibial myxedema (localized dermopathy)

body sensation, conjunctival redness, and periorbital edema. Fibrosis of extraocular muscles can cause diplopia. Rarely proptosis threatens vision by corneal exposure (due to incomplete lid closure) or compression of the optic nerve.

Diagnostic Testing

Hyperthyroidism should be suspected in any patient with compatible symptoms, as it is a readily treatable disorder that may become very debilitating.

- **Plasma TSH is the best initial diagnostic test,** as a TSH level >0.1 μU/mL excludes clinical hyperthyroidism. If plasma TSH is <0.1 μU/mL, **plasma free thyroxine (T_4)** should be measured to determine the severity of hyperthyroidism and as a baseline for therapy. If plasma free T_4 is elevated, the diagnosis of clinical hyperthyroidism is established.
  - If plasma TSH is <0.1 μU/mL but free T_4 is normal, the patient may have clinical hyperthyroidism due to **elevation of plasma triiodothyronine (T_3) alone (T_3 toxicosis);** plasma T_3 should be measured in this case.
  - TSH may also be suppressed by **severe nonthyroidal illness** (see Chapter 6). These patients have normal or low plasma free T_4 and low plasma T_3.
  - Finally, **mild (or subclinical) hyperthyroidism** may lower TSH to <0.1 μU/mL and, therefore, **suppression of TSH alone does not confirm that symptoms are caused by hyperthyroidism.**
- **Thyroid imaging with ultrasound or radionuclide scan is not useful in diagnosing hyperthyroidism.**

Differential Diagnosis

The cause of hyperthyroidism should be determined, since this affects the choice of therapy (Table 8-4). Differential diagnosis is based on:

- **Palpation of the thyroid.** Almost all hyperthyroid patients with a **diffuse nontender goiter** have Graves' disease, but this is also rarely due to postpartum or painless thyroiditis. Patients **without palpable thyroid enlargement** almost always have Graves' disease, but the possibility of factitious hyperthyroidism should be considered if there is no goiter. The diagnosis of toxic MNG or hyperthyroidism due to a thyroid adenoma is made by palpating multiple nodules or a single nodule. A painful, tender thyroid indicates subacute thyroiditis.
- **The presence of proptosis or pretibial myxedema,** which indicate Graves' disease (although many patients with Graves' disease lack these signs).
- **Recent pregnancy, neck pain, or iodine administration,** which suggest other causes.

TABLE 8-4	DIFFERENTIAL DIAGNOSIS OF HYPERTHYROIDISM
Type of goiter	**Diagnosis**
Diffuse, nontender goiter	Graves' disease or painless thyroiditis
Multiple thyroid nodules	Toxic multinodular goiter
Single thyroid nodule	Thyroid adenoma
Tender painful goiter	Subacute thyroiditis
Normal thyroid gland	Graves' disease, painless thyroiditis, or factitious hyperthyroidism

TABLE 8-5	DIFFERENTIAL DIAGNOSIS OF HYPERTHYROIDISM BASED ON RAIU	
Increased RAIU		**Decreased RAIU**
Graves disease		Subacute thyroiditis
Toxic multinodular goiter		Painless thyroiditis
Thyroid adenoma		Iodine-induced hyperthyroidism
		Factitious hyperthyroidism

RAIU, radioactive iodine uptake.

- Most cases are due to Graves' disease or toxic MNG, and the diagnosis is usually obvious from the clinical findings and palpation of the thyroid. In a few patients with a diffuse goiter or with no thyroid enlargement, **24-hour radioactive iodine uptake (RAIU,** Table 8-5) is needed to distinguish Graves' disease (in which RAIU is elevated) from diseases in which RAIU is low.

TREATMENT

- Some forms of hyperthyroidism (subacute or postpartum thyroiditis) are transient and require only symptomatic therapy.
- Three methods are available for definitive therapy (none of which controls hyperthyroidism rapidly): RAI, thionamides, and subtotal thyroidectomy. **During the initial phase of treatment, patients are followed by clinical evaluation and measurement of plasma free T$_4$.** Plasma TSH is useless in assessing the initial response to therapy, as it remains suppressed until after the patient becomes euthyroid.
- Regardless of the therapy used, all patients with Graves' disease require lifelong follow-up for recurrent hyperthyroidism or development of hypothyroidism.

Symptom Relief

A β-adrenergic antagonist (such as **atenolol** 25 to 100 mg daily) is used to relieve symptoms such as palpitations, tremor, and anxiety, until hyperthyroidism is controlled by definitive therapy, or until transient forms of hyperthyroidism subside. The dose is adjusted to alleviate symptoms and tachycardia, and then reduced gradually as hyperthyroidism is controlled. Verapamil at an initial dose of 40 to 80 mg orally tid can be used to control tachycardia in patients with contraindications to β-adrenergic antagonists.

Choice of Definitive Therapy in Graves' Disease

- **In Graves' disease, RAI therapy is the treatment of choice for almost all patients.** It is simple and highly effective, but it **cannot be used during pregnancy or lactation.**
- **Propylthiouracil (PTU) should be used to treat hyperthyroidism in pregnancy.**
- Long-term control of Graves' disease with thionamides is achieved in less than one-half of patients, and these drugs carry a small risk of life-threatening side effects. They are used in patients with Graves' disease who refuse RAI therapy.
- Thyroidectomy should be used in patients who refuse RAI therapy and who relapse or develop side effects with thionamide therapy.

Choice of Definite Therapy in Other Causes of Hyperthyroidism

- Toxic MNG and toxic adenoma should be treated with RAI (except in pregnancy).
- Transient forms of hyperthyroidism caused by thyroiditis should be treated symptomatically with atenolol.
- Iodine-induced hyperthyroidism is treated with methimazole and atenolol until the patient is euthyroid.
- Although treatment of some patients with amiodarone-induced hyperthyroidism with glucocorticoids has been advocated, **nearly all patients with amiodarone-induced hyperthyroidism respond well to thionamide therapy.**[2]

RAI Therapy

- A single dose of iodine-131 permanently controls hyperthyroidism in about 90% of patients, and further doses can be given if necessary. A **pregnancy test** is done immediately before therapy in potentially fertile women. A 24-hour RAIU is usually measured and used to calculate the dose.
- Thionamides interfere with RAI therapy and should be discontinued 3 to 7 days before treatment. If iodine therapy has been given, it should be discontinued at least 2 weeks before RAI therapy.
- Most patients with Graves' disease are treated with 8 to 10 mCi; treatment of toxic MNG requires higher doses.
- Several months are usually needed to restore euthyroidism. Patients are evaluated at 4- to 6-week intervals, with assessment of clinical findings and plasma free T_4. **If thyroid function stabilizes within the normal range,** the interval between follow-up visits is increased gradually to annual intervals. **If hypothyroidism develops,** thyroxine therapy is started.
- **If symptomatic hyperthyroidism persists after 6 months, RAI treatment is repeated.**
- **Side effects**
  - **Hypothyroidism** occurs in more than half of patients within the first year and continues to develop at a rate of approximately 3% per year thereafter.
  - Because of the release of stored hormone, a slight rise in plasma T_4 may occur in the first 2 weeks after therapy. This development is important only in **patients with severe cardiac disease,** which may worsen as a result. Such patients should be treated initially with thionamides to restore euthyroidism and to deplete stored hormone before treatment with RAI.
  - No convincing evidence has been found that RAI has a clinically important effect on the course of Graves' eye disease. It does not increase the risk of malignancy. No increase in congenital abnormalities has been found in the offspring of women who conceive after RAI therapy, and the radiation exposure to the ovaries is low, comparable to that from common diagnostic radiographs. Unwarranted concern for potential teratogenic effects should not influence physicians' advice to patients.

Thionamides

- **Methimazole** and **PTU** inhibit thyroid hormone synthesis by thyroid peroxidase.[3] PTU also inhibits extrathyroidal conversion of T_4 to T_3 by type 1 deiodinase. Once thyroid hormone stores are depleted (after several weeks to months), T_4 levels decrease.
- These drugs have no permanent effect on thyroid function. **In the majority of patients with Graves' disease, hyperthyroidism recurs within 6 months after therapy is discontinued.** Spontaneous remission of Graves' disease occurs in approximately

one-third of patients during thionamide therapy, and in this minority, no other treatment may be needed. Remission is more likely in mild hyperthyroidism of recent onset, and if the goiter is small.

- Because of a better safety profile, **methimazole should be used instead of PTU** except in specific situations (see below).[4]
- **Initiation of therapy.** Before starting therapy, patients must be warned of side effects and precautions. Usual starting doses are PTU, 100 to 200 mg orally tid, or methimazole, 10 to 40 mg orally daily; higher initial doses can be used in severe hyperthyroidism.
- **Follow-up.** Restoration of euthyroidism takes up to several months. Patients are initially evaluated at 4-week intervals with assessment of clinical findings and plasma free T_4. If plasma free T_4 levels do not fall after 4 to 8 weeks, the dose should be increased. Doses for PTU and methimazole, respectively, as high as 300 mg orally qid, or methimazole, 60 mg daily, may be required. Once the plasma free T_4 level falls to normal, the dose is adjusted to maintain plasma free T_4 within the normal range.
- There is no consensus on the optimal duration of therapy, but periods of 6 months to 2 years are most common. Patients must be monitored carefully for recurrence of hyperthyroidism after the drug is stopped.
- **Side effects** are most likely to occur within the first few months of therapy.
  - Minor side effects include rash, urticaria, fever, arthralgias, and transient leukopenia.
  - **Agranulocytosis** occurs in about 0.3% of patients treated with thionamides.
  - Other life-threatening side effects include **hepatitis,** vasculitis, and drug-induced lupus erythematosus. These complications usually resolve if the drug is stopped promptly, but fatal hepatitis is more common with PTU than methimazole.
  - **Patients must be warned to discontinue the drug immediately if jaundice or symptoms suggestive of agranulocytosis develop** (e.g., fever, chills, sore throat) and to contact their physician promptly for evaluation. Routine monitoring of the white blood cell (WBC) count is not useful for detecting agranulocytosis, which develops suddenly.

Subtotal Thyroidectomy

- This procedure provides long-term control of hyperthyroidism in most patients. Surgery may trigger a perioperative exacerbation of hyperthyroidism, and patients should be prepared for surgery by one of two methods.
  - **Methimazole** is given until the patient is nearly euthyroid. **Supersaturated potassium iodide (SSKI),** 80 mg (2 drops) orally bid, is then added 1 to 2 weeks before surgery. Both drugs are stopped postoperatively.
  - **Atenolol** (50 to 100 mg daily) is started 1 to 2 weeks before surgery. The dose of atenolol is increased, if necessary, to reduce the resting heart rate below 90 beats/minute and is continued for 5 to 7 days postoperatively. SSKI is dosed as indicated previously.
- Clinical findings and plasma free T_4 and TSH should be assessed 4 to 6 weeks after surgery. If thyroid function is normal, the patient is seen at 3 and 6 months, and then annually. If symptomatic hypothyroidism develops, thyroxine therapy is started. Mild hypothyroidism after subtotal thyroidectomy may be transient, and asymptomatic patients can be observed for an additional 4 to 6 weeks to determine whether hypothyroidism will resolve spontaneously. Hyperthyroidism persists or recurs in 3% to 7% of patients.
- **Complications** of thyroidectomy include **hypothyroidism** in 30% to 50% of patients and **hypoparathyroidism** in 3%. Rare complications include permanent

vocal cord paralysis, resulting from recurrent laryngeal nerve injury, and perioperative death. The complication rate appears to depend on the experience of the
surgeon.

SPECIAL CONSIDERATIONS

- **Mild (or subclinical) hyperthyroidism** is diagnosed when the plasma TSH is suppressed to <0.1 μU/mL, but the patient has no symptoms that are definitely caused
  by hyperthyroidism, and plasma levels of free T_4 and T_3 are normal. Because subclinical hyperthyroidism **increases the risk of atrial fibrillation in the elderly** and
  those with **heart disease;** and predisposes to **osteoporosis** in **postmenopausal
  women,** it should be treated in these patients. Asymptomatic young patients with
  mild Graves' disease can be observed at semiannual intervals for spontaneous resolution of hyperthyroidism, or the development of symptoms and increasing free T_4
  levels that warrant treatment.
- **Urgent therapy** is warranted when hyperthyroidism exacerbates heart failure or
  coronary artery disease and in rare patients with severe hyperthyroidism complicated by fever and delirium (thyroid storm).[5] Concomitant diseases should be
  treated intensively, and confirmatory tests should be obtained before therapy is
  started, including serum TSH and free T_4.
  - **PTU, 300 mg orally q6h,** should be started immediately. PTU is preferred over
    methimazole because it inhibits conversion of T_4 to T_3.
  - **Iodide (SSKI, 2 drops orally q12h)** should be started after the first dose of PTU,
    to inhibit thyroid hormone secretion rapidly.
  - **Propranolol,** 40 mg orally q6h (or an equivalent dose of a parenteral β-antagonist),
    should be given to patients with angina or myocardial infarction, and the dose
    should be adjusted to control tachycardia. Propranolol may benefit some patients
    with heart failure and marked tachycardia but can further impair left ventricular
    systolic function. In patients with clinical heart failure, propranolol should be
    given only with careful monitoring of left ventricular function.
  - Plasma free T_4 is measured every 3 to 7 days, and the doses of PTU and iodine
    are gradually decreased when free T_4 approaches the normal range. RAI therapy
    should be scheduled 2 weeks after iodine is discontinued.
- **Hyperthyroidism in pregnancy.**[6] Hyperthyroidism increases the risk of miscarriage,
  preeclampsia, premature labor, and low birth weight, so it must be controlled. If
  hyperthyroidism is suspected, plasma TSH should be measured. Plasma TSH
  declines in early pregnancy owing to the thyroid-stimulating effects of human chorionic gonadotropin (hCG), but rarely to <0.1 μU/mL. If TSH is <0.1 μU/mL, the
  diagnosis should be confirmed by measurement of plasma free T_4.
  - RAI therapy is contraindicated in pregnancy, and these patients should be treated
    with PTU. Methimazole is not used because it is associated with certain con-
    genital defects. The dose should be adjusted at 4-week intervals to maintain the
    plasma free T_4 near the upper limit of the normal range. The dose required often
    decreases in the later stages of pregnancy. It is important to avoid overtreatment,
    since PTU crosses the placenta and can cause fetal hypothyroidism.
  - Atenolol, 25 to 50 mg orally daily, can be used to relieve symptoms while await-
    ing the effects of PTU.
  - TSIs also cross the placenta and can cause fetal or neonatal hyperthyroidism. In
    pregnant women who have previously been treated with RAI or thyroidectomy

and are no longer hyperthyroid, measurement of plasma TSI in the third trimester helps assess the risk of neonatal hyperthyroidism.

○ Newborns should be monitored carefully for hyperthyroidism.

○ After delivery, methimazole should be substituted for PTU. Women treated with methimazole may safely breastfeed.

• **Treatment of Graves' ophthalmopathy.** Mild or moderate ophthalmopathy often resolves spontaneously and may require no treatment. Symptoms of conjunctival irritation respond to lubricant eye drops (e.g., Refresh eye drops) and ointment at bedtime (e.g., Refresh PM), which also protect against exposure keratitis. More severe ophthalmopathy, with the risk of visual loss, should be treated with glucocorticoids in consultation with an experienced ophthalmologist.

REFERENCES

1. Brent GA. Graves' disease. *N Engl J Med* 2008;358:2594–2605.
2. Osman F, Franklyn JA, Sheppard MC, et al. Successful treatment of amiodarone-induced thyrotoxicosis. *Circulation* 2002;105:1275–1277.
3. Drugs for thyroid disorders. *Treat Guidel Med Lett* 2009;7:57–64.
4. Cooper DS, Rivkees SA. Putting propylthiouracil in perspective. *J Clin endocrinol Metab* 2009;94:1881–1882.
5. Nayuk B, Burman K. Thyrotoxicosis and thyroid storm. *Endocrinol Metab Clin North Am* 2006;35:663–686.
6. Abalovich M, Amino N, Barbour LA, et al. Management of thyroid dysfunction during pregnancy and postpartum: An Endocrine society clinical practice guideline. *J Clin Endocrinol Metab* 2007;92:S1–S47.

Hypothyroidism

9

William E. Clutter

GENERAL PRINCIPLES

Hypothyroidism is the syndrome caused by thyroid hormone deficiency. It is common, especially in women, with a prevalence of about 2% (compared with 0.1% for men). The prevalence of subclinical hypothyroidism is about 7.5% in women and 3% in men, and increases with age. Congenital hypothyroidism is one of the most common congenital defects (about 1 in 5000 births).

Etiology

- **Primary hypothyroidism** (resulting from disease of the thyroid itself) accounts for more than 95% of cases (Table 9-1).
  - **Chronic lymphocytic thyroiditis** (**Hashimoto's disease**) is by far the most common cause. It is an autoimmune disorder in which the thyroid is damaged by cell-mediated immunity.
  - **Iatrogenic hypothyroidism** due to thyroidectomy or radioactive iodine (RAI, iodine-131) therapy is also common.
  - **Transient hypothyroidism** occurs in painless (or postpartum) thyroiditis and subacute thyroiditis, usually after a period of hyperthyroidism.
  - **Drugs that may cause hypothyroidism** (usually in patients with underlying autoimmune thyroiditis) include iodine-containing drugs such as **amiodarone,** lithium, interferon-α and interferon-β, interleukin-2, thalidomide, bexarotene, and sunitinib. Thionamide drugs used to treat hyperthyroidism can cause hypothyroidism if the dose is excessive.
- **Secondary hypothyroidism** due to thyroid-stimulating hormone (TSH) deficiency is uncommon but may occur in any disorder of the pituitary or hypothalamus, including surgery, trauma, or radiation to the area. However, it rarely occurs without other evidence of pituitary disease.
- Rare hemangiomas that express thyroid hormone deiodinase type 3 (which converts thyroxine [T_4] to inactive reverse triiodothyronine [rT_3]) have been reported to cause hypothyroidism, a syndrome called **consumptive hypothyroidism**.
- Thyroid hormone resistance caused by mutations in the thyroid hormone receptor-beta gene usually does not cause symptoms of hypothyroidism, since increased levels of thyroid hormone compensate for defective responsiveness.

Pathophysiology

- **Hashimoto's thyroiditis** (chronic lymphocytic thyroiditis) is much more common in women, and increases in prevalence with age. The disease gradually impairs the thyroid's ability to produce hormone, prompting a compensatory rise in TSH secretion. This additional stimulus maintains normal thyroid hormone levels for a time (a state called **subclinical hypothyroidism**). In many of these patients, hormone production eventually falls despite high TSH levels, and frank clinical hypothyroidism develops.

TABLE 9-1 CAUSES OF HYPOTHYROIDISM

Primary hypothyroidism
Chronic lymphocytic (Hashimoto's) thyroiditis
Radioactive iodine treatment or external neck radiation
Thyroidectomy
Transient (during recovery from painless thyroiditis or subacute thyroiditis)
Drugs
Severe iodine deficiency (not seen in the United States)
Congenital hypothyroidism (thyroid dysgenesis or genetic defects in thyroid
   hormone synthesis)
Secondary (central) hypothyroidism
Any pituitary or hypothalamic disease
Other
Consumptive hypothyroidism due to vascular tumors expressing deiodinase

Patients usually have antithyroid antibodies (**antithyroid peroxidase** and **antithyroglobulin**), but cellular immunity is more important in thyroid dysfunction. They may have autoimmune disease of other endocrine glands (such as Addison's disease), and often have a family history of either Hashimoto's or Graves' disease. There is lymphocytic infiltration of the thyroid, fibrosis, and variable degrees of follicular destruction. Depending on the extent of follicular damage and lymphocytic infiltration, it causes an **atrophic, impalpable thyroid** or a **firm, nontender diffuse goiter.** (Hashimoto's disease is also the most common cause of euthyroid goiter in the United States.)

- **Iatrogenic hypothyroidism** is a common complication of treatment for hyperthyroidism. After radioactive iodine therapy, it may occur quickly, or not until years later. Hypothyroidism always follows the complete or near-complete **thyroidectomy** done for thyroid cancer, and may occur after subtotal thyroidectomy for hyperthyroidism.
- Most cases of **congenital hypothyroidism** are caused by dysplasia or aplasia of the thyroid, with little or no detectable thyroid tissue. Rarely, genetic defects of hormone synthetic enzymes, or maternal treatment with antithyroid drugs or iodine cause congenital hypothyroidism with a goiter.
- **Drug-induced hypothyroidism** can occur during treatment of Graves' disease with **thionamides.** Occasionally, **iodine excess** or **lithium** (which inhibit thyroid hormone secretion) cause hypothyroidism, usually in patients with underlying autoimmune thyroiditis.
- Most cases of hypothyroidism are permanent, but **self-limited forms of thyroiditis** (painless lymphocytic thyroiditis and subacute thyroiditis) cause transient hypothyroidism, usually after a period of hyperthyroidism. Painless thyroiditis is most common in the postpartum period.
- In **secondary hypothyroidism** there are usually other pituitary hormone deficiencies, and since TSH is not elevated, there is no goiter.

DIAGNOSIS

Clinical Presentation

- Hypothyroidism causes a variety of symptoms, many of which are nonspecific (Table 9-2). It usually develops gradually, and the onset of symptoms is insidious.

TABLE 9-2	SYMPTOMS AND SIGNS OF HYPOTHYROIDISM
Symptoms	**Signs**
Cold intolerance	Delayed tendon reflex relaxation
Lethargy, fatigue	Facial and periorbital puffiness
Weight gain (modest)	Bradycardia
Dry skin, hair loss	Poor memory, dementia
Constipation	Nonpitting edema (myxedema)
Myalgias, arthralgias	Pleural and pericardial effusions
Menorrhagia	Carpal tunnel syndrome
Hoarseness	Deafness
	Hypoventilation
	Hypothermia

- The most specific findings are **cold intolerance** (feeling cold when others are comfortable) and **delayed relaxation of tendon reflexes.** Patients may or may not have a goiter. Other symptoms include mild weight gain (due to decreased metabolic rate), fatigue, somnolence, poor memory, constipation, menorrhagia and impaired fertility, myalgias, and hoarseness. Other signs include bradycardia, facial and periorbital edema, dry skin, and nonpitting edema (myxedema) that results from accumulation of glycosaminoglycans in interstitial spaces. **Hypothyroidism does not cause marked obesity.**
- Rare manifestations include hypoventilation, hypothermia, pericardial or pleural effusions, deafness, and carpal tunnel syndrome.
- Laboratory findings may include **hyponatremia** and elevated plasma levels of cholesterol, triglycerides, and creatine kinase. Primary hypothyroidism may cause hyperprolactinemia. The electrocardiogram (ECG) may show low voltage and T-wave abnormalities.

Diagnostic Testing

Hypothyroidism is common, readily treatable, and should be suspected in any patient with compatible symptoms, especially in the presence of a diffuse goiter or a history of RAI therapy or thyroid surgery.

- **In suspected primary hypothyroidism, plasma TSH is the best initial diagnostic test. A normal value excludes primary hypothyroidism, and a markedly elevated value (>20 μU/mL) confirms the diagnosis.** It is seldom necessary to measure thyroid autoantibodies, since Hashimoto's thyroiditis accounts for almost all spontaneous hypothyroidism.
- Mild elevation of plasma TSH (<20 μU/mL) may be caused by **nonthyroidal illness,** but usually indicates **mild (or subclinical) primary hypothyroidism,** in which thyroid function is impaired but increased secretion of TSH maintains plasma free T_4 levels within the reference range.
  - These patients may have nonspecific symptoms compatible with hypothyroidism and a mild increase in serum cholesterol and low-density-lipoprotein (LDL) cholesterol. They develop clinical hypothyroidism at a rate of about 2.5% per year.
  - In patients with mildly elevated plasma TSH, the test should be repeated with measurement of plasma free T_4 to confirm the diagnosis.

- **If secondary hypothyroidism is suspected because of evidence of pituitary disease** (e.g., a known sella turcica or hypothalamic mass, or a history of pituitary surgery, radiation, or trauma), **plasma free T$_4$ should be measured.** A low value is diagnostic of secondary hypothyroidism in this setting.
  - Plasma TSH levels are usually within the reference range in secondary hypothyroidism and cannot be used alone to make this diagnosis.
  - Patients with secondary hypothyroidism should be evaluated for other pituitary hormone deficits and the pituitary should be imaged with magnetic resonance imaging (MRI).

TREATMENT

- **Levothyroxine** is the drug of choice. The average replacement dose is 1.6 mcg/kg orally daily, and most patients require doses between 75 and 150 mcg daily. In elderly patients, the average replacement dose is lower. The need for lifelong treatment should be emphasized.
  - Levothyroxine should be taken 30 minutes before a meal, since dietary fiber and soy products interfere with its absorption. It should not be taken together with **medications that inhibit its absorption** including **calcium or iron supplements,** cholestyramine, sucralfate, and aluminum hydroxide.
  - **Other drug interactions that increase thyroxine clearance and dose requirement** include estrogen, rifampin, some anticonvulsants (carbamazepine, phenytoin, and phenobarbital), and some anticancer drugs (imatinib and bexarotene). Newer anticonvulsants have not been reported to cause this interaction. **Amiodarone** blocks conversion of T$_4$ to T$_3$, and also increases levothyroxine dose requirements.
- **Initiation of therapy.** Young, otherwise healthy adults should be started on 1.6 mcg/kg daily. This regimen gradually corrects hypothyroidism, since thyroxine has a half-life of 7 days, and several weeks are required to reach steady-state plasma levels of T$_4$. Symptoms begin to improve within a few weeks. In otherwise healthy **elderly patients,** the initial dose should be 50 mcg daily. Patients with **cardiac disease** should be started on 25 to 50 mcg daily and monitored carefully for exacerbation of cardiac symptoms.
- **Dose adjustment and follow-up**
  - **In primary hypothyroidism, the goal of therapy is to maintain plasma TSH within the normal range.** Plasma TSH should be measured 6 to 8 weeks after initiation of therapy. The dose of levothyroxine should be adjusted in 12 to 25 mcg increments at intervals of 6 to 8 weeks until plasma TSH level is normal. Thereafter, annual TSH measurement is adequate to monitor therapy. TSH should also be measured frequently in the **first trimester of pregnancy,** since the thyroxine dose requirement increases at this time (see Pregnancy section under Special Considerations).
  - **In secondary hypothyroidism, plasma TSH cannot be used to adjust therapy.** The goal of therapy is to **maintain the plasma free T$_4$ near the middle of the reference range.** The dose of levothyroxine should be adjusted at 6- to 8-week intervals until this goal is achieved. Thereafter, annual measurement of plasma free T$_4$ is adequate to monitor therapy.
- **Side effects.** Overtreatment produces **iatrogenic hyperthyroidism,** indicated by a subnormal TSH level, and should be avoided since it increases the risk of **osteoporosis** and **atrial fibrillation.**

- Coronary artery disease may be exacerbated by treatment of hypothyroidism. The dose of levothyroxine should be increased slowly, with careful attention to worsening angina, heart failure, or arrhythmias.
- In patients with concomitant **adrenal failure,** correction of hypothyroidism may exacerbate the symptoms and signs of adrenal failure.
- In patients with **pituitary disease** and secondary hypothyroidism, the pituitary–adrenal axis should be assessed and treatment of secondary adrenal failure started before treatment of hypothyroidism.

SPECIAL CONSIDERATIONS

Mild (or Subclinical) Hypothyroidism

- Patients with mild hypothyroidism should be treated with levothyroxine if any of the following are present:
  - symptoms compatible with hypothyroidism,[1]
  - a goiter,
  - hypercholesterolemia that warrants treatment,
  - pregnancy, or
  - the plasma TSH is >10 μU/mL.
- Untreated patients should be monitored annually, and levothyroxine should be started if symptoms develop or serum TSH increases to >10 μU/mL.

Pregnancy

Thyroxine dose requirement increases by an average of 50% in the first half of pregnancy owing to accelerated conversion of T_4 to reverse T_3 by placental deiodinase type 3.[2]

- In women with primary hypothyroidism, **plasma TSH level should be measured as soon as pregnancy is confirmed and monthly thereafter through the second trimester.**[3] The levothyroxine dose should be increased as needed to maintain plasma TSH level within the normal range.
- An alternative approach is to instruct patients to increase their levothyroxine dose by 1 to 2 pills per week as soon as pregnancy is confirmed, and to monitor and adjust the dose as above.[4]
- After delivery, the prepregnancy dose should be resumed.

Problems with Treatment

Treatment of most cases of hypothyroidism is simple and straightforward. Occasionally, it is difficult to achieve a levothyroxine dose that normalizes TSH level, or a dose that was adequate no longer maintains a normal TSH level. Common explanations for this include:

- **Poor or erratic medication compliance.** Directly observed therapy at weekly intervals may be necessary in some cases.
- **Drug interactions** (see Treatment section in this chapter).
- **Pregnancy,** in which the dose requirement increases in the first trimester.
- **Gradual failure of remaining endogenous thyroid function** after RAI treatment of hyperthyroidism.

Diagnosis of Hypothyroidism in Severely Ill Patients

In severe nonthyroidal illness, the diagnosis of hypothyroidism may be difficult (see Chapter 6).[5] Plasma total T_4 and free T_4 measured by routine assays may be low.

- Plasma TSH is the best initial diagnostic test. A normal TSH value is strong evidence that the patient is euthyroid, except when there is evidence of pituitary or hypothalamic disease or in patients treated with dopamine or high doses of glucocorticoids.
- Marked elevation of plasma TSH (>20 μU/mL) establishes the diagnosis of primary hypothyroidism.
- Moderate elevations of plasma TSH (<20 μU/mL) may occur in euthyroid patients with nonthyroidal illness and are not specific for hypothyroidism. Plasma free T_4 should be measured if TSH is moderately elevated, or if secondary hypothyroidism is suspected, and patients should be treated for hypothyroidism if plasma free T_4 is low. Thyroid function in these patients should be reevaluated after recovery from illness.

Emergent Therapy for Hypothyroidism is Rarely Necessary

Most patients with hypothyroidism and concomitant illness can be treated in the usual manner. However, hypothyroidism may impair survival in critical illness by contributing to hypoventilation, hypotension, hypothermia, bradycardia, or hyponatremia. Little evidence supports the contention that severe hypothyroidism alone causes coma or shock; most reports of myxedema coma predate recognition that nonthyroidal illness itself lowers thyroid hormone levels (see Section Diagnosis of Hypothyroidism in Severely Ill Patients in this chapter).

- Hypoventilation and hypotension should be treated intensively, along with any concomitant diseases. Confirmatory tests (plasma TSH and free T_4) should be obtained before thyroid hormone therapy is started in a severely ill patient.
- Levothyroxine, 50 to 100 mcg IV, can be given q6 to 8h for 24 hours, followed by 75 to 100 mcg IV daily until oral intake is possible. Replacement therapy should be continued in the usual manner if the diagnosis of hypothyroidism is confirmed. No clinical trials have determined the optimum method of thyroid hormone replacement, but this method rapidly alleviates thyroxine deficiency while minimizing the risk of exacerbating underlying coronary disease or heart failure.
- Such rapid correction is warranted only in extremely ill patients. Vital signs and cardiac rhythm should be monitored carefully to detect early signs of exacerbation of heart disease.
- Hydrocortisone, 50 mg IV q8h, is usually recommended during rapid replacement of thyroid hormone, because such therapy may precipitate adrenal crisis in patients with adrenal failure.

THYROIDITIS

General Principles

There are several types of thyroiditis that may cause hyperthyroidism, hypothyroidism, or a euthyroid goiter.[6]

- Autoimmune or Hashimoto's thyroiditis (See the Section Pathophysiology in this chapter)
- Painless thyroiditis (also known as postpartum or silent thyroiditis) is an autoimmune disorder that is most common in the first 6 months of the postpartum period. The incidence is believed to be approximately 10% in the United States.

○ It is characterized by a small, nontender diffuse goiter, and transient hyperthyroidism followed by hypothyroidism, although only one phase may be recognized clinically.

○ Hypothyroidism is usually transient, but may be permanent.

○ Hyperthyroidism results from follicular damage and release of stored hormone by a lymphocytic infiltrate. Consequently, **radioactive iodine uptake (RAIU) is very low.** Antithyroid peroxidase antibodies may be present.

○ The diagnosis should be suspected in women with symptoms of hyperthyroidism or hypothyroidism within 6 months of delivery. Plasma TSH and free T_4 should be measured to confirm the functional state. The hyperthyroid phase can be distinguished from Graves' disease by the absence of proptosis (which is seen only in Graves' disease), measurement of RAIU (if the patient is not nursing), and repeating thyroid function tests after several weeks to assess for spontaneous improvement.

○ Symptoms of hyperthyroidism should be treated with a β-**adrenergic antagonist.** Thionamides are not useful, since thyroid hormone synthesis is already suppressed.

○ Symptomatic hypothyroidism is treated with replacement therapy with levothyroxine for 2 to 3 months followed by discontinuation for 4 to 6 weeks and measurement of plasma TSH level. Women with a history of postpartum thyroiditis have a higher risk of developing hypothyroidism in later life.

• **Subacute thyroiditis** (also known as de Quervain's or granulomatous thyroiditis) is characterized by a painful, tender goiter and transient hyperthyroidism resulting from release of stored thyroid hormone, followed by transient hypothyroidism. It is the most common cause of thyroid pain. It frequently occurs after an upper respiratory tract infection and is thought to have a viral etiology.

○ Symptoms of hyperthyroidism occur in ~50% of patients and can be treated with a β-adrenergic antagonist.

○ Pain should be treated with nonsteroidal anti-inflammatory drugs (NSAIDs); corticosteroid treatment may be needed in severe cases.

○ Thionamides or RAI are not useful.

○ Transient hypothyroidism may be treated with levothyroxine for 3 to 6 months.

• **Acute infectious thyroiditis.** Infection of the thyroid by bacteria, fungi, mycobacteria, or parasites is rare. It may occur in immunosuppressed, elderly, or debilitated patients, or in patients with underlying thyroid disease. Patients are acutely ill, with fever, chills, dysphagia, anterior neck pain, and swelling. The thyroid is tender. Patients are usually biochemically euthyroid. Diagnosis is made by fine-needle aspiration, with Gram's staining and culture of the aspirate. Antibiotics and drainage of abscess are the mainstays of treatment.

• **Reidel's thyroiditis** is a very rare fibrosing thyroiditis that may be part of a systemic fibrosing process. Patients present with a painless, hard, fixed goiter. Patients are initially euthyroid, but hypothyroidism eventually develops. Treatment is primarily surgical, although therapy with glucocorticoids and methotrexate may be tried early in the course of the disease.

REFERENCES

1. Surks MI, Ortiz E, Daniels GH, et al. Subclinical thyroid disease. Scientific review and guidelines for diagnosis and management. *JAMA* 2004;291:228–238.

2. Alexander EK, Marqusee E, Lawrence J, et al. Timing and magnitude of increases in levo-thyroxine requirements during pregnancy in women with hypothyroidism. *N Engl J Med* 2004;351:241–249.
3. Abalovich M, Amino N, Barbour LA, et al. Management of thyroid dysfunction during pregnancy and postpartum: An Endocrine Society Clinical Practice Guideline. *J Clin Endocrinol Metab* 2007;92(Suppl):S1–S47.
4. Yassa L, Marqusee E, Fawcett R, et al. Thyroid hormone early adjustment in pregnancy (the THERAPY) trial. *J Clin Endocrinol Metab* 2010;95:3234–3241.
5. Adler SM, Wartofsky L. The nonthyroidal illness syndrome. *Endocrinol Metab Clin North Am* 2007;36:657–672.
6. Pearce EN, Farwell AP, Braverman LE. Thyroiditis. *N Engl J Med* 2003;348:2646–2655.

Adrenal Incidentaloma

10

Shunzhong Bao and Simon J. Fisher

GENERAL PRINCIPLES

Definition
- Adrenal incidentalomas are masses (>1 cm) found incidentally during radiographic imaging of the abdomen or chest. By definition, patients do not present for evaluation of signs or symptoms of adrenal diseases.
- This does not mean the patients do not have any symptoms or signs associated with it.

Epidemiology
- Using computed tomography (CT) scanning, the prevalence of adrenal incidentalomas in the general population is ~3%, and increases with age. In autopsy series, adrenal masses between 2 mm and 4 cm in size have been reported as high as 8.7%.[1]
- Bilateral masses were found in 10 to 15 percent of cases.

Etiology
- In one of the largest databases to date with 1004 adrenal incidentalomas, the National Italian Study Group has confirmed that the most common finding (85%) on evaluation with hormone testing is a nonfunctioning mass (cortical adenoma, myelolipoma, cyst, ganglioneuroma, or other).[2]
- Evaluation of the remaining masses revealed subclinical Cushing's syndrome (9.2%), pheochromocytoma (4.2%), aldosterone-secreting adenoma (1.6%), and a single virilizing tumor. Table 10-1 lists several common diagnoses associated with adrenal incidentalomas.

DIAGNOSIS

Clinical Presentation
- A thorough history for any symptoms of hormonal dysfunction and possibility of malignancy should be completed.
- Special effort should be made to elicit any subtle symptoms and physical examination signs suggesting specific hormonal hyperfunction or malignancy:
  - **Cushing's syndrome** (weight gain, moon facies, central obesity, supraclavicular fat pads, thinned skin, easy bruising, striae, acne, proximal muscle weakness, irregular menses, hirsutism, hypertension, diabetes, and vertebral compression fractures);
  - **Pheochromocytoma** (hypertension, paroxysms of headache, palpitations, anxiety attacks, perspiration, and/or pallor). About 15% patients with pheochromocytoma do not have hypertension.
  - **Aldosterone-secreting adenoma** (hypertension or hypokalemia);

TABLE 10-1	DIFFERENTIAL DIAGNOSIS OF ADRENAL INCIDENTALOMA

Benign

Nonhormone secreting
Nonfunctioning adenoma
Lipoma/myelolipoma
Cyst
Ganglioneuroma
Hematoma
Infection (tuberculosis, fungal)

Hormone secreting
Pheochromocytoma
Aldosterone-secreting adenoma
Subclinical Cushing's syndrome

Malignant
Adrenocortical carcinoma
Metastatic neoplasm
Lymphoma
Malignant pheochromocytoma

○ **Malignancy** (weight loss, history of primary nonadrenal cancers, lymphoma, and virilizing signs or symptoms suggestive of adrenocortical carcinoma).
○ A known history of malignancy makes metastasis to the adrenal gland more likely.

Diagnostic Criteria

In evaluating such a mass, the major concerns to address are:
• Is the mass benign or malignant?
• Does the mass secrete hormones, or is the mass nonfunctioning?

Diagnostic Testing

Laboratories
• Nearly all patients with an adrenal incidentalomas should be screened for subclinical Cushing's syndrome and pheochromocytoma. Hyperaldosteronism should be screened for in hypertensive patients. Patients with virilization should be screened for adrenocorticol carcinoma.
• Subclinical Cushing's syndrome: 2009 AACE/AAES Guidelines[3] suggest a **1 mg dexamethasone suppression test** to rule out subclinical Cushing's syndrome. Other screening tests that can be used are the midnight salivary cortisol level or a 24-hour urine cortisol level.
• Subclinical pheochromocytoma: screen with plasma metanephrine and normetanephrine or 24-hour urine metanephrine and normetanephrine.
• **Hyperaldosteronism:** serum potassium and plasma aldosterone concentration/plasma renin activity ratio (PAC/PRA) >20 is suggestive of hyperaldosteronism.
• A **dehydroepiandrosterone sulfate (DHEA-S) level** should be determined if virilizing signs or symptoms are present.
• Any positive results on these screening tests should prompt further evaluation. Please refer to chapters on Conn's syndrome (Chapter 13), Cushing's syndrome

(Chapter 14), and Pheochromocytoma (Chapter 15) for more detailed discussions of these tests and their interpretation.

Imaging

- **The probability of an adrenal mass being malignant directly correlates with its size.** Tumor diameters ranging from 3 to 6 cm have been proposed as cutoffs that should lead to surgical resection. A Mayo Clinic retrospective analysis of 342 adrenal masses removed over a 5-year period revealed that all adrenocortical carcinomas were ≥4 cm in diameter. In a larger retrospective series from Italy, a 4 cm cutoff was 93% sensitive for adrenocortical carcinoma, but 76% of lesions >4 cm were benign.
- CT scan may be useful in establishing whether an adrenal mass is benign or malignant. **A homogeneous adrenal mass <4 cm with smooth borders and an attenuation value <10 Hounsfield units strongly suggests a benign lesion.**[4,5]
- Diagnostic criteria are not as clear for lesions measuring 4 to 6 cm, but if they are hormonally inactive and have a clear benign appearance on CT scan, such lesions can be monitored. **Lesions >6 cm, regardless of appearance on CT scan, are more likely to be malignant, and surgical referral is warranted.** All lesions >4 cm with undeterminant imaging characteristics need to be referred for surgery.
- Magnetic resonance imaging (MRI) appears to be as effective as CT scanning in distinguishing benign and malignant masses,[5] with benign adenomas exhibiting signal drop on chemical shift imaging with intensity similar to that of T2-weighted images of the liver. Pheochromocytomas generally exhibit hyperintensity on T2-weighted imaging. Again, lesions >6 cm in diameter by MRI are more likely to be malignant, even if they have a benign appearance on MRI, and should prompt surgical referral.

Diagnostic Procedures

Fine-needle aspiration and tissue biopsy

- **Biopsy of the adrenal mass is generally not advised,** as it is rarely helpful.
- The major exception is a patient with a known extraadrenal primary malignancy. In this case, biopsy may help distinguish recurrence and metastasis of cancer from a benign adenoma.
- **Biopsy should be done only if pheochromocytoma has been ruled out** by biochemical testing, as biopsy of a pheochromocytoma can precipitate a hypertensive emergency.

TREATMENT

- At the completion of the clinical, biochemical, and radiologic evaluation described previously, any mass that suggests **primary adrenocortical malignancy** by size or by radiologic characteristics warrants surgical removal, as long as the patient is a good surgical candidate.
- **Metastatic cancer or a primary nonadrenal cancer,** such as lymphoma, generally no surgical removal is needed, but rather treatment of the primary cancer.
- Adrenal function is unlikely to be hindered by tumor invasion, because more than 70% to 80% of the gland function must be interrupted to pose any risk for adrenal crisis.
- **Pheochromocytomas** should be surgically removed (see Chapter 15 for a more detailed discussion).
- **Aldosterone-secreting adenomas** should be considered for surgical removal. However, it is not easy to differentiate between aldosterone-secreting adenomas and

primary adrenal hyperplasia. The distinction between these two is crucial, since aldosterone-secreting tumors are best treated surgically, while medical management is preferred for primary adrenal hyperplasia.

- Prior to surgical excision of an adrenal mass, it is important to exclude pheochromocytoma and to assess for excess cortisol secretion.
- The diagnoses of a hormonally hypersecreting adrenal mass and adrenocortical carcinoma are not mutually exclusive. It is common for adrenocortical carcinomas to release excessive cortisol.
- If there is any suspicion of excessive cortisol secretion, one should be aware of the possibility of adrenal crisis during or after the surgery. It has been reported several times in the literature that even mild cortisol hypersecretion of one adrenal gland may atrophy the contralateral adrenal gland.
- When the hyperfunctioning adrenal gland is removed, the atrophied gland may not be able to compensate in the setting of postsurgical recovery. These patients should be covered with stress-dose steroids during surgery and receive a corticotropin stimulation test after surgery to diagnose any resulting adrenal insufficiency.
- Patients who fail postoperative corticotropin stimulation testing may require months of glucocorticoid replacement before recovery of the hypothalamic-pituitary–adrenal axis. Thus, even if the size of the mass warrants its removal, the patient should still undergo a complete biochemical workup to rule out subclinical Cushing's syndrome or pheochromocytoma.

MONITORING/FOLLOW-UP

- If the history, physical examination, and hormonal and radiologic evaluations are not suggestive of either a primary adrenal carcinoma or a hypersecreting adenoma, then it is reasonable to conclude that the incidentaloma is benign, but follow-up is necessary.
- Patients should be evaluated annually with a thorough history and physical examination for development of overt signs of hypersecretion or malignancy.
- Schedules for follow-up by repeat radiologic imaging and biochemical analyses remain controversial.
- Imaging should be repeated in 3 to 6 months, and nodules that enlarge should be removed.[6] Nodules that remain stable in size are very unlikely to be malignant, and the risk of further imaging outweighs the benefits.[7]
- Biochemically, patients should be evaluated annually for at least 5 years.[3]

REFERENCES

1. Kloos RT, Gross MD, Francis IR, et al. Incidentally discovered adrenal masses. *Endocr Rev* 1995;16:460–484.
2. Mantero F, Terzolo M, Arnaldi G, et al. A survey on adrenal incidentaloma in Italy. Study Group on Adrenal Tumors of the Italian Society of Endocrinology. *J Clin Endocrinol Metab* 2000;85:637–644.
3. Zeiger MA, Thompson GB, Duh QY, et al. The American Association of Clinical Endocrinologists and American Association of Endocrine Surgeons medical guidelines for the management of adrenal incidentalomas. *Endocr Pract* 2009;15(Suppl 1):1–20.
4. Boland GW, Lee MJ, Gazelle GS, et al. Characterization of adrenal masses using unenhanced CT: An analysis of the CT literature. *AJR Am J Roentgenol* 1998;171:201–204.

5. Linwah Yip, Mitchell E. Tublin, Falcone JA, et al. The adrenal mass: Correlation of histopathology with imaging. *Ann Surg Oncol* 2010;17:846–852.
6. Nieman LK. Approach to the patient with an adrenal incidentaloma. *J Clin Endocrinol Metab* 2010;95:4106–4113.
7. Cawood TJ, Hunt PJ, O'Shea D, et al. Recommended evaluation of adrenal incidentalomas is costly, has high false-positive rates and confers a risk of fatal cancer that is similar to the risk of the adrenal lesion becoming malignant; time for a rethink? *Eur J Endocrinol* 2009;161 (4):513–527.

Adrenal Insufficiency

11

Zhiyu Wang and Kim Carmichael

GENERAL PRINCIPLES

- Adrenal insufficiency (AI) is a clinical syndrome arising from disruption of the normal hypothalamus–pituitary–adrenal (HPA) axis regulation of steroidogenesis.
- In 1855, Thomas Addison first described his eponymous syndrome, which was characterized by wasting and hyperpigmentation, and identified its cause as destruction of the adrenal gland.[1]

Classification

- **Primary AI** (**Addison's disease**) corresponds to dysfunction at the level of the adrenal gland from any cause.
- **Secondary AI** refers to ACTH deficiency. It can be due to dysfunction of either the hypothalamus or pituitary gland.

Epidemiology

- Chronic primary adrenal insufficiency has a prevalence of 90 to 140 per million and an incidence of 4.7 to 6.2 per million/year in Caucasian populations. The age at diagnosis peaks in the fourth decade of life.[2]
- Secondary adrenal insufficiency has an estimated prevalence of 150 to 280 per million with a peak age of diagnosis in the sixth decade of life.[2]
- Both conditions are more prevalent in women than in men.

Etiology

For a complete list of causes of adrenal insufficiency, see Table 11-1.

Primary AI

- When Thomas Addison described his initial case in 1855, tuberculosis was the most common etiology for primary AI, and it remains a major factor in the developing world.[3]
- Over the years, autoimmune destruction of the adrenal gland (autoimmune adrenalitis) has emerged as the leading cause of primary AI in the United States. It can be isolated or occur as part of an autoimmune polyglandular syndrome (APS, types I and II)[4] (see Chapter 36).
- Hereditary factors are increasingly recognized in primary AI.[5]
- Congenital adrenal hyperplasia causes functional abnormalities of adrenal steroid biosynthesis enzymes, leading to impaired cortisol synthesis (see Chapter 12).
- Other etiologies to consider for primary AI include the following:[2]
  - Disseminated tuberculosis, fungal infections, human immunodeficiency virus (HIV)-related opportunistic infections (most commonly cytomegalovirus [CMV]).
  - Bilateral adrenal hemorrhage associated with coagulopathies or sepsis.
  - Metastatic cancer involving more than 80% to 90% of the total adrenal mass.

TABLE 11-1   CAUSES OF ADRENAL INSUFFICIENCY

Primary (Adrenal)

Autoimmune (70%–90%)
  Isolated adrenal insufficiency
    (associated with HLA-DR3)
  Polyglandular autoimmune syndrome
    type I (mutation in the *AIRE gene*)
  Polyglandular autoimmune syndrome
    type II (associated with HLA-DR3)
Infectious and infiltrative
  Tuberculosis (7%–20%)
  Disseminated pseudomonas,
    histoplasmosis
  HIV and its opportunistic infections
    (CMV, *Mycobacterium avium* complex
    Cryptococcus, *Pneumocystis carinii*
    pneumonia, toxoplasmosis)
  Syphilis
  Amyloidosis
  Sarcoidosis
Metastatic carcinoma
  Lung, breast, colon cancer, melanoma
Medications
  Rifampin, phenytoin, barbiturates,
    ketoconazole, etomidate
Adrenal hemorrhage/infarction
  Meningococcal sepsis with Waterhouse–
    Friderichsen syndrome
  Primary antiphospholipid syndrome
  Disseminated intravascular coagulopathy
Genetic disorders
  Adrenoleukodystrophy (mutation in the
    ABCD1 gene)
  Congenital adrenal hyperplasia
    (deficiencies in steroidogenic acute
    regulatory protein, 21-hydroxylase,
    11-β-hydroxylase, 3-β-hydroxyl-Δ-5-
    steroid dehydrogenase)
  Mutations in *DAX-1* and *SF-1*
    transcription factors
  Smith–Lemli–Opitz syndrome (*DHCR7*
    gene mutation)
  Kearns–Sayre syndrome (mitochondrial
    DNA deletions)
  Familial glucocorticoid deficiency-Allgrove's
    syndrome (*AAAS* gene mutation)

Secondary (Pituitary or hypothalamus)

Prolonged use of exogenous
  glucocorticoids
Pituitary/hypothalamic tumors
  Pituitary adenoma
  Craniopharyngioma
  Rathke's cleft cyst
  Pituitary stalk lesions
Infectious and infiltrative
  Tuberculosis
  Histoplasmosis
  Neurosarcoidosis
  Metastasis
Infarction, hemorrhage/
  apoplexy
  Sheehan's syndrome
  Large intracranial artery
    aneurysms
Head trauma
Lymphocytic hypophysitis
Genetic pituitary abnormalities
  from mutations in *PROP-1*
  and other pituitary
  transcription factors
Isolated ACTH deficiency
Familial cortisol-binding
  globulin deficiency
Abrupt withdrawal of
  megesterol (a progestin with
  some glucocorticoid activity)

ACTH, adrenocorticotropic hormone; CMV, cytomegalovirus.

Adapted from Oelkers W. Adrenal insufficiency. *N Engl J Med* 1996;335:1206–1212; Arlt W, Allolio B. Adrenal insufficiency. *Lancet* 2003;361:1881–1893.

○ Some medications can also potentially precipitate symptomatic adrenal insufficiency in a person with limited adrenal reserve.
  ▪ Rifampin and phenytoin increase cortisol metabolism.
  ▪ Ketoconazole, aminoglutethimide, etomidate, and suramin decrease cortisol secretion by inhibiting cortisol biosynthesis.

Secondary AI

- Iatrogenic
  ○ Sudden cessation of exogenous glucocorticoid therapy is a common clinical problem and is the most frequent cause of secondary AI. Exogenous glucocorticoid administration via any route may lead to suppression of the HPA axis depending on the dose and duration of therapy.[6]
  ○ Megestrol acetate (Megace) can suppress the HPA axis to cause adrenal insufficiency; affected patients need to be supported with exogenous glucocorticoids until the axis recovers following discontinuation of megestrol acetate.[7]
- Hypothalamic-pituitary
  ○ Among patients with pituitary or hypothalamic disorders, a pituitary mass is usually associated with panhypopituitarism caused either by tumor growth or treatment with surgery or irradiation.
  ○ Other causes include autoimmune lymphocytice hypophysitis, infectious and infiltrative diseases, pituitary infarction or hemorrhage, and head trauma.
  ○ Isolated ACTH deficiency is rare.
  ○ Mutations of genes important for pituitary development or ACTH synthesis are also rare.

DIAGNOSIS

- Diagnosis of AI is critical but often difficult. It depends on a high index of clinical suspicion for the disease that is further corroborated by biochemical evidence.
- Despite the various testing options available, no single test classifies all patients accurately.
- The diagnosis of adrenal insufficiency requires clinical judgment, as more than one biochemical test is often needed. It is important to look for internal consistency among the various tests.

Clinical Presentation

- The clinical presentation of AI can be variable and is dependent on the level of the hypothalamic-pituitary–adrenal axis that is affected, as well as the rate and extent of loss of adrenal function.
- Patients may remain undiagnosed for quite some time until a significant physical stressor precipitates an adrenal crisis—an endocrine emergency.

Acute AI (Adrenal Crisis)

- Acute AI most often occurs in patients with primary AI. It is critical to recognize the clinical syndrome because acute adrenal crisis is an endocrine emergency that requires prompt treatment.[8]
- **Clinical features** include:
  ○ Usually precipitated by acute stress (surgery, infection, or bilateral adrenal hemorrhage).

○ Shock with severe volume depletion and hypotension that is out of proportion to the severity of the current illness.

○ May include nausea and vomiting with a history of weight loss and anorexia, abdominal pain ("acute abdomen" if the etiology is acute adrenal infarction or hemorrhage), fatigue, fever, confusion or coma, electrolyte abnormalities (especially hyperkalemia), and eosinophilia.

Chronic Primary Adrenal Insufficiency

• Chronic primary adrenal insufficiency is more insidious in its onset.[2]

• A significant illness can transform latent chronic primary AI into a life-threatening adrenal crisis. Hence, early recognition and diagnosis is essential.

• In its early stage, the **presenting symptoms may be nonspecific:**
  ○ Chronic malaise, generalized weakness, myalgias, weight loss;
  ○ Nausea, vomiting, anorexia, and chronic abdominal pain.

• Primary AI often leads to both glucocorticoid and mineralocorticoid deficiency.
  ○ Lack of feedback inhibition on the pituitary by cortisol leads to increased ACTH secretion, which stimulates the melanocortin receptor to upregulate melanin synthesis, and causes **generalized hyperpigmentation** of the skin and mucosa.
  ○ Mineralocorticoid deficiency results in renal salt wasting. Patients often present with salt craving, hyponatremia, hyperkalemia, as well as volume depletion and hypotension.
  ○ Adrenal androgen secretion is lost, which is clinically more apparent in women who may complain of loss of axillary and pubic hair, and impairment of wellbeing.

• Patients with autoimmune adrenalitis may have evidence of other autoimmune diseases such as hypo- or hyperthyroidism, type 1 diabetes, or vitiligo.

• Patients with longstanding adrenal insufficiency can also manifest psychiatric symptoms, ranging from impairment in memory to depression and psychosis.

Secondary AI

• Patients with secondary AI present with many of the same symptoms as chronic primary AI. They may rarely present acutely with pituitary apoplexy.

• In addition to AI symptoms, secondary AI patients may experience other pituitary hormone deficiency symptoms such as amenorrhea, decreased libido, or hypothyroidism. Mass effects (headaches or visual field defects) from a pituitary or hypothalamic tumor may also be present.

• In contrast to primary AI, secondary AI patients **do not manifest hyperpigmentation**, because their ACTH is not elevated.

• Secondary AI patients also have less prominent electrolyte abnormalities, volume depletion, and hypotension, because the renin–angiotensin–aldosterone system is usually intact.

Diagnostic Testing

• A multistep approach is needed to document:
  ○ Whether there is inadequate cortisol secretion by the adrenals.
  ○ Whether the cause of adrenal insufficiency is lack of ACTH.

• Once AI is documented, a cause should be sought and treated as appropriate.

Laboratory Studies

Testing for Inadequate Cortisol Secretion

Inappropriately low cortisol production is the *sine qua non* finding in the diagnosis of AI of any cause.

Basal Cortisol Measurements

- Basal cortisol levels of ≥19 mcg/dL rule out AI, whereas early morning (8 AM to 9 AM) cortisol values ≤3 mcg/dL are indicative of the disorder. All other patients need dynamic testing.[9]
- In interpreting the results, it is important to remember that estrogen therapy raise plasma corticosteroid-binding globulin and, therefore, cortisol concentrations.

Corticotropin Stimulation Tests

- The corticotropin stimulation tests are the most widely used dynamic tests to assess adrenal function.[9,10]
- The corticotropin (standard 250 mcg or low-dose 1 mcg) can be given intravenously or intramuscularly. Plasma cortisol is measured before and 30 and 60 minutes after corticotropin.
- Peak serum cortisol levels >18 mcg/dL (500 nmol/L) or, preferably, 20 mcg/dL (550 nmol/L), excludes primary adrenal insufficiency and severe chronic secondary adrenal insufficiency.
- The low-dose corticotropin stimulation test has been proposed as a more sensitive test, especially for mild secondary AI and after treatment with glucocorticosteroids. However, this concept remains controversial.[11,12]
- It is important to note that the corticotropin stimulation tests may be normal in recent-onset secondary AI.
  - Screening with the corticotropin stimulation test for AI after pituitary surgery should be done at least 4 to 6 weeks after the surgery, since adrenal atrophy develops only gradually after the onset of ACTH deficiency.
  - Furthermore, chronic partial secondary adrenal insufficiency may not be detected by the corticotropin stimulation test.
  - An insulin tolerance test (ITT) may be needed in these patients (see subsequent text).
- Most steroid replacements (e.g., cortisone, hydrocortisone, and prednisone) interfere with the radioimmunoassay for serum cortisol. Therefore, patients already receiving such replacement should have their dose delayed on the day of testing until after the cosyntropin stimulation test.
- If adrenal crisis is suspected, intravenous saline and dexamethasone, 4 mg IV q6h, should be started until the corticotropin stimulation test can be performed. In this acute setting, dexamethasone is the preferred glucocorticoid, because it does not cross-react with the cortisol in the assay and permits subsequent testing.

Insulin Tolerance Test

- ITT is regarded as the gold standard in the assessment of suspected secondary AI, since hypoglycemia is a powerful stressor that results in rapid activation of the HPA axis.[9]
- Intravenous insulin at a dose of 0.1 to 0.15 U/kg is given to achieve hypoglycemia. Plasma glucose and cortisol are measured at 0, 30, 45, 60, 90, and 120 minutes after insulin infusion.
- Adequate hypoglycemia of <40 mg/dL with neuroglycopenic symptoms is essential.
- Normal subjects have a plasma cortisol increase to at least 18 mcg/dL. Use of the higher cutoff point (≥20 mcg/dL) is preferable to avoid underdiagnosis of AI.
- During the test, close supervision is mandatory. Cardiovascular disease or a history of seizures are contraindications to performing this test.

Adrenal Function During Critical Illness
- Evaluating the HPA axis during critical illness can be challenging.[13]
- Cortisol levels vary broadly with disease severity.
  - Inappropriately low cortisol levels can be seen during critical illness with a structurally normal HPA axis ("relative" adrenal insufficiency).
  - Severely ill patients also have decreased cortisol-binding proteins, which leads to an increase in the ratio of free to bound serum cortisol.
- Recommendations from the American College of Critical Care Medicine have suggested that AI in critically ill patients is best diagnosed by a basal cortisol level of <10 mcg/dL or an incremental response <9 mcg/dL after standard 250 mcg corticotropin stimulation test.
- In light of these issues, there is currently no consensus regarding the precise diagnostic criteria in critical care settings.

Differentiating Primary and Secondary AI

Baseline ACTH Concentration[14,15]
- The cosyntropin stimulation test alone does not definitively differentiate between primary and secondary disease.
- A baseline ACTH level obtained at the same time as a basal cortisol level can be helpful in this regard. A disproportionately elevated baseline plasma ACTH level with a concurrently low basal serum cortisol suggests primary AI. On the other hand, secondary AI patients have low serum cortisol with a low or low-normal baseline plasma ACTH level.

CRH Stimulation Test
- The CRH stimulation test has utility for differentiating a pituitary from hypothalamic etiology of AI.[16]
- The plasma ACTH usually peaks at 15 to 30 minutes and cortisol value peaks 30 to 45 minutes following CRH administration in AI patients due to a hypothalamic, but not pituitary, etiology.
- CRH stimulation testing has limited usefulness due to its cost, availability, and limited data.

Renin and Aldosterone Concentrations
- Mineralocorticoids as well as glucocorticoids are usually affected in primary AI. Aldosterone levels are typically low, associated with elevated rennin activity in this setting.[17]
- In secondary AI, the rennin–angiotensin–aldosterone system can function normally.

Autoantibodies
- At the time of onset of clinically apparent autoimmune AI, adrenal antibodies are detected in more than 90% of patients. The presence of autoantibodies will often predate the onset of AI.[4] Abnormal antibodies are more common if there is associated vitiligo or alopecia.
- The presence of **adrenal cortex antibody (ACA)** and **21-hydroxylase (CYP21A2) antibody** is used to assist the diagnosis of autoimmune AI in clinical practice. The presence of both antibodies makes the diagnosis likely up to 99%.[18]
- A range of autoantibodies against other steroidogenic enzymes and other endocrine cells such as 17-α-hydroxylase antibodies, P450 side-chain cleavage antibodies and 3-β-hydroxysteroid dehydrogenase (3-β HSD) antibodies are also present in some patients.

- Evaluation of other endocrine gland dysfunction associated with autoimmune adrenal insufficiency may be sought by measuring serum calcium, islet cell antibodies, TSH, and tests of gonadal function. Consideration should also be made for vitamin B12 deficiency and autoimmune hepatitis or hemolytic anemia.
- In boys who have isolated primary adrenal insufficiency and neurologic symptoms, serum concentrations of very-long-chain fatty acids (>24 carbon chain length) should be measured to exclude adrenoleukodystrophy.[19]

Imaging
- **Radiologic imaging should only be performed once laboratory diagnosis of adrenal insufficiency is made.** An exception to this role is a case in which a patient is suspected of having a pituitary or hypothalamic tumor.[20]
- **MRI imaging** of the hypothalamic-pituitary region is superior to CT in most situations connected with secondary AI. Analysis of sagittal and coronal sections provides the most information.
- CT should be obtained if bone invasion or calcifications in a craniopharyngioma need to be demonstrated.
- CT and MRI are often used to image the adrenal glands as well. In autoimmune adrenalitis, imaging often reveals small or absent adrenal glands. Enlarged or calcified adrenals may suggest an infectious, hemorrhagic or malignant diagnosis.

Diagnostic Procedure
- CT-guided adrenal biopsy is not usually required except in the differential diagnosis of AI in patients with a presentation suspicious for metastases, in whom a known primary remains unidentified but pheochromocytoma has been excluded.[21]
- Adrenal biopsy may have additional diagnostic value in patient with other infiltrative etiologies.

TREATMENT

Acute Treatment
- Adrenal crisis is a life-threatening condition requiring immediate treatment. Therapy should not be delayed to perform diagnostic studies or await laboratory results.
- If there is no history suggestive of adrenal insufficiency, other causes of shock also need to be considered.
- Volume replacement using normal saline is essential to reverse hypotension and electrolyte abnormalities.
- While blood for serum cortisol, ACTH, and serum chemistry is drawn, "stress-dose" steroids should be started.
  - If the diagnosis is unclear, 4 mg IV dexamethasone (instead of hydrocortisone) should be given first, followed by corticotropin stimulation testing.
  - In patients with a clearly identified history of adrenal insufficiency, either dexamethasone (4 mg IV q12h) or hydrocortisone (50 to 100 mg IV q6–8h) can be given until their condition has stabilized.
  - Once the stressor has been alleviated, steroid doses can be tapered over 1 to 3 days to an oral maintenance daily dose.
- In the acute setting, mineralocorticoid replacement is not useful, as it takes several days for its sodium-retaining effects to become apparent; intravenous saline alone will suffice.

- Any signs or symptoms of adrenal crisis should resolve quickly, generally over the following 1 to 2 hours after glucocorticoid therapy.

Maintenance Treatment

- Maintenance therapy involves glucocorticoid replacement at physiologic levels. Many maintenance treatment regimens have been suggested.
  - Chronic therapy for patients with either primary or secondary adrenal insufficiency requires glucocorticoid replacement with **hydrocortisone** 15 to 30 mg/day PO or its equivalent (**prednisone** 4.0 to 7.5 mg/day PO).
  - The glucocorticoids can be administered in 1 to 3 divided doses. It is **generally best to give a single dose in the morning** to mimic the physiologic diurnal variation. If the patient thinks he or she could benefit from a split-dose regimen, usually the larger dose is given in the morning and the smaller dose later in the day.
  - **Treatment should be tailored (using the lowest dose possible) to the patient's symptoms** so as to avoid fatigue, weight loss, hyponatremia, and, in primary adrenal insufficiency, hyperpigmentation.
  - One should also **avoid the complications of excess glucocorticoid replacement**, such as weight gain, osteoporosis, and immune compromise.
  - Treatment surveillance is mainly based on clinical grounds, taking into account signs and symptoms potentially suggestive of over replacement or under-replacement. No laboratory assessment has proven to be reliable for monitoring replacement quality.
- Patients with primary adrenal insufficiency should also receive mineralocorticoid replacement. **Fludrocortisone** is given at a dose of 0.05 to 0.2 mg PO daily, and is titrated to the patient's symptoms of orthostasis, blood pressure normalization, normalization of potassium levels, and suppression of plasma renin activity to the middle to upper end of the normal range.
- Replacement of **dehydroepiandrosterone** (DHEA) has positive effects on wellbeing and mood in some patients with both primary and secondary AI.[22,23] Recommended doses are 25 to 50 mg daily in the morning. However, there is still lack of pharmaceutically controlled preparations and large-scale studies for DHEA therapy.

Treatment for Specific Situations

- Stress dosing
  - Supplementary glucocorticoid dosing should be based on the likelihood and degree of adrenal suppression, the degree of medical or surgical stress, and the cardiovascular and metabolic response to the therapy.
  - Patients and their families may be advised to increase the daily glucocorticoid dose during febrile illness, upper respiratory infection, nausea, vomiting, or any other undue physical stress.
  - In addition to aggressive hydration, the usual daily dose can initially be doubled and then doubled again if symptoms of AI persist. An injectable dexamethasone kit can be prescribed for home use. When the acute illness has resolved, patients may return to their usual daily replacement doses within 1 to 3 days.
  - If at any time there is uncertainty regarding the status or safety of the patient, the patient should be immediately brought to the nearest hospital for intravenous steroids.

- Perioperative dosing
  - During the perioperative and postsurgical period, inadequate steroid coverage may be manifested by signs and symptoms of impending adrenal crisis such as hypotension, nausea, vomiting, or fever.
  - Determining the appropriate coverage for surgical procedures is dependent on the complexity and duration of the procedure.
    - For minor procedures with local anesthesia and most radiologic studies, the patient's usual daily dose should suffice. This should NOT be withheld under any circumstances and if the patient is fasting a dose should be given parenterally.
    - For moderate procedures involving general anesthesia, patients should continue their usual daily steroid dose preoperatively and then receive hydrocortisone 25 mg IV q8h intravenously during the procedure.
    - For major operations involving cardiothoracic or abdominal cavities, patients should be given their baseline daily dose preoperatively and then receive hydrocortisone 50 mg IV q8h during the procedure.
    - Glucocorticoid can usually be rapidly tapered to usual dose over 1 to 2 days.[24]
- Secondary adrenal insufficiency.
  - There is no need for mineralocorticoid replacement. However, other pituitary hormone deficiencies may need to be replaced.
- Thyroid disease
  - If a patient is concurrently diagnosed with both adrenal insufficiency and hypothyroidism, the patient must first receive adequate glucocorticoid replacement before initiating thyroid hormone therapy to avoid precipitating adrenal crisis.
  - In patients with adrenal insufficiency and unresolved hyperthyroidism, glucocorticoid replacement should be doubled or tripled, since hyperthyroidism increases cortisol clearance.[2]
- Pregnancy
  - Increased cortisol-binding globulin, antimineralocorticoid action of increased progesterone, and increased plasma renin activity are characteristic physiologic changes that occur in the later stages of pregnancy.
  - Therefore, in the third trimester, glucocorticoid replacement doses may need to be doubled. Fludrocortisone is adjusted according to blood pressure and serum potassium level.
  - During labor, adequate normal saline hydration and hydrocortisone 25 mg IV q6h should be administered. At the time of delivery, or if labor is prolonged, hydrocortisone should be administered intravenously in a dose of 100 mg q6h or as a continuous infusion.
  - After delivery, the dose can be tapered rapidly to maintenance within 2 to 3 days.[2]

PATIENT EDUCATION

- All patients with adrenal insufficiency should obtain a **medical-alert bracelet** indicating the diagnosis of steroid dependence, and a physician's number to call.
- In addition, every patient should have with them **prefilled syringes of dexamethasone** (4 mg/mL in saline solution); the patient and one or more responsible family or household members should be instructed on how to inject the dexamethasone in case of emergency (e.g., massive blood loss, inability to maintain oral intake, or presence of any of the symptoms of adrenal crisis).
- Instruction should also include the need to be brought to medical attention immediately in presence of symptoms of adrenal crisis.

REFERENCES

1. Addison T. *On the constitutional and local effects of disease of the supra-renal capsules.* London: Samuel Highley; 1855.
2. Arlt W, Allolio B. Adrenal insufficiency. *Lancet* 2003;361(9372):1881–1893.
3. Carey RM. The changing clinical spectrum of adrenal insufficiency. *Ann Intern Med* 1997; 127(12):1103–1105.
4. Betterle C, Dal Pra C, Mantero F, et al. Autoimmune adrenal insufficiency and autoimmune polyendocrine syndromes: Autoantibodies, autoantigens, and their applicability in diagnosis and disease prediction. *Endocr Rev* 2002;23(3):327–364.
5. Bornstein SR. Predisposing factors for adrenal insufficiency. *N Engl J Med* 2009;360(22): 2328–2339.
6. Krasner AS. Glucocorticoid-induced adrenal insufficiency. *JAMA* 1999;282(7):671–676.
7. Chidakel AR, Zweig SB, Schlosser JR, et al. High prevalence of adrenal suppression during acute illness in hospitalized patients receiving megestrol acetate. *J Endocrinol Invest* 2006; 29(2):136–140.
8. Bouillon R. Acute adrenal insufficiency. *Endocrinol Metab Clin North Am* 2006;35(4):767–775, ix.
9. Grinspoon SK, Biller BM. Clinical review 62: Laboratory assessment of adrenal insufficiency. *J Clin Endocrinol Metab* 1994;79(4):923–931.
10. May ME. Adrenocortical insufficiency – clinical aspects. In: Vaughan ED Jr, Carey RM, eds. *Adrenal Disorders.* New York: Thieme Medical, 1989:171–189.
11. Magnotti M, Shimshi M. Diagnosing adrenal insufficiency: Which test is best–the 1-microg or the 250-microg cosyntropin stimulation test? *Endocr Pract* 2008;14(2):233–238.
12. Suliman AM, Smith TP, Labib M, et al. The low-dose ACTH test does not provide a useful assessment of the hypothalamic-pituitary-adrenal axis in secondary adrenal insufficiency. *Clin Endocrinol (Oxf)* 2002;56(4):533–539.
13. Marik PE, Pastores SM, Annane D, et al. Recommendations for the diagnosis and management of corticosteroid insufficiency in critically ill adult patients: Consensus statements from an international task force by the American College of Critical Care Medicine. *Crit Care Med* 2008;36(6):1937–1949.
14. Wallace I, Cunningham S, Lindsay J. The diagnosis and investigation of adrenal insufficiency in adults. *Ann Clin Biochem* 2009;46(Pt 5):351–367. Epub 2009 Aug 12.
15. Blevins LS Jr, Shankroff J, Moser HW, et al. Elevated plasma adrenocorticotropin concentration as evidence of limited adrenocortical reserve in patients with adrenomyeloneuropathy. *J Clin Endocrinol Metab* 1994;78(2):261–265.
16. Orth DN. Corticotropin-releasing hormone in humans. *Endocr Rev* 1992;13(2):164–191.
17. Salvatori R. Adrenal insufficiency. *JAMA* 2005;294(19):2481–2488.
18. Falorni A, Laureti S, Nikoshkov A, et al. 21-hydroxylase autoantibodies in adult patients with endocrine autoimmune diseases are highly specific for Addison's disease. Belgian Diabetes Registry. *Clin Exp Immunol* 1997;107(2):341–346.
19. Mosser J, Douar AM, Sarde CO, et al. Putative X-linked adrenoleukodystrophy gene shares unexpected homology with ABC transporters. *Nature* 1993;361(6414):726–730.
20. Oelkers W. Adrenal insufficiency. *N Engl J Med* 1996;335(16):1206–1212.
21. Grumbach MM, Biller BM, Braunstein GD, et al. Management of the clinically inapparent adrenal mass ("incidentaloma"). *Ann Intern Med* 2003;138(5):424–429.
22. Hunt PJ, Gurnell EM, Huppert FA, et al. Improvement in mood and fatigue after dehydroepiandrosterone replacement in Addison's disease in a randomized, double blind trial. *J Clin Endocrinol Metab* 2000;85(12):4650–4656.
23. Johannsson G, Burman P, Wirén L, et al. Low dose dehydroepiandrosterone affects behavior in hypopituitary androgen-deficient women: A placebo-controlled trial. *J Clin Endocrinol Metab* 2002;87(5):2046–2052.
24. Coursin DB, Wood KE. Corticosteroid supplementation for adrenal insufficiency. *JAMA* 2002;287(2):236–240.

Adult Congenital Adrenal Hyperplasia

12

Judit Dunai and Kim Carmichael

GENERAL PRINCIPLES

- Congenital adrenal hyperplasia (CAH) consists of a group of autosomal recessive genetic disorders characterized by functional abnormalities of adrenal steroid biosynthetic enzymes, leading to impaired cortisol biosynthesis, and a compensatory increase in serum adrenocorticotropic hormone (ACTH).[1–3]
- High ACTH levels induce hyperplastic changes of the dysfunctional adrenal tissue and increase production of virilizing steroids with little or no increase in cortisol production.
- Classic CAH is responsible for most cases of pseudohermaphroditism in females and about 50% of all cases of ambiguous genitalia.
- A spectrum of phenotypes is observed. A severe form with concurrent aldosterone deficiency results in salt wasting, and a form with apparently normal aldosterone biosynthesis leads to various degrees of virilization. Together, these are called classic CAH. Milder, nonclassic forms that maybe asymptomatic are often associated with postnatal androgen excess.[1]

Epidemiology

- About 95% of cases result from **21-hydroxylase deficiency**.
- Five to eight percent of cases are due to **11-β-hydroxylase deficiency**, which is the second most common enzyme deficiency and is characterized by virilization and low-renin hypertension. For details on this topic, please refer to an excellent review by Nimkarn and New[4] as discussion of CAH in this chapter is limited to 21-hydroxylase deficiency.
- The incidence of classic 21-hydroxylase deficiency is thought to be 1 per 14,000 births.
  - The carrier frequency is 1 in 60.
  - The majority of cases of classic CAH are discovered during childhood; however, better understanding of the genetics and pathophysiology of CAH has led to frequent discoveries of its milder, nonclassic forms during adulthood.
- The overall incidence of nonclassic CAH is not known but appears to be 0.1% to 0.2% in the general population. 11-β-hydroxylase deficiency occurs in 1 per 100,000 births.[4]

Etiology

- **Deficient cortisol production** is the key aberration in CAH, and mastery of the adrenal steroid biosynthesis pathway is essential to understanding the pathogenesis of the disease and the rationale behind treatment (Fig. 12-1).
- Differing mutations occurring in **CYP21A2**, the gene encoding 21-hydroxylase (P450c21) affect the severity and expression of the disease.[5]

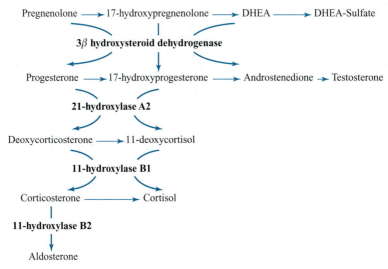

FIGURE 12-1 The adrenal steroid biosynthesis pathway.

- Mutations associated with large reductions in enzyme activity result in severe deficiencies of aldosterone and cortisol, whereas mutations associated with milder reductions result in less severe hormone abnormalities and a nonclassic course.
- Some patients with nonclassic CAH have one allele of the 21-hydroxylase gene with a "severe" mutation and one allele with a "mild" mutation. Thus, the severity of the phenotype in compound heterozygotes is determined by the less severe mutation.[1]
- The reduction in cortisol levels stimulates ACTH release by the pituitary, in turn causing increased production of cortisol precursors, such as progesterone and 17-OH progesterone (17-OHP), which may be metabolized to androgen precursors (see Fig. 12-1).

Classification

- Three-fourths of patients with classic CAH are **"*salt wasters*,"** as they have no 21-hydroxylase activity and produce insufficient aldosterone to retain sodium.
- The remaining one-fourth of patients, who produce low but detectable enzyme activity, retain enough ability to produce aldosterone, and, although virilized, do not sodium waste, and so are known as **"*simple virilizers*."**
- Those who retain 20% to 60% of enzymatic activity typically present in adulthood with more subtle, nonclassic forms, and acute adrenal crisis is uncommon.[3]
- Patients with classic 21-hydroxylase deficiency are at high risk for development of adrenal insufficiency without exogenous glucocorticoid administration.

DIAGNOSIS

Clinical Presentation

- **Classic 21-hydroxylase deficiency** presents at birth or within several weeks of birth with hypotension as a result of adrenal insufficiency.

- **Simple virilizing 21-hydroxylase deficiency** is usually diagnosed shortly after birth in females owing to external genital abnormalities (clitoral enlargement, fusion of the labial folds, formation of urogenital sinus), but for boys the diagnosis can be delayed for years until signs of androgen excess develop.
- The symptoms of nonclassic 21-hydroxylase deficiency may be subtle or even absent. It can present at any age after birth usually with hyperandrogenic symptoms such as cystic acne, hirsutism, infertility, and irregular menses. These symptoms can wax and wane over time. Males with nonclassic CAH may experience infertility and acne.
- In children of both sexes, nonclassic CAH may be diagnosed during a work-up for premature pubarche or accelerated linear growth with advanced bone age.
- The **differential diagnosis for nonclassic CAH in adults** is limited but includes **polycystic ovarian syndrome, virilizing adrenal or ovarian tumors, and exogenous anabolic steroid use.**

Physical Examination

- In nonclassic CAH females, hyperandrogenic features dominate the physical examination. Hirsutism is the single most common symptom, followed by oligomenorrhea and acne.[1]
- Men might present with small testes compared to the phallus, oligospermia, infertility, and short stature.
- Final adult height may be reduced owing to premature closure of epiphyses due to androgen excess.

Diagnostic Testing

- **Classic 21-hydroxylase deficiency is characterized by significantly elevated levels of 17-OHP** in infancy, with varying degrees of virilization that may not become apparent until later in childhood.
- Screening newborns for CAH minimizes delay in diagnosis and reduces morbidity from adrenal crisis. A few nonclassic CAH cases are detected by newborn-screening, but most are missed because of borderline or normal 17-OHP.

Hormonal Evaluation

- Early morning 17-OHP levels should be drawn during the follicular phase in women. A **17-OHP of <200 ng/dL makes CAH unlikely,** and a **value >400 ng/dL has been reported to have 100% specificity and 90% sensitivity.**[6]
  - The gold standard for hormonal diagnosis is the cosyntropin stimulation test, which should be done for values between 200 ng/dL and 400 ng/dL.
    - 250 mcg of synthetic ACTH is administered IV and plasma concentrations of 17-OHP is measured at baseline and at 60 minutes after the drug is given; reference values for the local laboratory should be obtained. **Patients with nonclassic CAH will usually have 17-OHP values >1000 ng/dL.**[1]
    - Plasma cortisol is measured at baseline and at 30 minutes after stimulation.
    - If the post-ACTH cortisol level is <20 mcg/dL, the patient should be made aware of the need to take additional glucocorticoids during times of physiologic stress. Please see Chapter 11 for details on diagnosing adrenal insufficiency.
- Genotyping should only be done if cosyntropin stimulation results are equivocal and for purposes of genetic counseling.[7]
- First-degree family members of affected patients should be screened for CAH because of the potential absence of clinical signs and potential harm that may result if a patient does not receive therapy.

TREATMENT

Medical Therapy

- The goal of therapy in CAH is to both correct the deficiency in cortisol secretion and to suppress ACTH overproduction.
- Therapy consists of a balance between sufficient glucocorticoid replacement to suppress the overproduction of androgens and to prevent adrenal crises in classic cases, while avoiding complications related to glucocorticoid excess.
- **Treatment for classic "salt-wasting" CAH** is glucocorticoid and mineralocorticoid replacement and sodium chloride supplementation.[1]
- **Treatment of adults with *nonclassic* 21-hydroxylase deficiency** should only be undertaken for infertility or hyperandrogenism that is unacceptable to the patient. There are no reports of death from adrenal insufficiency as a result of nonclassic CAH in the medical literature; therefore, stress dose steroids are usually not required unless subnormal cortisol response was demonstrated during cosyntropin stimulation. See Chapter 11 for details on diagnosis and management of adrenal insufficiency.
- **Hydrocortisone is the preferred treatment in children** because of improved clinical outcomes with respect to final adult height.
  - Typical dose is 10 to 15 mg/m^2/day of hydrocortisone in two or three divided doses.
- After completion of linear growth, long-acting glucocorticoids are preferred.
  - Dex**amethasone** (Decadron) given in the evening (0.25 mg) is often considered to be the most effective treatment in adults and can reduce hirsutism and irregular menstruation within months.[1]
- Aldosterone biosynthetic defect is clinically apparent only in the salt-wasting form. However, **subclinical aldosterone deficiency** is present in all forms and can be **evaluated by the aldostetrone to plasma renin activity (PRA) ratio**.
  - All patients with elevated PRA or decreased aldosterone to PRA ratio benefit from mineralocorticoid therapy and adequate dietary sodium supplementation.[1]
  - Maintenance of sodium balance reduces vasopressin and ACTH levels, allowing the use of lower glucocorticoid doses.
  - Sensitivity to mineralocorticoids may vary over time, and the need for mineralocorticoid replacement should be reassessed periodically.

COMPLICATIONS

- Unfortunately, treatment outcome in CAH is often suboptimal either due to incomplete suppression of hyperandrogenism or, conversely, due to overtreatment-induced hypercortisolism. Both of these can result in decreased final adult height, 1.7 to 2.0 SD below the average in the normal population.[2]
- Final adult height may be improved in children with advanced bone age, predicted to be at least one standard deviation below midparental target height, with the use of growth hormone and luteinizing hormone releasing hormone agonists.[8]
- For management of adrenal crisis in classic, salt-wasting CAH (see Chapter 11).

MONITORING

- Monitoring the effects of steroid replacement is crucial. 17-OHP levels are relatively resistant to suppression by glucocorticoids, and thus, a normal 17-OHP level often represents overtreatment. Overtreatment can cause iatrogenic Cushing's syndrome and lead to reduced bone mineral density.

- 17-OHP levels should be maintained at the upper end of normal to mildly supranormal levels. Androstenedione levels are more sensitive to suppression and may be a better indicator of replacement dosing, with a goal of keeping the androstenedione levels in the upper one-third of normal range.
- Mineralocorticoid replacement may be monitored by following blood pressure and potassium levels.
- Elevated renin levels or hypotension may signify insufficient mineralocorticoid replacement.
- Adrenal imaging should be reserved only for those with an atypical clinical or biochemical course. There is insufficient data to recommend routine screening for adrenal masses.
- Pregnancy in classic CAH should be managed by an endocrinologist experienced in this area. Women with nonclassic CAH generally do not require glucocorticoid therapy during pregnancy. Treatment of prenatal CAH is regarded as experimental.[1]
- Discussion of prenatal counseling, diagnosis, and treatment of CAH is beyond the scope of this chapter, and the reader is referred to the following reviews.[1,9,10]

REFERENCES

1. Speiser PW, Azziz LS, Baskin LG, et al. Congenital adrenal hyperplasia due to steroid 21-hydroxilase deficiency: An endocrine society clinical practice guideline. *J Clin Endocrinol Metab* 2010;95:4133–4160.
2. Merke DP, Bomstein S. Congenital adrenal hyperplasia. *Lancet* 2005;365:2125–2136.
3. Speiser PW, White PC. Congenital adrenal hyperplasia. *N Eng J Med* 2003;349:776:88.
4. Nimkarn S, New MI. Steroid 11beta- hydroxylase deficiency congenital adrenal hyperplasia. *Trends Endocrinol Metab* 2008;19(3):96–99.
5. Krone N, Arlt W. Genetics of congenital adrenal hyperplasia. *Best Pract Res Clin Endocrinol Metab* 2009;23(2):181–192.
6. Azziz R, Hincapie LA, Knochenhauer ES, et al. Screening for 21-hydroxylase-deficient nonclassic adrenal hyperplasia among hyperandrogenic women: A prospective study. *Fertil Steril* 1999;72(5):915–925.
7. Torok D, Halasz Z, Garami M, et al. Limited value of serum steroid measurements in identification of mild form of 21-hydroxylase deficiency. *Exp Clin Endocrinol Diabetes* 2003; 111:27–32.
8. Lin-Su K, Vogiatzi MG, Marshall I, et al. Treatment with growth hormone and luteinizing hormone releasing hormone analog improves final adult height in children with congenital adrenal hyperplasia. *J Clin Endocrinol Metab* 2005;90(6):3318–3325.
9. Nimkarn S, New MI. Congenital adrenal hyperplasia due to 21-hydroxylase deficiency: A paradigm for prenatal diagnosis and treatment. *Ann N Y Acad Sci* 2010;1192:5–11.
10. Nimkarn S, New MI. Prenatal diagnosis and treatment of congenital adrenal hyperplasia. *Horm Res* 2007;67:53–60.

Conn's Syndrome

13

Mariko Johnson and Thomas J. Baranski

GENERAL PRINCIPLES

Definition

Primary aldosteronism, also known as Conn's syndrome, is defined as inappropriate (renin-independent) overproduction of aldosterone. Primary aldosteronism must be distinguished from secondary aldosteronism, which is appropriate (renin-dependent) increased production of aldosterone in response to relative hypovolemia as is seen in renovascular hypertension and with diuretic therapy.

Classification

Distinguishing between unilateral and bilateral disease is of utmost importance because it determines therapy. Unilateral disease is confined to a single adrenal gland and is usually treated with surgery. Bilateral disease is present in both adrenal glands and is usually treated medically.

Epidemiology

The true prevalence of primary aldosteronism is not known. Older literature had suggested a low prevalence of <1% in hypertensive patients. More recent literature suggests a prevalence of up to 10% in hypertensive patients.[1]

Etiology

Primary aldosteronism can be caused by several adrenal disorders:
- Aldosterone-producing adenoma (APA)
- Adrenal gland hyperplasia (unilateral or bilateral)
- Aldosterone-secreting adrenal cortical carcinoma (ACC)
- Aldosterone-secreting ovarian tumor
- Familial hyperaldosteronism

Pathophysiology

Aldosterone is produced in the zona glomerulosa and is synthesized and released in response to renin-dependent production of angiotensin II. However, serum potassium, adrenocorticotropic hormone (ACTH), dopamine, and atrial natriuretic peptide (ANP) also affect its production and secretion. Aldosterone-induced sodium retention and potassium wasting do not lead to generalized edema or profound hypokalemia because of "aldosterone escape," in which an increase in urinary sodium and decrease in urinary potassium excretion counteract the acute effects of excess aldosterone. This phenomenon is thought to be mediated by increased secretion of ANP induced by hypervolemia, decreased abundance of the thiazide-sensitive NaCl cotransporter, and pressure natriuresis.

DIAGNOSIS

Clinical Presentation

The classic findings in primary aldosteronism are hypertension and hypokalemia. However, it is now understood that **the most common presentation of primary aldosteronism is normokalemic hypertension.** Hypertension is usually, but not always, present[2], but hypokalemia is present in less than half of confirmed cases.[1,3]

History

Symptoms related to hypokalemia, such as muscle weakness and cramping, can occur. Other symptoms are nonspecific and may include headache, fatigue, palpitations, and polyuria. A careful medication history is important, as many antihypertensives can interfere with diagnostic testing, as can licorice ingestion or use of chewing tobacco. A family history of early onset primary aldosteronism, hypertension, or cerebrovascular events should raise suspicion for familial hyperaldosteronism.

Physical Examination

There are no specific physical findings in primary aldosteronism, though hypertension is present in the majority of cases.

Diagnostic Criteria

The diagnosis of primary aldosteronism is based on the demonstration of renin-independent overproduction of aldosterone.

Differential Diagnosis

- **Adrenal gland hyperplasia and aldosterone-secreting adenomas account for the majority of cases of primary aldosteronism.** Other causes are rare and account for <3% of cases.
- APAs account for approximately one-third of cases of primary aldosteronism. They are seen on occasion in multiple endocrine neoplasia type 1.
- Adrenal gland hyperplasia, also known as idiopathic hyperaldosteronism (IHA), accounts for approximately two-thirds of cases of primary aldosteronism and may affect one or both adrenal glands.
- Aldosterone-secreting ACC is rare, and only a subset of these tumors will secrete aldosterone. These tumors often come to attention as a result of pain from local invasion or cosecretion of cortisol and/or adrenal androgens, which lead to symptoms of Cushing's syndrome and/or virilization.
- Aldosterone-secreting ovarian tumor as a cause of primary aldosteronism is extremely rare.
- Familial hyperaldosteronism
  - Familial hyperaldosteronism (FH) type 1, also called glucocorticoid-remediable aldosteronism (GRA), is inherited in an autosomal-dominant fashion and is usually associated with bilateral adrenal hyperplasia. It is caused by recombination between the promoter regions of 11-β-hydroxylase (*CYP11B1*) and the coding regions of 18-hydroxylase (*CYP11B2*), such that in the chimeric gene, ACTH (rather than renin or serum potassium) drives the expression of aldosterone synthase and aldosterone production. In contrast to most patients with primary aldosteronism who develop hypertension between the third and fifth decades, GRA patients develop hypertension at birth or in early childhood. Patients with

GRA are usually normokalemic because their aldosterone release has the same circadian pattern as that of ACTH, and, therefore, aldosterone secretion is above normal for only part of the day. However, these patients can develop marked hypokalemia when treated with thiazide diuretics. Patients with GRA also tend to have an increased prevalence of early cerebrovascular complications, especially hemorrhagic strokes from ruptured intracerebral aneurysms.

○ Familial hyperaldosteronism type 2 is ACTH independent and leads to the occurrence of APA, IHA, or both, in an autosomal-dominant pattern. Although the exact genetic defect is unknown, a locus on chromosome 7p22 has been implicated.

Diagnostic Testing

Diagnostic testing for primary aldosteronism aims to establish renin-independent aldosterone excess and determines whether the source is unilateral or bilateral via the three-step algorithm shown in Figure 13-1:

• Screening for renin-independent aldosterone production
• Confirmation of renin-independent aldosterone production
• Localization of aldosterone production

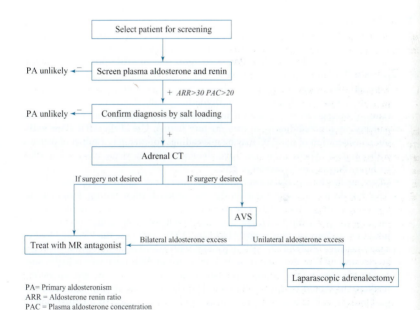

PA= Primary aldosteronism
ARR = Aldosterone renin ratio
PAC = Plasma aldosterone concentration
CT = Computed tomography
AVS = Adrenal vein sampling
MR = Mineralocorticoid receptor

FIGURE 13-1 Approach to the patient with suspected primary aldosteronism. Adapted from Funder JW, Carey RM, Fardella C, et al. Case detection, diagnosis, and treatment of patients with primary aldosteronism: an endocrine society clinical practice guideline. *J Clin Endocrinol Metab* 2008;93(9):3266–3281.

Laboratories

- **Screening for renin-independent hyperaldosteronism** is recommended in patient groups with a relatively high prevalence, including patients with:
  ○ Moderate to severe hypertension (blood pressure >160–179/100–109 mm Hg)
  ○ Drug-resistant hypertension
  ○ Hypertension of any stage associated with spontaneous or diuretic-induced hypokalemia
  ○ Hypertension associated with adrenal incidentaloma
  ○ Hypertension with a family history of early-onset hypertension or cerebrovascular accident at an early age (<40 years)
  ○ Hypertension and a first-degree relative with primary aldosteronism[4]
- Screening for GRA via PCR-based genetic testing should be considered in patients with confirmed primary aldosteronism and any of the following:
  ○ Onset prior to 20 years of age
  ○ Family history of primary aldosteronism
  ○ Personal or family history of stroke prior to age 40[4]
- Clinicians should ensure that potassium is replete, sodium intake is liberalized, and certain interfering substances are discontinued for at least 4 weeks before proceeding with screening. Interfering medications include diuretics (particularly mineralocorticoid receptor antagonists such as spironolactone) and products derived from licorice root, such as chewing tobacco.
- **The two tests ordered for biochemical screening for primary hyperaldosteronism are the plasma aldosterone concentration (PAC) and the plasma renin activity (PRA). The aldosterone renin ratio (ARR) can be calculated from these two values and is equal to PAC/PRA. A PAC > 20 ng/dL and an ARR >30 (units are ng/dL per ng/mL/hour) used together have a 90% sensitivity and specificity for primary hyperaldosteronism.**[5] Using these values as screening cutoffs is reasonable, though they are not universally agreed upon. Borderline results should be interpreted with caution; testing can be repeated if interference from medications is suspected or patients can proceed directly to confirmatory testing. **Use of the ARR alone without consideration of the PAC may be misleading.** For example, a subset of patients with essential hypertension may have elevated ratios by virtue of very low PRA without concomitant elevation in PAC.
- Many medications (particularly antihypertensives) can interfere with the PAC or ARR but do not necessarily need to be discontinued before testing. However, the results of testing should always be interpreted after taking into account potential interference (see Table 13-1). For example, angiotensin-converting enzyme (ACE) inhibitors and angiotensin receptor blockers (ARBs) may raise the PRA and lead to a false-negative result for the ARR in patients with primary aldosteronism. However, an elevated ARR in the context of ACE inhibitor or ARB treatment is highly suggestive of primary aldosteronism. If a false screening result is suspected, interfering medications should be discontinued and hydralazine, verapamil, or alpha adrenergic blockers such as doxazosin used to control blood pressure. An interpretation of the possible combinations of PAC and PRA can be found in Table 13-2.
- **Confirmation of renin-independent hyperaldosteronism** is made by documenting nonsuppression of aldosterone during sodium loading. Oral and intravenous sodium loading tests are the most commonly used confirmatory tests. The principle underlying testing is that an increase in intravascular volume should decrease renin release and subsequent aldosterone production in patients without primary aldosteronism. Sodium loading may lead to volume overload, especially in patients with

| TABLE 13-1 | MEDICATIONS THAT MAY AFFECT SCREENING FOR PRIMARY ALDOSTERONISM | | |

Medications	Effect on PAC	Effect on PRA	Effect on ARR
Diuretics	↑	↑↑	↓
Beta blockers, alpha-2 agonists, NSAIDs, renin inhibitors	↓	↓↓	↑
ACE inhibitors, ARBs, Ca-channel blockers, renin inhibitors	↓	↑↑	↓

PAC, plasma aldosterone concentration; PRA, plasma renin activity; ARR, aldosterone renin ratio; NSAID, non-steroidal anti-inflammatory drug; ACE, angiotensin-converting enzyme; ARB, angiotensin receptor blocker; Ca, calcium.

Adapted from Funder JW, Carey RM, Fardella C, et al. Case detection, diagnosis, and treatment of patients with primary aldosteronism: an endocrine society clinical practice guideline. *J Clin Endocrinol Metab* 2008;93(9):3266–3281.

compromised left ventricular function or renal failure, and must be closely monitored. Potassium should be adequately replaced prior to initiation of either test.

○ **Oral sodium loading test**

The patient is instructed to consume 6 g/day of sodium, either from dietary sources or sodium chloride tablets. Potassium must be measured daily and replaced as needed, because sodium loading in patients with primary aldosteronism leads to potassium wasting. A 24-hour urine collection is started no sooner than the third day and assayed for urine aldosterone, sodium, and creatinine. Urine aldosterone excretion >12 to 14 mcg per 24 hours confirms nonsuppressibility of aldosterone. Adequacy of sodium loading is documented by urinary excretion of sodium >200 mEq/day.[4]

| TABLE 13-2 | DIFFERENTIAL DIAGNOSIS FOR HYPERTENSION AND HYPOKALEMIA | | |

↑ PAC and ↓ PRA	↑ PRA and ↑ PAC	↓ PRA and ↓ PAC
Primary aldosteronism	**Secondary aldosteronism**	**Mineralocorticoid excess states**
Aldosterone-producing adrenal adenomas	Renal artery stenosis	17-α-hydroxylase deficiency
Idiopathic hyperaldosteronism	Renin-secreting tumor	17-, 20-hydroxlyase deficiency
Glucocorticoid-remediable aldosteronism	Malignant hypertension	11-β-hydroxylase deficiency
Primary adrenal hyperplasia	Chronic renal disease	Deoxycorticosterone-secreting tumors
	Aortic coarctation	
	Aortic stenosis	

PAC, plasma aldosterone concentration; PRA, plasma renin activity.

○ **Intravenous sodium loading test**

Two liters of normal saline are infused intravenously over 4 hours into the recumbent patient. Potassium repletion should be confirmed before but does not need to be monitored during saline infusion. A PAC >10 ng/dL at 4 hours confirms and a PAC <5 ng/dL refutes the diagnosis of primary aldosteronism. A PAC between 5 ng/dL and 10 ng/dL is considered a "grey zone."[4]

○ **Alternate tests**

The protocols for alternate tests including the fludrocortisone suppression test and captopril challenge test are detailed elsewhere.[4] The use of the fludrocortisone suppression test is limited by the need for inpatient admission for monitoring purposes. The captopril suppression test is an acceptable but less standardized alternative if sodium loading is contraindicated as in heart or renal failure.

Imaging and Diagnostic Procedures

Localization of aldosterone production is essential to direct therapy in patients with primary aldosteronism who desire a surgical cure, because only patients with unilateral disease are likely to derive benefit from surgery. As a rule, imaging is not a reliable way to distinguish unilateral from bilateral disease but should be performed to identify tumors likely to be malignant. Adrenal vein sampling (AVS) remains the localization procedure of choice for patients seeking a surgical cure.

• **Adrenal imaging**

A computed tomography (CT) of the adrenal glands should be performed to identify adrenocortical carcinoma, which tends to be large (>4 cm) and has a characteristic CT appearance. A magnetic resonance imaging (MRI) study can be substituted if CT is contraindicated. Imaging should not be used alone to localize aldosterone production because it cannot reliably distinguish between a unilateral and a bilateral source. For example, IHA and a nonfunctioning adrenal incidentaloma may coexist. In these cases, a unilateral adrenal mass would be detected on imaging, but the source of aldosterone excess would be bilateral. Conversely, APAs may be too small to be detected by CT. In that situation, the presence of "normal" adrenal glands might incorrectly imply a bilateral source of aldosterone excess. Concordance between CT and AVS is only approximately 50%.[6,7]

• **Adrenal vein sampling**

AVS is expensive, invasive, and technically difficult, but is 95% sensitive and 100% specific for detection of unilateral disease.[6] Almost all patients will require AVS to localize the source of aldosterone excess. Patients with GRA are an exception to this rule since their disease is always bilateral. Some groups also make an exception for patients younger than age 40 with a solitary unilateral adenoma because nonfunctioning adenomas are less common in this age group.[6,8] AVS involves catheterization of the bilateral adrenal veins. A continuous cosyntropin infusion (50 mcg/hour) may be begun 30 minutes before catheterization and continued throughout the procedure. The infusion stimulates aldosterone production, thereby minimizing the effect of stress-induced fluctuations on aldosterone production, avoiding the problem of sampling when an APA might be hormonally silent, and maximizing the cortisol gradient between the adrenal vein and vena cava, which is used to confirm successful placement of the catheter. Blood samples from bilateral adrenal veins and a single peripheral vein are then obtained for the measurement of plasma aldosterone and cortisol. Right and left adrenal aldosterone concentrations should be divided by their respective cortisol concentrations to correct for dilutional effects. The right and left cortisol corrected aldosterone levels can then be compared.

A lateralization ratio of more than 4:1 is indicative of unilateral aldosterone excess. A ratio of <3:1 suggests a bilateral source. A ratio between 3:1 and 4:1 is inconclusive. An adrenal/peripheral vein cortisol ratio of 10:1 confirms successful adrenal vein catheterization.

- **Other tests**
  Other ancillary tests can be used in cases where AVS is unsuccessful, though none have been validated. As such, many clinicians avoid them altogether and instead repeat AVS or decide between surgical and medical therapy on the basis of clinical evidence or imaging. The postural stimulation test (in which a paradoxical fall in PAC occurs from a supine 8 AM sample to a sample obtained after 4 hours of upright posture in the presence of an APA) is used rarely. Adrenal scintigraphy with a ^{131}I-labeled cholesterol analog and measurement of plasma 18-hydroxycorticosterone levels are no longer used in most centers.

TREATMENT

Surgical resection is the treatment of choice for unilateral disease. Medical therapy is the treatment of choice for bilateral disease or for patients with unilateral disease who are poor surgical candidates.

Medications

- **Spironolactone** (12.5–400 mg orally daily) is the primary mineralocorticoid receptor antagonist used in the treatment of primary aldosteronism. Although doses up to 400 mg daily have traditionally been used, recent guidelines suggest a maximum dose of 100 mg.[4] Spironolactone is rapidly effective in correcting hypokalemia, but its antihypertensive effects may not be apparent for several weeks. Antiandrogenic side effects, including gynecomastia, erectile dysfunction, impotence, and decreased libido in men and menstrual irregularities in women, limit its tolerability.
- **Eplerenone** (25–50 mg orally twice daily) is a new highly selective mineralocorticoid receptor antagonist currently approved for treatment of essential hypertension. It has 60% of the potency of spironolactone but has fewer side effects due to its extremely low binding affinity for both the androgen and progesterone receptors. The improved tolerability of eplerenone needs to be weighed against its greater cost and the lack of clinical trials thus far supporting its use in primary aldosteronism.
- **Amiloride** (5–20 mg orally daily) and **triamterene** (100–150 mg orally twice daily) are potassium-sparing diuretics that block the aldosterone-sensitive sodium channel in the collecting tubules. They are less efficacious than the mineralocorticoid receptor antagonists but can be considered as adjunct therapy or as monotherapy if other agents are poorly tolerated. Since these agents do not block the aldosterone receptor itself, they do not prevent the deleterious effects of aldosterone on the cardiovascular system. Side effects include dizziness, fatigue, and nausea.
- **Dexamethasone** (0.125 mg orally at bedtime, titrated as needed) and **prednisone** (2.5 mg orally at bedtime, titrated as needed) are the glucocorticoids of choice in the treatment of GRA and work by partially suppressing ACTH secretion by the pituitary. They should not be used for treatment of primary aldosteronism due to other causes. Dexamethasone and prednisone are preferable to hydrocortisone due to their longer half lives and should be given at bedtime to suppress the early morning ACTH surge. The lowest effective dose should be used to minimize risk for iatrogenic Cushing's syndrome. Treatment with a glucocorticoid alone may not be

sufficient to normalize blood pressure and the addition of a mineralocorticoid receptor antagonist may be required.

- Other antihypertensive agents may need to be used in combination with a mineralocorticoid receptor antagonist if blood pressure remains uncontrolled.

Surgical Management

- Laparoscopic total adrenalectomy performed by an experienced surgeon is the treatment of choice for unilateral disease because it may eliminate the need for antihypertensive medication, reduce the number of antihypertensives needed, and correct endogenous aldosterone overproduction. Laparoscopic adrenalectomy is associated with shorter hospital stays and lower morbidity than an open approach. Partial adrenalectomy should not be performed because AVS cannot determine whether a single APA or unilateral hyperplasia is the cause of aldosterone excess.
- Preoperative management goals are adequate blood pressure control and correction of hypokalemia. Typically, an aldosterone receptor antagonist is recommended prior to surgery.
- Postoperative management can be guided by PAC, which should be measured to confirm surgical cure shortly after surgery. Serum potassium should be followed, as hypokalemia corrects quickly after adrenalectomy, and supplements should be discontinued. Mineralocorticoid antagonists should be discontinued and other antihypertensive therapy reduced as tolerated based on blood pressure. Maximum improvement in blood pressure is usually achieved in the first 6 months after surgery, but blood pressure can continue to fall for up to 1 year.[4] Since aldosterone production in the remaining adrenal gland can initially be suppressed, a sodium-rich diet and weekly monitoring of serum potassium levels are recommended for the first month after surgery.

COMPLICATIONS

Studies have indicated that long-term exposure to aldosterone excess may lead to structural damage of both the cardiovascular system[9] and kidneys[10,11] that is independent of blood pressure. Patients with primary aldosteronism are not only at increased risk for surrogate endpoints such as left ventricular hypertrophy[12] and diastolic dysfunction,[13] but they are also at increased risk for hard cardiovascular endpoints[14] as compared to patients with essential hypertension. Aldosterone has also been implicated in the development of endothelial dysfunction[15] and arterial stiffness.[16] Glomerular filtration rate and urinary albumin excretion are both higher in patients with primary aldosteronism than in patients with essential hypertension, and long-term follow-up of these patients suggests that these parameters are reversible with appropriate treatment of the aldosterone excess.[17]

OUTCOME/PROGNOSIS

- Although blood pressure improves and serum potassium levels normalize in most patients with surgically treated primary aldosteronism, the presence of preexisting essential hypertension, end-organ damage, changes in vascular tone, or nephrosclerosis may contribute to postoperative hypertension, which persists in between 40% and 70% of patients despite complete correction of the hyperaldosteronism.[18–20]

- Factors that predict an increased chance for surgical cure include the following: presence of an APA, preoperative response to spironolactone, younger age (<44 years), shorter duration of hypertension (<5 years), preoperative use of fewer anti-hypertensives (≤2 agents), higher preoperative ARR, and a family history of hypertension in no more than one first-degree relative.[19,20]
- Clinical trial evidence as to whether treatment of aldosterone excess in primary aldosteronism reduces morbidity and/or mortality is not currently available.

REFERENCES

1. Mulatero P, Stowasser M, Loh KC, et al. Increased diagnosis of primary aldosteronism, including surgically correctable forms, in centers from five continents. *J Clin Endocrinol Metab* 2004;89(3):1045–1050.
2. Kono T, Ikeda F, Oseko F, et al. Normotensive primary aldosteronism: Report of a case. *J Clin Endocrinol Metab* 1981;52(5):1009–1013.
3. Rossi GP, Bernini G, Caliumi C, et al. A prospective study of the prevalence of primary aldosteronism in 1,125 hypertensive patients. *J Am Coll Cardiol* 2006;48(11):2293–300.
4. Funder JW, Carey RM, Fardella C, et al. Case detection, diagnosis, and treatment of patients with primary aldosteronism: An endocrine society clinical practice guideline. *J Clin Endocrinol Metab* 2008;93(9):3266–3281.
5. Weinberger MH, Fineberg NS. The diagnosis of primary aldosteronism and separation of two major subtypes. *Arch Intern Med* 1993;153(18):2125–2129.
6. Young WF, Stanson AW, Thompson GB, et al. Role for adrenal venous sampling in primary aldosteronism. *Surgery* 2004;136(6):1227–1235.
7. Nwariaku FE, Miller BS, Auchus R, et al. Primary hyperaldosteronism: Effect of adrenal vein sampling on surgical outcome. *Arch Surg* 2006;141(5):497–502; discussion 02–3.
8. Tan YY, Ogilvie JB, Triponez F, et al. Selective use of adrenal venous sampling in the lateralization of aldosterone-producing adenomas. *World J Surg* 2006;30(5):879–885; discussion 86–87.
9. Rocha R, Funder JW. The pathophysiology of aldosterone in the cardiovascular system. *Ann N Y Acad Sci* 2002;970:89–100.
10. Greene EL, Kren S, Hostetter TH. Role of aldosterone in the remnant kidney model in the rat. *J Clin Invest* 1996;98(4):1063–1068.
11. Hollenberg NK. Aldosterone in the development and progression of renal injury. *Kidney Int* 2004;66(1):1–9.
12. Rossi GP, Sacchetto A, Visentin P, et al. Changes in left ventricular anatomy and function in hypertension and primary aldosteronism. *Hypertension* 1996;27(5):1039–1045.
13. Rossi GP, Sacchetto A, Pavan E, et al. Remodeling of the left ventricle in primary aldosteronism due to Conn's adenoma. *Circulation* 1997;95(6):1471–1478.
14. Milliez P, Girerd X, Plouin PF, et al. Evidence for an increased rate of cardiovascular events in patients with primary aldosteronism. *J Am Coll Cardiol* 2005;45(8):1243–1248.
15. Taddei S, Virdis A, Mattei P, et al. Vasodilation to acetylcholine in primary and secondary forms of human hypertension. *Hypertension* 1993;21(6 Pt 2):929–933.
16. Blacher J, Amah G, Girerd X, et al. Association between increased plasma levels of aldosterone and decreased systemic arterial compliance in subjects with essential hypertension. *Am J Hypertens* 1997;10(12 Pt 1):1326–1334.
17. Sechi LA, Novello M, Lapenna R, et al. Long-term renal outcomes in patients with primary aldosteronism. *JAMA* 2006;295(22):2638–2645.
18. Meyer A, Brabant G, Behrend M. Long-term follow-up after adrenalectomy for primary aldosteronism. *World J Surg* 2005;29(2):155–159.
19. Celen O, O'Brien MJ, Melby JC, et al. Factors influencing outcome of surgery for primary aldosteronism. *Arch Surg* 1996;131(6):646–650.
20. Sawka AM, Young WF, Thompson GB, et al. Primary aldosteronism: Factors associated with normalization of blood pressure after surgery. *Ann Intern Med* 2001;135(4):258–261.

Cushing's Syndrome

14

Scott Goodwin and Julie Silverstein

GENERAL PRINCIPLES

Definition
- Cushing's syndrome is a clinical condition resulting from prolonged exposure to excessive glucocorticoids from either endogenous or exogenous sources.
- The most common cause of Cushing's syndrome is from the administration of exogenous glucocorticoids.

Classification
Cushing's syndrome can be divided into two categories based on pathophysiology: ACTH-dependent or ACTH-independent (see Table 14-1).
- **ACTH-dependent** hypercortisolism is the most common cause of endogenous Cushing's syndrome and may be due to an ACTH-secreting pituitary tumor, an ectopic ACTH syndrome, or an ectopic-corticotropin-releasing hormone (CRH) syndrome.
  - When Cushing's syndrome is secondary to an ACTH-secreting pituitary adenoma, it is called **Cushing's disease**, which was originally described by Harvey Cushing in 1932.[1] ACTH secretion from the pituitary adenoma stimulates the over-production of glucocorticoids from the adrenal glands.
  - Ectopic-ACTH syndromes lead to bilateral adrenocortical hyperplasia and hyperfunction. Small cell carcinoma of the lung is the most common cause of ectopic ACTH secretion.
  - In ectopic CRH syndrome, CRH secretion by the primary tumor causes hyperplasia of pituitary corticotrophs, consequent hypersecretion of ACTH, bilateral adrenal hyperplasia, and finally cortisol hypersecretion.[2] It is extremely rare.
- **ACTH-independent** forms of Cushing's syndrome are due to exogenous glucocorticoids or primary adrenal disorders. Examples include adrenal adenomas, carcinomas, and nodular adrenal hyperplasias.

Epidemiology
Cushing's syndrome is exceedingly rare with an annual incidence of only 0.7 to 2.4 per million and is slightly more common in women than men.[1]

Associated Conditions
- **Carney's complex** is an autosomal-dominant syndrome characterized by micronodular adrenal hyperplasia and pituitary adenomas, testicular and thyroid tumors, cardiac atrial myxomas, pigmented lentigines, blue nevi, and schwannomas.
- **McCune–Albright syndrome** is characterized by hypercortisolism from hyperplastic adrenal macronodules, as well as café-au-lait spots and polyostotic fibrous dysplasia.[2,3]

98

TABLE 14-1	CAUSES OF CUSHING'S SYNDROME
Diagnosis	**% of Patients**
ACTH-dependent	
Cushing's disease (pituitary hypersecretion of ACTH)	70
Ectopic ACTH syndrome (nonpituitary tumors)	10
Ectopic CRH syndrome (nonhypothalamic tumors causing pituitary hypersecretion of ACTH)	<1
ACTH-independent	
Adrenal adenoma	10
Adrenal carcinoma	5
Micronodular hyperplasia	1
Macronodular hyperplasia	<2
Pseudo-Cushing's syndrome	
Major-depressive disorder	1
Alcoholism	<1

Adapted from Aron DC, Findling JW, Tyrrell JB. Glucocorticoids & adrenal androgens. In: Gardner DG, Shoback D, eds. *Greenspan's Basic and Clinical Endocrinology.* 8th ed. New York, NY: McGraw-Hill Companies, 2007:346–395.

DIAGNOSIS

Clinical Presentation

- Patients present with a wide spectrum of manifestations ranging from subclinical to overt symptoms, depending on the underlying etiology, and the duration and intensity of excess glucocorticoid production.
- The signs and symptoms of this syndrome are often nonspecific and there are inherent limitations in the diagnostic testing, making the diagnosis of Cushing's syndrome one of the most challenging in endocrinology.
- Some of the findings suggestive of Cushing's syndrome are presented below (also see Table 14-2). However, it is important to note that none of them are truly pathognomonic of the syndrome, requiring a high degree of clinical suspicion to diagnose Cushing's syndrome.[1,2]
  - **Progressive central obesity** involving the abdomen, face, and neck (buffalo hump, moon facies, supraclavicular fat pads, and exophthalmos from retroorbital fat deposition).
  - **Metabolic complications** include glucose intolerance (owing to stimulation of gluconeogenesis by cortisol and peripheral insulin resistance caused by obesity), and hypertension (through poorly understood multifactorial etiologies), both of which confer increased cardiovascular risk, a major cause of morbidity and death in patients with Cushing's syndrome.[1] Severe hypertension and hypokalemia are more commonly seen in patients with ectopic ACTH syndrome because the very high serum cortisol levels overwhelm the capacity of the 11-β-hydroxysteroid dehydrogenase type 2 enzyme, which oxidizes cortisol to inactive cortisone in renal tubules, thereby resulting in activation of mineralocorticoid receptors.[2]

TABLE 14-2	SYMPTOMS AND SIGNS IN PATIENTS WITH CUSHING'S SYNDROME	
Sign/symptom	**% of Patients**	
Truncal obesity	95	
Facial fullness	90	
Gonadal dysfunction (decreased libido)	90	
Skin atrophy and bruising	80	
Menstrual irregularity	80	
Hypertension	75	
Hirsutism, acne	75	
Mood disorders	70	
Muscle weakness	65	
Diabetes or glucose intolerance	60	
Osteopenia, osteoporosis, fractures	50	

Adapted from Newell-Price J, Bertagna X, Grossman AB, et al. Cushing's syndrome. *Lancet* 2006;367:1605–1617; Newell-Price J, Bertagna X, Grossman AB, et al. Cushing's syndrome. *Lancet* 2006;367:1605–1617.

○ **Dermatologic manifestations** include skin atrophy (thinning of the stratum corneum), fragile skin with easy bruisability, wide purple striae (due to the stretching of fragile skin), cutaneous fungal infections, and hyperpigmentation (in ectopic ACTH syndrome).

○ **Reproductive changes** include menstrual irregularities, hirsutism, oily facial skin with acne, and other signs of virilization (temporal balding, deepening voice), especially in women with adrenal carcinoma.

○ **Musculoskeletal manifestations** are proximal myopathy, muscle wasting (resulting from the catabolic effects of excess glucocorticoid on skeletal muscle), and osteoporosis (caused by decreased bone formation, increased bone resorption, and decreased intestinal and renal calcium reabsorption). Vertebral compression fractures, pathologic fractures of the rib or long bones, and aseptic necrosis of the femoral heads may also be present.

○ **Neuropsychiatric changes** can include labile mood, agitated depression, anxiety, panic attacks, mild paranoia, impaired short-term memory and cognition, and insomnia.

Differential Diagnosis

• **Pseudo-Cushing's syndrome** is characterized by mild hypercortisolism and may be difficult to distinguish from true Cushing's syndrome.

○ Causes include depression, alcoholism, medications, obesity, psychiatric illness, stress/trauma/acute illness, and states of elevated cortisol-binding protein (pregnancy, estrogen therapy).[4,5]

○ The distinguishing feature of this disorder is that the laboratory and clinical findings of hypercortisolism disappear if the primary process is successfully treated.[4,5]

• The metabolic syndrome which is characterized by central obesity, hypertension, and glucose intolerance may mimic Cushing's syndrome.

• The polycystic ovarian syndrome may present with menstrual irregularities and hyperandrogenism (hirsutism, acne) which can be features of Cushing's syndrome.

Diagnostic Testing

- The biochemical diagnosis of Cushing's syndrome involves **three critical steps**:
  - (1) Documenting the presence of hypercortisolism (Does the patient have Cushing's syndrome?)
  - (2) Determining if the cortisol excess is ACTH-independent or ACTH-dependent (Does the patient have primary adrenal disease or an ACTH-secreting tumor?)
  - (3) Determining the source of the ACTH in the ACTH-dependent form (Does the patient have Cushing's disease or ectopic ACTH syndrome?)
- *Does the patient have Cushing's syndrome?*
  - The **24 hour urine free cortisol** measurement is one of the most frequently utilized tests for the diagnosis of Cushing's syndrome. The patient can be assumed to have Cushing's syndrome if basal urinary cortisol excretion is 3 to 4 times higher than the normal range on at least two separate occasions. The evaluation can then proceed to the next step of establishing the cause for the hypercortisolism. If it is equivocally increased—that is, above the upper limit of normal, but not quite 3 to 4 times as much—the patient needs to be reevaluated after several weeks or undergo further testing (see subsequent text and Table 14-3).[6–8]
  - The **1 mg overnight dexamethasone suppression test** is another commonly used screening test. Unfortunately, this test is associated with a high false-positive rate (Table 14-4) and it should not be used as the sole criterion for making the diagnosis of Cushing's syndrome. Some authors suggest obtaining a dexamethasone level at the same time as cortisol. A low dexamethasone level suggests noncompliance, individual variation in dexamethasone metabolism, or drug effects on dexamethasone metabolism.[6–8]
  - Some endocrinologists prefer to use the 48 hour, 2 mg/day **low-dose dexamethasone suppression test** (LDDST) as a screening test in patients who have conditions associated with overactivation of the HPA axis (e.g., in patients with certain psychiatric conditions, obesity, alcoholism, or diabetes mellitus) because in some studies it has been shown to have a higher specificity than the 1 mg test.[6]
  - The **late evening salivary cortisol** is another validated screening test with distinct advantages: it is noninvasive, saliva is easily collected, cortisol is stable in saliva even at room temperature for several days, and it can be performed by the patient at home.[6,9]
  - The **CRH after-dexamethasone test** may be useful to differentiate patients with Cushing's from those with pseudo-Cushing's syndrome. Compared to patients with Cushing's syndrome, depressed patients continue to show a suppressed plasma cortisol (<1.4 mcg/dL) even after CRH infusion, which reflects preserved sensitivity of ACTH secretion to dexamethasone suppression.[6]
- **Does the patient have ACTH-independent or ACTH-dependent Cushing's syndrome?**
  - This question can be answered by measuring **plasma ACTH levels and basal serum cortisol.**[1,6]
  - Undetectable or low levels of ACTH (<5 pg/dL) in a patient with a serum cortisol concentration >15 mcg/dL characterizes a primary adrenal source (ACTH-independent Cushing's syndrome). If ACTH-independent Cushing's syndrome is suspected, thin-section computed tomography (CT) or magnetic resonance imaging (MRI) of the adrenal glands looking for an adrenal mass is indicated.
  - ACTH levels >15 pg/dL typically indicate an ACTH-dependent cause, and the next step involves a search for the source of the high ACTH (pituitary vs. nonpituitary).

TABLE 14-3 BIOCHEMICAL TESTS FOR ESTABLISHING HYPERCORTISOLISM

Test	Protocol	Measurements	Interpretation	Sensitivity (%)	Specificity (%)
1 mg overnight DST 24-Hour UFC	Dex, 1 mg PO at 11 PM 24 hour urine collection	8 AM plasma cortisol Cortisol, creatinine	Normal, <1.8 mcg/dL Values 3- to 4-fold higher than the upper limit of normal suggest Cushing's syndrome	98 95–100	70–80 98
2-Day LDDST (urine)	Dex, 0.5 mg PO q6h for 48 hrs (last dose 6 AM)	24 hour urine for cortisol, creatinine during last 24 hour of dex administration.	UFC >36 mcg/day suggests Cushing's syndrome	56–69	74–100
2-Day LDDST (serum)	Dex, 0.5 mg PO q6h for 48 hours (last dose 6 AM)	Plasma cortisol 2 hours after last dose of dex	Normal <1.8 mcg/dL	>95%	>95%
CRH/dex	Same as LDDST with first dose dex given at noon; CRH, 1 mcg/kg IV at 8 AM after last dose of dex	Plasma cortisol 15 min after CRH injection	Cortisol >1.4 mcg/dL suggests Cushing's syndrome	100	100
Late-evening salivary cortisol	11 PM sample	Salivary cortisol	Value <1.45 ng/mL excludes Cushing's syndrome	92–100	93–100
Midnight plasma cortisol	Indwelling catheter and hospitalization recommended	Midnight plasma cortisol	Cortisol >7.5 mcg/dL if awake or >1.8 mcg/dL if sleeping, suggests Cushing's syndrome	83–96	96–100

CRH, corticotrophin-releasing hormone; UFC, urine free cortisol; dex, dexamethasone; DST, dexamethasone suppression test; LDDST, low-dose dexamethasone suppression test.

TABLE 14-4	CAUSES OF FALSE-POSITIVE AND FALSE-NEGATIVE BIOCHEMICAL TESTS FOR CUSHING'S SYNDROME	
Test	**False-positive**	**False-negative**
1 mg overnight DST; 2-day LDDST	Error with timing of dex administration Meds increasing metabolism of dex Decreased absorption of dex Hypercortisolemia without Cushing's syndrome Pseudo-Cushing's syndrome	Chronic renal failure (GFR <30 mL/min) Increased sensitivity of the HPA axis to dex
24-hour UFC	High fluid intake Interference with carbamazepine in the HPLC assay Hypercortisolemia without Cushing's syndrome Pseudo-Cushing's syndrome	Cyclic Cushing's Early Cushing's Chronic renal failure Interference with fibrate-class of drugs
Midnight plasma cortisol; Late-evening salivary cortisol	Stress from hospitalization or blood draw Critically ill patients Patients with depression Brushing teeth before obtaining sample Touching swab with hands	Cyclic Cushing's

dex, dexamethasone; UFC, urine free cortisol; DST, dexamethasone suppression test; LDDST, low-dose dexamethasone suppression test; HPLC, high-performance liquid chromatography.

Adapted from Biller BMK, Grosman AB, Stewart PM, et al. Treatment of ACTH-dependent Cushing's syndrome: A consensus statement. *J Clin Endocrin Metab* 2008;2007–2734; Nieman LK, Biller BMK, Findling JW, et al. The dianosis of Cushing's syndrome: An endocrine society clinical practice guideline. *J Clin Endocrinol Metab* 2008;93:1526–1540.

○ An ACTH level in the 5 to 15 pg/dL range is considered indeterminate and should be repeated. If the ACTH level remains consistently in the indeterminate range, a **CRH-stimulation test** can be performed. After CRH infusion, if the peak ACTH response is blunted (<10 pg/dL), an ACTH-independent (adrenal) cause is likely. However, if there is >50% increase in mean plasma cortisol from baseline after CRH infusion, an ACTH-dependent cause is then more likely.

• **Does the patient have Cushing's disease or ectopic ACTH syndrome?**
  ○ There can be considerable overlap in ACTH levels between patients with Cushing's disease and ectopic ACTH syndrome, but the distinction between the two is critical as it significantly influences treatment. Several tests can be utilized to aid in the differentiation between pituitary Cushing's disease and nonpituitary (ectopic) ACTH syndrome (see Table 14-5).

TABLE 14-5	TESTS TO DIFFERENTIATE CUSHING'S DISEASE FROM ECTOPIC ACTH SYNDROME			
Test	Protocol	Interpretation	Sensitivity (%)	Specificity (%)
2-day HDDST	Collect 24 hour urine for UFC, creatinine; give dex, 2 mg PO q6h for 48 hours; re-collect urine during last 24 hours of dex administration	Suppression of UFC >90% compared to baseline suggests Cushing's disease	83	100
8 mg overnight dex	Measure plasma cortisol at 8 AM; give dex, 8 mg p.o. at 11 PM; re-draw blood for plasma cortisol next morning at 8 AM	Suppression of plasma cortisol by >50% compared to baseline suggests Cushing's disease	92	100
CRH	Place an indwelling venous catheter 2 hours prior to testing. Give CRH 1 mcg/kg i.v. bolus at 8 AM; draw plasma ACTH at −5, −1 minute before CRH and +15, +30 minutes after CRH	Increase of ACTH (mean of +15 and +30 minute values) by 35% greater than baseline (mean of −5 and −1 minute) suggests Cushing's disease	93	100
IPSS	Simultaneous bilateral inferior petrosal sinus sampling and peripheral sampling for ACTH before and after CRH, 100 mcg i.v.	Basal petrosal: peripheral ACTH ratio ≥2 or post-CRH petrosal: peripheral ACTH ratio ≥3 suggests Cushing's disease	97–100	100

ACTH, adrenocorticotropic hormone; CRH, corticotrophin-releasing hormone; dex, dexamethasone; HDDST, high-dose dexamethasone suppression test; IPSS, inferior petrosal sinus sampling; UFC, urine free cortisol.

Adapted from Biller BMK, Grosman AB, Stewart PM, et al. Treatment of ACTH-dependent Cushing's syndrome: A consensus statement. *J Clin Endocrin Metab* 2008;2007–2734; Nieman LK, Biller BMK, Findling JW, et al. The dianosis of Cushing's syndrome: An endocrine society clinical practice guideline. *J Clin Endocrinol Metab* 2008;93:1526–1540.

○ **The high-dose dexamethasone suppression test (HDDST)** takes advantage of the fact that high doses of glucocorticoids partially suppress ACTH secretion from most corticotroph pituitary adenomas whereas most non-pituitary tumors associated with ectopic ACTH are resistant to feedback inhibition (exceptions include carcinoid tumors of the bronchus, thymus, and pancreas). The high-dose test can be administered as a standard 2-day test (2 mg, every 6 hours × 8 doses) or as a single overnight 8 mg dose (see Table 14-5). If the urine free cortisol suppresses >90%, or the plasma cortisol suppresses >50% from baseline, Cushing's disease is most likely. An MRI of the pituitary gland should be obtained next.[1,6]

○ **Inferior petrosal sinus sampling (IPSS)** is an invasive procedure that involves measuring the central-to-peripheral ACTH gradient and may be useful when the source of ACTH production (i.e., pituitary vs. ectopic) remains elusive despite other non-invasive testing (i.e., when there is cortisol suppression on HDDST [suggesting Cushing's disease] in the setting of a negative pituitary MRI). See Table 14-5 for more details.[1,2]

○ **[111]In-octreotide** or **pentetreotide scintigraphy** can detect some ectopic ACTH-secreting tumors, although neither is specific for ACTH-secreting tumors.

TREATMENT

• Treatment is based on the source of the hypercortisolism, so the need for an accurate diagnosis cannot be overemphasized. The goal of treatment is to reverse the clinical manifestations of hypercortisolemia by decreasing cortisol secretion to normal levels.

• In **exogenous Cushing's syndrome**, gradual withdrawal of the glucocorticoid is important because most patients on long-term therapy will have some degree of HPA-axis suppression with resultant adrenal insufficiency if therapy is abruptly discontinued.

• In **ACTH-independent Cushing's syndrome**, adrenal imaging by either CT or MRI will demonstrate unilateral or bilateral disease. Patients should be referred for **adrenalectomy**. During and after unilateral adrenalectomy, patients should receive glucocorticoid replacement until the HPA axis recovers from the prolonged suppressive effects of glucocorticoid excess. Patients with bilateral adrenalectomy require lifelong glucocorticoid and mineralocorticoid replacement.[10,11]

• In **Cushing's disease**, a **transsphenoidal microadenectomy** is the treatment of choice for patients with a clearly circumscribed microadenoma. In other cases, subtotal resection of the anterior pituitary may be performed. Patients with incomplete resection of the tumor may undergo repeat surgery or pituitary irradiation with either conventional radiation or stereotactic radiation with the ^{60}Co gamma knife. Pituitary irradiation may not control the hypercortisolemia for months to years, and patients require medical therapy until the full effects of the radiation are seen. Surgical cure with transsphenoidal adenomectomy can be assessed on postoperative day 2 to 3 with morning cortisol and ACTH levels, which are undetectable with successful complete resection of the tumor. During and after transsphenoidal resection of the adenoma, patients require glucocorticoid replacement until recovery of the HPA axis.[11]

• **Ectopic ACTH–dependent Cushing's syndrome** should be confirmed with imaging studies, including CT, MRI, and/or scintigraphy. Tumors that can be localized by imaging studies should be removed surgically. If the source is an occult tumor or if there is metastatic disease, medical treatment is required. Bilateral adrenalectomy may be performed in refractory cases.[11]

Medications[1,10,11]

- **Ketoconazole** is an antifungal agent that inhibits 17 to 20 lyase, 11-β-hydroxylase, and cholesterol side-chain cleavage enzyme. It is usually the first-line medication. Its cortisol-reducing effects are dose-dependent and can be seen rapidly. The major side effect is liver toxicity. Other side effects include gynecomastia, impotence, and gastrointestinal symptoms. Doses range from 200 to 1200 mg orally daily in 2 to 3 divided doses.
- **Mitotane** inhibits cholesterol side-chain cleavage enzyme and 11-β-hydroxylase. Mitotane induces permanent destruction of adrenocortical cells and, therefore, can be used to achieve medical adrenalectomy as an alternative to surgical adrenalectomy. Glucocorticoid replacement is started at initiation of mitotane treatment. Mineralocorticoid treatment may eventually be required. Side effects are generally dose dependent and include gastrointestinal symptoms, weakness, lethargy, leukopenia, gynecomastia, and hypercholesterolemia. Doses start at 0.5 grams orally at bedtime and are increased slowly to 2 to 3 g/day in 3 to 4 divided doses for a total of 6 to 9 months.
- **Metyrapone** inhibits 11-β-hydroxylase. Major side effects include increased androgens, hypertension, and hypokalemia through increased 11-deoxycorticosterone. Doses range from 250 to 1000 mg orally, given every 6 hours. Lower doses of 500 to 750 mg orally daily can be used when given in combination with ketoconazole and/or aminoglutethimide.
- **Aminoglutethimide** is an anticonvulsant that inhibits the cholesterol side-chain cleavage enzyme. The usual dose is 250 mg 2 to 3 times a day. Side effects include gastrointestinal upset, lethargy, ataxia, hypothyroidism, headache, bone marrow suppression, and skin rash. It is not as effective for monotherapy as ketoconazole or metyrapone, and thus is frequently used in combination with other agents.
- Other agents with limited or modest anti-corticosteroid capabilities include Mifepristone (RU486), somatostatin receptor ligands (Octreotide, Lanreotide, Pasireotide), Etomidate, and dopamine receptor agonists (Bromocriptine or Cabergoline).

SPECIAL CONSIDERATIONS

- **Nelson's syndrome** can occur in patients with Cushing's disease (pituitary adenoma) who have refractory disease and are treated with bilateral adrenalectomy. It results in enlargement of the pituitary and extreme elevations in serum ACTH levels. The patient develops hyperpigmentation associated with the high ACTH levels. Pituitary irradiation before bilateral adrenalectomy may prevent this syndrome.[11]
- There have been rare cases of Cushing's syndrome during pregnancy. **Pregnant patients** may be treated effectively with transsphenoidal surgery for Cushing's disease.[12] Bilateral adrenalectomy may also be performed. Metyrapone and aminoglutethimide may be used during pregnancy, but mitotane and ketoconazole, which are teratogenic, are contraindicated.[11]

PROGNOSIS

- Untreated Cushing's syndrome is often fatal, with most deaths resulting from cardiovascular/thromboembolic complications or bacterial/fungal infections. Effective therapy, either by surgical cure or by pharmacologic control of hypercortisolism, leads to gradual improvement in the symptoms and signs of Cushing's syndrome over a period of 2 to 12 months. Hypertension, glucose intolerance, osteoporosis, and psychiatric symptoms generally improve but may not resolve completely.[2,13]

- Cure rates after transsphenoidal surgery for Cushing's disease range from 80% to 90%, depending on the various criteria used to define a cure. Cure is likely if the patient develops hypocortisolism in the first few days to weeks after surgery. Postoperative random plasma cortisol levels of <2 mcg/dL have been used to designate remission and a low recurrence rate of approximately 10% in 10 years.[11] Remission is also achieved in an additional 45% to 80% of patients undergoing pituitary irradiation after unsuccessful pituitary surgery.[11] Most patients are rendered hypoadrenal for months to years after the procedure. During this period, they require glucocorticoid replacement therapy.

- The HPA axis must be evaluated 6 to 12 months after surgery to determine the potential need for lifetime exogenous steroid replacement therapy. Patients with panhypopituitarism subsequent to surgery require lifetime monitoring and titration of hormone replacement therapy.[11]

- Patients with adrenal adenomas and benign ACTH-secreting tumors that can be completely resected can be cured. However, patients with ectopic ACTH secretion or adrenocortical carcinoma may have a poor prognosis associated with the underlying malignancy. These patients are rarely cured, but the hypercortisolemia can be controlled with medications or bilateral adrenalectomy.[13]

REFERENCES

1. Pivonello R, DeMartino MC, DeLeo M, et al. Cushings syndrome. *Endocrinol Metab Clin N Am* 2008;37:135–149.
2. Aron DC, Findling JW, Tyrrell JB. Glucocorticoids & adrenal androgens. In: Gardner DG, Shoback D, eds. *Greenspan's Basic and Clinical Endocrinology.* 8th ed. New York, NY: McGraw-Hill Companies, 2007:346–395.
3. Biller BMK, Grosman AB, Stewart PM, et al. Treatment of ACTH-dependent Cushing's syndrome: A consensus statement. *J Clin Endocrin Metab* 2008;2007–2734.
4. Newell-Price J, Bertagna X, Grossman AB, et al. Cushing's syndrome. *Lancet* 2006;367: 1605–1617.
5. Yanovski JA, Cutler GB Jr, Chrousos GP, et al. ACTH-releasing hormone stimulation following low-dose dexamethasone administration: A new test to distinguish Cushing's syndrome from pseudo-Cushing's states. *JAMA* 1993;269:2232–2238.
6. Nieman LK, Biller BMK, Findling JW, et al. The dianosis of Cushing's syndrome: An endocrine society clinical practice guideline. *J Clin Endocrinol Metab* 2008;93:1526–1540.
7. Giraldi FP, Ambrogio AG, DeMartin M, et al. Specificity of first-line tests for the diagnosis of Cusings syndrome: Assessment in a large series. *J Clin Endocrinol Metab* 2007;92:4123–4129.
8. Elmamin MB, Murad MH, Mullan R, et al. Accuracy of diagnostic tests for Cushing's syndrome: A systemic review and metaanalyses. *J Clin Endocrinol Met* 2008;93:1553–1562.
9. Kirk LF, Hash RB, Katner HP, et al. Cushing's disease: Clinical manifestations and diagnostic evaluation. *Am Fam Physician* 2000;62:1119–1127.
10. Gross BA, Mindea SA, Pick AJ, et al. Medical management of Cushing disease. *Neurogurg Focus* 2007;23:1–6.
11. Aron DC, Schnall AM, Sheeler LR. Cushing's syndrome and pregnancy. *Am J Obstet Gynecol* 1990;162:244–252.
12. Sonino N, Zielezny M, Fava GA, et al. Risk factors and long-term outcome in pituitary-dependent Cushing's disease. *J Clin Endocrinol Metab* 1996;81:2647–2652.
13. Fassnacht M, Eder M, Allolio B. Clincal management of adrenocortical carcinoma. *Best practice & research clinical endocrinology & metabolism* 2009:23;273–289.

Pheochromocytoma

Prajesh M. Joshi and Simon J. Fisher

15

GENERAL PRINCIPLES

- Pheochromocytoma refers to a tumor arising from catecholamine-producing chromaffin cells in the adrenal medulla. Similar catecholamine-producing tumors that occur within sympathetic and parasympathetic ganglia are classified as extraadrenal paragangliomas.
- Although adrenal and extraadrenal tumors can present in a similar fashion, it is important to differentiate between them not only for anatomical and surgical reasons, but also because they have distinct characteristics such as association with malignancy and genetic predisposition to various syndromes.
- The term *pheochromocytoma* comes from the Greek words *phaios,* meaning "dusky," and *chromo,* meaning "color." The first description of a pheochromocytoma is credited to Frankel, who reported finding bilateral adrenal tumors on autopsy in an 18-year-old woman in 1886.
- For educational purposes, the "rule of tens" has historically been used to describe pheochromocytoma as being 10% malignant, 10% extraadrenal, 10% familial, and 10% in children. However, with enhanced detection capabilities and genetic screening, emerging evidence has made many changes to this "rule."

Definition

- Pheochromocytomas are neuroendocrine tumors arising from catecholamine-producing chromaffin cells of the adrenal medulla.[1]
- Tumors arising from extraadrenal chromaffin tissue (sympathetic or parasympathetic paraganglioma) are referred to as extraadrenal paragangliomas.[2]
- Extraadrenal pheochromocytomas are most commonly located in the carotid body of the head and neck, in the mediastinum (1%), close to the inferior vena cava and abdominal aorta alongside the sympathetic ganglia, in the organ of Zuckerkandl (7% to 10%), and near the urinary bladder.[3,4]

Classification

- Pheochromocytomas can be classified into adrenal (90%) and extraadrenal tumors (9% to 23%).[5,6]
- Adrenal tumors are usually benign and secrete both epinephrine and norepinephrine in at least half of all cases. Extraadrenal paragangliomas are either sympathetic, which secrete norepinephrine and/or dopamine and have a more aggressive, metastatic nature, or are parasympathetic, which are mostly silent tumors.
- Pheochromocytomas can also be classified as sporadic (solitary, unilateral, and intraadrenal tumors) or familial (also typically intraadrenal, but often multicentric and bilateral).

Epidemiology

- The prevalence of pheochromocytoma in patients with hypertension is 0.1% to 0.6%[7]
- Approximately 5% of all asymptomatic adrenal incidentalomas >1 cm in size are pheochromocytomas.[8]
- Most pheochromocytomas are sporadic, but up to 25% have been reported as hereditary.
- Its prevalence in MEN (multiple endocrine neoplasia) 2A syndrome presenting with medullary thyroid cancer is approximately 42%.[9]
- Prevalence of pheochromocytoma metastases is up to 5% in adrenal pheochromocytoma. The rate of metastases increases to 33% for extraadrenal tumors.

Etiology

- Pheochromocytomas can occur in the context of autosomal dominant hereditary syndromes. The hereditary basis for pheochromocytomas is more frequent than previously thought, with an estimated prevalence of 24%.[7]
- Germline mutations in various genes have been identified to be responsible for familial pheochromocytomas: *RET* proto-oncogenes in MEN 2; tumor suppressor genes such as *VHL* in von Hippel–Lindau syndrome and *NF1* in von Recklinghausen's disease; and genes encoding the B and D subunits of mitochondrial succinate dehydrogenase (*SDHB* and *SDHD*, respectively) in familial nonsyndromic paragangliomas and pheochromocytomas. Mutation of the succinate dehydrogenase subunit C has only been reported in parasympathetic paragangliomas thus far.[10] More recently, germline mutation of *FP/TMEM127* has been associated with pheochromocytoma but not paraganglioma.[11]

Pathophysiology

- Improved knowledge of catecholamine metabolism under normal and disease states associated with elevated catecholamine release provides better understanding of pheochromocytoma and the utility and limitations of biochemical tests for its diagnosis.
- Norepinephrine released from sympathetic nerves acts locally and is metabolized locally so that only a small proportion enters the bloodstream. In contrast, adrenomedullary cells secrete catecholamines directly into the bloodstream.
- Most of the norepinephrine produced and released by sympathetic nerves is metabolized within the nerves by monoamine oxidase (MAO) to dihydroxyphenylglycol (DHPG).
- Catechol-O-methyltransferase (COMT) in extraneuronal cells, such as smooth muscle cells or liver cells, metabolizes norepinephrine to normetanephrine (epinephrine to metanephrine), and DHPG formed in nerves is converted to 3-methoxy-4-hydroxy-phenylglycol (MHPG). Sympathetic nerves lack COMT.
- Vanillylmandelic acid (VMA), the major end product of norepinephrine and epinephrine metabolism, is produced almost exclusively from metabolism by the liver of circulating catecholamines and their metabolites. The majority of VMA is derived from circulating DHPG and MHPG, most of which is derived from neuronal norepinephrine metabolism, which explains why VMA is a relatively insensitive marker for pheochromocytoma.
- Approximately 90% of metanephrines and up to 40% of normetanephrines are formed from metabolism of epinephrine and norepinephrine within the adrenals before release into the circulation, making it the single largest source in the body.[12,13]

- Over 94% of elevated plasma normetaneprhines and metanephrines are derived from metabolism of catecholamines by COMT within the tumor cells independent of catecholamine release, which gives support to rationale for measuring metanephrines and normetanephrines in diagnosing pheochromocytoma.[14]

DIAGNOSIS

Clinical Presentation

History

- Patients with pheochromocytoma often experience a characteristic paroxysm or crises caused by the release of catecholamines.
- The **classic symptomatic triad** includes episodes of **headache, sweating,** and **palpitations.**[6] In the presence of hypertension, this triad is found to be 91% sensitive and 94% specific for pheochromocytoma (Table 15-1).[15]
- **Hypertension is the most common feature** and occurs in more than 90% of patients and is paroxysmal in 25% to 50%.[17]
- Headache may vary in duration and intensity and can occur in up to 80% to 90% of symptomatic patients, with palpitations occurring in 64%.[6] Generalized sweating is present in up to 57% of patients. **Other less frequent symptoms** include pallor, dyspnea, generalized weakness, blurry vision, panic attacks, weight loss, polyuria, polydipsia, constipation, and unexplained cardiopulmonary dysfunction.

TABLE 15-1	SYMPTOMS AND SIGNS IN PATIENTS WITH PHEOCHROMOCYTOMA[16]
Symptoms	**Signs**
Headache (80%)	Hypertension (often severe)
Sweating (71%)	Postural hypotension
Palpitations (64%)	Resting tachycardia
Pallor (42%)	Fever
Nausea (42%)	Perspiration
Tremor (31%)	Pallor (especially of the face and chest)
Weakness/fatigue (28%)	Tremor
Anxiety (22%)	Abdominal mass
Epigastric pain (22%)	Hypertension and paroxysmal symptoms after abdominal palpation
	Hypertensive retinopathy
	Retinal angiomas (von Hippel–Lindau syndrome)
	Hyperplastic corneal nerves (slit lamp exam, MEN2B)
	Marfanoid body habitus; mucosal neuromas (MEN2B)
	Thyroid nodule (MEN2A or 2B)
	Café-au-lait spots (neurofibromatosis)

Adapted from Thomas JE, Rooke ED, Kvale WF. The neurologist's experience with pheochromocytoma. A review of 100 cases. *JAMA* 1966;197:754–758.

- Patients with pheochromocytoma **may also be completely asymptomatic**. In a Mayo Clinic series of 150 patients, ~10% of patients with a pheochromocytoma were discovered incidentally on abdominal computerized technology (CT) scanning. Another series from the Cleveland Clinic of 33 patients showed that nearly 58% of patients diagnosed with adrenal pheochromocytoma were asymptomatic and their adrenal tumors were an incidental finding on imaging done for other reasons.[18] Therefore, the diagnosis of pheochromocytoma requires a high index of suspicion, especially in patients with one or more of the following:
  - ○ Refractory hypertension and/or onset of hypertension before 20 years of age;
  - ○ Non-exertional palpitations, spells, diaphoresis, headache, or tremor;
  - ○ Familial syndrome (e.g., MEN2, NF1, VHL) or a family history of pheochromocytoma;
  - ○ Incidental adrenal mass with imaging characteristics consistent with pheochromocytoma (marked enhancement on contrast CT or high-signal intensity on T2-weighted magnetic resonance imaging [MRI]);
  - ○ Hypertensive response during anesthesia and surgery;
  - ○ Idiopathic dilated cardiomyopathy.
- Paroxysms associated with pheochromocytoma may be precipitated by displacement of abdominal contents (e.g., lifting or palpation). Typically, paroxysms last 30 to 40 minutes and occur with sufficient frequency for an event to be observed within 1 to 2 days. Paroxysms tend to increase in frequency and severity over time. Blood pressure can be elevated, often to alarming levels, when measured during a paroxysm.
- Several medications may precipitate a **hypertensive crisis** in the setting of pheochromocytoma (Table 15-2). These drugs should be avoided until pheochromocytoma has been excluded or resected or the patient has been premedicated with a α-adrenergic antagonist.

Physical Examination

- **Hypertension** is the most common physical examination finding in pheochromocytoma. It is usually severe, refractory to conventional therapy, and associated with signs of end-organ damage such as proteinuria or retinopathy; however, it may also resemble essential hypertension in the absence of paroxysms.

TABLE 15-2	DRUGS THAT MAY PRECIPITATE HYPERTENSIVE CRISIS IN THE SETTING OF PHEOCHROMOCYTOMA

Decongestants
Tricyclic antidepressants
MAO inhibitors
Phenothiazines
β-Blockers
Metoclopramide
Atropine
Glucagon
Cosyntropin (ACTH)
Radiographic contrast
Droperidol

—
ACTH, adrenocorticotropic hormone; MAO, monoamine oxidase.

• Rare presentations include episodic hypotension (when the tumor secretes only epinephrine) or rapid cyclic fluctuations of blood pressure. (See Table 15-1 for more symptoms and signs of pheochromocytoma.)

Diagnostic Criteria

Definitive diagnosis of pheochromocytoma is made by a biochemical evaluation followed by anatomical and functional imaging to localize the tumor.

Differential Diagnosis[7]

• Endocrine: hyperthyroidism, carcinoid, hypoglycemia, medullary thyroid carcinoma, mastocytosis, menopausal symptoms
• Cardiovascular: heart failure, arrhythmias, ischemic heart disease, baroreflex failure
• Neurologic: migraine, stroke, meningioma, postural orthostatic tachycardia syndrome (POTS)
• Miscellaneous: porphyria, panic disorder or anxiety, use of sympathomimetic drugs, MAO inhibitors, clonidine withdrawal, illicit drugs (i.e., cocaine).

Diagnostic Testing

There are **two essential components** to the diagnosis of pheochromocytoma: (a) **biochemical confirmation**, and subsequently (b) **anatomic localization of the tumor.**

Laboratories

• Diagnosis of pheochromocytoma requires biochemical evidence of excessive catecholamine production by the tumor, which is achieved by measurements of catecholamines and certain catecholamine metabolites in plasma or urine (see Table 15-3).

TABLE 15-3	PERFORMANCE CHARACTERISTICS OF BIOCHEMICAL ASSAYS FOR PHEOCHROMOCYTOMA	
Test	**Sensitivity (%)**	**Specificity (%)**
NIH series[19]		
Plasma		
Free metanephrines	99	89
Catecholamines	84	81
24 hour urine		
Fractionated metanephrines	97	69
Total metanephrines	77	93
Catecholamines	86	88
Vanillylmandelic acid	64	95
Mayo series[20]		
Plasma free metanephrines	97	85
24 hour urine total metanephrines and catecholamines	90	98
Perry et al.[21]		
Urine fractionated metanephrines	97	91

- The potentially fatal consequences of a missed diagnosis necessitate the need for a laboratory test with high degree of sensitivity. Plasma free metanephrines and urinary fractionated metanephrines have been shown to offer the highest sensitivity for diagnosis of pheochromocytoma, and the current consensus statements from the First International Symposium on Pheochromocytoma recommend measurements of **plasma free metanephrines** or **urinary fractionated metanephrines**, or both as the initial test.[2] A summary of the performance characteristics of the plasma and urine tests is presented in Table 15-3.

- Dietary factors, drugs, or inappropriate sampling conditions can interfere with biochemical testing (see Table 15-4).[7] These confounders can be avoided by fasting and abstaining from beverages containing caffeine (even partially decaffeinated beverages) overnight before blood draws. Patients should also be placed supine for at least 20 minutes before sampling to avoid false positive results. Acetaminophen is known

TABLE 15-4 FACTORS INTERFERING WITH BIOCHEMICAL TESTING

Stimulation of endogenous catecholamines	Exogenous catecholamines	Drugs that alter catecholamine metabolism	Drugs that interfere with biochemical assays
• Emotional and physical stress (surgery, trauma) • Drug withdrawal (alcohol, clonidine) • Drugs (vasodilators, caffeine, nicotine, theophylline, ephedrine, amphetamines) • Hypoglycemia • Obstructive sleep apnea • Myocardial ischemia • Stroke	• Bronchodilators • Appetite suppressants • Decongestants	• β-Blockers (falsely increases urine catecholamines and metanephrines) • Phenoxybenzamine (falsely increases plasma and urine norepinephrine and normetanephrine) • Tricyclic antidepressants (falsely increases plasma and urine norepinephrine and normetanephrine) • Levodopa • Theophylline • MAO-inhibitors	• Labetalol, sotalol[†] • Acetaminophen[#] • Clofibrate • Quinidine

[†]Interference only with the spectrophotometric assay for metanephrines; catecholamines measured by HPLC and metanephrines by mass spectrometry are not affected.

[#]Plasma free metanephrines measured by HPLC are not affected.

Diuretics, ACE inhibitors, and SSRIs generally do not interfere with the biochemical tests.

ACE, angiotensin-converting enzyme; HPLC, high performance liquid chromatography; MAO, monoamine oxidase.; SSRI, selective serotonin uptake inhibitors.

to interfere with analytic method during assaying of plasma free metanephrines, hence its avoidance is recommended to avoid false results.[22] Tricyclic antidepressants and phenoxybenzamine are major causes of false-positive results on urinary and plasma normetanephrine and norepinephrine.[23]

- The high degree of sensitivities of these biochemical tests means that negative test results essentially rule out pheochromocytoma; however, a positive test does not always reliably indicate presence of the disease. Most true positive results can be distinguished from false positives by the magnitude of increases in test results above the reference range. Rather than values slightly above normal, biochemical parameters are typically elevated more than two- to threefold above normal when a pheochromocytoma is present.

- Although there is no consensus on whether plasma or urine measurements are preferred, given 97% to 99% sensitivity, plasma metanephrines are the best initial test in patients with high pretest probability of disease (MEN2, von Hippel-Lindau syndrome, and previously surgically cured pheochromocytomas). Normal plasma normetanephrine (NMN) and metanephrine (MN) levels essentially rule out a diagnosis of pheochromocytoma except in patients with small and microscopic tumors (<1 cm) and those with dopamine-secreting tumors. However, given an 85% to 89% specificity, elevated plasma NMN and MN levels, unless markedly increased (two- to threefold above normal), need to be further confirmed with more specific tests such as 24-hour urine metanephrines and catecholamines (98% specific).[20]

- Before repeating the tests, careful consideration of the various causes of false-positive results from medications and other factors is warranted (Table 15-4).

- The much-improved biochemical assays for catecholamines and their metabolites have made pharmacologic stimulation and suppression tests for pheochromocytoma largely unnecessary. However, the clonidine suppression test and glucagon stimulation test are occasionally helpful. The clonidine suppression test may be useful when plasma catecholamines are elevated but nondiagnostic. A decrease in plasma norepinephrine by >50% is the normal expected response to clonidine suppression, whereas consistently elevated levels suggest pheochromocytoma. False-positive results can occur in patients taking tricyclic antidepressants or beta-blockers. A more than three fold rise in plasma norepinephrine after administration of glucagon diagnoses pheochromocytoma with high specificity, but the test has low sensitivity. Premedication with a α-adrenergic blocker is necessary to limit the potential pressor response to norepinephrine.[23]

Electrocardiography

Signs of left ventricular hypertrophy can be seen in EKG due to persistent hypertension.

Imaging

- **Radiologic evaluation should be initiated only after catecholamine excess has been confirmed biochemically.** In situations of a high-pretest probability, less compelling biochemical evidence might justify imaging studies.

- Based on the First International Symposium on Pheochromocytoma, there was no consensus on CT scan or MRI as the preferred imaging for initial localization of a tumor.

- Because ~95% of pheochromocytomas are intraabdominal, an abdominal CT or MRI scan is usually obtained first.

- CT has high sensitivity of 85% to 94% for detecting adrenal pheochromocytoma (90% for extraadrenal, metastatic, or recurrent pheochromoccytoma) but a specificity of only 29% to 50%. Following an unenhanced CT with contrast-enhanced and delayed contrast-enhanced CT imaging for adrenal lesions improves sensitivity to 98% and specificity to 92%.[24] If the CT is negative in a biochemically positive pheochromocytoma, the next step is MRI.
- Pheochromocytomas usually appear round or oval, with clear margins, usually >3 cm in diameter with heterogeneous texture punctuated by cystic areas on imaging studies. Due to their low lipid content, their unenhanced CT density is >10 Hounsfield units (HU) and the contrast washout is <50% at 10 minutes.[25]
- Chemical shift MRI is used to differentiate adrenal masses based on presence/absence of fat similar to the CT. The hypervascularity of pheochromocytoma makes them appear characteristically bright, with a high signal intensity on T2 sequences and no signal loss on opposed phase images. MRI has high sensitivity in detecting adrenal diseases (93% to 100%), but its specificity has been reported to be around 50%.[26]
- Functional imaging should always be performed after anatomic imaging (regardless of whether CT and MRI are positive or negative) to localize the primary tumor and rule out multifocal tumors or metastases.
- For many years, metaiodobenzylguanidine (MIBG) has been used for diagnostic imaging in pheochromocytoma because of its resemblance to norepinephrine, with ^{123}I-MIBG being superior to ^{131}I-MIBG.[27,28]
- An octreotide scan (^{111}In-octreotide) is insensitive (<30%) but may detect tumors in unusual locations when MIBG scans are negative, especially metastatic pheochromocytoma. Octreotide scans have been shown to be better than ^{123}I-MIBG scan in detecting malignant/metastatic pheochromocytoma (87% vs. 57% of lesion).
- All rapidly metabolizing cells take up glucose, so imaging with FDG-PET is nonspecific for pheochromocytoma but may be good for localizing dedifferentiated and/or rapidly growing pheochromocytoma tumors. Adrenal tumors associated with a VHL gene mutation, extraadrenal paragangliomas, and metastatic paragangliomas are best imaged by [18F] FDA PET.

Diagnostic Procedures

Genetic screening is currently recommended for patients diagnosed with pheochromocytoma before age 50 years, bilateral adrenal tumors, multiple paragangliomas, or who have a family history of pheochromocytoma or paraganglioma.[7]

TREATMENT

- **Surgical resection is the definitive therapy for pheochromocytoma.[29]**
- Removing a pheochromocytoma is a high-risk surgical procedure, and an experienced surgeon–anesthesiologist team is required. In addition, patients must undergo appropriate medical preparation to control the effects of excessive adrenergic stimulation and prevent intraoperative hypertensive crisis. An endocrinologist or other physician experienced in the management of pheochromocytoma should supervise preoperative therapy.
- Pheochromocytomas have traditionally been resected through a transabdominal approach. However, refinements in radiologic localization have permitted an increase

- Diagnosis is still made on the basis of elevated plasma and/or urinary fractionated metanephrines and anatomic localization by MRI. Nuclear scintigraphy and stimulation tests are considered unsafe during pregnancy.
- Women should be prepared for surgery with phenoxybenzamine followed by β-blockade as necessary for tachycardia. Although phenoxybenzamine is considered to be safe for the fetus, it does cross the placenta and can cause perinatal depression and transient hypotension.
- If the diagnosis of pheochromocytoma is made before 24 weeks of gestation, surgical resection is usually performed. After 24 weeks of gestation, medical management is continued until fetal maturation (as close to term as possible), at which time combined cesarean delivery and tumor resection are performed.

MONITORING/FOLLOW-UP

- Long-term follow-up is indicated in all patients, even in those apparently cured. Catecholamines and metanephrines should be rechecked 1 week after surgery to assess the adequacy of tumor resection by monitoring for a return to the laboratory reference range. If the levels are normal and the patient remains asymptomatic, biochemical screening should be performed annually for the next 5 years and biannually thereafter. Biochemical testing should also be performed if symptoms suspicious for pheochromocytoma recur.
- Patients with familial tumor syndromes, bilateral tumors, or paragangliomas should be monitored annually.

OUTCOME/PROGNOSIS

- In a large surgical series, overall perioperative mortality and morbidity rates were 2.4% and 24%, respectively. Surgical removal of a pheochromocytoma does not always lead to long-term cure of pheochromocytoma or hypertension, even in patients with a benign tumor. In one series, pheochromocytoma recurred as a benign or malignant tumor in 14% of patients with an apparently benign tumor at the time of surgical resection.
- Hypertension-free survival in patients without recurrence was 74% at 5 years and 45% at 10 years. Survival does not appear to be affected by the site of the tumor. Patients with malignant pheochromocytoma have a 5-year survival of ~40%. Recurrence is more likely in patients with familial pheochromocytoma/paraganglioma, right-sided adrenal tumors, and extraadrenal tumors.[34]

REFERENCES

1. Dluhy RG, Lawrence JE, Williams GH. Endocrine hypertension. In: Larsen PR, Kronenberg HM, Melmed S, et al., eds. *Williams Textbook of Endocrinology*, 10th ed. Philadelphia, PA: WB Saunders; 2003:552–585.
2. Pacak K, Eisenhofer G, Ahlman H, et al. Pheochromocytoma: Recommendations for clinical practice from the First International Symposium. *Nat Clin Pract Endocrinol Metab* 2007;3:92–102.
3. O'Riordain DS, Young WF Jr, Grant CS, et al. Clinical spectrum and outcome of functional extra adrenal paraganglioma. *World J Surg* 1996;20:916–921.

4. Ling D, Lee JKT. The adrenals. In: Lee JKT, Sagel SS, Stanley FJ, eds. *Computer Body Tomography with MRI Correlation,* 2nd ed. New York, NY: Raven Press; 2012:827–849.

5. Whalen RK, Althausen AF, Daniels GH. Extra-adrenal pheochromocytoma. *J Urol* 1992;147:1–10.

6. Bravo EL, Tagle R. Pheochromocytoma: State-of-the-art and future prospects. *Endocr Rev* 2003;24:539–553.

7. Lenders JW, Eisenhofer G, Mannelli M, et al. Pheochromocytoma. *Lancet* 2005; 366:665–675.

8. Young WF Jr. Management approaches to adrenal incidentalomas: A view from Rochester, Minnesota. *Endocrinol Metab Clin North Am* 2000;29:159–185.

9. Howe JR, Norton JA, Wells SA Jr. Prevalence of pheochromocytoma and hyperparathyroidism in multiple endocrine neoplasia type 2A: Results of long-term follow-up. *Surgery* 1993;114:1070–1077.

10. Karagiannis A, Mikhailidis DP, Vasilios GA, et al. Pheochromocytoma: An update on genetics and management. *Endocr Relat Cancer* 2007;14:935–956.

11. Yao L, Schiavi F, Cascon A, et al. Spectrum and prevalence of FP/TMEM127 gene mutations in pheochromocytomas and paragangliomas. *JAMA* 2010;304:2611–2619.

12. Eisenhofer G, Friberg P, Pacak K, et al. Plasma metadrenalines: do they provide useful information about sympatho-adrenal function and catehcholamine metabolism? *Clin Sci (Lond)* 1995;88:533–542.

13. Eisenhofer G, Rundquist B, Aneman A, et al. Regional release and removal of catecholamines and extraneuronal metabolism to metanephrines. *J Clin Endocrinol Metab* 1995; 80:3009–3017.

14. Eisenhofer G, Keiser H, Friberg P, et al. Plasma metanephrines are markers of pheochromocytoma produces by catecho-O-methyltransferase within tumors. *J Clin Endocrinol Metab* 1998;83:2175–2185.

15. Plouin PF, Degoulet P, Tugaye A, et al. Screening for phaeochromocytoma: In which hypertensive patients? A semiological study of 2585 patients, including 11 with phaeochromocytoma. *Nouv Presse Med* 1981;10:869–872.

16. Thomas JE, Rooke ED, Kvale WF. The neurologist's experience with pheochromocytoma. A review of 100 cases. *JAMA* 1966;197:754–758.

17. Bravo EL. Pheochromocytoma: New concepts and future trends. *Kidney Int* 1991;40:544–556.

18. Motta-Ramirez GA, Remer EM, Herts BR, et al. Comparison of CT findings in symptomatic and incidentally discovered pheochromocytomas. *AJR Am J Roentgenol* 2005;185:684–688.

19. Lenders JW, Pacak K, Walther MM, et al. Biochemical diagnosis of pheochromocytoma: Which test is best? *JAMA* 2002;287:1427–1434.

20. Sawka AM, Jaeschke R, Singh RJ, et al. A comparison of biochemical tests for pheochromocytoma: Measurement of fractionated plasma metanephrines compared with the combination of 24-hour urinary metanephrines and catecholamines. *J Clin Endocrinol Metab* 2003;88:553–558.

21. Perry CG, Sawka AM, Singh R, et al. The diagnostic efficacy of urinary fractionated metanephrines measured by tandem mass spectrometry in detection of pheochromocytoma. *Clin Endocrinol* 2007;66:703–708.

22. Lenders JW, Eisenhofer G, Armando I, et al. Determination of metanephrines in plasma by liquid chromatography with electrochemical detection. *Clin Chem* 1993;39:97–103.

23. Eisenhofer G, Goldstein DS, Walther MM, et al. Biochemical diagnosis of pheochromocytoma: How to distinguish true- from false-positive test results. *J Clin Endocrinol Metab* 2003;88:2656–2666.

24. Ilias I, Pacak K. Current approaches and recommended algorithm for the diagnostic localization of pheochromocytoma. *J Clin Endocrinol Metab* 2004;89:479–491.

25. Young WF Jr. The incidentally discovered adrenal mass. *N Eng J Med* 2007;356:601–610.

26. Francis IR, KOrobkin M. Pheochromocytoma. *Radiol Clin North Am* 1996;34:1101–1112.

27. Nielsen JT, Nielsen BV, Rehling M. Location of adrenal medullary pheochromocytoma by I-123 metaiodobenzylguanidine SPECT. *Clin Nucl Med* 1996;21:695–699.

28. Van der Harst E, de Herder WW, Bonjer HJ, et al. [¹²³I] Metaiodobenzylguanidine and [¹¹¹In] octreotide uptake in benign and malignant pheochromocytomas. *J Clin Endocrinol Metab* 2001;86:685–693.

29. Ulchaker JC, Goldfarb DA, Bravo EL, et al. Successful outcomes in pheochromocytoma surgery in the modern era. *J Urol* 1999;161:764–767.

30. Pacak K. Preoperative management of the pheochromocytoma patient. *J Clin Endocrinol Metab* 2007;92:4069–4079.

31. Hull CJ. Pheochromocytoma: diagnosis, preoperative preparation and anesthetic management. *Br J Anaesth* 1986;58:1453–1468.

32. Goldstein RE, O'Neill JA Jr, Holcomb GW 3rd, et al. Clinical experience over 48 years with pheochromocytoma. *Ann Surg* 1999;229:755–764.

33. Bruynzeel H, Feelders RA, Groenland THN, et al. Risk Factors for Hemodynamic Instability during Surgery for Pheochromocytoma. *J Clin Endocrinol Metab* 2010;95:678–685.

34. Plouin PF, Chatellier G, Fofol I, et al. Tumor recurrence and hypertension persistence after successful pheochromocytoma operation. *Hypertension* 1997;29:1133–1139.

Amenorrhea

16

Sara Chowdhury and Amy E. Riek

GENERAL PRINCIPLES

- The menstrual cycle is determined by interactions between the hypothalamic-pituitary–ovarian (HPO) axis and the uterus.
- At the level of the ovary, the menstrual cycle is divided into the follicular phase and luteal phase. Growth of a dominant ovarian follicle and ovulation occurs during the follicular phase. After ovulation, the luteal phase begins in which the ovary secretes hormones that are needed for the embryo to implant in the uterus.
- Disturbance of complex hormonal feedback loops at any level—the hypothalamus, pituitary, ovary, or uterus—can lead to disruption of the normal menstrual cycle, including cessation of menses.

Hypothalamic-Pituitary–Ovarian Axis

- The hypothalamus secretes gonadotropin-releasing hormone (GnRH), which stimulates the release of luteinizing hormone (LH) and follicle-stimulating hormone (FSH) from the anterior pituitary gland.
- During the late luteal phase, GnRH is secreted in a slow pulsatile manner (pulses every 90 to 120 minutes) by neurons with inherent rhythmic behavior, known as the "pulse generator." This favors FSH secretion. Subsequently, FSH stimulates ovarian follicles to develop. The follicle with the most FSH receptors becomes the dominant follicle. The maturing follicle secretes estradiol in response to FSH.
- Estradiol production in the ovary occurs according to the two-cell theory, which involves interaction between the theca and granulosa cells of the follicle. The theca cells surrounding the follicles produce androgens, which are aromatized to estradiol by neighboring granulosa cells. Increasing levels of estradiol provide negative feedback to the pituitary to suppress FSH.
- Estradiol is also involved in a positive feedback loop that increases the frequency of GnRH pulses to every 60 minutes (during the follicular phase) and it acts directly on the pituitary to stimulate LH secretion.
- LH causes further increases in estradiol production by the ovary which is a factor in increasing pituitary sensitivity to GnRH. This heightened sensitivity results in a rapid rise in LH production, the LH surge, which stimulates ovulation. The LH surge lasts approximately 50 hours. About 36 hours after the LH surge, ovulation occurs and the oocyte is released from the dominant follicle at the surface of the ovary.
- Progesterone levels start increasing just before ovulation. After ovulation, the theca and granulosa cells in the ruptured follicle differentiate and together form the corpus luteum, which continues to secrete progesterone.
- The exact mechanism that stops the LH surge is not known. However, it is postulated that the increase in progesterone levels provides a negative feedback loop to

decrease GnRH pulsatility (every 3 to 5 hours), which inhibits further LH secretion by the pituitary but favors FSH synthesis.

- FSH stimulates estrogen production during the luteal phase, which occurs similar to the two cell theory as described above. FSH has little influence on progesterone production. Progesterone levels rise and peak around day 8 of the luteal phase, which lasts about 14 days total.
- In absence of pregnancy, the corpus luteum starts to regress (luteolysis). This causes an abrupt decline in progesterone levels and also a decrease in estadiol levels. The decrease in these hormones causes an increase in GnRH pulsatility, which results in the start of another menstrual cycle.

The Uterus

- Throughout the menstrual cycle, the endometrium responds to hormones secreted from the ovaries.
- Estrogens secreted during the follicular phase stimulate the proliferative phase of the endometrium. The proliferative phase starts with menses and ends with ovulation.
- After ovulation, progesterone and estrogen secreted during the luteal phase corresponds to the secretory phase of the endometrium. This phase promotes several changes in the endometrium to prepare for implantation.
- If there is no implantation of an embryo, the endometrium enters the degenerative phase as a result of progesterone and estrogen decline during luteolysis. The reduction of these hormones results in sloughing of the endometrium and the onset of menses.
- If implantation takes place, the embryo secretes human chorionic gonadotropin (hCG). This maintains progesterone secretion by the corpus luteum and is essential for the continuation of pregnancy.

Physiology

- **Puberty** is characterized by the onset of regular menstrual cycles and development of secondary sexual features. The average time between the onset of **thelarche** (breast development) and **menarche** (onset of menses) is 2 years.
- The age of menarche is variable depending on genetic and socioeconomic factors. The mean age of menarche in the United States is approximately 12.8 years. There are differences in the age of menarche among racial groups.
- An average adult menstrual cycle lasts approximately 28 days and usually has little cycle variability between the ages of 20 and 40 years.
- There is considerably more variation in a woman's menstrual cycle for the first 5 to 7 years after menarche and for the last 10 years before menopause.
- The mean age of **menopause** in the United States is 51 years, but may occur earlier in smokers, nulliparity, or those with a family history of early menopause. It is common in the preceding 2 to 8 years before menopause to have irregular menses and breakthough bleeding, since the normal ovulatory cycle is interspersed with anovulaory cycles of varying length. Cessation of menses before age 40 is generally considered premature menopause.

Definitions

- **Amenorrhea** is the absence of menses or abnormal cessation of menses. This can be a temporary, intermittent, or a permanent condition.

- Patients should be evaluated if they meet the following criteria[1].
  - ○ No menses by age 14 in the absence of growth or development of secondary sexual characteristics.
  - ○ No menses by age 16 regardless of the presence of secondary sexual characteristics.
  - ○ In previously menstruating women, the absence of menses for an interval of time equal to three previous cycles or 6 months.
- **Oligomenorrhea** is defined as <9 menstrual cycles a year.

Classification

- Traditionally, amenorrhea has been classified as primary or secondary.
  - ○ **Primary amenorrhea** describes patients who have never menstruated.
  - ○ **Secondary amenorrhea** describes patients who previously menstruated, but have subsequently stopped.
- The classical distinction serves little practical purpose as the differential diagnoses between the two are very similar. However, epidemiologic data are presented below according to the traditional classification.
- The **new approach is to group causes of amenorrhea based on the level of involvement in the regulatory system.**[1,2]
  - ○ Disorders of the genital outflow tract and uterus
  - ○ Disorders of the ovary
  - ○ Disorders of the pituitary
  - ○ Disorders of the hypothalamus
  - ○ Other endocrine causes

Epidemiology

The prevalence of amenorrhea not resulting from pregnancy, lactation, or menopause is 3% to 4%.[3]

Etiology

- There are several potential causes amenorrhea as listed in Table 16-1.
- The **most common causes of amenorrhea** are polycystic ovary syndrome (PCOS), hypothalamic amenorrhea, hyperprolactinemia, and ovarian failure.[3]
- Women who do not menstruate within 3 months after the discontinuation of oral contraceptives should be evaluated for amenorrhea.
- The most common etiologies by the traditional classification of **primary amenorrhea** are[4]
  - ○ Chromosomal abnormalities causing gonadal dysgenesis (premature depletion of all ovarian oocytes and follicles [50%])
  - ○ Hypothalamic causes (20%)
  - ○ Congenital anatomic lesions of reproductive organs (20%)
  - ○ Pituitary causes (5%)
  - ○ Other (5%)—combination of enzyme deficiencies, receptor mutations, polycystic ovary syndrome
- Once pregnancy is excluded, the most common areas that are affected in the traditional classification of **secondary amenorrhea** are[3,5]
  - ○ Ovaries (40%)
  - ○ Hypothalamus (35%)
  - ○ Pituitary (19%)
  - ○ Uterus (5%)
  - ○ Other (1%)

TABLE 16-1 ETIOLOGIES OF AMENORRHEA

Disorders of genital outflow tract and uterus
Müllerian agenesis
Androgen insensitivity syndrome
Imperforate hymen
Transverse vaginal septum/cervical atresia
Asherman's syndrome
Cervical stenosis

Ovarian causes
Gonadal dysgenesis: Turner syndrome (45,XO), Mosaic Turner syndrome, Swyer syndrome (46,XY), 46,XX gonadal dysgenesis
Premature ovarian failure: idiopathic, chemotherapy, radiation, mumps oophoritis, fragile X permutations, structural and numerical chromosomal abnormalities, autoimmune
Enzymatic deficiencies: galactosemia, 17a-hydroxylase deficiency, aromatase deficiency, 17,20-lyase deficiency

Pituitary causes
Prolactinoma
Other pituitary tumors
Empty sella syndrome
Pituitary infarction (Sheehan's syndrome)
Infiltrative diseases: lymphocytic hypophysitis, hemochromatosis
Radiation
Surgery
FSH or LH receptor mutations
Panhypopituitarism

Hypothalamic causes
Functional hypothalamic amenorrhea (exercise, anorexia nervosa, weight loss, stress, chronic disease, depression)
Congenital GnRH deficiency: idiopathic hypogonadotropic hypogonadism, Kallmann syndrome
Infiltrative diseases: sarcoidosis, lymphoma, Langerhans' cell histiocytosis, hemochromatosis
Infection: tuberculosis, syphilis, encephalitis/meningitis
Tumors (craniopharyngioma, germinoma, hamartoma, etc.)
GnRH receptor mutations

Other endocrine causes
Hyperprolactinemia
Thyroid disorders
Cushing's syndrome
Polycystic ovary syndrome
Nonclassic congenital adrenal hyperplasia
Adrenal tumors with androgen overproduction
HAIR-AN (hyperandrogenism, insulin resistance, acanthosis nigricans) syndrome

Physiologic causes
Pregnancy
Lactation
Menopause
Constitutional delay of puberty

- If patients are of typical age (>40 years) and/or with usual associated symptoms (e.g., hot flashes, vaginal dryness), then physiologic menopause should be considered.

Selected Disorders

- **Turner syndrome** is a chromosomal abnormality caused by the absence of an X chromosome (45,XO). Patients have normal development of the external female genitalia, uterus, and fallopian tubes until puberty, at which time there is failure of sexual maturation owing to lack of estrogen because the ovaries are replaced with fibrous tissue.
- **Swyer's syndrome** (46,XY) is characterized by individuals with normal karyotype, gonadal dysgenesis, and female genitalia. The most frequent gene defect in these individuals is a mutation in the *SRY* gene (sex-determining region of the Y chromosome). Since the frequency of gonadal tumors is high, gonads should be removed at the time of diagnosis.
- **Müllerian agenesis**, also known as vaginal agenesis, results in congenital absence of a vagina and abnormal uterine development. Affected individuals are phenotypically and genetically female. Physical findings are a shortened or absent vagina and small masses resembling a rudimentary uterus or absence of a uterus. This disorder is associated with urogenital abnormalities in 1/3 of patients, such as horseshoe kidney, pelvic kidney, and unilateral renal agenesis.
- **Androgen insensitivity syndrome** (AIS) (also known as testicular feminization) is characterized by a 46,XY karyotype. Patients appear as women and breast development occurs during puberty form peripheral conversion of testostertone to estradiol. The uterus, fallopian tubes, and the upper third of the vagina are absent. It is caused by a defect in the androgen receptor that results in resistance to the actions of testosterone. It presents similar to Müllerian agenesis, but patients with complete AIS lack pubic hair. The testes can often be palpated in the labia or inguinal region and should be surgically removed after puberty due to an increased risk of malignancy.
- **Idiopathic hypogonadotropic hypogonadism** (IHH) is congential GnRH deficiency that can be inherited or occur sporadically. If it is associated with anosmia, Kallmann's syndrome should be suspected. These disorders cause amenorrhea owing to absence of GnRH secretion from the hypothalamus.
- **Functional hypothalamic amenorrhea** excludes pathologic disease. It is marked by abnormal GnRH secretion, resulting in low or low-normal levels of serum FSH and LH, absent LH surge, anovulation, and a state of estrogen deficiency. Three main causes are stress, exercise, or weight loss.
- **Hyperandrogenism** from any source can lead to amenorrhea due to chronic anovulation. These disorders include late-onset congenital adrenal hyperplasia, Cushing's syndrome, PCOS (see Chapter 20), exogenous androgen use, or adrenal tumors.
- **Premature ovarian failure** (POF) is characterized by amenorrhea, estrogen deficiency, and elevated FSH in patients younger than 40 years of age. Ovarian function may fluctuate. Up to 40% of women with POF may have other autoimmune endocrinopathies such as autoimmune thyroiditis, type 1 diabetes mellitus, hypoparathyroidism, myasthenia gravis, and, very rarely, Addison's disease (see Chapter 36).
- **Hyperprolactinemia** can result from a prolactin-secreting pituitary tumor, disruption of the pituitary stalk, medications, or increased thyrotropin-releasing hormone

release due to hypothyroidism. Prolactin is thought to suppress GnRH secretion which leads to amenorrhea.

DIAGNOSIS

Clinical Presentation

History

Important elements to obtain as part of the history include the following:

- Age of menarche
- Frequency and length of previous menstrual cycles
- Sexual activity
- Number of pregnancies and any complications
- Family history of pubertal development, menarche, and menstrual history (e.g., constitutional delay of puberty)
- Family history of genetic defects
- Weight changes, dietary habits
- Exercise regimen
- Psychosocial stressors
- Prescription medication or illicit drug use
- Gynecologic surgery/instrumentation or infection
- History of chemotherapy, central nervous system (CNS), or pelvic radiation
- Symptoms of estrogen deficiency (e.g., hot flashes, vaginal dryness, decreased libido)
- Symptoms of endocrine diseases (e.g., hypothyroidism, galactorrhea)
- Symptoms of mass effect (e.g., headache, visual disturbance)
- History of anosmia (Kallmann's syndrome)
- Cyclic abdominal pain and breast changes (outflow obstruction or Müllerian agenesis)

Physical Examination

- It is important to include weight, height, breast examination, and pelvic examination.
- Review of the growth chart may indicate constitutional delay of growth and puberty.
- In cases of primary amenorrhea, assess Tanner stage and the presence or absence of secondary sexual characteristics.
- Short stature, webbed neck, and widely spaced nipples should raise suspicion of Turner syndrome.
- A blind or absent vagina with breast development suggests Müllerian agenesis, transverse vaginal septum (pubic hair present), or AIS (minimal or no pubic hair).
- Patients with hirsutism or male-pattern hair loss should have a free serum testosterone level checked. Signs of virilization (deepening of the voice, clitoromegaly, increased muscle mass) on physical examination should always prompt further evaluation for an androgen-secreting tumor.
- Central obesity, supraclavicular fat pads, easy bruising, skin thinning, proximal muscle weakness, glucose intolerance, and hypertension should raise the suspicion of Cushing's syndrome.
- Acanthosis nigricans is associated with insulin resistance, a feature of PCOS, and HAIR-AN syndrome (hyperandrogenism insulin resistant acanthosis nigricans).

Diagnostic Testing

- Figure 16-1 provides an algorithm for the diagnostic workup of amenorrhea, listing the most common causes.
  - ○ Work-up of secondary amenorrhea starts with a measurement of β-hCG to rule out pregnancy.
  - ○ **Rule out pregnancy** by checking **β-hCG.**
  - ○ Other basic laboratory tests should include **thyroid-stimulating hormone (TSH), prolactin (PRL),** and **FSH.** Serum estradiol levels can fluctuate significantly in all disorders and must be interpreted with caution and based on the clinical scenario.
  - ○ **Elevated FSH levels** (hypergonadotropic amenorrhea ~ 40% of cases) suggests an ovarian etiology and gonadal failure.[6]
    - In primary amenorrhea with the absence of secondary sexual characteristics, a karyotype analysis should be performed to rule out a chromosomal abnormality such as Turner syndrome (45,XO), POF (46,XX), or to assess for the presence of an occult Y chromosome, which is associated with an increased risk for gonadal tumors.

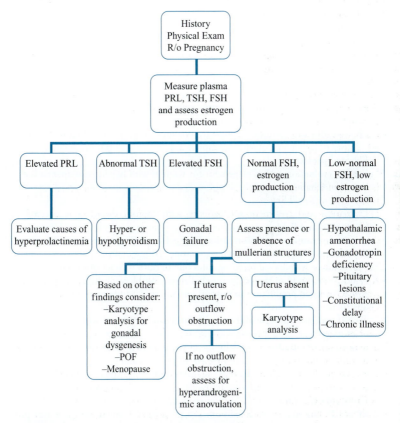

FIGURE 16-1 Diagnostic algorithm for amenorrhea.

- In women under age 30 years with POF, a karyotype analysis should also be performed to assess for mosaic Turner's syndrome and other various chromosomal abnormalites.[3]
- Other causes for ovarian failure such as ovarian tumors, prior trauma, pelvic radiation, and chemotherapy should be evaluated.
  - **Normal FSH levels** (normogonadotropic amenorrhea ~30% of cases)[6]
    - In primary amenorrhea, normal gonadotropins with evidence of estrogen production (breast development) could point to anatomic defects (i.e., Müllerian agenesis, AIS) or outflow tract obstruction (i.e., imperforate hymen, vaginal septum, cervical, or vaginal agenesis).
    - **In primary amenorrhea**, a **pelvic ultrasound** should be performed to confirm the presence of a uterus and Müllerian structures. Absence of Müllerian structures should prompt further evaluation with a karyotype analysis and serum testosterone level.
    - In secondary amenorrhea, if there is a history of uterine infection or instrumentation, the possibility of outflow obstruction (Asherman's syndrome) should be addressed (see progestin challenge test below).
  - **Low or low-normal FSH levels** (hypogonadotropic amenorrhea ~30% of cases)[6]
    - Low gonadotropin levels point to a central etiology (hypothalamic or pituitary pathology), and a cranial MRI is indicated in most cases to rule out a hypothalamic or pituitary lesion before other etiologies are considered.
    - In primary amenorrhea, the most common cause is constitutional delay of puberty (10% of cases). Other causes are hypothalamic or pituitary disorders, idiopathic GnRH deficiency, Kallman's syndrome, or functional hypothalamic amenorrhea.
    - In secondary amenorrhea, the most common cause is functional hypothalamic amenorrhea. Panhypopituitarism secondary to space-occupying lesions, infiltrative diseases, pituitary apoplexy, previous surgery, or radiation are other causes of hypogonadotropic amenorrhea with low estrogen production.
  - **Elevated prolactin**
    Further evaluation and management for women with hyperprolactinemia is discussed in Chapter 2.
  - **Elevated or low TSH**
    Evaluation and treatment for patients with thyroid disorders is covered in Chapters 8 and 9.
- Assess uterine outflow tract obstruction is by performing a **progestin challenge test**. The patient is prescribed medroxyprogesterone, 10 mg orally daily for 10 days and the presence of withdrawal bleeding rules out an outflow tract obstruction.
  - Failure to respond to the progestin challenge with bleeding suggests either inadequate estrogen production to support endometrial proliferation or outflow tract obstruction.
  - To differentiate these possibilities, the challenge is repeated with a combination of estrogen and progesterone (conjugated equine estrogen [Premarin] 1.25 mg orally daily or estradiol 2 mg daily for 21 days followed by progesterone as noted, or with progesterone added during days 12 to 21). Failure to bleed in response to this combination regimen strongly suggests outflow obstruction and should lead to anatomic investigation by hysterosalpingogram or hysteroscopy.
  - Unfortunately, withdrawal bleeding correlates poorly with estrogen status and should be interpreted with caution. Up to 20% of women with estrogen production and amenorrhea will have no withdrawal bleeding, thus a false-positive

result. Up to 40% to 50% of women with disorders causing low estrogen production will have withdrawal bleeding, giving a false-negative result.[3]

- In the presence of hirsutism and other signs of androgen excess such as acne, seborrhea, and alopecia, causes of hyperandrogenic anovulation should be evaluated.
  - **Polycystic ovary syndrome** is the most common cause of hyperandrogenic anovulation, but it **is a diagnosis of exclusion** (see Chapter 20).
  - A **17-hydroxyprogesterone level** should be measured to rule out **nonclassic congenital adrenal hyperplasia** (CAH); 21-hydroxylase deficiency is the most common cause of nonclassic CAH (see Chapter 12).
  - **Testosterone and dehydroepiandrosterone sulfate (DHEA-S)** should be measured, and, if elevated (total testosterone, >200 ng/dL; DHEA-S, >600 mcg/dL), appropriate imaging should be ordered to evaluate for the presence of an adrenal or ovarian tumor.
  - **Cushing's syndrome** can be ruled out with a **1 mg overnight dexamethasone suppression test** or **24-hour urine free cortisol** (see Chapter 14).

TREATMENT

- Treatment of amenorrhea is **directed at correcting the underlying etiology** when possible and, if desired by the patient, **helping to achieve fertility**. Another aim is to **prevent complications**, such as osteoporosis.
- **Patients with primary amenorrhea** should be counseled about the underlying cause and their potential for achieving sexual maturation, induction of menses, and reproduction. Induction of puberty should be pursued under the direction of a specialist because the timing of menarche can greatly affect epiphyseal closure and final adult height.
- **Patients with congenital anatomic abnormalities** may require surgical correction. Patients with Y chromosomal material and residual testes should have their testes excised after puberty owing to the increased risk of testicular cancer after age 25.[7]
  - Women with gonadal dysgenesis or failure can now carry a pregnancy on their own with the use of donor oocytes and new assisted reproductive technologies.
  - For women with ovaries but no uterus, their own oocytes can be used and the embryos can be transferred to a gestational carrier.
- Ovulation and fertility can often be restored in **patients with hypothalamic amenorrhea** through administration of **pulsatile GnRH therapy**. GnRH is injected every 1 to 2 hours by a programmable pump to simulate endogenous pulsatile GnRH secretion. Treatment with pulsatile GnRH achieves fertility in ~90% of women after six cycles and carries a low risk of multiple pregnancies.[8]
- **Patients with anovulation due to pituitary disease** do not respond to GnRH therapy and require therapy with exogenous gonadotropins if fertility is desired. Pure recombinant FSH and LH can be used in an effort to achieve fertility, but this should be done only under the direction of an experienced specialist. Patients should be warned that the chances of having a multiple pregnancy with this method are high.
- Correcting the precipitating factors for functional hypothalamic disorders usually restores the normal menstrual cycle. In patients with amenorrhea caused by eating disorders or excessive exercise, a modest increase in caloric intake or decrease in athletic training can restore regular menses.

- Oral contraceptives may decrease bone turnover and preserve bone density. Adequate calcium and vitamin D should also be recommended.
- Patients with either hypothalamic or pituitary disease who do not desire fertility and patients with secondary ovarian failure can simply be treated with hormone replacement therapy until the age of menopause, at which time continuing hormone replacement becomes controversial and will need to be addressed on an individual basis.
  - **Every woman should be counseled about the potential risks of hormone replacement therapy** such as increased incidence of stroke, thromboembolic events, and breast cancer.
  - Smoking cessation should be advised before the initiation of oral contraceptive agents because of the increased risk of deep venous thrombosis.
- Specific therapy for PCOS is discussed in Chapter 20, and is aimed at controlling hirsutism, resuming menstruation, achieving fertility, and avoiding long-term sequelae of PCOS (glucose intolerance, endometrial hyperplasia, and possibly cardiovascular complications).
- Management for patients with hyperprolactinemia or prolactinoma is discussed in Chapter 2.

REFERENCES

1. Fritz MA, Speroff L. Amenorrhea. *Clinical Gynecologic Endocrinology and Infertility* 8th ed. Philadelphia: Lippincott Williams and Wilkins; 2011:435–493.
2. Rosen MP, Cedars MI. Female reproductive endocrinology and infertility. In: Gardner D, Shoback D, eds. *Greenspan's Basic and Clinical Endocrinology,* 9th ed. McGraw Hill; 2011:423–477.
3. Current evaluation of amenorrhea. The practice committee of the American Society of Reproductive medicine. *Fertil Steril* 2006;86(suppl 4):S148–S155.
4. Reindollar RH, Byrd JR, McDonough PG. Delayed sexual development: A study of 252 patients. *Am J Obstet Gynecol* 1981;140:371.
5. Reindollar RH, Novak M, Tho SP, et al. Adult-onset amenorrhea: A study of 262 patients. *Am J Obstet Gynecol* 1986;155:531.
6. Baird DT. Amenorrhea. *Lancet* 1997;350:275–279.
7. Krasna IH, Lee ML, Smilow P, et al. Risk of malignancy in bilateral streak gonads: The role of the Y chromosome. *J Pediatr Surg* 1992;27:1367.
8. Martin KA, Hall JE, Adams JM, et al. Comparison of exogenous gonadotropins and pulsatile gonadotropin-releasing hormone for induction of ovulation in hypogonadotropic amenorrhea. *J Clin Endocrinol Metab* 1993;77:125.

Gynecomastia

17

Scott Goodwin and Simon J. Fisher

GENERAL PRINCIPLES

Definition

Gynecomastia is a glandular enlargement of the male breast that is often asymmetrical or unilateral and may be tender.[1]

Classification

- Gynecomastia commonly occurs during the neonatal period, in puberty, with aging, and as a side effect of several medications.
- Gynecomastia can be divided into two large categories: physiologic or pathologic gynecomastia.
  - **Physiologic gynecomastia** occurs in the presence of normal fluctuations in hormonal levels observed at different ages. Treatment is typically not necessary, as the gynecomastia often resolves spontaneously.
    - Transient gynecomastia occurs in 60% to 90% of newborns due to high levels of circulating estrogen during pregnancy and typically regresses within 2 to 3 weeks after birth.[1]
    - Pubertal gynecomastia usually occurs in adolescents between the ages of 13 and 14 years, regresses within 18 months, and is uncommon after age 17. Gynecomastia results from transient imbalance of estrogen–androgen levels during puberty as estradiol concentrations rise to adult levels before testosterone concentrations.[1]
    - Gynecomastia of aging can occur in otherwise healthy older males in their 50s to 80s and is related to decreased testosterone synthesis leading to a relative increase in the estrogen-to-androgen ratio. Aging-associated increased body fat also contributes to gynecomastia via increased adipose tissue aromatization of testosterone to estradiol and of androstenedione to estrone.[1]
  - **Pathologic gynecomastia** is due to a congenital or acquired disease causing an imbalance of estrogen to androgen hormones in the circulation.
    - In contrast to women, estrogen is the only hormone that promotes breast growth and development in men.
    - Fundamentally, the pathogenesis of gynecomastia results from an increase in the estrogen-to-androgen ratio, which occurs via excessive estrogen production, deficient androgen production, increased estrogen precursors available for peripheral conversion, blockage of androgen receptors, and/or increased binding of androgen to sex-hormone binding globulin.

Etiology

The common causes of gynecomastia are summarized in Table 17-1.

TABLE 17-1 CAUSES OF GYNECOMASTIA

Physiologic causes
Neonatal period
Puberty
Aging

Pathologic causes
Decreased production/action of androgens: primary (Klinefelter's syndrome, trauma, viral orchitis) or secondary hypogonadism, enzymatic defects in testosterone synthesis, androgen resistance
Increased estrogen production: adrenal, testicular, or ectopic carcinoma producing estrogen or hCG, true hermaphroditism
Systemic illness: chronic liver or kidney disease, thyrotoxicosis, malnutrition, refeeding after starvation
Drugs: antiandrogens (spironolactone, finasteride), estrogens and their analogs, growth hormone, gonadotropins, calcium channel blockers, ACE inhibitors, amiodarone, digoxin, tricyclic antidepressants, haloperidol, diazepam, omeprazole, cimetidine, ranitidine, alkylating agents, antiretroviral agents, methotrexate, imatinib, phenytoin, phenothiazines, ketoconazole, isoniazid, metoclopramide, heroin, marijuana, methadone, alcohol, amphetamines, androgens, and anabolic steroids
Idiopathic

ACE, angiotensin-converting enzyme; hCG, human chorionic gonadotropin

Associated Conditions

- Conditions that decrease the production and effect of androgens[2]:
  - In **primary hypogonadism** there is a deficiency in testosterone production that leads to a compensatory increase in LH release and enhanced aromatization of testosterone to estradiol, resulting in relative estrogen excess, thereby producing gynecomastia.
    - Primary hypogonadism can be due to testicular disorders such as trauma, infections, vascular insufficiency, infiltrative disorders, congenital abnormalities (such as Klinefelter's syndrome), or enzymatic defects in the testosterone biosynthesis pathway.
  - **Secondary hypogonadism** can also be associated with gynecomastia, although this is less common. In secondary hypogonadism, the pituitary gland fails to produce LH, leading to decreased testosterone secretion, but the adrenal cortex continues to produce estrogen precursors that are aromatized in extraglandular tissues. The net effect is an estrogen–androgen imbalance, which can sometimes lead to excess production of breast tissue.
  - In **androgen insensitivity syndrome** there is ineffective testosterone action due to defects in or absence of intracellular androgen receptors in target tissues. Therefore, genotypic male patients appear as phenotypic females with breasts that resemble those of a normal woman.
- Conditions that increase the production of estrogen[2]:
  - Certain tumors secrete estrogen, causing patients to develop gynecomastia. Examples include Leydig and Sertoli cell tumors and feminizing adrenocortical carcinomas.

○ Patients with true hermaphroditism may have gynecomastia due to increased estrogen production from the ovarian component of their gonads.
○ Germ cell tumors of the testes or bronchogenic carcinomas can secrete human chorionic gonadotropin (hCG), which in turn stimulates Leydig cell aromatase activity leading to increased conversion of androgen precursors to estrone and estradiol, resulting in gynecomastia.
• Drugs can cause gynecomastia via several mechanisms[3] (Table 17-1):
○ Analogs of estrogen and gonadotropins directly increase estrogenic activity in the plasma.
○ Antiandrogens, such as spironolactone (Aldactone), block androgen receptors, thereby increasing the relative estrogen-to-androgen ratio.
○ Some drugs, such as alkylating agents and ketoconazole (Nizoral), suppress testosterone biosynthesis leading to increases in the estrogen-to-androgen ratio.
○ Other drugs induce gynecomastia by as yet unidentified mechanisms.
• Systemic illnesses have been associated with gynecomastia[2]:
○ Cirrhosis: roughly two-thirds of patients with cirrhosis have gynecomastia due to increased production of androstenedione from the adrenals as well as enhanced aromatization of androgens to estrone and estradiol.
○ End-stage kidney disease: as many as 50% of patients with end-stage renal disease on hemodialysis have gynecomastia as a result of Leydig cell dysfunction, leading to decreased testosterone levels.
○ Gynecomastia has also been associated with malnutrition, refeeding syndrome, and thyrotoxicosis.

DIAGNOSIS

Clinical Presentation

• True gynecomastia is characterized by a symmetric ridge of glandular tissue, is rubbery to firm in consistency, and contains a fibrous-like cord. Pseudogynecomastia presents with no discrete mass.[1]
• Key elements in the history include a detailed medication list, the timing of the onset, presence of breast pain, and symptoms of systemic illnesses such as liver disease, renal disease, or thyrotoxicosis.
• Physical examination should focus on breast and testicular exams as well as an assessment for virilization.

Differential Diagnosis

• Gynecomastia is caused by excessive estrogen action or an increased estrogen-to-androgen ratio. True gynecomastia needs to be differentiated from breast cancer and pseudogynecomastia.
○ **Pseudogynecomastia** occurs commonly in obese men and is characterized by adipose tissue deposition without glandular proliferation.[4]
○ **Male breast cancer** is rare and is generally unilateral and eccentric in location rather than symmetric to the nipple and may be associated with skin changes.[5]

Laboratory Evaluation

In the biochemical workup of gynecomastia, testosterone, estradiol, LH, prolactin, TSH, and hCG levels are measured to differentiate among various etiologies.[6]

- Interpretation of abnormal plasma **LH** and **testosterone** levels: an elevated LH and low testosterone are seen in primary hypogonadism. If both LH and testosterone levels are low, secondary hypogonadism is likely, provided prolactin levels are normal. If prolactin is elevated in this setting, it implies that hyperprolactinemia is the cause of the hypogonadism. An elevation of both LH and testosterone levels characterizes androgen resistance in the presence of normal thyroid function. Elevated LH and testosterone in the presence of a suppressed TSH level suggests hyperthyroidism as a cause for the gynecomastia.
- An elevated **β-hCG** level suggests an hCG-secreting neoplasm. Further evaluation should include testicular ultrasound to rule out testicular germ-cell tumors. If the patient has a normal testicular ultrasound, then a chest radiograph or abdominal computed tomography (CT) scan is necessary to localize an extragonadal germ cell tumor or bronchogenic carcinoma.
- An elevated **estradiol** level should be investigated with testicular ultrasound to rule out a Leydig or Sertoli cell tumor. If the ultrasound is normal, an adrenal CT scan or magnetic resonance imaging (MRI) is indicated to rule out an adrenal neoplasm. Workup should include a 24-hour urinary 17-ketosteroids level, which are elevated in adrenocortical carcinoma. If the adrenal imaging studies are negative, workup should focus on causes of increased extraglandular aromatase activity.
- If none of the above workup is revealing, a diagnosis of **idiopathic gynecomastia** may be entertained.

TREATMENT

- The approach to treatment depends on the etiology of the gynecomastia. Depending on the condition, appropriate treatments could include observation, surgery, and/or medical therapy. When an underlying cause for gynecomastia is identified, treatment of that condition typically resolves the gynecomastia.
- If the patient is taking medications associated with gynecomastia, discontinuation of the offending drugs is appropriate. Resultant symptomatic improvement generally confirms the diagnosis of drug-induced gynecomastia.
- A more conservative approach with periodic follow-up is appropriate if gynecomastia is asymptomatic and discovered during routine examination in a patient with no underlying disease and not taking medications associated with gynecomastia.

Nonpharmacologic Therapy
Observation is the initial step for most peripubecent males and for most men after stopping any potentially offending medications.

Medical Therapy
- Medical therapy is most effective during the earlier phases of gynecomastia. Medical therapy is usually reserved for men with severe painful gynecomastia while surgery is being contemplated.
- Several classes of medications have been studied, but none are currently approved by the FDA for treatment of gynecomastia.
  - **Selective estrogen receptor modulators (SERMs),** such as Tamoxifen 10 mg orally twice a day or Raloxifene 60 mg daily, have been used and shown to be effective for patients with painful gynecomastia.[6,7] However, these medications do not result in complete regression of breast tissue. Additionally, use of these

agents is associated with adverse side effects such as headache, nausea, impotence, and loss of libido, and patients tend to relapse after the medication has been discontinued.

○ Testosterone replacement is only useful in hypogonadal men. It has no utility in eugonadal men and, in some cases, could actually worsen gynecomastia due to aromatization of the additional testosterone to estradiol.

Surgical Management

Surgery is indicated if there is continued growth, tenderness, malignancy, cosmetic problems, or severe psychological problems or if the underlying cause cannot be corrected.[8]

REFERENCES

1. Braunstein GD. Gynecomastia. *N Engl J Med* 2007;357:1229–1237.
2. Wilson JD, Aiman J, MacDonald PC. The pathogenesis of gynecomastia. *Adv Intern Med* 1980;25:1–32.
3. Thompson DF, Carter JR. Drug-induced gynecomastia. *Pharmacotherapy* 1993;13:37–45.
4. Yazici M, Sahin M, Bolu E, et al. Evaluation of breast enlargement in young males and factors associated with gynecomastia and pseudogynecomastia. *Ir J Med Sci* 2010;179:575–583.
5. Volpe CM, Raffetto JD, Collure DW, et al. Unilateral male breast masses: Cancer risk and their evaluation and management. *Am Surg* 1999;65:250–253.
6. Gikas P, Mokbel K. Management of gynaecomastia: An update. *Int J Clin Pract* 2007;61:1209–1215.
7. Lawrence SE, Faught KA, Vethamuthu J, et al. Beneficial effects of raloxifene and tamoxifen in the treatment of pubertal gynecomastia. *J Pediatr* 2004;145:71–76.
8. Cordova A, Moschella F. Algorithm for clinical evaluation and surgical treatment of gynaecomastia. *J Plast Reconstr Aesthet Surg* 2008:61;41–49.

Hirsutism

18

Mariko Johnson and Kim Carmichael

GENERAL PRINCIPLES

Definition
- **Hirsutism** is the development of excessive androgen-dependent terminal body hair in a male distribution in a woman.
- True hirsutism needs to be differentiated from **hypertrichosis**, a condition in which there is an increase in androgen-independent total body hair.

Epidemiology
Hirsutism affects 5% of women of reproductive age and is commonly accompanied by other cutaneous manifestations such as acne and temporal hair loss.[1]

Etiology
- Hirsutism is caused by increased androgen production by the ovaries or adrenal glands or increased target-organ responsiveness to androgen.
- Although it may be a normal variant of hair growth, hirsutism can also be the first sign of a serious endocrine disorder.

Pathophysiology
- Androgens are necessary for the growth of sexual hair and transform vellus hair into terminal hair in sex-specific areas. Vellus hairs are fine, soft, and nonpigmented. Terminal hairs are thick, coarse, and pigmented.
- The growth cycles of terminal hairs are nonsynchronous and last approximately 4 months. Results of hormonal therapy for hirsutism may not be apparent for 6 months due to the long duration of the growth cycle.
- The levels of circulating androgens do not always correlate with the extent of hirsutism. Local conversion of testosterone to the more potent dihydrotestosterone and variability in sensitivity of the hair follicle to androgen also affect hair growth. Therefore, hirsutism can occur in the presence of normal circulating androgen levels.

DIAGNOSIS

The clinician should keep in mind the following **three goals in the approach to the patient with hirsutism:**
- Determine the underlying etiology, excluding rare but serious conditions first.
- Assess the degree of hirsutism in terms of objective measures and hirsutism-related patient distress.
- Assess reproductive goals, since hormonal treatment cannot be used in patients seeking pregnancy.

Clinical Presentation

History

- Most women with hirsutism have either the idiopathic form or polycystic ovary syndrome (PCOS). However, it is very important to exclude rare but serious causes of hirsutism such as androgen-secreting neoplasms or other underlying endocrinopathies.
- The following **clinical features** are **suggestive of an ovarian or adrenal neoplasm:**
  - Virilization (voice deepening, increased muscle mass, clitoromegaly, breast atrophy)
  - Late onset of symptoms (during or after the third decade of life)
  - Rapid progression of hirsutism
  - Significant elevations in levels of androgen
- Hirsutism can be seen in serious endocrine disorders such as Cushing's syndrome, thyroid dysfunction, hyperprolactinemia, severe insulin-resistance syndromes, or acromegaly. However, all of these disorders usually present with other typical disease-specific manifestations and are not a cause of isolated hirsutism.
- Even if no symptoms of a serious endocrine disorder are elicited, a full history including age of onset, distribution of hair growth, rapidity of progression, and associated features such as acne or temporal balding should be sought.
- A **menstrual history** is very important in the differential diagnosis of hirsutism. The presence of irregular menses distinguishes PCOS from idiopathic hirsutism. Irregular menses that are *acquired* with an onset after menarche may suggest one of the less common endocrinopathies listed since irregular menses due to PCOS usually present at menarche.
- A **weight history** should also be elicited since gradual weight gain over time is more consistent with and can worsen hirsutism due to PCOS, whereas rapid weight gain may suggest Cushing's syndrome.
- Certain **medications** can cause hirsutism, including oral contraceptives containing androgenic progestins, danazol, anabolic or androgenic steroids, and valproic acid.
- A fraction of women presenting with hirsutism will have nonclassic congenital adrenal hyperplasia (CAH), which may be suggested by ethnic background or family history.
- Clinicians should always **assess the degree to which patients are distressed by their hirsutism**, since idiopathic hirsutism that does not cause patient distress does not require treatment.
- Clinicians should always **discuss reproductive goals**, since hormonal treatments cannot be used in patients seeking pregnancy.

Physical Examination

- Physical examination should include measurement of **height, weight,** and **blood pressure** and calculation of **body mass index.**
- An **objective assessment of hair distribution and quality of hair** should be documented. A simple scoring scale can be used, such as the modified scale of Ferriman and Gallwey in which a score of 0 to 4 is given for each of the nine androgen-dependent sites (see Figure 18-1).
- **Skin** should be examined for acne, seborrhea, temporal balding, acanthosis nigricans, striae, abnormal thickness, or bruising.
- **Signs of virilization** such as deepening of the voice, increased muscle mass, and clitoromegaly should be carefully sought.

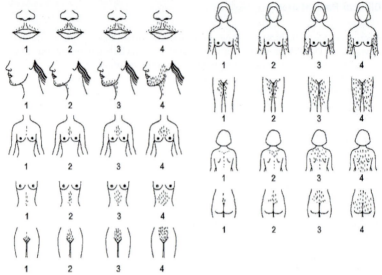

FIGURE 18-1 Modified Ferriman–Gallwey scale for assessing hirsutism. (Modified from Hatch, et al. Hirsutism: Implications, etiology, and management. *Am J Obstet Gynecol* 1981;140:815–830.)

Diagnostic Criteria

- A Ferriman–Gallwey score ≥8 has traditionally defined hirsutism, since 95% of white and black women of reproductive age have a score <8 (see Figure 18-1).
- The Ferriman–Gallwey score has several limitations, the most important of which are
  - "Normal" hair growth varies by ethnic group. Women of Mediterranean origin tend to have more hair, whereas Asian women have less hair in androgen-dependent areas.
  - Previous cosmetic treatments may not allow for accurate assessment of hair growth.
  - The scale does not reflect the degree of distress the hirsutism causes an individual patient.
- Therefore, clinicians should not be dogmatic in their approach and should instead focus their effort on uncovering and treating serious disorders that cause hirsutism. Once an underlying condition has been excluded, the clinician can focus on the cosmetic concerns of the individual patient.

Differential Diagnosis

- Causes of hirsutism are listed in Table 18-1 and fall into the following general categories:
- Polycystic ovary syndrome
  PCOS is the most common cause of hyperandrogenism in women of reproductive age. The criteria for diagnosis are menstrual irregularity and clinical or biochemical evidence of hyperandrogenism. Hirsutism usually develops within the first several years after menarche. Insulin resistance is thought to play a role in this disorder by promoting ovarian hyperandrogenism. Insulin and androgens also decrease the sex hormone–binding globulin (SHBG) concentration, thereby increasing the free

TABLE 18-1 CAUSES OF HIRSUTISM

Common causes
PCOS
Idiopathic

Other causes (less common)
Ovarian
Ovarian neoplasms
Ovarian hyperthecosis
Severe insulin resistance syndromes

Adrenal
Classic and nonclassic congenital adrenal hyperplasia
Adrenal neoplasms
Cushing's syndrome
Glucocorticoid resistance

Drugs
Androgenic progestins, anabolic and androgenic steroids, danazol, valproic acid

Other endocrine disorders
Hyperprolactinemia, acromegaly, hypothyroidism

Pregnancy-related hyperandrogenism
Luteoma of pregnancy, hyperreactio luteinalis, fetal aromatase deficiency

—

PCOS, polycystic ovary syndrome.

Adapted from Bulun SE, Adashi, E.Y. The Physiology and Pathology of the Female
Reproductive Axis. In: Kronenberg HM, Melmed, S., Polonsky, K.S., Larsen, P.R., editor.
Williams Textbook of Endocrinology. 11th ed. Philadelphia, PA: Saunders/Elsevier, 2008.

testosterone level. The clinical features, diagnosis, and management of PCOS are discussed in Chapter 20.

• **Idiopathic hirsutism**
Idiopathic hirsutism can be diagnosed when regular menses, normal serum androgen levels, and no identifiable underlying disorder are present. It may represent a mild form of PCOS, but the absence of irregular menses distinguishes this disorder from PCOS.

• **Ovarian neoplasms**
Androgen-secreting tumors of the ovary usually occur later in life and progress rapidly. Sertoli–Leydig cell tumors, hilus-cell tumors, and granulosa-theca cell tumors are a few examples.

• **Adrenal neoplasms**
Adrenal neoplasms can secrete dehydroepiandrosterone sulfate (DHEA-S), dehydroepiandrosterone (DHEA), androstenedione, cortisol (Cushing's syndrome), and in rare instances, testosterone.

• **Congenital adrenal hyperplasia**
CAH usually presents at birth or in early infancy, but late-onset or nonclassic forms of CAH present at puberty with hirsutism and menstrual irregularity. The nonclassic form of CAH is usually due to 21-hydroxylase deficiency and results in excessive production of 17-hydroxyprogesterone and androstenedione.

• **Other causes**
Certain medications, conditions associated with pregnancy, and other endocrinopathies are rare causes of hirsutism (see Table 18-1).[2]

Diagnostic Testing

- Patients with isolated mild hirsutism do not require testing for elevated androgen levels.
- Patients with moderate or severe hirsutism, or hirsutism of any degree associated with symptoms compatible with PCOS or an androgen-secreting neoplasm, should be evaluated for androgen excess. These symptoms include
  - ○ Signs of virilization
  - ○ Rapid progression of hirsutism
  - ○ Menstrual irregularity
  - ○ Acanthosis nigricans
  - ○ Central obesity
- Patients with features of an underlying endocrine disorder should be evaluated for that disorder.

Laboratory Studies

- **Serum testosterone**
  Serum testosterone can be measured either as total or free testosterone and provides the best overall estimate of androgen production in hirsute women. Free testosterone, the biologically active form, is typically elevated in women with androgen excess even when total levels are within the normal range. Therefore, free testosterone is the most sensitive test for androgen excess, but reliability of the assay (particularly radioimmunoassays) is variable. Testing for total testosterone is widely available and better standardized. Serum total testosterone is often >200 ng/dL in women with androgen-secreting tumors.[1] Patients with PCOS or idiopathic hirsutism typically have normal or slightly elevated levels of testosterone.
- **Serum dehydroepiandrosterone sulfate**
  Measuring DHEA-S is indicated to rule out adrenal androgen excess when signs of virilization are present or symptoms are abrupt in onset and rapidly progressive. Women with androgen-secreting adrenal tumors typically have DHEA-S levels >700 mcg/dL.[1]
- **Serum prolactin**
  Prolactin can be measured in women with hirsutism and irregular menstrual cycles to rule out hyperprolactinemia.
- **Serum thyroid stimulating hormone**
  Thyroid stimulating hormone (TSH) can be measured in women with hirsutism and irregular menstrual cycles to rule out hypothyroidism.
- **Serum 17-hydroxyprogesterone**
  Measurement of 17-hydroxyprogesterone is useful to differentiate between late-onset CAH and PCOS. Testing in women of Hispanic, Yugoslav, or Eastern European Jewish origin may have a higher yield due to increased prevalence. Because oral contraceptives and/or antiandrogens are the first-line treatments for hirsutism due to late onset CAH and PCOS,[3] formal diagnosis of late onset CAH may not be necessary unless pregnancy is desired.
- **Screening tests for Cushing's syndrome**
  Cushing's syndrome and PCOS can present in a similar fashion with hirsutism, irregular menses, and weight gain. Screening tests for Cushing's syndrome include the low dose dexamethasone suppression test, 24-hour urine collection for free cortisol, or measurement of late-night salivary cortisol. For a full description of these tests, see Chapter 14.
- **Other tests**
  Tests to rule out insulin resistance syndromes or acromegaly may also be warranted in the appropriate clinical setting.

Imaging

Radiologic studies, such as pelvic ultrasound and abdominal CT and MRI, are indicated only if a tumor is suspected.

TREATMENT

- Treatment for hirsutism should focus first on identification of treatable underlying disorders. For idiopathic hirsutism or hirsutism due to PCOS, an underlying etiology is not yet well defined.
- Patients may be treated systemically with medications and/or locally with direct hair removal according to patient preference.
- The response to pharmacologic therapy is slow, and a trial of at least 6 months should be given before doses are changed or new medications are added.
- None of the pharmacologic treatments for hirsutism result in permanent hair removal, and hirsutism generally recurs with discontinuation of therapy.

Medications

- **Hormonal treatment for hirsutism should only be considered in women not desiring pregnancy.**
- Oral contraceptives are the first-line medical therapy for hirsutism in most cases. If response is inadequate after 6 months of treatment with oral contraceptives, an antiandrogen can be added. **Because of their teratogenic potential, antiandrogens should never be used in premenopausal women unless adequate contraceptive measures are used.** Other agents are not considered first-line agents for hirsutism.
- **Oral contraceptives**
  - Combination estrogen–progestin oral contraceptives are the best first-line agents in patients who do not desire pregnancy.
  - A preparation that contains ethinyl estradiol in conjunction with a progestin with minimal androgenic activity (desogestrel or norgestimate) or antiandrogenic activity (drosperinone) should be selected.
  - Oral contraceptives act to reduce hirsutism through a variety of mechanisms. They cause a suppression of luteinizing hormone (LH) release, leading to decreased ovarian androgen production; an increase in SHBG levels, thereby lowering the free testosterone level; and a mild reduction in adrenal androgen production, and they slightly inhibit the binding of androgen to its receptor.
- **Antiandrogens**
  - **Spironolactone** (100 to 200 mg orally daily) can decrease the effect of androgens by blocking the androgen receptor. When used in combination with an oral contraceptive, both androgen levels and action are decreased. Spironolactone can cause hyperkalemia, and a potassium level should be checked after initiation of therapy and with dose titration. Menstrual irregularity can be prevented by concomitant use of oral contraceptives.
  - **Finasteride** (5 mg orally daily) competitively inhibits 5-α-reductase and can also be used to treat hirsutism by reducing dihydrotestosterone levels.
  - **Flutamide** is not FDA approved for treatment of hirsutism, and its use is limited as it can cause hepatotoxicity.[3] Topical antiandrogens are not currently recommended due to inconclusive data regarding their efficacy. Cyproterone acetate is an antiandrogen widely available worldwide but not currently available in the United States.

- **Gonadotropin-releasing hormone (GnRH) agonists**
  GnRH agonists inhibit ovarian androgen production by inhibiting gonadotropins. The ensuing estrogen deficiency can be treated with a combination estrogen–progestin pill. The GnRH agonist–oral contraceptive combination is more cumbersome, more expensive, and has not been shown to be more efficacious than the antiandrogen–contraceptive combination. Therefore, it should only be used as second-line therapy in cases of severe hirsutism, and bone density should be monitored during treatment.[3]

- **Glucocorticoids**
  - Glucocorticoids, which suppress adrenal androgen production, are no longer considered a first-line treatment option for hirsutism due to nonclassical CAH, as oral contraceptive pills and antiandrogens may be more efficacious and have a better side effect profile.[3]
  - Glucocorticoids can be used as a second-line treatment for hirsutism in CAH patients with a poor response to, intolerance of, or contraindication to oral contraceptives and/or antiandrogens.[3]
  - Dexamethasone (0.2 to 0.5 mg) or prednisone (5 to 10 mg) should be taken at bedtime to suppress the nocturnal surge of ACTH.

- **Insulin-lowering drugs**
  The benefits of the insulin-sensitizing drugs (metformin and the thiazolinediones) in treating hirsutism are not well established and as such cannot be recommended for treatment of idiopathic hirsutism.[3] However, metformin is often prescribed to treat the metabolic derangements of PCOS.

- **Other**
  Topical eflornithine applied twice daily can be used for treatment of facial hirsutism.

Other Nonpharmacologic Therapies

Nonpharmacologic treatment should be considered in all patients, either as the sole treatment or as an adjunct to drug therapy. Weight loss should be encouraged in overweight or obese women, as it can lower androgen levels and improve hirsutism. Bleaching, waxing, shaving, depilatories, electrolysis, and laser treatment are all ways of removing undesired hair. Electrolysis and laser treatment can be expensive, time consuming, and painful but can have long-lasting effects.

PATIENT EDUCATION

Pharmacologic treatment for hirsutism can be expected to reduce, not eliminate, terminal hair growth. Realistic goals of treatment should be explained to patients beginning treatment for hirsutism.

REFERENCES

1. Rosenfield RL. Clinical practice. Hirsutism. *N Engl J Med* 2005;353:2578–2588.
2. Bulun SE, Adashi, EY. The Physiology and Pathology of the Female Reproductive Axis. In: Kronenberg HM, Melmed S, Polonsky KS, Larsen PR, eds. *Williams Textbook of Endocrinology.* 11th ed. Philadelphia, PA: Saunders/Elsevier, 2008: chapter 16.
3. Martin KA, Chang RJ, Ehrmann DA, et al. Evaluation and treatment of hirsutism in premenopausal women: An endocrine society clinical practice guideline. *J Clin Endocrinol Metab* 2008;93:1105–1120.

Male Hypogonadism

19

Shunzhong Bao and Stephen J. Giddings

GENERAL PRINCIPLES

Symptoms of male hypogonadism depend on the age of the patient at the onset of disease.[1] The production of an adequate amount of testosterone is necessary for the development of external genitalia and secondary sexual characteristics in children and adolescents. In adults, androgen production is necessary for the maintenance of lean body mass, bone mass, libido, sexual function, and spermatogenesis.[1-3] Men with a total testosterone level less than ~300 ng/dL often develop symptoms and signs of hypogonadism that can have long-term clinical effects.

Definition

Male hypogonadism is defined as the **failure of the testes to produce testosterone, sperm, or both.**

Classification

- Hypogonadism is classified as primary, secondary, and combined primary and secondary hypogonadism.
- **Primary hypogonadism** is caused by failure of the testis (hypergonadotropic hypogonadism).
- **Secondary hypogonadism** is caused by defects at the hypothalamic-pituitary level (hypogonadotrophic hypogonadism).
- The **combined form,** manifested by both testicular and hypothalamic-pituitary defects, may occur with hemochromatosis, sickle cell disease, thalassemia, glucocorticoid treatment, alcoholism, and DAX-1 mutations, and in older men.
- **Late-onset of hypogonadism** is a distinct clinical syndrome associated with age, which is characterized by symptoms of and a deficiency in serum testosterone levels.[4]
- Rarely, hypogonadism can be due to defects at the receptor level as seen in androgen-resistance syndromes, which are characterized by resistance to the effects of testosterone.

Epidemiology

- Four to 5 million men in the United States have hypogonadism.
- In longitudinal studies, as men advance in age, total testosterone declines. Serum testosterone declines at ~1% to 2% a year after age 30. It is estimated that 30% to 40% of men older than 65 years of age, and 79% to 80% of men older than age 80 have hypogonadism.[1,5,6]

Etiology

Primary Hypogonadism

- **Developmental defects**
  - ○ **Klinefelter's syndrome** is the most common congenital defect causing male hypogonadism (1 in 1000 males). Clinical features include small, firm testis; varying degrees of impaired sexual development; azoospermia; gynecomastia; and elevated gonadotrophins. The underlying defect is the presence of an extra X chromosome, 47, XXY being the most common. Diagnosis is confirmed by karyotype analysis.[7]
  - ○ The 46,XY/XO karyotype (mosaic for loss of Y chromosome) clinically presents with a broad spectrum from Turner syndrome to mixed gonadal dysgenesis (MGD), male pseudohermaphroditism (MPH), or phenotypically normal male. The gonads vary from streak to normal testes. If both a streak gonad and a dysgenetic testis ("mixed gonadal dysgenesis") are found, there is at least a 20% risk of developing gonadoblastoma. Therefore, gonadectomy should be performed.[8,9]
  - ○ Mutations in genes encoding testosterone synthesis and secretion can lead to a decrease or absence of testeosterone secretion. This occurs in the first trimester of pregancy, leading to incomplete virilization.
- **Acquired diseases**
  - ○ **Mumps** is the most common infection affecting the testis and may lead to infertility and reduced testosterone levels.
  - ○ **Radiation** affects both spermatogenesis and testosterone production. Impaired testosterone production is caused by reduced blood flow to the testis. The extent of damage to Leydig cells is directly related to the dose of radiation and inversely related to age.[10]
  - ○ **Drugs** such as ketoconazole (Nizoral), spironolactone (Aldactone), and cyproterone interfere with testosterone synthesis. Enzyme-inducing drugs, such as phenytoin (Dilantin) and carbamazepine (Carbatrol), can lower bioavailable testosterone, raise SHBG and LH levels, and decrease metabolic clearance. Ethanol ingestion reduces testosterone levels by inhibiting the synthesis of testosterone and impairing the hypothalamic-pituitary axis. Cyclophosphamide and other alkylating agents can induce infertility. Spironolactone, cyproterone, cimetidine, and omeprazole compete for the androgen receptor causing gynecomastia and impotence.[1,11]
  - ○ Systemic illnesses, such as renal failure (testicular failure, hyperprolactinemia), liver failure (both testicular failure and inhibition of the hypothalamic-pituitary axis), sickle cell disease, chronic illness, thyrotoxicosis, HIV, and immune disorders can lead to hypergonadotrophic hypogonadism.

Secondary Hypogonadism

- **Congenital disorders**
  - ○ **Idiopathic hypogonadotropic hypogonadism** (IHH) is a rare heterogeneous disorder caused by isolated GnRH deficiency.
    - Affected individuals present in teenage years because of deficient sexual maturation. They have a normal male phenotype at birth because maternal human chorionic gonadotropin (hCG) stimulates normal sexual differentiation in the first trimester.
    - Affected individuals have impaired phallic development characterized by microphallus at birth owing to lack of testosterone production in the final trimester. Clinical features include delayed bone age (typically not beyond 11 to 12 years in

males), osteopenia, eunuchoid body proportions, gynecomastia, and delayed puberty. These patients have low testosterone and LH levels.

- Male patients with testes ≥4 cm have incomplete IHH, but those with testes <4 cm have complete IHH. Gonadotropin and testosterone values cannot differentiate between the two disorders.
- IHH must be differentiated from delay of puberty, and the diagnosis cannot be made until patients are >18 years of age. Pulsatile GnRH treatment induces full pubertal development.
- Karyotype analysis is not recommended unless multiple congenital anomalies are present or if there is a suspicion of Prader–Willi syndrome (deletion of 15q11–q13). IHH has been associated with mutation in KAL1 (X-linked recessive), GNRHR (autosomal recessive), and FGFR1 (autosomal dominant).

○ **Kallmann's syndrome** is characterized by hypogonadotropic hypogonadism and hyposmia with or without other nongonadal anomalies. Some patients with the X-linked form have a deletion of the KAL1 gene located on short arm of the X chromosome, which prevents migration of GnRH neurons to the brain from the olfactory placode during embryogenesis. Patients may also have midfacial clefting, renal agenesis, and neurologic abnormalities (deafness, cerebellar dysfunction, mental retardation, eye abnormalities).[11]

○ Secondary hypogonadism can also occur in Laurence–Moon syndrome and Bardet–Biedl syndrome.

○ Androgen receptor dysfunction causes incomplete virilization in 46XY males, who have bilateral testes and normal testosterone production. The diagnosis should be considered in girls with inguinal or labial masses, women with primary amenorrhea, adolescent girls who become virilized and develop clitoromegaly, adolescent boys who have persistent gynecomastia and fail to undergo puberty, and adult males with undervirilization or infertility associated with azoospermia or severe oligospermia.

○ In addition, hypogonadotropic hypogonadism can be caused by impaired development of the pituitary gland. Mutations in the PROP1 gene result in absence of several pituitary hormones, including growth hormone, thyroid-stimulating hormone (TSH), prolactin, and gonadotropins. PROP1 encodes a protein expressed in the embryonic pituitary necessary for function of POU1F1, which codes for a pituitary transcription factor. HESX1 gene mutations result in septooptic dysplasia, which may include poor development of the pituitary.[12]

- **Acquired disorders**
  ○ Any disease that affects the hypothalamic-pituitary axis by one of the following mechanisms leads to hypogonadotropic hypogonadism.
    - Hypothalamus—impairs GnRH secretion.
    - Pituitary stalk—inhibits GnRH from reaching the pituitary gland.
    - Pituitary gland—directly impairs LH and FSH secretion.
  ○ **Mass lesions** of the pituitary or hypothalamus preferentially affect gonadotropins. In many patients with space-occupying lesions, adrenocorticotropic hormone (ACTH) and TSH are unaffected. Gonadotropin deficiency may result from a space-occupying lesion of the sella, either by destroying the pituitary gland or by interrupting the nerve fibers that bring GnRH to the hypophyseal circulation. Patients present with headaches, visual disturbances, and variable manifestations of hypopituitarism.
  ○ **ACTH-producing tumors** can cause impotence, decreased libido, and infertility. Testosterone levels are low, and GnRH-stimulated LH concentrations are suppressed.

- **Prolactinoma** affects pulsatile GnRH secretion, subsequently causing hypogonadism. Men have low testosterone levels and attenuated pulsatile LH secretion. Treatment with dopamine agonists can normalize prolactin levels and restore sexual function.
- **Infiltrative diseases** such as Langerhans' cell histiocytosis and sarcoidosis may involve the hypothalamus and pituitary gland, thereby causing hypogonadism. Hemochromatosis can cause selective gonadotropin deficiency owing to deposition of iron in the pituitary cells.
- **Leydig cell tumors** and **adrenal tumors** produce estradiol, leading to gynecomastia and gonadotropin deficiency. hCG secreted by choriocarcinoma can increase estradiol levels and suppress gonadotropins.
- **Trauma** severing the pituitary stalk, postinfectious lesions of the central nervous system (CNS), vascular abnormalities of the CNS, critical illness, chronic narcotic administration, exogenous steroids, brain irradiation, and pituitary apoplexy are some other causes of secondary hypogonadism. Traumatic brain injury may cause temporary or persistent pituitary hypofunction of one or several axes (up to 68.5%).[13,14] The most commonly affected is the pituitary gonadal axis (up to 22.7% in some series). This is followed in frequency by growth hormone deficiency (~18.2%) and ACTH and TSH (both 5% or less).[15]
- **Excessive exercise** can cause hypothalamic hypogonadism in men similar to exercise-induced hypothalamic amenorrhea in women. Serial measurement of testosterone levels has been proposed as one means of screening for overtraining syndromes in elite male athletes.
- **Chronic opiate use** may also suppress the pituitary–gonadal axis and result in profound suppression of testosterone. This effect may be ameliorated by participation in substance abuse programs or by switching to buprenorphine.
- **Primary hypothyroidism** can cause hyperprolactinemia and hypogonadism (due to elevated thyrotropin-releasing hormone [TRH]).

Pathophysiology

- The testis functions as part of the hypothalamic-pituitary–gonadal axis. A hypothalamic pulse generator resides in the arcuate nucleus, which releases gonadotropin-releasing hormone (GnRH) into the hypothalamic-pituitary portal system.
- In response to these pulses of GnRH, the anterior pituitary secretes the gonadotropins—follicle-stimulating hormone (FSH) and luteinizing hormone (LH)—which in turn stimulate gonadal activity.
- LH and FSH control testosterone production by Leydig cells and spermatozoa production by seminiferous tubules. GnRH, LH, and FSH secretion is controlled by negative feedback from the testis by testosterone and inhibin B. Testosterone is the major product of Leydig cells. LH stimulates the testis in a pulsatile manner, resulting from the pulsatile GnRH secretion by the hypothalamus. An adult testis produces approximately 7 mg of testosterone daily. FSH is necessary for seminiferous tubule growth. FSH and LH control seminiferous tubule production of sperm. The action of LH is through local secretion of testosterone. Both FSH and testosterone are required to stimulate spermatogenesis quantitatively.
- LH secretion is negatively regulated by testosterone, estradiol, and dihydrotestosterone (DHT). FSH is under the negative influence of inhibin B and testosterone. They are stimulated in a pulsatile fashion by GnRH.

- Sixty percent of testosterone is transported in plasma bound to sex hormone–binding globulin (SHBG), 1% to 3% is free, and the remainder is bound to albumin. Both free testosterone and albumin-bound testosterone are bioavailable.[16]
- Circulating SHBG levels (and, therefore, total testosterone) can be increased in chronic hepatitis, hyperthyroidism, HIV infection, estrogen use, and anticonvulsant use. Reduction in SHBG level is associated with aging, obesity, low-protein states (nephrotic syndrome), hypothyroidism, hyperinsulinism, and glucocorticoid use.[17–20]
- Approximately 6% to 8% of testosterone is converted to more potent DHT by 5-α-reductase in prostate, testis, liver, kidney, and skin. A small proportion (0.2%) of testosterone is converted to estradiol by aromatase.
- The actions of testosterone are the combined effects of testosterone, plus its active androgenic (DHT) and estrogenic (estradiol) metabolites.[1]
- The testosterone-receptor complex is responsible for gonadotropin regulation, stimulation of spermatogenesis, and virilization of the Wolffian ducts, whereas the DHT-receptor complex mediates virilization of the external genitalia during embryogenesis and most of the virilization that occurs at male puberty. Estradiol inhibits gonadotropin secretion and promotes epiphyseal maturation in the adolescent male.
- Hypogonadism may occur if the hypothalamic-pituitary–gonadal axis is interrupted at any level.[7]
- Primary hypogonadism results if the testis does not produce the amount of sex steroid sufficient to suppress secretion of LH and FSH to normal levels.
- Secondary hypogonadism may result from failure of the hypothalamic GnRH pulse generator or from inability of the pituitary to respond with secretion of LH and/or FSH.
- Most commonly, secondary hypogonadism is observed as one aspect of multiple pituitary hormone deficiencies resulting from malformations or lesions of the pituitary that are acquired postnatally.

DIAGNOSIS

- Diagnosis is based on a thorough history, physical examination, and laboratory data. The general scheme for assessment of hypogonadism is outlined in Figure 19-1.
- Testosterone levels are high in the morning and reach nadir in the afternoon. The magnitude of this diurnal rhythm decreases with age. In men 30 to 40 years old, testosterone levels were 20% to 25% lower at 1600h than 0800h, compared to 10% difference in men 70 years old.[21] Although diurnal variation is less, older men who are thought to have low testosterone by virtue of an afternoon measurement should be retested with a morning testosterone measurement.
- Late-onset hypogonadism is a distinct entity. The diagnosis is still controversial since testosterone levels naturally decline with age. There is no cut off of testosterone level for diagnosis. Generally speaking, the diagnosis is made based on total testosterone levels that are lower than the limit of young normal range in context of symptoms or signs suggesting hypogonadism.[2,22] There is a consensus that patients with serum total testosterone levels below 230 ng/dL will usually benefit from testosterone replacement.[2,22]

Clinical Presentation

- Clinical features depend on whether the impairment involves spermatogenesis or testosterone secretion, or both. It also depends on the time of onset of the defect. Impaired spermatogenesis typically leads to reduced sperm count and testicular size.

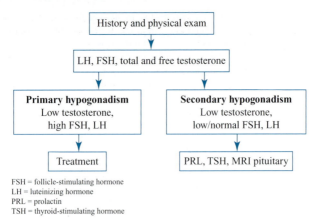

FSH = follicle-stimulating hormone
LH = luteinizing hormone
PRL = prolactin
TSH = thyroid-stimulating hormone

FIGURE 19-1 Algorithm for assessment of hypogonadism. FSH, follicle-stimulating hormone; LH, luteinizing hormone; PRL, prolactin; TSH, thyroid-stimulating hormone.

- Reduced testosterone production during the first trimester of pregnancy leads to partial virilization—ranging from severe deficiency causing posterior labial fusion to mild deficiency resulting in hypospadias. Complete lack of testosterone during this period results in female external genitalia (both clitoris and labia).
- If the defect occurs during the third trimester, it leads to micropenis and cryptorchidism.
- If testosterone production is inhibited before puberty, males will fail to initiate (average age 14) or complete puberty (completed in 3 to 4 years).
- Postpubertal deficit leads to decreased libido, muscle mass, hair growth, energy, mood, concentration, hematocrit, and bone mass. Decreased libido and fatigue are most readily experienced, whereas other symptoms take years to manifest. Long-standing hypogonadism in males manifests with decreased facial hair growth (female hair distribution) and development of fine wrinkles at the corners of the mouth and eyes.
- Hypogonadism has been associated with several comorbid conditions, including metabolic syndrome, diabetes, dyslipidemia, sleep apnea, and erectile dysfunction.
- Primary hypogonadism is more common than the secondary form and is more likely to be associated with a decrease in sperm production than in a decrease in testosterone production.
- Primary hypogonadism is more likely to be associated with gynecomastia. Supranormal serum FSH and LH levels stimulate testicular aromatase to increase the conversion of testosterone to estradiol, resulting in elevated levels of estradiol relative to testosterone.

History
- History should include developmental milestones, with emphasis on sexual development, current symptoms, and information pertaining to possible causes. History of ambiguous genitalia; micropenis; cryptorchidism; failed or delayed puberty; or decrease in libido, sexual function, and/or energy gives clues regarding time of onset of the hypogonadism.
- Inquiry should be made into the rapidity of onset and progression of the symptoms, presence or absence of early morning erections, and changes in voice, muscle strength, or hair growth.

- Ask about history of headache, visual problems, symptoms suggestive of kidney or liver disease, depression, thyroid disease, drug abuse, chemotherapy, radiation therapy, and anosmia.
- History of ethanol abuse, opiate abuse, history of brain trauma injury, and medication history can yield important clues regarding the etiology of the disease.
- Patients should also be screened for sleep apnea symptoms. It is unknown if obstructive sleep apnea precedes testosterone deficiency or is a clinical manifestation of it.
- Inquire about history of other comorbid diseases such as metabolic syndrome, diabetes, osteoporosis, bone fracture, and coronary artery disease.

Physical Examination

- A complete physical examination should be done to look for the presence of eunuchoid proportions (a lower body segment [floor to pubis] that is more than 2 cm longer than upper body segment [pubis to crown], and an arm span that is more than 5 cm longer than height), other developmental anomalies, visual problems, abnormal hair distribution, and gynecomastia.[1]
- Examination of the external genitalia should include measuring testicular size (normal, 4 to 7 cm) and volume (normal, 15 to 30 mL) and Tanner stage for adolescents. Consistency of the testicle should also be noted. Typically, firm testes are associated with Klinefelter's syndrome owing to hyalinization or fibrosis. Small, rubbery testes are characteristically found in prepubertal males, whereas postpubertal testicular atrophy results in a soft or mushy consistency. Gynecomastia may be present, as may increased body fat and reduced muscle mass.
- Physical findings are not always present in adults, since some secondary sexual characteristics, such as reduced muscle mass, may take years to develop. In such instances, appropriate laboratory evaluation may be helpful.

Diagnostic Criteria

The history and physical examination will suggest hypogonadism and laboratory data will reveal an unequivocal lower level of testosterone, usually <300 ng/dL. Further categorization into a diagnosis of primary, secondary, or combined hypogonadism is necessary. The diagnosis of late onset of hypogonadism is made in a similar manner.

Differential Diagnosis

Patients with other diseases may present with similar signs and symptoms. Patients with headaches, visual problems, galactorrhea, papilledema, or optic disc pallor should raise concern for a pituitary tumor. Malaise, fatigue, anorexia, and weight loss are seen in hypopituitarism.

Diagnostic Testing

Laboratories

- **Initial laboratory evaluation** should include (preferably morning between 8 AM and 10 AM) **testosterone, FSH, LH, and prolactin levels.** Presence of low testosterone with elevated FSH and LH denotes primary hypogonadism, whereas low testosterone and low or normal FSH and LH levels indicate secondary hypogonadism.
- A man with total testosterone levels below 300 ng/dL is likely hypogonadal, but levels need to be repeated. Levels between 200 and 400 ng/dL should be repeated with measurement of free testosterone. Diurnal variations in the levels of testosterone need to be considered when interpreting results. As men age, there may be less diurnal

variation, but sampling time may still be important in some individuals. Thus, it is preferable to obtain an AM level after one low testosterone level measurement.

- **Measuring free testosterone** becomes important when an abnormality affecting SHBG levels is suspected. Obesity may cause a decrease in sex hormone–binding globulin, thereby causing a lowered total testosterone but normal free testosterone.
- **Semen analysis** is the best means of analyzing sperm count and is typically ordered for men who desire fertility. It should be performed after 1 to 3 days of sexual abstinence and examined within 2 hours of specimen collection. Sperm are analyzed for number, motility, and morphology. Typically, normal semen analysis parameters are $>20 \times 10^6$ sperm per mL, $>50\%$ progressive motility, and $>30\%$ normal morphology (lower limits are permissible for patients desiring artificial reproductive technology). Abnormal results might be caused by recent fever, trauma, or drug exposure that can transiently impair spermatogenesis.
- Subnormal sperm count and supranormal serum FSH in the setting of normal serum testosterone concentration and normal LH concentration indicate damage to seminiferous tubules (resulting in loss of inhibin feedback on FSH secretion), whereas testosterone production by Leydig cells remains normal.
- If secondary hypogonadism is suspected, a **prolactin level, TSH, free thyroxine (T_4), and cortisol** (8 AM level or cosyntropin stimulation testing) should be performed.
- Other laboratory tests may be indicated if HIV, ESRD, hemochromatosis, Langerhans' cell histiocytosis, or sarcoidosis is suggested.

Imaging

Magnetic resonance imaging (MRI) is indicated if a low testosterone level and low LH or elevated prolactin level is found. If other pituitary hormones are abnormal or if visual field abnormalities or other neurologic abnormalities are present, an MRI of the pituitary gland must be ordered to rule out a lesion. If an MRI is contraindicated, although of inferior quality, a head computed tomography (CT) scan with and without contrast could be performed to visualize larger lesions.

TREATMENT

Medications

- **Testosterone** should be administered only to men who are hypogonadal, as evidenced by symptoms and signs consistent with androgen deficiency and a distinctly subnormal serum testosterone concentration. Increasing the serum testosterone in a man who has symptoms suggestive of hypogonadism but has normal testosterone concentrations will typically not relieve those symptoms.
- Treatment for both primary and secondary hypogonadism consists of replacing testosterone. The following are initial dose and preparation recommendations.
  - Testosterone enanthate/cypionate intramuscular injections, 75 to 100 mg weekly or 150 to 200 mg every 2 weeks
  - Testosterone gel (Androgel or Testim), 2.5 to 5 g applied topically to upper arm or other covered area each day
  - Transdermal testosterone (Androderm), 5 mg patch daily
  - Scrotal patch, 6 mg patch daily (hair needs to shaved and adhesive may not last 24 hours)
  - Buccal tablet (Striant), 30 mg twice daily

- Generally, the gels are the most costly, whereas patches and injectable esters are the least expensive. The possibility of skin transfer of the gel to a female partner or children in close contact is possible and needs to be avoided by washing thoroughly before close contact.[2]

Other Nonpharmacologic Therapies

- Therapeutic lifestyle changes are also indicated in treating male hypogonadism. It is still controversial if physical inactivity, alcohol, and smoking decrease testosterone levels. However, physical inactivity leads to obesity, which increases SHBG, while alcohol and smoking have detrimental effects on seminal parameters.
- **Urgent surgical correction is needed if cryptorchidism is found.**
- A pituitary or hypothalamus mass might need surgical or radiation therapy or medical therapy for prolactinoma.

SPECIAL CONSIDERATIONS

- Patients with secondary hypogonadism desiring fertility can be treated with pulsatile GnRH or gonadotropins with hCG. Spermatogenesis can also be stimulated by GnRH in men who have secondary hypogonadism from hypothalamic disease. Replacement of GnRH in a physiologic manner will cause secretion of LH and FSH, which in turn will stimulate the testes to produce testosterone and sperm. hCG stimulates the testes to make testosterone and is especially useful in stimulating both testosterone and sperm production. FSH is typically not used, since it is extremely costly and LH and hCG alone can stimulate spermatogenesis.[2,23,24]
- Use of gonadotropins in conjunction with artificial reproductive technologies is also a consideration.
- Some experts also suggest considering short-term testosterone therapy as an adjunctive therapy in HIV-infected men with low testosterone levels and weight loss to promote weight maintenance and gains in lean body mass and muscle strength,[2] or for hypogonadal men receiving high doses of glucocorticoids to promote preservation of lean body mass and bone mineral density.[2]

MONITORING/FOLLOW-UP

- Serum testosterone measurements are helpful to assess the adequacy of treatment and should be checked 2 to 3 months after initiating treatment. They should be measured midway between injections in patients receiving injectable testosterone. The dosage should be adjusted to maintain total testosterone levels in the mid-normal range (400 to 700 ng/dL). In patients treated with a testosterone patch, levels should be checked 3 to 12 hours after application. With use of the gel or buccal tablets, serum levels of testosterone can be measured at any time and should be in the mid- or low-normal range.
- In postpubertal men, it is reasonable to **treat with the minimum amount of testosterone that alleviates symptoms** of decreased libido, impaired sexual function, and energy levels.
- In primary hypogonadism, normalization of serum LH can be used as a surrogate marker to determine the adequacy of therapy.
- Assessment of effectiveness is very reasonable after 3 months of treatment. If there is no improvement in symptoms and signs, the treatment should be terminated.

- **Assessment of bone density** at 2-year intervals is advised in hypogonadal men and serum testosterone measurements should be obtained in all men with less than normal bone mineral density.[12]
- Transdermal testosterone patches can be associated with skin rash and itching and may require application of corticosteroid cream. Men treated with testosterone injections will have wide swings of plasma testosterone levels and can develop emotional and physiologic effects. These include breast tenderness, hyperactivity at peak levels, and at the nadir fatigue, depression, or anger. Thus, it is advisable to start at lower doses, especially in older men, and then titrate upward to reduce mood fluctuations. Buccal preparations can cause gingival irritation, taste perversion, and bitter taste.
- Patients receiving testosterone should be **monitored for potential side effects**, including benign prostatic hyperplasia, prostate cancer, erythrocytosis, and the development or worsening of sleep apnea. Other minor effects are acne/oily skin and reduced sperm production/infertility.
- **Digital rectal examination (DRE) and measurement of prostate-specific antigen (PSA)** should be performed in all men 50 years or older before initiation of testosterone therapy and at 3 to 6 months, and then annually thereafter. African Americans and any man with a history of prostate cancer in a first-degree relative should be monitored after age 40. Some experts recommend that patients should be promptly referred for a prostate biopsy if a nodule is palpated by DRE or if the PSA is elevated >1.4 ng/mL and PSA increasing at a rate >0.4 ng/dL/year. Discontinuation of therapy may be warranted.[21] However, the use of PSA as a screening and following up for prostate cancer is still very controversial. The benefits and risks should be thoroughly discussed with patients.
- The **hemoglobin and hematocrit** should be monitored after 3 to 6 months and then yearly to screen for the development of erythrocytosis. If the hemotocrit increases to above 54%, testosterone replacement needs to be held until the hematocrit decreases to a safe level. The patient may need to be further evaluated for hypoxia and sleep apnea.[2]
- **Obstructive sleep apnea** may worsen. Symptoms of obstructive sleep apnea such as daytime drowsiness or witnessed apnea should be evaluated at each visit.

OUTCOME/PROGNOSIS

- Normalizing testosterone levels typically leads to improvement in symptoms and normal virilization in men in 3 to 6 months.
- Dramatic improvements in muscle mass and bone density may be seen in the first year of treatment.
- Typically, by 24 months, men with osteopenia/osteoporosis reach and maintain normal bone mineral density.
- Increases in lean body mass, prostate volume, erythropoiesis, energy, and sexual function occur within the first 6 months.
- Ten percent of patients with IHH (including Kallmann syndrome), previously thought to require lifelong therapy, were found to have sustained remission of IHH after discontinuation of hormonal therapy. Therefore, it is reasonable to try brief discontinuation of hormonal therapy to assess reversibility of hypogonadotropic hypogonadism after full virilization is achieved.[25]
- A 30-year retrospective study from Japan showed long-term administration of hCG/hMG for 12 to 240 months (average 56 +/– 11) resulted in sperm production in

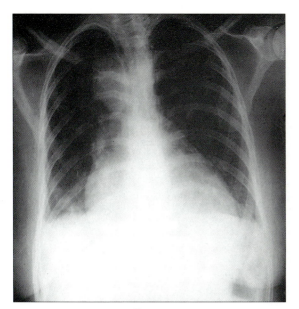

◀ 14
This patient presents with acute, central chest pain radiating through to the back. What is the abnormality and how would you confirm the diagnosis?

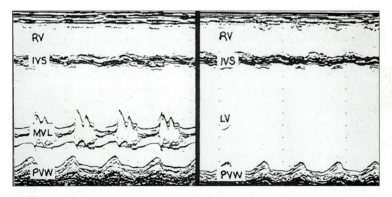

▲ 15

i. Describe the findings on this M-mode echocardiogram.
   (RV = right ventricle; LV = left ventricle; PVW = posterior ventricular wall; IVS = interventricular septum; MVL = mitral valve leaflets.)

ii. List three conditions that lead to this abnormality.

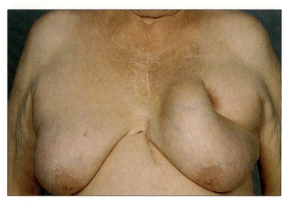

▲ **16**
This patient had a permanent pacemaker implant 10
years earlier.
i.   What is the abnormality due to?
ii. What is the major complication?
iii. What is the important part of treatment?

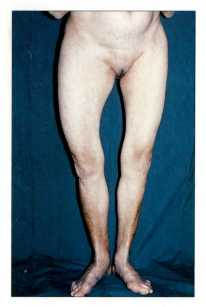

◀ **17**
This patient presented with
breathlessness. What is the cause?

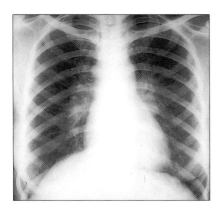

◀ **18**
This chest X-ray is taken from a 27-year-old woman who presented with a Stokes-Adams attack. She was found to be in complete heart block.
i. What abnormalities are seen on the X-ray?
ii. What is the likely diagnosis?
iii. What other cardiac manifestations are seen in this condition?

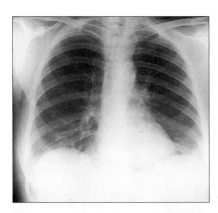

◀ **19**
This patient had a routine medical examination, including a chest X-ray, for an insurance company.
i. What abnormality is seen?
ii. What is its significance?

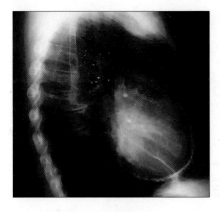

◀ **20**
i. Describe the abnormality on this X-ray.
ii. List five possible causes.

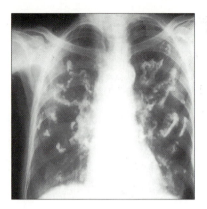

◀ **21**
This chest X-ray is from a 60-year-old man with progressive breathlessness. He was found to have finger clubbing.
i. Describe the abnormality.
ii. What is the diagnosis?

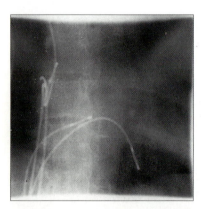

◀ **22**
This radiographic image was taken during a procedure performed on a young man with a history of palpitations.
i. What procedure did the patient undergo?
ii. List the most common complications.

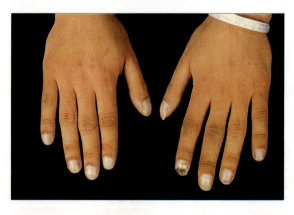

◀ **23**
i. What abnormalities are seen in these hands?
ii. What is the likely cause?

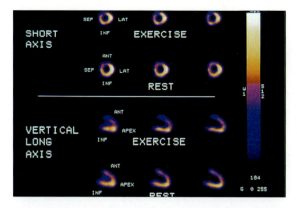

◀ 24
Describe the
abnormalities on
this image.

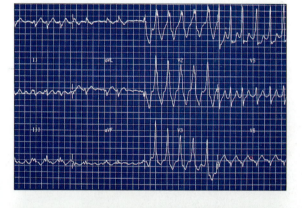

◀ 25
This ECG is from
a 20-year-old
woman with a
two year history
of palpitations.
i. Describe the
    ECG features.
ii. What is the
    likely
    diagnosis?

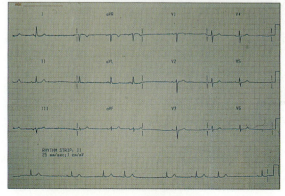

◀ 26
Describe the
findings on this
ECG.

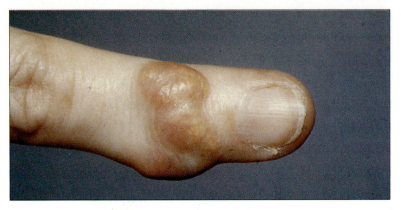

▲ 27

This 45-year-old man has insulin dependent diabetes mellitus.

i. What is the lesion seen in this patient's finger?

ii. What is the incidence of coronary artery disease in this type of patient?

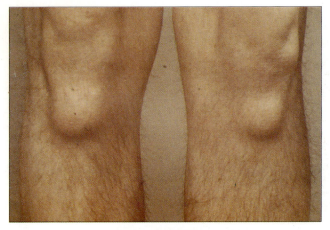

▲ 28

This 25-year-old man was found to have a cholesterol level of 13 mmol/l with a normal triglyceride level.

i. What are the lesions?

ii. What is the inheritance pattern?

○ Obesity causing increased vitamin D deposits in fat but decreased bioavailability for other tissues.
- **Increased catabolism**
  ○ Anticonvulsants, glucocorticoids, highly active anti-retroviral therapy (HAART), and transplant antirejection medications.
- **Decreased synthesis of 25(OH)D**
  ○ Liver cirrhosis (proportional to disease severity—25(OH)D <16 ng/mL found in approximately 66% of patients with Child–Turcotte–Pugh class B or C and 96% of patients awaiting liver transplantation).[9]
- **Increased urinary loss of 25(OH)D**
  ○ Nephrotic syndrome (via loss of 25(OH)D bound to DBP in urine).
- **Decreased synthesis of 1,25(OH)$_2$D**
  ○ Chronic kidney disease (CKD) [via hyperphosphatemia-mediated decrease in 1α-hydroxylase activity in early stages, tubular destruction and reduced substrate 25(OH)D availability in late stages, 25(OH)D <30 ng/mL present in 87.5% stage V CKD patients].[10]
- **Rickets**
  ○ Heritable disorders (vitamin D–dependent rickets types I, II, III; X-linked hypophosphatemic rickets; autosomal dominant hypophosphatemic rickets; autosomal-recessive hypophosphatemic rickets).
  ○ Acquired disorders: tumor-induced osteomalacia.
- **Increased conversion of 25(OH)D to 1,25(OH)$_2$D**
  ○ Primary hyperparathyroidism [via PTH-induced tubular 1α-hydroxylase acceleration of 25(OH)D to conversion; vitamin D insufficiency reported in 53% and vitamin D deficiency (25(OH)D <12 ng/mL) in 27%].[11]
  ○ Granulomatous disorders [sarcoidosis, tuberculosis, and lymphoma; via cytokine induction of macrophage 1α-hydroxylase, converting 25(OH)D to 1,25(OH)$_2$D].
- **Accelerated metabolism**
  ○ Hyperthyroidism

Risk Factors

- In the absence of the disease states described above, any factor that impairs skin production or dietary intake of vitamin D can contribute to vitamin D deficiency.
- The median dietary intake of vitamin D varies from 160 IU/day to 396 IU/day for various populations in the United States assessed by NHANES 2005–2006.[12] Total-body sun exposure for 15 minutes easily provides 10,000 IU vitamin D per day for a Caucasian adult, or 50 to 100 times the average food intake of vitamin D.[13] Therefore, food intake is not a critical source to maintain vitamin D levels in those with adequate sun exposure.
- Many factors reduce vitamin D synthesis in the skin, including time spent indoors, use of sunscreens due to greater awareness of skin cancer, higher latitude, winter season, higher melanin content of the skin, and age-related decline in epidermal 7-DHC. For example, sunscreen with sun protection factor (SPF) of eight reduces vitamin D$_3$ production by about 98%. The concentration of previtamin D in the skin reaches equilibrium in Caucasians within 20 minutes of UV exposure, but it takes 3 to 6 times longer for dark-skinned people to reach the equilibrium concentration.[13]
- Therefore, the following environmental factors represent risk factors for vitamin D deficiency in otherwise healthy people:
  ○ Premature birth

- ○ Pigmented skin
- ○ Low sunshine exposure
- ○ Breast-feeding
- ○ Use of sunscreen
- ○ Indoor activities
- ○ Obesity
- ○ Advanced age
- ○ Seasons
- ○ Latitudes further from the equator

Prevention

- The most efficient way to maintain vitamin D levels is through moderate sun exposure. As described above, total-body sun exposure for 15 minutes easily provides 10,000 IU vitamin D per day for a Caucasian adult.[13]
- Few commonly consumed foods are naturally good sources of vitamin D. Fish is the primary natural food source of dietary vitamin D_3; wild salmon (3.5 oz) provides 600 to 1000 IU. The same amount of mackerel, sardine, or tuna fish provides between 200 and 300 IU, whereas cod liver oil (1 tsp) provides between 600 and 1000 IU and egg yolks 20 IU of vitamins D_2 and D_3. Few sources of vitamin D_2 are regularly eaten; sun-dried shiitake mushrooms provide a good source of vitamin D_2.[5]
- In the United States, the major dietary source is fortified foods. For example, a glass (8 oz) of fortified milk, orange juice, yogurt; 3 oz of fortified cheese; or a serving of fortified breakfast cereal each provides 100 IU vitamin D_3.[5]
- Infants who are nourished exclusively by nursing must get vitamin D supplements or sun exposure to ensure adequate intake because breast milk is a poor source of this vitamin.

Associated Conditions

Bone Effects of Vitamin D

- As a person becomes 25(OH)D deficient, intestinal absorption of calcium and phosphorus decrease, serum ionized calcium levels drop, and a compensatory synthesis and secretion of PTH is stimulated (secondary hyperparathyroidism). Increased plasma PTH levels maintain serum calcium levels by enhancing renal production of 1,25(OH)$_2$D, by increasing bone turnover and bone loss, and by promoting tubular calcium reabsorption and phosphate excretion. Increased 1,25(OH)$_2$D induces intestinal absorption of calcium and phosphorus and stimulates osteoclast activity, which increases the availability of calcium and phosphorus in the blood.[8]
- **Rickets or osteomalacia** caused by deficiency of vitamin D, calcium, or phosphorus can impair normal mineralization of bone. In children, inadequate mineralization of the osteoid and cartilage in the growth plates causes rickets, a disease characterized by widening at the end of the long bones, prominent costochondral junctions (rachitic rosary), deformations in the skeleton including frontal bossing, and deformities of the lower limbs causing bowed legs and knocked knees. In adults, failure to mineralize the bone matrix is termed osteomalacia, a disease characterized by generalized bone pain, muscle weakness, waddling gait, and pseudofractures, a classical radiologic feature characterized by areas of cortical lucency with surrounding sclerosis in the long bones.
  - ○ **Vitamin D–dependent rickets/osteomalacia**

- **Nutritional rickets/osteomalacia.** Vitamin D deficiency is most commonly seen in infants with prolonged breast-feeding who do not receive vitamin D supplementation or adequate exposure to sunlight. All infant formulas in the United States are fortified with at least 400 IU/L of vitamin D. The American Academy of Pediatrics recommends vitamin D supplementation to all infants who receive <1 L (or 1 quart) of vitamin D–fortified formula to ensure total daily intake of 400 IU.[14] Nutritional rickets/osteomalacia is also seen in elderly people with dark skin and with limited exposure to sunlight. Patients will have low serum calcium and phosphorus and high PTH levels. In adults, ergocalciferol doses of 50,000 IU weekly for 8 to 10 weeks along with calcium supplementation of 1000 mg/day has been used for rickets treatment.[15] Serum calcium, phosphorus, alkaline phosphatase, and urine calcium/creatinine ratios are measured before and 4 weeks after initiation of therapy, and every 3 months thereafter. Radiographs are obtained to document healing of rachitic changes.
- **Vitamin D–dependent rickets type I,** also called pseudovitamin D deficiency rickets, usually manifests before 2 years of age. It has an autosomal-recessive inheritance and is linked to chromosome 12q14. It is caused by a defect in renal tubular 1α-hydroxylase enzymes that convert 25(OH)D into the active $1,25(OH)_2D$. Serum calcium levels are usually low or normal, 25(OH)D levels are normal or high, $1,25(OH)_2D$ levels are low, and PTH is high secondary to hypocalcemia. Serum phosphorus is usually low owing to high PTH and low $1,25(OH)_2D$ levels. Treatment involves replacement with calcitriol $(1,25[OH]_2D)$, and the aim of therapy is to maintain serum calcium, phosphorus, alkaline phosphatase, and PTH levels within normal limits.
- **Vitamin D–dependent rickets type II,** also called hereditary vitamin D–resistant rickets, is very rare. It has autosomal-recessive inheritance and is associated with end-organ resistance to calcitriol, resulting from mutations in the gene that encodes the VDR. Affected children are normal at birth, but metabolic bone disease presents early within the first 2 years of life. Serum calcium is low, PTH is high, 25(OH)D is normal to high, and $1,25(OH)_2D$ is normal to high. Treatment involves high doses of calcitriol and calcium. Long-term central venous infusion of calcium is an alternative for severely resistant patients.
- **Vitamin D–independent rickets/osteomalacia**
  - **X-linked hypophosphatemic rickets** is an X-linked dominant genetic disorder (Xp22). It is caused by a defect in PHEX (phosphate-regulating endopeptidase), which lyses a circulating factor that causes renal phosphate losses. Patients with this disorder also have defective $1,25(OH)_2D$ synthesis secondary to low levels of plasma phosphorus. Patients have low $1,25(OH)_2D$, low phosphorus, normal calcium, and normal PTH levels. Treatment includes supplementation with phosphorus and vitamin D.
  - **Autosomal-dominant hypophosphatemic rickets** results from a mutation in fibroblast growth factor (FGF23) that causes increased levels of this phosphatonin leading to large renal losses of phosphate. FGF23 directly inhibits renal 1α-hydroxylase and, therefore, $1,25(OH)_2D$ synthesis. The clinical manifestations and treatment are similar to X-linked hypophosphatemic rickets.
  - **Autosomal-recessive hypophosphatemic rickets** results from a homozygous mutation in dentin matrix protein 1 (DMP1), which is made in the osteocytes. DMP1 inhibits secretion or production of FGF23, and mutation results in release of the inhibition of FGF23, thereby causing phosphaturia and osteomalacia. Clinical features are similar to those of autosomal-dominant rickets.

- ■ **Tumor-induced osteomalacia** is characterized by increased production of phosphatonins by sclerosing tumors of mesenchymal origin. Patients have increased renal phosphate losses and a compensatory rise in $1,25(OH)_2D$ synthesis. Treatment includes repletion of phosphorus, tumor resection, and somatostatin analogs.
- ■ **Hypophosphatemia with hypercalciuria** is a result of an autosomal-recessive defect in type 2c Na-PO4 cotransport in the renal proximal tubule. Patients have low phosphorus and a compensatory rise in vitamin D, which causes increased intestinal calcium absorption and hypercalciuria. Treatment includes phosphorous supplementation.

- **Osteoporosis**
  - Osteoporosis is a systemic disorder characterized by decreased bone mass and microarchitectural deterioration of bone tissue, leading to bone fragility and increased susceptibility to fractures of the hip, spine, and wrist. Secondary hyperparathyroidism has been proposed as the principal mechanism connecting vitamin D deficiency with the pathogenesis of decreased BMD and osteoporosis.
  - Despite the fact that higher serum 25(OH)D concentrations are associated with higher BMD in all population subgroups (NHANES III), the ability of vitamin D supplements to prevent fractures continues to be debated. Vitamin D and calcium supplementation (1000 mg of calcium and 800 IU of vitamin D per day) significantly reduced the risk of hip fractures by 43% and nonvertebral fractures by 32% among 3270 postmenopausal women who were vitamin D–deficient (mean 25(OH)D, 16 ng/mL) and increased 25(OH)D levels to 42 ng/mL after treatment.[16] In a recent meta-analysis, vitamin D supplementation (700 to 800 IU) reduced hip fractures by 26% and nonvertebral fractures by 23%, compared to subjects without vitamin D supplementation.[17] In contrast, a subgroup analysis of the Women's Health Initiative (WHI) reported that the supplementation of 36,282 postmenopausal women for 7 years with vitamin D_3 (400 IU) and calcium carbonate (1000 mg) failed to prevent hip fractures despite slight improvement in hip BMD in the treated group when compared to placebo. Several issues have been raised regarding this study that limit its interpretation, including lower rates of adherence to therapy, higher calcium intake at baseline in study participants, and perhaps the selection of a suboptimal vitamin D_3 supplement. In the WHI study, the serum 25(OH)D increased by only ~2.8 ng/mL.[18] The randomized trial of vitamin D and calcium for the secondary prevention of osteoporosis related fractures in the elderly (RECORD) showed no prevention of a second fracture for patients receiving 1000 mg/day of calcium and 800 IU/day of vitamin D_3.[19] However, multiple questions have been raised altering the interpretation of these results. First, the placebo group was allowed to receive calcium and vitamin D regardless of the intervention. Second, there was poor compliance with the regimen. Reports of compliance in the first year were 60% and 47% in the second year. Third, the achieved mean 25(OH)D concentrations were only 24.8 ng/mL in the vitamin D treatment group. When hip fractures were shown to improve with vitamin D, the optimal fracture prevention occurred when 25(OH)D concentrations achieved were 36 to 40 ng/mL. These concentrations were reached only in trials that gave 700 to 800 IU/day of vitamin D_3 to subjects with mean baseline concentrations between 17 and 31 ng/mL. Therefore, optimal fracture prevention may require intakes of >700 to 800 IU/day vitamin D_3 in populations with baseline 25(OH)D concentrations <17 ng/mL.[17,20]

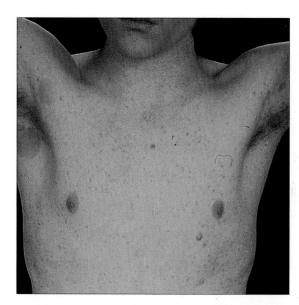

◀ 29

This 50-year-old
man was found to
have raised blood
pressure.
i. What
   abnormality is
   seen?
ii. What is the
    likely diagnosis?

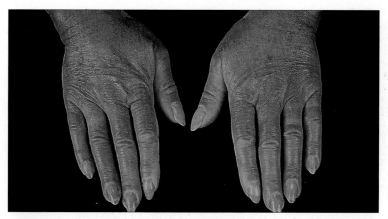

▲ 30
This 48-year-old woman presented with breathlessness over a period of 12
months.
i. What do her hands show?
ii. What is the likely diagnosis?
iii. What is the cause of her breathlessness?

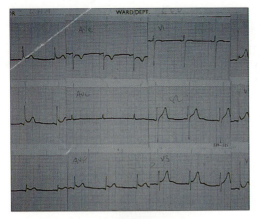

◀ 31

This ECG is from a 28-year-old man who presented with a recent history of malaise and fever, associated with chest pain.

i. Describe the abnormality on the ECG.

ii. What other cardiological investigations should be carried out?

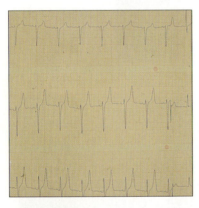

◀ 32

This rhythm strip is from a patient with chronic renal failure.

i. What is the abnormality of the rhythm strip?

ii. What is it due to?

iii. What are the complications associated with it?

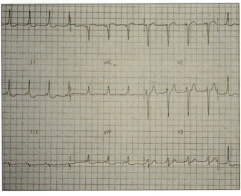

◀ 33

This ECG is from a 22-year-old woman with a history of palpitations.

i. Describe the abnormalities.

ii. What is the diagnosis?

iii. What is the cause of her palpitations?

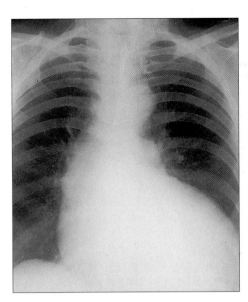

◀ 34

This chest X-ray is of a 27-year-old man who presented with exertional dyspnoea, vague chest pain and one episode of syncope. He had an older brother who died suddenly of an unknown cause.

i. Describe the abnormalities.
ii. What is the diagnosis?
ii. What other investigations should be carried out?

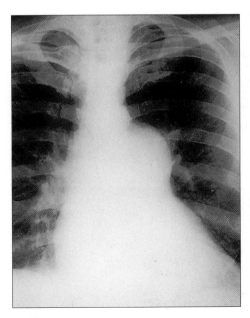

◀ 35

This chest X-ray is of a 68-year-old man who presented to his doctor with a slight cough.

i.   Describe the abnormality.
ii. What is the diagnosis?
iii. What investigations would confirm it?

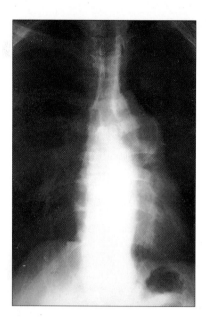

36

A 42-year-old man presented with a history of breathlessness. Cardiac auscultation revealed a 'continuous' murmur, loudest in the left first and second intercostal spaces. There was also a mid-diastolic murmur in the apex.

i. Describe the cardiac findings on the X-ray.

ii. What is the underlying condition?

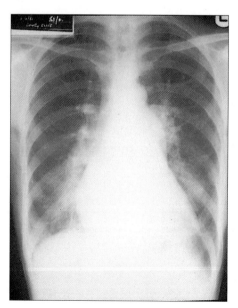

37

This chest X-ray is from a 57-year-old man with a two year history of progressive breathlessness.

i. Describe the abnormalities.

ii. What is the likely diagnosis?

Non-calcemic Actions of Vitamin D

- A growing body of evidence from both rodent models and humans suggests that maintaining optimal vitamin D stores is important for overall health and not just bone health. Although much of the data are correlational at this point, the weight of the evidence suggests that vitamin D deficiency may lead to worsening of known risk factors for cardiovascular disease. The outcomes of prospective randomized controlled clinical trials will be essential.
- **Type 2 diabetes mellitus (DM)**
  - The prevalence of hypovitaminosis D is higher in women with type 2 diabetes. Analysis of NHANES III and the Workforce Diabetes Study confirmed that patients with 25(OH)D levels >30 ng/mL have about one-third the risk of developing diabetes or impaired glucose tolerance when compared with those with vitamin D levels <24 ng/mL.[21,22] Studies in rodents have suggested that vitamin D deficiency may lead to impaired insulin secretion and to insulin resistance. In humans, the insulin sensitivity index, as assessed by hyperinsulinemic-hyperglycemic clamps, improves in direct relationship with ambient levels of vitamin D; moreover, interventional studies in vitamin D–deficient subjects have shown improved insulin sensitivity in glucose-intolerant subjects after replacement of vitamin D.[23] However, several interventional trials found no effect of vitamin D supplementation on glucose metabolism.[24,25]
- **Type 1 diabetes mellitus**
  - Type 1 DM is recognized as a T-cell–mediated autoimmune disease. Vitamin D compounds are known to suppress T-cell activation and to alter the antigen-presenting capacity of macrophages and dendritic cells, as well as modulate their cytokine release. These actions may protect beta cells against autoimmune injury. Several epidemiologic studies have described a correlation between geographic latitude and the incidence of type 1 diabetes.[26] A previous study has shown that 25(OH)D levels are lower in patients newly diagnosed with type 1 diabetes compared to healthy controls. The Diabetes Autoimmunity Study in the Young (DAISY) reported that the presence of autoantibodies to islet cells inversely correlated with maternal dietary vitamin D intake during pregnancy. In addition, in patients with rickets, the incidence of childhood diabetes is 3 times higher than the incidence in healthy children.[27] Case-control studies have shown that treatment of children with 400 IU or less vitamin D per day did not reduce the risk of developing type 1 DM.[28] However, the only prospective study based on the assessment of vitamin D intake during infancy (of 10,821 children) showed that vitamin D supplementation in infants with doses of 2000 IU/day for a year decreased the risk of developing type 1 DM by 80% by the age of 30 years.[29] Additional studies are needed to determine whether vitamin D should be started during pregnancy and to determine the ideal vitamin D doses without side effects.
- **Hypertension**
  - Interventional studies suggest that vitamin D replacement decreases blood pressure. In an 8-week treatment study consisting of oral calcium and vitamin D_3 replacement in elderly women with vitamin D deficiency, plasma 25(OH)D levels increased to ≥25 ng/mL and systolic blood pressure (SBP) decreased significantly, by 13 mm Hg, compared with the calcium-only treated control group.[30] UVB exposure by skin-tanning sessions increased plasma 25(OH)D levels to 40 ng/mL and decreased blood pressure in mildly hypertensive patients.[31] However, oral administration of 1,25(OH)$_2$D has not shown consistent blood pressure effects, possibly due to discrepancies in the population plasma vitamin D status, as well as different vitamin D doses and duration of the vitamin D replacement.

○ Vitamin D suppresses the renin–angiotensin system. In animal models, vitamin D downregulates renin gene promoter activity independent of calcium metabolism. Mice lacking the VDR exhibit hypertension and cardiac hypertrophy due to increased renin expression and plasma angiotensin II production.[32] Oral administration of vitamin D in spontaneously hypertensive rats decreased blood pressure as well as improved endothelial cell–dependent vasodilation.[33,34] In humans, there is an inverse relationship between vitamin D levels and plasma renin levels. Interventional studies with oral synthetic vitamin D replacement lowered plasma renin in nondiabetic vitamin D–deficient patients.[35] This evidence supports the conceptual relationship between vitamin D and the renin–aldosterone system in essential hypertension and the beneficial effect of vitamin D supplementation on blood pressure.

• **Cardiovascular disease**
  ○ Vitamin D not only alters the hormones involved in the pathophysiology of hypertension and diabetes, but it also has a direct effect on the vasculature. The expression of VDRs and the activation of vitamin D by the 1α-hydroxylase enzyme in endothelial and vascular smooth muscle cells suggest the importance of vitamin D in vascular cell metabolism.[36,37] Vitamin D deficiency is more prevalent in patients with peripheral vascular disease, and vitamin D levels are inversely correlated with vascular resistance in hypertensive patients. Cardiovascular events are more prevalent during winter months and at increased geographic latitudes where average serum vitamin D levels are the lowest.[38]
  ○ Epidemiologic studies have found an association between vitamin D insufficiency, reflected by low serum 25-hydroxyvitamin D levels, and higher rates of CVD morbidity[39,40] and mortality.[41–43] Controversy regarding the effects of vitamin D on cardiovascular disease stems from several interventional trials including the WHI.[44,45] In a randomized controlled trial, 2686 men and women aged 65 or older were randomly assigned to receive either 100,000 IU of oral vitamin D every 4 months or matching placebo (an average of 833 IU/day). After 5 years of followup, there were no significant differences in the incidence of ischemic heart disease or stroke. In the WHI, 36,282 postmenopausal women were randomized to vitamin D (400 IU) and calcium carbonate (1000 mg) daily versus placebo for 7 years. The intervention failed to prevent coronary or cerebrovascular disease when compared to those in the placebo group. As mentioned above, however, there were limitations to this study and well-designed medical trials with appropriate doses of vitamin D supplementation are required to clarify the effects of vitamin D in cardiovascular disease.[46–48]

• **Immunity**
  ○ The VDR is present in macrophages and T lymphocytes. $1,25(OH)_2D$ acts as an immune system modulator, preventing excessive expression of inflammatory cytokines and increasing the "oxidative burst" potential of macrophages.[49] Most importantly, vitamin D stimulates antimicrobial peptides (cathelicidin and beta-defensin 2) that exist in neutrophils, monocytes, natural killer cells, and in epithelial cells lining the respiratory tract, where they play a major role in protecting against bacteria, viruses, and fungi. African Americans, known to have increased susceptibility to tuberculosis (TB), are reported to have low serum levels of 25(OH)D and inefficient induction of cathelicidin expression. Adding vitamin D to serum from African Americans increased cathelicidin production by macrophages and accelerated rates of TB-microbe killing. Cathelicidin and beta-defensin 2 display broad-spectrum antimicrobial activity, including antiviral

activity, and have been shown to inactivate the influenza virus.[50] Volunteers inoculated with live attenuated influenza virus during winter are more likely to develop fever and serologic evidence of an immune response compared to those inoculated during summer, suggesting a correlation between vitamin D levels and the recurrent seasonality of the influenza epidemics.[51] Increased vitamin D levels by UV radiation and cod liver reduces the incidence of respiratory infections in children.[52] This suggests that differences in the ability to produce vitamin D may contribute to susceptibility or resistance to microbial infection.

- **Antiproliferative effects**
  ○ The active vitamin D metabolite, in addition to regulating calcium–phosphate homeostasis and bone mineralization, induces in vitro cell cycle arrest, differentiation, and apoptosis in a variety of cancer cells.[53] Patients with genetic VDR polymorphisms, specifically the *Bsm I* genotype bb, have twice the incidence of colon, prostate, and breast cancer. The VDR *FokI* polymorphism modifies prostate cancer risk; men with the less functional *FokI* ff genotype are more susceptible to this cancer in the presence of low 25(OH)D levels.[54]
  ○ The Health Professionals Follow-up Study, a prospective cohort study, found a 17% reduction in total cancer incidence and a 29% reduction in total cancer mortality for every 10 ng/dL increase in serum 25(OH)D level.[55] However, data from NHANES III did now show any association between 25(OH)D level and total cancer mortality.[56] Results from several interventional trials with osteoporosis as the primary outcome and cancer risk determined by secondary analysis of safety data have been conflicting, but these have all relied upon subjects notifying the investigators of their diagnosis. Therefore, interventional trials of vitamin D with cancer risk and cancer mortality as a primary outcome are needed to clarify this possible relationship.
  ○ In **colon cancer**, the evidence of an association with vitamin D is substantial. Most studies that have examined circulating 25(OH)D concentrations and subsequent risk of colorectal cancer or adenoma found a lower risk associated with higher 25(OH)D concentrations. In the recent analysis of the Nurses' Health Study, colon cancer risk negatively correlated with 25(OH)D concentrations; patients with 25(OH)D concentrations of 39.9 ng/mL had approximately half the relative risk (RR) of developing colon cancer (RR, 0.53; confidence interval [CI] 0.27 to 1.04) compared to patients with levels <16 ng/mL. Benefit from higher 25(OH)D concentrations was observed for older women with cancer at the distal colon and rectum, but was not evident for those at the proximal colon. In a prospective study of 1954 men, vitamin D intake of 233 to 652 IU/day decreased the relative risk of developing colon cancer by half compared to men with a vitamin D intake <6 to 94 IU/day. The WHI found that women at enrollment who had low blood vitamin D levels (<12.4 ng/mL) had a greater than two-fold risk of bowel cancer compared to those with vitamin D levels >23.4 ng/mL, but there was no evidence that treatment with calcium (1000 mg/day) and vitamin D (400 IU/day) reduced bowel cancer occurrence over the 7 years of follow-up.[54,57–59] Based on these and previous studies, the estimated optimal serum 25(OH)D concentrations associated with reduced incidence of colonic adenomas are 30 to 35 ng/mL, though further interventional trials are needed.
  ○ In **prostate cancer**, epidemiologic and laboratory data support the role of vitamin D in the growth and differentiation of human prostatic cells.[60] In a Finnish study, prostate cancer incidence was assessed in 18,966 men, ages 40 to 57, over 14 years. Those with 25(OH)D levels below 16 ng/mL had a 70% higher incidence

rate of prostate cancer than those with levels 16 ng/mL or above. For younger men with 25(OH)D levels below 16 ng/mL, the incidence of prostate cancer was 3.5 times higher than for those with levels of 16 ng/mL or above, and the incidence of invasive cancer was 6.3 times higher. A few small phase II trials showed evidence that $1,25(OH)_2D$ alone or in combination with antimitotic chemotherapy decreases prostate cancer progression, but further studies are needed.

○ In **breast cancer**, combined analysis of 1760 women from two trials reporting risk of breast cancer by quintiles of 25(OH)D showed that a 50% reduction of breast cancer risk was associated with 25(OH)D levels of 50 ng/mL compared to those with levels of 10 ng/mL.[61] In addition, women in the lowest quartile of serum $1,25(OH)_2D$ had a risk of breast cancer 5 times higher than those in the highest quartile.[62] Low $1,25(OH)_2D$ levels were also associated with faster progression of metastatic breast cancer.[63] Animal studies confirmed that $1,25(OH)_2D$ inhibits breast cancer, but interventional studies in humans are still pending.[64]

• **Myopathy**
○ Muscle weakness is a common clinical feature in patients with vitamin D deficiency. It may affect fracture risk by altering the susceptibility to falls. Combined evidence from five studies including 1237 patients showed that vitamin D intake reduced the risk of falling by 22% (OR, 0.78; 95% CI, 0.64 to 0.92). In a recent double-blinded study, elderly ambulatory subjects taking 700 IU vitamin D plus 500 mg calcium had a 46% decreased risk of falling compared to those taking placebo. Fall reduction was most pronounced in less active women. Poor physical performance and a greater decline in physical performance in 1234 older men and women were found when serum 25(OH)D concentrations were below 20 ng/mL. Hypovitaminosis D myopathy may be present even before biochemical signs of bone disease develop. Full normalization of hypovitaminosis D myopathy demands high-dose vitamin D treatment for 6 months or more. There is also evidence that idiopathic low back pain in patients with vitamin D deficiency markedly improves when levels are restored. Low levels of 25(OH)D are also common in patients with fibromyalgia and chronic refractory nonspecific musculoskeletal pain.[20]

• **Rheumatoid arthritis**
○ Rheumatoid arthritis (RA) is one of the most common chronic inflammatory diseases and affects about 1% of the population in the United States. Epidemiologic studies have reported low serum levels of vitamin D and its metabolites in patients with RA.[65] Small interventional studies in RA with high-dose oral alfacalcidol (form of vitamin D) therapy showed a positive effect on disease activity in 89% of the patients, and only 11% of patients showed no improvement.[66] In psoriatic arthritis, oral administration of $1,25-(OH)_2D_3$ showed an improvement in disease symptoms.[67] In the Iowa Women's Health Study, women who received less <200 IU of vitamin D in their diets each day were 33% more likely to develop rheumatoid arthritis than women who received more.[65] These results provide evidence that VDR ligands can be of potential clinical use for the treatment of RA.

• **Multiple sclerosis**
○ Epidemiologic data correlate the geographic location and the prevalence of MS. In women, the Nurses' Health Study and Nurses' Health Study II results confirm a protective effect of vitamin D on the risk of multiple sclerosis (MS). The relative risk of developing MS was decreased by 60% when comparing women with an intake of ≥400 IU/day with women not taking supplemental vitamin D.[68,69] No prospective studies have addressed this hypothesis.

DIAGNOSIS

Clinical Presentation

History
- The majority of cases of vitamin D deficiency are largely asymptomatic unless severe enough to lead to rickets in children or osteomalacia in adults.
- Therefore, clinical suspicion should be high in any patient presenting with comorbid diseases or environmental factors that place them at higher risk for vitamin D deficiency (see Sections Etiology and Risk Factors).

Physical Exam
Physical exam is typically unremarkable unless progression to rickets or osteomalacia has occurred (see Section Associated Conditions).

Diagnostic Testing

Laboratories
- 25(OH)D is the major circulating form of vitamin D and serum levels increase in proportion to cutaneous synthesis and dietary intake of vitamin D, thus representing the best indicator of vitamin D status. Classification of vitamin D status is described in Section Classification.
- Previous reports suggest that IDS RIA or ADVANTAGE CPBA system assays for 25(OH)D might not detect vitamin D_2 levels, which will give misleading results and could lead to misdiagnosis and subsequent dangerous consequences for the patient. Lab-specific assay characteristics should be verified prior to treatment.[70,71]

TREATMENT

Medications

- The vitamin D dose depends on the target concentration of 25(OH)D desired. New clinical research indicates that the vitamin D intake used to prevent rickets is much lower than the requirement for prevention of osteoporosis related bone fractures, cancer, and improvement of the metabolic abnormalities described previously. However, **the ideal oral intake of vitamin D that provokes healthy effects without side effects has not been completely elucidated.**
- Vitamin D is available in two forms for supplementation: **ergocalciferol** (vitamin D_2) made from yeast fat exposed to UV light and **cholecalciferol** (vitamin D_3) obtained from animal fat. Some data has shown that vitamin D_2 is one-third less potent than vitamin D_3 and has a shorter duration of action relative to vitamin D_3 (<14 days).[72] However, recent evidence found that a daily dose of 1000 IU of vitamin D_2 daily was as effective as 1000 IU of vitamin D_3 in maintaining 25-hydroxyvitamin D_3 levels.[73] The half-life of 25(OH)D in the circulation is reported to be approximately 1 month in humans. Conventional pharmacology indicates it should take at least four half-lives before a drug's equilibrium is achieved.[4] Increased responsiveness to vitamin D administration is seen more in thin patients with low vitamin D levels at baseline using low vitamin D doses and long duration of vitamin D supplementation. An increased dose of vitamin D does not increase the plasma 25(OH)D levels proportionally. Previous studies indicate that 75% or more of the molecules of vitamin D that enter to the body are catabolized and excreted without

becoming 25(OH)D. Generally, 100 IU/day for 8 months increases 25(OH)D levels by 1 ng/mL.[4]

- The **current recommendations,** based on the assumption that young and middle-aged adults are more likely than older adults to be exposed to sunlight, are as follows: **400 IU/day for infants, 600 IU/day for children and adults up to age 70 years, and 800 IU/day for those older than 70 years.** These doses are adequate to reach the current recommended 25(OH)D level of 20 ng/mL in the majority of adults. Subgroups of the population such as obese individuals, pregnant women, and patients with nephrotic syndrome and chronic renal failure require 1000 to 2000 IU of vitamin D_3 daily or 50,000 IU of vitamin D_2 every 2 weeks to prevent vitamin D deficiency during the winter months. The Food and Nutrition Board guidelines specify 4000 IU vitamin D_3 as the highest vitamin D intake that healthy adults can consume without risking toxicity.[3]

- In the United States, the only pharmaceutical preparation of vitamin D is vitamin D_2. **The recommended dose of ergocalciferol to treat vitamin D deficiency is 50,000 IU every week for 8 weeks.** If the patient does not achieve 25(OH)D levels >30 ng/mL, then another 8 weeks of therapy is recommended. If the 25(OH)D levels are >30 ng/mL, then follow with maintenance therapy of 50,000 IU every other week or once a month depending on the etiology of the vitamin D deficiency. In patients with obesity, nephrotic syndrome, or malabsorption, or in patients taking anticonvulsants, glucocorticoids, HAART (AIDS treatment), and transplant antirejection medications, ergocalciferol loading doses (50,000 IU/week) should be administered for longer periods (8 to 12 weeks). If 25(OH)D levels are still <30 ng/mL after a loading dose, repeat for another 8 to 12 weeks of treatment. Maintenance doses in this special subgroup of patients should be 50,000 IU every week or every other week.[5]

- Another way to replace vitamin D is to administer it as a single large dose, either orally or through injection. This approach, known as stoss therapy, should be closely monitored by an experienced physician.[74]

Other Nonpharmacologic Therapies

Sun exposure very efficiently forms vitamin D_3. In summer months, total-body sun exposure for 15 to 30 minutes in Caucasian adults generates about 250 mcg (10,000 IU) of vitamin D_3/day, with no signs of vitamin D–induced intoxication. In a randomized control study in a psychogeriatric nursing home, exposure to UV irradiation with half of the minimal erythematous dose on 1000 cm^2 of the back 3 times per week for 12 weeks increased plasma 25(OH)D to the same levels as those who received oral 400 IU/day of vitamin D_3. Exposure of face, forearms, and hands (total exposed skin area was 426 ± 32 cm^2) to sunlight for 15 minutes and calcium supplementation may be safe and effective in increasing BMD and reducing the risk of fracture in chronically hospitalized elderly women with Alzheimer's disease. Most tanning beds emit 2% to 6% UVB radiation. In patients with malabsorption, tanning-bed exposure is a potential source of vitamin D supplementation.[5]

COMPLICATIONS

- **Multiple medications can interact with vitamin D.** Cholestyramine, Colestipol, mineral oil, Orlistat, and Olestra (a fat substitute) reduce vitamin D absorption. Administration of ketoconazole 300 to 1200 mg daily in healthy men for 7 days decreased serum 1,25(OH)$_2$D levels. Anticonvulsants, glucocorticoids, HAART

(AIDS treatment), and transplant antirejection medications activate the destruction of 25(OH)D and 1,25(OH)$_2$D to inactive compounds.

- **Hypersensitivity** to vitamin D supplementation can occur in patients with primary hyperparathyroidism, sarcoidosis, TB, or lymphoma. In primary hyperparathyroidism, production of 1,25(OH)$_2$ is persistently upregulated by high PTH concentrations, and 1,25(OH)$_2$D concentrations correlate directly with serum 25(OH)D. However, the current data provide preliminary evidence that vitamin D repletion in patients with mild primary hyperparathyroidism does not promote an increase in serum calcium and has beneficial effects by decreasing PTH levels and bone turnover.[11] We recommend assessment of plasma calcium and urinary calcium/creatinine ratio (see Section Monitoring) in the first 2 weeks of the vitamin D replacement and then monthly during replacement.
- **Vitamin D toxicity**
  - ○ Toxicity is extremely rare and generally occurs by accidental or uninformed consumption of very high doses of vitamin D. Toxicity occurred with ingestion of more than 40,000 IU/day, which reflects 4 times the maximum vitamin D (10,000 IU) acquired by sunshine exposure. Concentrations of 1,25(OH)$_2$D are not increased by vitamin D intoxication but free 1,25(OH)$_2$D levels are generally high.[3,75]
  - ○ **Hypercalcemia** (>11 mg/dL) is the main criterion for vitamin D–induced toxicity. The **clinical manifestations** include anorexia, nausea and vomiting, hypotonicity, lethargy, constipation, generalized pain, conjunctivitis, fever, chills, thirst, and weight loss. Hypercalcemia can result in a loss of the urinary concentrating mechanism of the kidney tubule, resulting in polyuria and polydipsia. The prolonged ingestion of excessive amounts of vitamin D and the accompanying hypercalcemia can result in metastatic calcification of soft tissues—including the kidney, blood vessels, heart, and lungs—and increased risk for nephrolithiasis.
  - ○ The only **treatment for vitamin D toxicity** is to decrease the hypercalcemia by forcing a negative calcium balance. Glucocorticoids, intravenous saline, furosemide, calcitonin, or a bisphosphonate has been used. Because vitamin D is stored in fat, vitamin D intoxication may persist for weeks after vitamin D ingestion is terminated. The elimination half-life of vitamin D is about 3 weeks to 1 month. Persistent treatment with corticosteroid or an oral bisphosphonate for this period is required.

MONITORING/FOLLOW-UP

The most sensitive clinical index of safety during vitamin D replacement is measurement of urinary calcium. This is measured by **morning calcium-to-creatinine ratio** (normal values are <1 mmol/mmol or <0.35 mg/mg in a well-hydrated patient). An elevated calcium-to-creatinine ratio increases the risk for nephrolithiasis, and increased caution in replacement dosing, hydration, and monitoring should be exercised. However, hypercalciuria cannot be excluded if the urinary creatinine concentration is >40 mg/dL.[76] Given that during vitamin D replacement serum 25(OH)D is at the plateau concentration by 1 month, we suggest an assessment of serum calcium and urine calcium-to-creatinine ratio 2 to 4 weeks after starting vitamin D replacement therapy. We recommend repeating these studies monthly for 1 or 2 months because the plateau of 25(OH)D concentration may be slightly underestimated in some cases.

REFERENCES

1. Dusso AS, Brown AJ, Slatopolsky E. Vitamin D. *Am J Physiol Renal Physiol* 2005;289:F8–28.
2. Lips P. Vitamin D physiology. *Prog Biophys Mol Biol* 2006;92:4–8.
3. Ross AC, Taylor CL, Yaktine AL, et al. *Dietary reference intakes for calcium and vitamin D.* Washington, DC: National Academy of Sciences; 2010.
4. Vieth R. Vitamin D supplementation, 25-hydroxyvitamin D concentrations, and safety. *Am J Clin Nutr* 1999;69:842–856.
5. Holick MF. Vitamin D deficiency. *N Engl J Med* 2007;357:266–281.
6. Gutierrez OM, Farwell WR, Kermah D, et al. Racial differences in the relationship between vitamin D, bone mineral density, and parathyroid hormone in the National Health and Nutrition Examination Survey. *Osteoporos Int* 2010. Last accessed: 12/21/10 http://www.springerlink.com.
7. Harris SS, Soteriades E, Coolidge JA, et al. Vitamin D insufficiency and hyperparathyroidism in a low income, multiracial, elderly population. *J Clin Endocrinol Metab* 2000;85:4125–4130.
8. Favus M. *Primer on the metabolic bone disease and disorders of mineral metabolism.* Philadelphia, PA: Lippincott-Raven Publishers; 1996.
9. Crawford BA, Labio ED, Strasser SI, et al. Vitamin D replacement for cirrhosis-related bone disease. *Nat Clin Pract Gastroenterol Hepatol* 2006;3:689–699.
10. LaClair RE, Hellman RN, Karp SL, et al. Prevalence of calcidiol deficiency in CKD: A cross-sectional study across latitudes in the United States. *Am J Kidney Dis* 2005;45:1026–1033.
11. Grey A, Lucas J, Horne A, et al. Vitamin D repletion in patients with primary hyperparathyroidism and coexistent vitamin D insufficiency. *J Clin Endocrinol Metab* 2005;90:2122–2126.
12. Bailey RL, Dodd KW, Goldman JA, et al. Estimation of total usual calcium and vitamin D intakes in the United States. *J Nutr* 2010;140:817–822.
13. Holick MF. Vitamin D: A D-Lightful health perspective. *Nutr Rev* 2008;66:S182–S194.
14. Wagner CL, Greer FR. Prevention of rickets and vitamin D deficiency in infants, children, and adolescents. *Pediatrics* 2008;122:1142–1152.
15. Hollis BW, Wagner CL. Normal serum vitamin D levels. *N Engl J Med* 2005;352:515–516.
16. Chapuy MC, Arlot ME, Duboeuf F, et al. Vitamin D3 and calcium to prevent hip fractures in the elderly women. *N Engl J Med* 1992;327:1637–1642.
17. Bischoff-Ferrari HA, Willett WC, Wong JB, et al. Fracture prevention with vitamin D supplementation: A meta-analysis of randomized controlled trials. *JAMA* 2005;293:2257–2264.
18. Jackson RD, LaCroix AZ, Gass M, et al. Calcium plus vitamin D supplementation and the risk of fractures. *N Engl J Med* 2006;354:669–683.
19. Grant AM, Avenell A, Campbell MK, et al. Oral vitamin D3 and calcium for secondary prevention of low-trauma fractures in elderly people (randomised evaluation of calcium or vitamin D, RECORD): A randomised placebo-controlled trial. *Lancet* 2005;365:1621–1628.
20. Bischoff-Ferrari HA, Giovannucci E, Willett WC, et al. Estimation of optimal serum concentrations of 25-hydroxyvitamin D for multiple health outcomes. *Am J Clin Nutr* 2006; 84:18–28.
21. Scragg R, Holdaway I, Singh V, et al. Serum 25-hydroxyvitamin D3 levels decreased in impaired glucose tolerance and diabetes mellitus. *Diabetes Res Clin Pract* 1995;27:181–188.
22. Scragg R, Sowers M, Bell C. Serum 25-hydroxyvitamin D, diabetes, and ethnicity in the Third National Health and Nutrition Examination Survey. *Diabetes Care* 2004;27:2813–2818.
23. Chiu KC, Chu A, Go VL, et al. Hypovitaminosis D is associated with insulin resistance and beta cell dysfunction. *Am J Clin Nutr* 2004;79:820–825.
24. Pittas AG, Lau J, Hu FB, et al. The role of vitamin D and calcium in type 2 diabetes. A systematic review and meta-analysis. *J Clin Endocrinol Metab* 2007;92:2017–2029.
25. Avenell A, Cook JA, MacLennan GS, et al. Vitamin D supplementation and type 2 diabetes: A substudy of a randomised placebo-controlled trial in older people (RECORD trial). *Age Ageing* 2009;38:606–609.
26. Karvonen M, Jantti V, Muntoni S, et al. Comparison of the seasonal pattern in the clinical onset of IDDM in Finland and Sardinia. *Diabetes Care* 1998;21:1101–1109.

27. Fronczak CM, Baron AE, Chase HP, et al. In utero dietary exposures and risk of islet auto-immunity in children. *Diabetes Care* 2003;26:3237–3242.

28. Vitamin D supplement in early childhood and risk for Type I (insulin-dependent) diabetes mellitus. The EURODIAB Substudy 2 Study Group. *Diabetologia* 1999;42:51–54.

29. Hypponen E, Laara E, Reunanen A, et al. Intake of vitamin D and risk of type 1 diabetes: A birth-cohort study. *Lancet* 2001;358:1500–1503.

30. Pfeifer M, Begerow B, Minne HW, et al. Effects of a short-term vitamin D(3) and calcium supplementation on blood pressure and parathyroid hormone levels in elderly women. *J Clin Endocrinol Metab* 2001;86:1633–1637.

31. Krause R, Buhring M, Hopfenmuller W, et al. Ultraviolet B and blood pressure. *Lancet* 1998;352:709–710.

32. Li YC, Kong J, Wei M, et al. 1,25-Dihydroxyvitamin D(3) is a negative endocrine regulator of the renin-angiotensin system. *J Clin Invest* 2002;110:229–238.

33. Borges AC, Feres T, Vianna LM, et al. Recovery of impaired K+ channels in mesenteric arteries from spontaneously hypertensive rats by prolonged treatment with cholecalciferol. *Br J Pharmacol* 1999;127:772–778.

34. Borges AC, Feres T, Vianna LM, et al. Effect of cholecalciferol treatment on the relaxant responses of spontaneously hypertensive rat arteries to acetylcholine. *Hypertension* 1999; 34:897–901.

35. Li YC. Vitamin D regulation of the renin-angiotensin system. *J Cell Biochem* 2003;88:327–331.

36. Towler DA, Clemens TL. Vitamin D and cardiovascular medicine. In: Feldman D, Glorieux FHPJW, eds. *Vitamin D.* Boston, MA: Elsevier Academic Press; 2005:899–913.

37. Norman PE, Powell JT. Vitamin D, shedding light on the development of disease in peripheral arteries. *Arterioscler Thromb Vasc Biol* 2005;25:39–46.

38. Holick MF. Sunlight and vitamin D for bone health and prevention of autoimmune diseases, cancers, and cardiovascular disease. *Am J Clin Nutr* 2004;80:1678S–1688S.

39. Wang TJ, Pencina MJ, Booth SL, et al. Vitamin D deficiency and risk of cardiovascular disease. *Circulation* 2008;117:503–511.

40. Giovannucci E, Liu Y, Hollis BW, et al. 25-hydroxyvitamin D and risk of myocardial infarction in men: A prospective study. *Arch Intern Med* 2008;168:1174–1180.

41. Wang AY, Lam CW, Sanderson JE, et al. Serum 25-hydroxyvitamin D status and cardiovascular outcomes in chronic peritoneal dialysis patients: A 3-y prospective cohort study. *Am J Clin Nutr* 2008;87:1631–1638.

42. Dobnig H, Pilz S, Scharnagl H, et al. Independent association of low serum 25-hydroxyvitamin D and 1,25-dihydroxyvitamin d levels with all-cause and cardiovascular mortality. *Arch Intern Med* 2008;168:1340-1349.

43. Pilz S, Dobnig H, Fischer JE, et al. Low vitamin D levels predict stroke in patients referred to coronary angiography. *Stroke* 2008;39:2611–2613.

44. Trivedi DP, Doll R, Khaw KT. Effect of four monthly oral vitamin D3 (cholecalciferol) supplementation on fractures and mortality in men and women living in the community: Randomised double blind controlled trial. *BMJ* 2003;326:469.

45. Hsia J, Heiss G, Ren H, et al. Calcium/vitamin D supplementation and cardiovascular events. *Circulation* 2007;115:846–854.

46. Wang L, Manson JE, Song Y, et al. Systematic review: Vitamin D and calcium supplementation in prevention of cardiovascular events. *Ann Intern Med* 2010;152:315–323.

47. Guallar E, Miller ER 3rd, Ordovas JM, et al. Vitamin D supplementation in the age of lost innocence. *Ann Intern Med* 2010;152:327–329.

48. Pittas AG, Chung M, Trikalinos T, et al. Systematic review: Vitamin D and cardiometabolic outcomes. *Ann Intern Med* 2010;152:307–314.

49. Mathieu C, Adorini L. The coming of age of 1,25-dihydroxyvitamin D(3) analogs as immunomodulatory agents. *Trends Mol Med* 2002;8:174–179.

50. Liu PT, Stenger S, Li H, et al. Toll-like receptor triggering of a vitamin D-mediated human antimicrobial response. *Science* 2006;311:1770–1773.

51. Cannell JJ, Vieth R, Umhau JC, et al. Epidemic influenza and vitamin D. *Epidemiol Infect* 2006;134:1129–1140.

52. Cannell JJ, Vieth R, Willett W, et al. Cod liver oil, vitamin A toxicity, frequent respiratory infections, and the vitamin D deficiency epidemic. *Ann Otol Rhinol Laryngol* 2008;117: 864–870.

53. Bouillon R, Eelen G, Verlinden L, et al. Vitamin D and cancer. *J Steroid Biochem Mol Biol* 2006;102:156–162.

54. Garland CF, Garland FC, Gorham ED, et al. The role of vitamin D in cancer prevention. *Am J Public Health* 2006;96:252–261.

55. Giovannucci E, Liu Y, Rimm EB, et al. Prospective study of predictors of vitamin D status and cancer incidence and mortality in men. *J Natl Cancer Inst* 2006;98:451–459.

56. Freedman DM, Looker AC, Chang SC, et al. Prospective study of serum vitamin D and cancer mortality in the United States. *J Natl Cancer Inst* 2007;99:1594–1602.

57. Feskanich D, Ma J, Fuchs CS, et al. Plasma vitamin D metabolites and risk of colorectal cancer in women. *Cancer Epidemiol Biomarkers Prev* 2004;13:1502–1508.

58. Wactawski-Wende J, Kotchen JM, Anderson GL, et al. Calcium plus vitamin D supplementation and the risk of colorectal cancer. *N Engl J Med* 2006;354:684–696.

59. Jenab M, Bueno-de-Mesquita HB, Ferrari P, et al. Association between pre-diagnostic circulating vitamin D concentration and risk of colorectal cancer in European populations: A nested case-control study. *BMJ* 2010;340:b5500.

60. Chen TC, Holick MF. Vitamin D and prostate cancer prevention and treatment. *Trends Endocrinol Metab* 2003;14:423–430.

61. Garland CF, Gorham ED, Mohr SB, et al. Vitamin D and prevention of breast cancer: Pooled analysis. *J Steroid Biochem Mol Biol* 2007;103:708–711.

62. Janowsky EC, Lester GE, Weinberg CR, et al. Association between low levels of 1,25-dihydroxyvitamin D and breast cancer risk. *Public Health Nutr* 1999;2:283–291.

63. Mawer EB, Walls J, Howell A, et al. Serum 1,25-dihydroxyvitamin D may be related inversely to disease activity in breast cancer patients with bone metastases. *J Clin Endocrinol Metab* 1997;82:118–122.

64. Anderson LN, Cotterchio M, Vieth R, et al. Vitamin D and calcium intakes and breast cancer risk in pre- and postmenopausal women. *Am J Clin Nutr* 2010;91:1699–1707.

65. Merlino LA, Curtis J, Mikuls TR, et al. Vitamin D intake is inversely associated with rheumatoid arthritis: Results from the Iowa Women's Health Study. *Arthritis Rheum* 2004;50: 72–77.

66. Andjelkovic Z, Vojinovic J, Pejnovic N, et al. Disease modifying and immunomodulatory effects of high dose 1 alpha (OH) D3 in rheumatoid arthritis patients. *Clin Exp Rheumatol* 1999;17:453–456.

67. Huckins D, Felson DT, Holick M. Treatment of psoriatic arthritis with oral 1,25-dihydroxyvitamin D3: A pilot study. *Arthritis Rheum* 1990;33:1723–1727.

68. Munger KL, Levin LI, Hollis BW, et al. Serum 25-hydroxyvitamin D levels and risk of multiple sclerosis. *JAMA* 2006;296:2832–2838.

69. Munger KL, Zhang SM, O'Reilly E, et al. Vitamin D intake and incidence of multiple sclerosis. *Neurology* 2004;62:60–65.

70. Binkley N, Krueger D, Cowgill CS, et al. Assay variation confounds the diagnosis of hypovitaminosis D: A call for standardization. *J Clin Endocrinol Metab* 2004;89:3152–3157.

71. Hollis BW. Editorial: The determination of circulating 25-hydroxyvitamin D: No easy task. *J Clin Endocrinol Metab* 2004;89:3149–3151.

72. Armas LA, Hollis BW, Heaney RP. Vitamin D2 is much less effective than vitamin D3 in humans. *J Clin Endocrinol Metab* 2004;89:5387–5391.

73. Holick MF, Biancuzzo RM, Chen TC, et al. Vitamin D2 is as effective as vitamin D3 in maintaining circulating concentrations of 25-hydroxyvitamin D. *J Clin Endocrinol Metab* 2008;93:677–681.

74. Heikinheimo RJ, Inkovaara JA, Harju EJ, et al. Annual injection of vitamin D and fractures of aged bones. *Calcif Tissue Int* 1992;51:105–110.

75. Orbak Z, Doneray H, Keskin F, et al. Vitamin D intoxication and therapy with alendronate (case report and review of literature). *Eur J Pediatr* 2006;165:583–584.

76. Wills MR. The urinary calcium-creatinine ratio as a measure of urinary calcium excretion. *J Clin Pathol* 1969;22:287–290.

Osteoporosis

25

Amy E. Riek, Kathryn Diemer, and Roberto Civitelli

GENERAL PRINCIPLES

- Osteoporosis is the most common metabolic bone disorder in humans, and the spectrum of osteoporosis and low bone mass affects more than 43 million people in the United States[1] and 200 million worldwide.[2] Approximately 2 million osteoporotic fractures occur each year in the United States, with significant associated morbidity and mortality, particularly related to hip fractures, and economic costs are projected to reach $25 billion by 2025.[3]
- Significant advances in diagnostic testing since the early 1990s have made osteoporosis relatively easy to diagnose. Multiple pharmacotherapeutic agents are available that enhance bone density and decrease the rates of fracture at various clinical sites.
- A significant percentage of patients with osteoporosis, including those who have already experienced fractures, are not appropriately diagnosed and treated.

Definition

Osteoporosis, which literally means "porous bone," is a disorder characterized by low bone mass and microarchitectural deterioration of bone that leads to a decrease in bone mass, enhanced bone fragility, and a consequent increase in the risk of fractures.[4]

Classification

- Clinically, osteoporosis may be diagnosed on the basis of any fragility or low-trauma fracture (fall from standing height or less or a bone that breaks under conditions that normally would not cause fracture), regardless of bone mineral densitometry testing.
- The World Health Organization (WHO) has established osteoporosis by criteria based on bone densitometry testing. The T-score is the difference, in standard deviation units, between a patient's bone mineral density (BMD) and that of a young adult reference mean (see Bone Mineral Density Testing in this chapter). Diagnostic categories are based on the **lowest T-score out of the lumbar spine, total hip, and femoral neck** (not individual vertebrae or Ward's triangle).[5]
  ○ **Normal:** BMD within 1 SD of the young adult reference mean (T ≥ −1.0)
  ○ **Low bone bass ("osteopenia"):** BMD between 1 and 2.5 SDs below the young adult reference mean (−2.5 < T < −1.0)
  ○ **Osteoporosis:** BMD ≥ 2.5 SDs below the young adult reference mean (T ≤ −2.5)
  ○ **Established or severe osteoporosis:** BMD ≥ 2.5 SDs below the young adult reference mean (T ≤ −2.5) and the presence of one or more fragility fractures
- The WHO classification was established in postmenopausal women and thus does not apply to premenopausal women or younger men (but can be applied to

perimenopausal women and men >50 years). In premenopausal women and men <50 years, the diagnosis of osteoporosis cannot be made based on BMD alone, and these patients should have their bone density classified by Z-scores (compared to age-matched reference mean).[6]

○ **"Within the expected range for age"**: BMD within 2.0 SDs of the reference mean (Z > –2.0)

○ **"Below the expected range for age"**: BMD ≥ 2.0 SDs below the reference mean (Z ≤ –2.0)

• T-scores should be based on a Caucasian, gender-specific reference mean, and Z-scores should be based on a gender- and race-specific reference mean.[6]

Epidemiology

• Approximately 8 million women and 2 million men in the United States have osteoporosis, and an additional 34 million have low bone mass and are at risk for the development of osteoporosis.[1]

• The prevalence of low bone mass and progression to osteoporosis increases with age, from 54% and 4%, respectively, in women age 50 to 59 years, to 43% and 52% in those age 80 to 85 years.[7]

• There are racial/ethnic differences in prevalence as reported on older women from recent NHANES 2005–2006 data, with low bone mass and osteoporosis reported in 52% and 11%, respectively, of non-Hispanic white older women, 36% and 7% of non-Hispanic black women, and 38% and 10% of Mexican American women.[8]

Pathophysiology

• Total bone mineral content in adults is dependent on peak bone mass achieved during early adulthood and level of bone remodeling. Bone remodeling takes place throughout childhood and adulthood and is a result of the balance of concurrent bone resorption and new bone formation. Osteoporosis can result from either inadequate bone mass accrual in the first 2 to 3 decades of life and failure to achieve expected peak bone mass or from increased bone remodeling and bone loss with age.[9]

• Peak bone mass is generally reached at approximately age 25 to 30 and is primarily determined by genetic factors, including race and gender. However, potentially modifiable environmental and metabolic conditions, such as nutritional status, calcium intake, physical activity level, tobacco use, hormonal deficiencies, and other medical comorbidities, can also affect the level of peak bone mass achieved.[9]

• Black women and men typically achieve higher levels of peak bone mass than white women, which is a key contributor to the lower rates of osteoporosis and fractures in these groups. Men typically have a BMD that is 8% to 18% greater at different sites than women. However, such difference is in most part accounted for by the fact that male bones are larger than female bones, resulting in higher BMD values, as detected by dual-energy X-ray absorptiometry (DXA). Adults who do not achieve their predicted peak bone mass are at risk of developing osteoporosis at an earlier age.[9]

• When the rate of bone resorption exceeds that of bone formation, the overall increased rate of bone turnover leads to a net loss of bone mass. Men and women slowly begin to lose peak bone mass at a rate of ~0.5% to 1% per year starting at approximately age 35. The rate of net bone loss is increased after menopause in

TABLE 25-1	RISK FACTORS FOR OSTEOPOROSIS AND FRACTURES

Female sex
White race
Advanced age
Personal history of a fracture
Family history of osteoporosis/fracture in a first-degree relative
Small body habitus/low body weight (<127 lb)
Sedentary lifestyle/lack of physical activity
Tobacco use
Excessive alcohol intake (>2 drinks/day)
Insufficient intake of calcium or vitamin D
Excessive caffeine intake
Ovarian failure or early (medical or surgical) menopause (age <45 years)

women, as estrogen deficiency enhances osteoclast activity via loss of estrogen inhibition of osteoclastogenic factors. This accelerated rate of bone loss is most prominent in areas of trabecular bone, such as the spine, and may result in a rate of loss of bone mass of 3% to 5% per year for up to 10 years. The rate of bone loss in areas with more cortical bone, such as the hips, tends to be delayed and less rapid. Because men achieve a higher peak bone mass initially and do not usually go through a rapid period of bone loss, in the absence of secondary disorders, bone loss does not tend to reach levels that increase the risk for fractures until age 65 to 70.[9]

Risk Factors

- Multiple risk factors have been shown to be independently associated with low bone mass (Table 25-1). Some of these risk factors are modifiable and are important to address in a regimen to prevent or treat osteoporosis.[10]
- There are also many chronic medical conditions and medications that are risk factors for causing secondary osteoporosis (Table 25-2).[10]
- Osteoporotic fractures typically result from falls in adults with low bone density. As such, risk factors for falling independent of those for low bone mass are important contributors to morbidity from osteoporotic fractures (Table 25-3).[10]

Prevention

- Most patients with osteoporosis are asymptomatic until they develop fractures. Regardless whether a diagnostic test for osteoporosis is requested, prevention strategies should focus on reduction of risk factors (Tables 25-1 and 25-2).
- Based on the prevalence of the condition, accessibility of diagnostic testing, and available treatment options, several national societies have issued guidelines for identifying subjects at risk of fragility (low trauma) fractures (Table 25-4).[10–12] In general, all groups agree that women who present with fragility fractures in the absence of trauma should be tested, but opinions vary on whether and under which conditions adults without fractures should be tested. **Most U.S. guidelines support bone density testing all women over age 65**, with **some supporting testing all men over age 70**, regardless of risk factors. In younger adults, testing is typically recommended in the presence of previous fractures or risk factors for osteoporosis. Of note, although the majority of data on the diagnosis and treatment of osteoporosis

TABLE 25-2 CAUSES OF SECONDARY OSTEOPOROSIS

Endocrine disorders
Acromegaly
Amenorrhea (primary or secondary
   amenorrhea of any cause)
Anorexia
Cushing's syndrome/hypercortisolism
Diabetes mellitus, type 1
Hyperparathyroidism
Hyperprolactinemia
Hyperthyroidism
Hypogonadism (primary or
   secondary)
Porphyria

Genetic/collagen disorders
Ehlers–Danlos
Glycogen storage diseases
Homocystinuria
Hypophosphatasia
Osteogenesis imperfect

Gastrointestinal/hepatic disorders
Celiac disease
Chronic cholestatic liver disease
Chronic malabsorptive conditions
Cirrhosis
Gastric bypass/gastrectomy
Hemochromatosis
Inflammatory bowel disease

Hematologic disorders
Amyloidosis
Leukemia/lymphoma
Mastocytosis
Multiple myeloma

Infectious diseases
HIV/AIDS

Metabolic/nutritional disorders
Alcoholism
Hyperhomocystinemia
Hypocalcemia
Vitamin D deficiency

Pulmonary disorders
Chronic obstructive pulmonary
   disease

Renal disorders
Chronic kidney disease (of any
   cause)
Renal tubular acidosis

Rheumatologic disorders
Ankylosing spondylitis
Rheumatoid arthritis

Medications
Aluminum
Cyclosporine
Dilantin
Glucocorticoids
Gonadotropin agonists (e.g., Lupron)
Heparin (prolonged use)
Methotrexate
Phenobarbital
Phenothiazines
Protease inhibitors
Thyroxine (excessive replacement)

TABLE 25-3 RISK FACTORS FOR FALLING

History of falls
Dementia
Impaired vision
Poor physical condition/frailty
Foot problems or inappropriate footwear
History of stroke or Parkinson's disease
Environmental hazards
Use of benzodiazepines, anticonvulsants, or anticholinergic medications

TABLE 25-4 RECOMMENDED TESTING GUIDELINES FOR OSTEOPOROSIS

Group	Recommended in all women, regardless of risk factors?	Recommended in adult women with risk factors?	Recommended in all men, regardless of risk factors?	Recommended in adult men with risk factors?
National Osteoporosis Foundation	Yes, age 65	Yes, if postmenopausal with fractures or risk factors, if any age with high risk condition or medication	Yes, age 70	Yes, if age >50 with fractures or risk factors, if any age with high risk condition or medication
American Association of Clinical Endocrinologists	Yes, age 65	Yes, if postmenopausal with risk factors, esp. with low body weight (<57.6 kg) or family history of hip/spine fracture, if any age with fragility fracture	No	No
U.S. Preventative Services Task Force	Yes, age 65	Yes, if age 60–64, esp. with low body weight (<70 kg) or no estrogen	No	No

is in white women, the recommendations for screening for osteoporosis are irrespective of race.

Associated Conditions

Osteoporotic fractures

- **Fragility fractures are the primary cause of morbidity and mortality in adults with osteoporosis.** The most common sites for osteoporotic fractures are the hip, the spine, and the distal radius (forearm or wrist). Approximately 1.5 million osteoporotic fractures occur each year in the United States, including 700,000 vertebral fractures, 300,000 hip fractures, 200,000 wrist fractures, and 300,000 other fractures.[9]
- In white women age 65 to 85, it is estimated that 90% of all vertebral fractures, 90% of all hip fractures, 70% of all forearm fractures, and 50% of all other fractures are attributable to osteoporosis. The corresponding rates in black women are 80% for vertebral fractures, 80% for hip fractures, 60% for forearm fractures, and 40% for all other fractures. In both races, a smaller percentage of fractures can be attributed to osteoporosis in women younger than age 65, but a larger percentage can be attributed to osteoporosis in women older than 85.[13]
- A 50-year-old white woman has an approximately 40% risk of experiencing an osteoporotic fracture during her lifetime (compared to the 23% risk in a man), including a 15% risk of a having a vertebral fracture, a 17% risk of having a hip fracture, and a 16% risk of having a wrist fracture. With the anticipated aging of the population, osteoporotic fractures are predicted to increase several-fold worldwide by 2050.[14]
- **Hip fractures are the most devastating cause of morbidity and mortality attributable to osteoporosis.** Mortality rates in the first year following fracture are 20%, and an additional 50% lose daily functioning, resulting in only 30% of patients regaining their prefracture level of function. Many patients lose independence and require long-term care. Treatment of hip fractures and their associated complications is responsible for the majority of the cost of treating osteoporosis, estimated at $14 billion in 1995 and $17 billion in 2001.[9]
- Vertebral fractures are also associated with significant morbidity and mortality. **Vertebral fractures tend to be more occult than hip fractures,** with only one-third presenting clinically. As opposed to hip and wrist fractures, most vertebral fractures are not related to acute trauma and can result from routine everyday activities. Up to 20% of patients require hospitalization, and vertebral fractures are associated with chronic back pain, loss of height, and kyphosis. Multiple vertebral fractures can result in the development of restrictive lung disease or gastrointestinal complications that have been shown to decrease quality of life across several domains. Most important, long-term prospective studies have shown that vertebral fractures, whether symptomatic or not, are associated with a 15% to 30% increased rate of overall mortality, including increased risk of mortality secondary to all cancers, specifically lung cancer.[9,15]
- **Prior osteoporotic fracture represents the greatest risk factor for future fracture** with relative risk ranging from 1.4 to 4.4 depending on the site of initial fracture.[16]

DIAGNOSIS

Clinical Presentation

Most patients with osteoporosis are asymptomatic until they develop fractures. As such, the history and physical examination are usually not sufficiently sensitive until the advanced stages of disease to make a diagnosis of osteoporosis in the absence of diagnostic testing. However, a complete assessment of the patient's history and physical findings may suggest a high likelihood of low bone mass, the presence of an occult fracture, or of other modifiable risk factors even before bone density is assessed. A thorough history will also identify exposure to medications or the presence of diseases that are known to affect bone metabolism.[17] Men are more likely than women to have secondary osteoporosis. Recent findings suggest that a **laboratory evaluation, including serum testosterone, is recommended in men,** as 75% of men had a secondary cause of their osteoporosis.[18]

History
The primary focus should include all risk factors for low bone mass, fracture, and falling to address prevention strategies (Tables 25-1 through 25-3).

Physical Examination
The physical exam should include assessment of findings suggestive of fracture and/or disability contributing to fracture risk:
- Loss of height
- Kyphosis
- Chest deformity
- Rib-pelvis overlap
- Respiratory difficulty
- Protuberant abdomen and GI symptoms
- Impaired ambulation

Diagnostic Criteria
See Classification Section.

Diagnostic Testing
Laboratories
- Laboratory assessment of asymptomatic postmenopausal women with osteoporosis led to identification of a secondary etiology in 47%.[17] **Laboratory analysis on all patients should include**
  ○ Chemistry panel, including calcium, phosphorus, creatinine
  ○ Hepatic function panel including liver transaminases, alkaline phosphatase, total protein, albumin
  ○ 25-OH vitamin D (25(OH)D)
- Further testing as clinically indicated could include
  ○ Intact PTH
  ○ 24-hour urine for calcium and creatinine
  ○ Thyroid function tests
  ○ Serum or urine protein electrophoresis
  ○ 24-hour urine for cortisol
  ○ Antibodies for assessment of celiac disease
  ○ Testosterone (men only)
- **Bone turnover markers are rarely used in the diagnosis of osteoporosis.** Although they do have some utility in predicting fracture risk in population-based studies,[19] their high biologic and analytical variability limit their diagnostic usefulness in individual subjects. They could be used after initiation of antiresorptive treatment as indicators of adherence to treatment.

○ Markers of bone formation: serum alkaline phosphatase and osteocalcin
○ Markers of bone resorption: serum C-telopeptide (CTX) and urine N-telopeptide (NTX)

Imaging
• **Bone mineral density testing**
  ○ The **standard of care for diagnosis and evaluation of adults for osteoporosis** is to assess BMD. Several radiologic tests are available to measure BMD, including central and peripheral dual energy X-ray absorptiometry (DXA), central and peripheral quantitative computed tomography (QCT), and quantitative ultrasonography (QUS).
  ○ Decreased BMD is a strong predictor of subsequent fracture. On average, the risk of fracture approximately doubles for each 1 SD decrease in the T-score. Although decreased bone density at one site allows the diagnosis of osteoporosis to be made and increases the risk for fracture at all sites, the best predictor of fracture at a specific site is the bone density at that site. This is most important at the hip, which is the fracture site most associated with morbidity and mortality. For each 1 SD decrease in hip BMD, the risk of hip fractures increases by 2.6-fold, that of vertebral fractures by 1.8-fold, that of wrist fractures by 1.4-fold, and the risk of all fractures increases by 1.5-fold. The risk of a subsequent hip fracture associated with decreased BMD at other sites is somewhat lower.[20,21]
  ○ **Central (includes torso, pelvis, proximal femurs) DXA**
    ■ DXA imaging, the current standard method for bone density testing, requires a low level of radiation exposure (approximately one-tenth that of a traditional X-ray) and has excellent precision and reproducibility.[6]
    ■ The **recommended sites to measure are the spine and the proximal femur**, with the distal radius being an alternate possibility. BMD results are calculated as the bone mineral content divided by the area of bone measured (g/cm^2). In the lumbar spine, measurements are generally made at the L1, L2, L3, and L4 vertebrae and vertebrae-specific and total L1–L4 spine BMD data are given. At the hip, measurements are made in three different areas: at the femoral neck, the greater trochanter, and the intertrochanteric area, which includes part of the proximal diaphysis. A total proximal femur BMD is also calculated as the sum of bone mineral content of all three areas divided by the total area. An area roughly corresponding to the Ward's triangle is no longer used for diagnostic purposes. The femoral neck BMD, composed almost equally of cortical and trabecular bone, is a very good predictor of fracture risk; whereas the total proximal femur BMD is generally used for monitoring changes.[6]
    ■ Results of BMD testing are then reported in comparison to reference ranges and normalized to the standard deviation of the reference population. The **T-score** represents the difference, in SD units, between the patient's BMD and the average peak BMD of young healthy adults of the same gender, while the **Z-score** represents the patient's BMD in SDs after subtracting the average BMD of adults of the same age and gender. The T-score and Z-score are interpreted as described in the Classification section. A critical consideration to keep in mind is that T-scores (and Z-scores) are technique-specific; since different normative databases are used, T-scores obtained from different methods for assessing bone density are not comparable. For estimation of fracture risk and diagnosis of osteoporosis, only central DXA T-scores are used. As described in the Classification section, the lowest of total spine, total proximal femur, or femoral neck BMD determines the diagnosis of low bone mass or osteoporosis.[6]

- Several important factors should be considered with respect to sites for DXA. For a full assessment of a patient's bone mass and more accurate determination of fracture risk, bone density testing should be obtained of both the spine and hip. Nonetheless, since in the early postmenopausal period bone loss occurs more rapidly in the spine, this site is often more helpful in women younger than 65 or within 15 years of menopause. Furthermore, vertebral fractures are the most common type of fracture in this age group. **In older subjects, the bone density of the spine may be falsely elevated by osteoarthritis of the spine or vascular calcification,** so bone density of the hip is often more clinically useful, especially since hip fractures become more of a clinical concern. Adults with primary hyperparathyroidism lose bone most rapidly in the distal radius, so this site would be preferred in this circumstance. Finally, patients with a prior fracture should not have the fracture site included in DXA assessment, as BMD will be falsely elevated.[6]
  ○ **Quantitative CT scanning** can be performed by any commercially available CT scanner. Similarly to central DXA, it measures BMD of the hip and spine and has a similar ability to predict fractures. Unlike DXA, it is a measure of volumetric density and reports results in g/cm^3. It, therefore, may have utility in patients at extremes of size (extremely thin or extremely obese) and is less affected by superimposed osteoarthritis. However, quantitative CT scanning is more expensive, requires a larger dose of radiation, and is not frequently used clinically.[22] Furthermore, based on the criteria of the National Osteoporosis Foundation, it cannot be used for the diagnosis of osteoporosis or low bone mass.[10]
  ○ **Peripheral (extremities excluding the proximal femurs) bone density testing** can be performed with DXA, QCT, or QUS. Sites that can be measured include the forearm, finger, and heel. The primary benefits of peripheral bone densitometry techniques are the portability of the equipment and the ability of the tests to be performed in a primary care office. While these modalities have been shown to be predictive of fractures, there are no universally accepted diagnostic criteria for the variety of machines available, and the precision of the machines does not allow their use for monitoring response to therapy. Peripheral testing has not been fully endorsed for use in the diagnosis of osteoporosis, but if peripheral testing is performed, abnormal results should be followed up with a central DXA to establish or confirm the diagnosis.[23]
- **Conventional radiography (plain films)** is generally an unreliable marker of bone mass, as 30% of bone must be lost before changes are evident on X-ray. If osteopenia is suggested by radiographs, bone densitometry should be performed to confirm low bone mass.[24]

TREATMENT

- **Indications for treatment**[10]
  ○ All adults with osteoporotic fractures
  ○ All adults over age 50 with DXA T-score ≤ −2.5 of the femoral neck or spine (osteoporosis)
  ○ All adults over age 50 with DXA T-score between −1.0 and −2.5 (low bone mass) with 10-year risk for hip fracture ≥3% or major osteoporotic fracture ≥20%
    - The WHO Fracture Risk Assessment Tool (FRAX) was recently developed to estimate 10-year fracture risk and is available at www.sheffield.ac.uk/FRAX. This algorithm integrates age, gender, ethnicity, geographic locality, weight, height, personal and family fracture history, tobacco use, glucocorticoid use,

diagnosis of rheumatoid arthritis, alcohol use, and femoral neck BMD to produce an estimated fracture risk in patients with a diagnosis of low bone mass. However, it has not been validated in currently or previously treated patients, and it cannot be used for treatment monitoring.[25]

○ **All patients should be evaluated for risk factors for osteoporosis.** The nonpharmacologic and lifestyle recommendations (see Lifestyle/Risk Modification section) should be suggested to all adults, including those who do not meet the criteria for specific pharmacologic therapy for osteoporosis, to prevent the development of osteoporosis.

Medications

First Line
- For information about osteoporosis medications, see Tables 25-5 and 25-6.
- **Aminobisphosphonates: alendronate (Fosamax), Risedronate (Actonel, Atelvia), Ibandronate (Boniva), and Zoledronic acid (Reclast).** The aminobisphosphonates have a chemical structure that resemble pyrophosphate and are powerful inhibitors of osteoclast-mediated bone resorption. All agents have been shown to **improve bone density** at 3 years at various sites in the skeleton and **decrease the rates of hip and vertebral fractures** (except ibandronate, which has only been shown to decrease vertebral fractures).[26–34]

  ○ **Oral aminobisphosphonates** approved by the FDA for the treatment of osteoporosis include **alendronate, risedronate, and ibandronate,** with dosing regimens ranging from daily to monthly. Alendronate is available with supplemental vitamin D, and risedronate is available with supplemental calcium. Oral aminobisphosphonates are poorly absorbed and **should be taken early in the morning with a glass of water followed by at least 30 minutes without recumbency, food, or other medications** to prevent retention of the pills in the esophagus. Recently approved Atelvia may be taken with breakfast, but still requires 30 minutes without recumbency. Antacids and calcium limit their absorption. In the randomized, placebo-controlled trials with alendronate, risedronate, and ibandronate, there was no significant difference in the rate of gastrointestinal side effects between the agents and placebo, and more recent once-weekly and once-monthly dosing regimens have improved compliance. However, in clinical practice, about 10% of patients have gastrointestinal distress, and severe erosive esophagitis related to pill "reflux" is a rare but serious complication. Recently, concerns have been raised regarding a possible increased risk of esophageal cancer, but this is rare and causative data are conflicting. **However, oral formulations should not be given to those with Barrett's esophagus or gastrointestinal disease.**[35]

  ○ **Intravenous formulations** approved by the FDA for osteoporosis include **ibandronate and zoledronic acid,** with dosing every 3 or 12 months, respectively. The infusion can cause an acute phase "flu-like" reaction in some patients, but this is tempered by pretreatment with acetaminophen.[36] Aminobisphosphonates are cleared by the kidney, and renal failure has been reported with intravenous formulations, so **creatinine should be checked prior to each infusion.** This association has not been demonstrated with ibandronate, so this may be a preferred choice in patients with chronic kidney disease, but **GFR <30 mL/minute (<35 mL/minute for zoledronic acid) is a contraindication to treatment.**[37] Atrial fibrillation has been found to be associated with zoledronic acid administration in one trial, but this has not been confirmed in any other trials with the same or other aminobisphosphonates.[27]

TABLE 25-5   AVAILABLE AGENTS AND DOSING FOR OSTEOPOROSIS

Agent	FDA approved for Prevention	Dose for prevention	FDA approved for treatment	Dose for treatment
Alendronate (Fosamax)	Yes	5 mg PO daily 35 mg PO weekly	Yes	10 mg PO daily 70 mg PO weekly
Risedronate (Actonel, Atelvia)	Yes	5 mg PO daily 35 mg PO weekly 75 mg PO on two consecutive days monthly 150 mg PO monthly	Yes	5 mg PO daily 35 mg PO weekly 75 mg PO on two consecutive days monthly 150 mg PO monthly
Ibandronate (Boniva)	Yes	2.5 mg PO daily 150 mg PO monthly	Yes	2.5 mg PO daily 150 mg PO monthly 4 mg IV every 3 months
Zoledronate (Reclast)	Yes	5 mg IV every 2 years	Yes	5 mg IV yearly
Raloxifene (Evista)	Yes	60 mg PO daily	Yes	60 mg PO daily
Estrogen (alone or with progesterone; multiple combinations available	Yes	Variable, typically 0.625 mg PO daily conjugated estrogen	No	Not applicable
Calcitonin (Miacalcin)	No	Not applicable	Yes	200 IU intranasally daily
Teriparatide (Forteo)	No	Not applicable	Yes	20 mcg SQ daily
Denosumab (Prolia)	No	Not applicable	Yes	60 mg SQ every 6 months

TABLE 25-6 AVAILABLE AGENTS FOR OSTEOPOROSIS: IMPACT ON BONE MINERAL DENSITY (BMD) AND FRACTURES

Agent	Increase in BMD of spine	Increase in BMD of hip	Decrease in rate of vertebral fractures	Decrease in rate of hip fractures	Decrease in rate of nonvertebral fractures
Alendronate (Fosamax)	6%–13%	4%–7%	40%–55%	50%–55%	20%–47%
Risedronate (Actonel, Atelvia)	5%–11%	2%–5%	40%–60%	40%–60%	20%–40%
Ibandronate (Boniva)	3%–5%	2%–5%	50%–60%	Studies not powered	Studies not powered
Zoledronate (Zometa, Reclast)	4%–7%	3%–6%	70%	41%	25%
Raloxifene (Evista)	3%	2%	30%–50%	Not significant	Not significant
Teriparatide (Forteo)	8%–14%	3%–5%	65%–70%	Studies not powered	53%
Denosumab (Prolia)	9%	6%	63%	40%	20%
Estrogen/hormone replacement therapy[a]	4%–7%	2%–4%	34%–40%	34%–36%	24%–27%
Calcitonin (Miacalcin)	1%–2%	No change	33%	Not significant	Not significant
Strontium Ranelate	14%	8%	40%	36%	Not studied

[a]Data for estrogen-/hormone-replacement therapy are from studies in postmenopausal women and not in women with known osteoporosis.

○ **Osteonecrosis of the jaw** is a rare complication of treatment, occurring in 1/10,000 to 1/100,000 patients, usually related to oral bone trauma and infection. Patients receiving high cumulative intravenous doses, typically in the setting of malignancy, are at increased risk, but at the doses of aminobisphosphonates used for osteoporosis osteonecrosis of the jaw is extremely rare. Defining its real incidence is complicated by the often inconsistent definition of the syndrome. Nonetheless, current recommendations are to **delay the initiation of amino-bisphosphonates until after any planned oral surgery and avoid oral surgery as much as possible while on these medications.**[38]

○ Recently, reports of subtrochanteric fractures, also called "atypical femoral fractures," have emerged in patients exposed to aminobisphosphonates. These are non-traumatic, transverse or slightly oblique, non-union fractures of the subtrochanter or femoral diaphysis sometimes called "chalk-stick" fractures. While the cause of these fractures is not entirely clear, they may be related to underlying abnormal bone quality. Whether they are caused or prevented by aminobisphosphonates remains to be seen, as these fractures also occur in subjects who have not received these drugs. A link to prolonged inhibition of bone turnover has been postulated but not demonstrated. Even assuming that atypical femoral fractures are a complication of therapy, it is estimated that at most 1 occurs for every 100 "routine" hip fractures prevented. Nonetheless, because of these increased concern about long-term effects of bisphosphonates on bone mineralization and turnover, in subjects with less severe osteoporosis (no prior fracture or T-score $\geq$ –3.5) a drug holiday of <2 years following 5 years of aminobisphosphonate treatment does not appear to increase fracture risk. **If an atypical fracture occurs, the aminobisphosphonate should be discontinued, with consideration of initiation of alternative therapies.**[39]

○ Other contraindications to aminobisphosphonates include drug class hypersensitivity and hypocalcemia.

• **Raloxifene (Evista)** is an orally formulated selective estrogen receptor modulator that is approved by the FDA for the treatment of osteoporosis. It exhibits pro-estrogenic effects on certain tissues and anti-estrogenic effects on other tissues, exhibiting beneficial effects on bone by blocking the activity of cytokines that stimulate osteoclast-mediated bone resorption. Raloxifene has been shown in randomized controlled trials lasting up to 3 to 4 years to **improve BMD** at the spine and the hip and to **decrease the rate of new vertebral fractures.**[40] Raloxifene has not been found to have a significant impact on hip or total nonvertebral fractures. Therefore, the ideal candidate for raloxifene is a woman who has predominantly decreased BMD at the spine with more preserved levels of bone density at the hip, especially a woman who cannot tolerate an aminobisphosphonate.

○ Raloxifene decreases total cholesterol and low-density lipoprotein (LDL) cholesterol in a manner similar to estrogen, but does not raise high-density lipoprotein (HDL) cholesterol and triglycerides as estrogen does. Raloxifene does not reduce hot flashes. It does **increase the risk of deep venous thrombosis and pulmonary embolism** in a fashion similar to estrogen, which is thus a contraindication to its use. However, raloxifene does not stimulate the endometrium or breast and does not increase the risk of endometrial hyperplasia or cancer or breast cancer. In fact, a significant decrease in estrogen receptor–positive breast cancer as a secondary end point was found in a large clinical trial with raloxifene.[41,42]

○ Because of the adverse cardiovascular events associated with estrogen use, the RUTH study was performed to study the cardiovascular impact of raloxifene. This randomized controlled trial of postmenopausal women with coronary heart disease (CHD) or risk factors for CHD were followed for 5.6 years with no significant difference in the risk of primary coronary events between the raloxifene and placebo groups. The study did show a decrease in the risk of breast cancer, but an increased risk of venous thromboembolism and fatal strokes in the treatment arm, although total all-cause mortality was similar between groups. Therefore, these risks need to be weighed against the benefits of reducing vertebral fractures and the risk of breast cancer in women considered for raloxifene therapy.[41]

- **Teriparatide** (Forteo) is a recombinant formulation of the active 34 N-terminal peptide portion of parathyroid hormone, and it is FDA-approved for osteoporosis. Although continuous exposure to PTH (as in patients with primary hyperparathyroidism) leads to increased bone resorption, intermittent exposure has been shown to stimulate bone formation. Teriparatide is the first bone "anabolic" agent introduced for clinical use; unlike pharmacologic agents that decrease bone resorption, teriparatide works by stimulating new bone formation. Its mechanism of action is not completely clear, but it has been shown to act at different steps in the osteoblast differentiation program, including recruitment of new osteoblasts, stimulating the activity of existing osteoblasts, and prolonging their survival.[43]

  ○ Teriparatide is administered by daily subcutaneous injections, at a dose of 20 mcg, and increases BMD at the spine and hip by 19 months to a greater extent than any of the aminobisphosphonates. It also decreases vertebral fractures and total nonvertebral fractures, but hip fracture improvement has not yet been demonstrated.[44]

  ○ Because of its significant cost, teriparatide should generally be **reserved for patients with severe or established osteoporosis**, particularly those who cannot tolerate or have not responded well to bisphosphonates. Mild hypercalcemia develops within 4 to 6 hours after injection, but serum calcium returns within the normal range thereafter. High doses of teriparatide in rats resulted in an increased rate of osteosarcoma, though this has not been seen in human trials. Teriparatide thus carries a **black-box warning about osteosarcoma** and is **contraindicated in those with preexisting hypercalcemia, metastatic bone disease, or increased risk for osteosarcoma** (Paget's disease, prior radiation therapy to bone, open epiphyses). Treatment is not recommended for >2 years.[43]

- **Denosumab (Prolia)** is the most recently FDA-approved drug for the treatment of osteoporosis. Receptor activator of nuclear factor kappa B ligand (RANKL) is released by osteoblasts and is essential to stimulate the differentiation of osteoclasts. Denosumab is a monoclonal antibody against RANKL, thus inhibiting osteoclast bone resorption. In fact, it is the most powerful inhibitor of bone resorption among the drugs used in osteoporosis. Similar to other bone resorption inhibitors, denosumab also decreases osteoblast-mediated bone formation, because bone resorption and formation are so tightly coupled. Denosumab is administered by subcutaneous injection of 60 mg every 6 months.[45]

  ○ In a study of postmenopausal women with severe osteoporosis (23% with prior fracture and average spine T-score –2.8), denosumab improved BMD in the total hip, femoral neck, and spine at 3 years compared to placebo. Additionally, the relative risk of fracture was reduced by 68% for vertebral, 40% for hip, and 20% for nonvertebral fractures. The risk reduction in vertebral fracture was independent of age, baseline bone turnover, baseline BMD, baseline fractures, and prior treatments for osteoporosis. These reductions are comparable to those of zoledronic acid and teriparatide.[46]

  ○ Adverse effects reported with denosumab include skin infections, eczema and/or rash, and pancreatitis. As with all antiresorptive medications, hypocalcemia and drug hypersensitivity are contraindications. Osteonecrosis of the jaw has been reported with denosumab in two cases after more than 3 years of treatment. No "atypical" fractures have emerged in any denosumab trials do far.[45] Denosumab is not cleared by the kidney, so adjustment for renal failure is not necessary. However, in 38% of patients, bone biopsy at 3 years showed no tetracycline labeling, suggestive of virtually absent bone formation.[47] Given the risk of low turnover bone disease in patients with chronic kidney failure, extreme caution should be taken as the long-term effects of denosumab in this population are unclear. Denosumab is approved for patients with osteoporosis at high risk of fractures, and in those who are intolerance or insensitive to other therapies.

Second Line
- **Estrogen/hormone replacement therapy (HRT)** is **FDA-approved only for the prevention of osteoporosis** and improves bone density by inhibiting osteoclast activity. Little of the clinical data assessing the impact of estrogen have been in women with documented osteoporosis. As a result, most of the data on estrogen are more appropriate to interpret for prevention rather than treatment of osteoporosis.
  - Estrogen alone or in combination with progestin improves BMD in the spine and hip at 3 years in recently postmenopausal women.[48] The WHI demonstrated that combination estrogen–progesterone replacement therapy decreases the rate of total fractures, vertebral fractures, hip fractures, and other osteoporotic fractures by 24%, 34%, 34%, and 23%, respectively.[49]
  - Extraskeletal effects of HRT are numerous. In the WHI, although the rate of colon cancer was decreased by 37%, the overall rate of adverse events, including a 29% increase in CHD, a 41% increase in stroke, a 111% increase in deep venous thrombosis/pulmonary embolism, and a 26% increase in breast cancer, exceeded the benefits, including fracture reduction. Similar rates of fracture reductions were found in the estrogen-alone group in women of the WHI who previously had a hysterectomy, with fewer of the adverse effects seen in the combination estrogen/progesterone group. Additionally, no increased risk cardiovascular disease was demonstrated in women within 10 years of menopause.[50]
  - Little prospective data actually exist in patients with known osteoporosis; only one published small trial found a decrease in vertebral fractures with transdermal estrogen.[51] Based on the lack of data in treating known osteoporosis and the balance of adverse events shown in the WHI, HRT has largely fallen out of favor for the prevention or treatment of osteoporosis. In women considering HRT for relief of menopausal symptoms, it should be used in the lowest effective doses for the shortest possible time period, and these women may gain benefit in BMD and fracture risk. However, other treatments should be strongly considered first for osteoporosis prevention in women with no other indication for HRT.
- **Calcitonin (Miacalcin)** is an endogenous peptide that enhances BMD by **inhibiting osteoclast activity**. Calcitonin is available in both subcutaneous and intranasal forms, but the intranasal route has been most studied. The daily intranasal formulation is approved by the FDA for osteoporosis in women who are at least 5 years postmenopause.
  - The beneficial effects on BMD of the spine are generally less with calcitonin than with most of the other agents available to treat osteoporosis, with no differences with placebo after 2 years. Minimal to no impact has been seen on BMD of the hip. In the Prevent Recurrences of Osteoporotic Fracture (PROOF) study, only the 200 IU/day dose was found to decrease vertebral fractures after 5 years, and there was no significant decrease in hip or nonvertebral fractures.[52]

○ Calcitonin is typically a second- or third-line agent for the treatment of osteoporosis and is primarily reserved for patients with either contraindications to or intolerable side effects from other agents, particularly bisphosphonates. It can rarely cause nasal irritation and epistaxis. However, intranasal calcitonin has been found to be **beneficial in treating the pain of acute vertebral compression fractures.**[53]

- **Unapproved medications**
  ○ **Strontium ranelate**, a strontium salt of ranelic acid, is approved in an oral formulation for the treatment of osteoporosis in more than 70 other countries, primarily in Europe. Strontium has been shown to reduce the risk of vertebral fractures by 40%, with hip fracture reductions of 36% in an older subgroup of patients. It was well tolerated with no significant adverse events reported. However, its mechanism of action remains puzzling, as there is no strong evidence that it affects bone remodeling in any way, and whether its stimulatory action on the calcium sensing receptor contributes to the beneficial effect on fracture prevention is unclear.[54] Strontium ranelate is not currently approved by the FDA, but strontium citrate is available in the US in over-the-counter food supplements. However, this preparation has no fracture data. It should be noted that strontium is retained in the mineral phase of bone, and since the atom has a higher X-ray absorbance than calcium, exposure to strontium leads to a spurious increase in bone density using DXA.
  ○ **Hydrochlorothiazide (HCTZ)** is a thiazide diuretic typically used to treat hypertension that is not approved for the treatment of osteoporosis. However, it is recognized that HCTZ treatment increases BMD, and a large population cohort study found that adults taking thiazide diuretics experienced significantly fewer hip fractures, especially if they had been receiving treatment for >1 year.[55] This was traditionally thought to be by inhibiting the thiazide-sensitive sodium chloride co-transporter (NCC) in the distal tubule, which promotes reabsorption of calcium from the urine, making HCTZ an effective treatment for hypercalciuria, which can contribute to low bone mass. More recently, the NCC was found to be expressed in human osteoblasts, and thiazides were shown to stimulate osteoblast differentiation, suggesting these drugs may have an additional direct bone-forming effect.[56] Hypercalcemia and other electrolyte disturbances are the primary adverse effects of HCTZ and especially need to be monitored in the elderly.

Combination Therapy
- Several different combination regimens of dual antiresorptive agents have been studied with variable results. Adding alendronate or risedronate to regimens of patients already taking hormone-replacement therapy (HRT) has shown additive effects on bone density. Similar results were found by adding raloxifene to alendronate. However, these studies only demonstrated impact on BMD and have not been large enough or long enough to assess fracture risk.[57] In the absence of such data, the increased adverse effects and cost of treating need to be considered before initiating dual therapy with these agents.
- With the addition of teriparatide to medications for osteoporosis, the most promising drug combination was speculated to be teriparatide with an aminobisphosphonate, as these potent drugs have different mechanisms of effect and could potentially work synergistically. However, subsequent clinical data have contradicted this. Several studies, including one in men,[58] have found that combination therapy with teriparatide and alendronate is less effective than teriparatide alone at improving

BMD and increasing new bone formation.[59] More promise has been shown with sequential treatment, and in a recent study, BMD improvements with one year of teriparatide therapy were maintained or improved with subsequent alendronate but lost if therapy was not followed by an aminobisphosphonate.[60] Therefore, the typical approach currently is to immediately start an aminobisphosphonate following discontinuation of teriparatide treatment to maintain the improved bone strength.

Lifestyle/Risk Modification

Lifestyle modifications are crucial to osteoporosis treatment and prevention. Adults with osteoporosis should be encouraged to **stop smoking** and **avoid excessive alcohol intake.** Dietary and activity modifications should be made as described below.

Diet

- Adequate intake of calcium is essential to achieve peak bone mass in early adulthood and to maintain bone mass throughout postmenopausal life.[61] Vitamin D increases calcium absorption in the intestine and calcium reabsorption in the kidney. Vitamin D is supplied both in the diet and in the conversion from skin precursors in the presence of sunlight. Elderly adults, especially those who are chronically ill or institutionalized, have a high prevalence of vitamin D deficiency, as they have limited exposure to sunlight.[62] The majority of clinical trials have found that **supplementation with calcium and vitamin D** has a modest beneficial effect on BMD. Most important, one study of elderly women in nursing homes found that supplementation with calcium and vitamin D decreased the rate of hip and other fractures.[63] Additionally, a meta-analysis found that supplementation with 700 to 800 IU of vitamin D demonstrated decreased risk of hip and nonvertebral fracture in elderly adults.[64]
- **Calcium**
  ○ The recommended daily intake varies somewhat in different consensus guidelines, but in general is at least **1000 mg daily of elemental calcium in adults under age 50** and **1200 mg daily of elemental calcium in adults over age 50.**[9,10] **Foods rich in calcium** include milk, yogurt, cheeses, sardines, and fortified juices. The average daily calcium intake in adults from nondairy foods is 250 mg/day. For dairy products, on average, 8 ounces of milk, 6 ounces of yogurt, or 1.5 ounces of cheese contain 300 mg of elemental calcium.[9]
  ○ Essentially all of the clinical trials in adults with osteoporosis that have included dietary assessments of calcium intake have found that the dietary calcium intake of most adults is significantly below recommended levels.[61] As such, most adults both with and without osteoporosis require calcium supplementation. There are a multitude of calcium supplements available, most as either calcium carbonate or calcium citrate. It is important to realize that the recommendations for calcium are for elemental calcium and that **many over-the-counter calcium supplements are labeled by the amount of calcium carbonate (40% elemental) or citrate (21% elemental) per pill.** Calcium salts are best absorbed with meals.
  ○ A recent meta-analysis of 15 clinical trials of calcium supplementation (without vitamin D) in older adults that assessed cardiovascular outcomes found an increased risk of myocardial infarction with calcium supplementation. The implications of this analysis are yet to be fully understood, but currently it seems prudent to advise patients to optimize calcium intake from dietary sources rather than from supplementation whenever possible.[65]

8. Looker AC, Melton LJ 3rd, Harris TB, et al. Prevalence and trends in low femur bone density among older US adults: NHANES 2005–2006 compared with NHANES III. *J Bone Miner Res* 2010;25:64–71.

9. Bone Health and Osteoporosis: A Report of the Surgeon General. Rockville, MD: U.S. Department of Health and Human Services, Office of the Surgeon General; 2004.

10. Clinician's Guide to Prevention and Treatment of Osteoporosis. Washington, DC: National Osteoporosis Foundation; 2010.

11. Screening for osteoporosis in postmenopausal women: Recommendations and rationale. *Ann Intern Med* 2002;137:526–528.

12. Hodgson SF, Watts NB, Bilezikian JP, et al. American Association of Clinical Endocrinologists medical guidelines for clinical practice for the prevention and treatment of postmenopausal osteoporosis: 2001 edition, with selected updates for 2003. *Endocr Pract* 2003;9:544–564.

13. Melton LJ 3rd, Thamer M, Ray NF, et al. Fractures attributable to osteoporosis: Report from the National Osteoporosis Foundation. *J Bone Miner Res* 1997;12:16–23.

14. Cummings SR, Melton LJ. Epidemiology and outcomes of osteoporotic fractures. *Lancet* 2002;359:1761–1767.

15. Kado DM, Browner WS, Palermo L, et al. Vertebral fractures and mortality in older women: A prospective study. Study of Osteoporotic Fractures Research Group. *Arch Intern Med* 1999;159:1215–1220.

16. Klotzbuecher CM, Ross PD, Landsman PB, et al. Patients with prior fractures have an increased risk of future fractures: A summary of the literature and statistical synthesis. *J Bone Miner Res* 2000;15:721–739.

17. Tannenbaum C, Clark J, Schwartzman K, et al. Yield of laboratory testing to identify secondary contributors to osteoporosis in otherwise healthy women. *J Clin Endocrinol Metab* 2002;87:4431–4437.

18. Ryan CS, Petkov VI, Adler RA. Osteoporosis in men: The value of laboratory testing. *Osteoporos Int* 2010. Last accessed 12/12/10 http://www.springerlink.com./content/t511307167178676/fulltext.pdf

19. Garnero P, Hausherr E, Chapuy MC, et al. Markers of bone resorption predict hip fracture in elderly women: The EPIDOS Prospective Study. *J Bone Miner Res* 1996;11:1531–1538.

20. Cummings SR, Black DM, Nevitt MC, et al. Bone density at various sites for prediction of hip fractures. The Study of Osteoporotic Fractures Research Group. *Lancet* 1993;341:72–75.

21. Marshall D, Johnell O, Wedel H. Meta-analysis of how well measures of bone mineral density predict occurrence of osteoporotic fractures. *BMJ* 1996;312:1254–1259.

22. Genant HK, Engelke K, Fuerst T, et al. Noninvasive assessment of bone mineral and structure: State of the art. *J Bone Miner Res* 1996;11:707–730.

23. Brunader R, Shelton DK. Radiologic bone assessment in the evaluation of osteoporosis. *Am Fam Physician* 2002;65:1357–1364.

24. Haller J, Andre MP, Resnick D, et al. Detection of thoracolumbar vertebral body destruction with lateral spine radiography. Part II: Clinical investigation with computed tomography. *Invest Radiol* 1990;25:523–532.

25. Kanis JA, Johnell O, Oden A, et al. FRAX and the assessment of fracture probability in men and women from the UK. *Osteoporos Int* 2008;19:385–397.

26. Black DM, Cummings SR, Karpf DB, et al. Randomised trial of effect of alendronate on risk of fracture in women with existing vertebral fractures. Fracture Intervention Trial Research Group. *Lancet* 1996;348:1535–1541.

27. Black DM, Delmas PD, Eastell R, et al. Once-yearly zoledronic acid for treatment of postmenopausal osteoporosis. *N Engl J Med* 2007;356:1809–1822.

28. Chesnut IC, Skag A, Christiansen C, et al. Effects of oral ibandronate administered daily or intermittently on fracture risk in postmenopausal osteoporosis. *J Bone Miner Res* 2004;19: 1241–1249.

29. Cummings SR, Black DM, Thompson DE, et al. Effect of alendronate on risk of fracture in women with low bone density but without vertebral fractures: Results from the Fracture Intervention Trial. *JAMA* 1998;280:2077–2082.

30. Harris ST, Watts NB, Genant HK, et al. Effects of risedronate treatment on vertebral and nonvertebral fractures in women with postmenopausal osteoporosis: A randomized controlled

trial. Vertebral Efficacy with Risedronate Therapy (VERT) Study Group. *JAMA* 1999; 282:1344–1352.

31. Liberman UA, Weiss SR, Broll J,et al. Effect of oral alendronate on bone mineral density and the incidence of fractures in postmenopausal osteoporosis. The Alendronate Phase III Osteoporosis Treatment Study Group. *N Engl J Med* 1995;333:1437–1443.

32. McClung MR, Geusens P, Miller PD, et al. Effect of risedronate on the risk of hip fracture in elderly women. Hip Intervention Program Study Group. *N Engl J Med* 2001;344: 333–340.

33. Reginster J, Minne HW, Sorensen OH, et al. Randomized trial of the effects of risedronate on vertebral fractures in women with established postmenopausal osteoporosis. Vertebral Efficacy with Risedronate Therapy (VERT) Study Group. *Osteoporos Int* 2000;11:83–91.

34. Reid IR, Brown JP, Burckhardt P, et al. Intravenous zoledronic acid in postmenopausal women with low bone mineral density. *N Engl J Med* 2002;346:653–661.

35. Wysowski DK. Reports of esophageal cancer with oral bisphosphonate use. *N Engl J Med* 2009;360:89–90.

36. A once-yearly IV bisphosphonate for osteoporosis. *Med Lett Drugs Ther* 2007;49:89–90.

37. Perazella MA, Markowitz GS. Bisphosphonate nephrotoxicity. *Kidney Int* 2008;74: 1385–1393.

38. Khosla S, Burr D, Cauley J, et al. Bisphosphonate-associated osteonecrosis of the jaw: Report of a task force of the American Society for Bone and Mineral Research. *J Bone Miner Res* 2007;22:1479–1491.

39. Shane E, Burr D, Ebeling PR, et al. Atypical subtrochanteric and diaphyseal femoral fractures: Report of a task force of the American Society for Bone and Mineral Research. *J Bone Miner Res* 2010;25:2267–2294.

40. Ettinger B, Black DM, Mitlak BH, et al. Reduction of vertebral fracture risk in postmenopausal women with osteoporosis treated with raloxifene: Results from a 3-year randomized clinical trial. Multiple Outcomes of Raloxifene Evaluation (MORE) Investigators. *JAMA* 1999;282:637–645.

41. Barrett-Connor E, Mosca L, Collins P, et al. Effects of raloxifene on cardiovascular events and breast cancer in postmenopausal women. *N Engl J Med* 2006;355:125–137.

42. Delmas PD, Bjarnason NH, Mitlak BH, et al. Effects of raloxifene on bone mineral density, serum cholesterol concentrations, and uterine endometrium in postmenopausal women. *N Engl J Med* 1997;337:1641–1647.

43. Teriparatide (forteo) for osteoporsis. *Med Lett Drugs Ther* 2003;45:9–10.

44. Neer RM, Arnaud CD, Zanchetta JR, et al. Effect of parathyroid hormone (1-34) on fractures and bone mineral density in postmenopausal women with osteoporosis. *N Engl J Med* 2001;344:1434–1441.

45. Lewiecki EM. Treatment of osteoporosis with denosumab. *Maturitas* 2010;66:182–186.

46. Cummings SR, San Martin J, McClung MR, et al. Denosumab for prevention of fractures in postmenopausal women with osteoporosis. *N Engl J Med* 2009;361:756–765.

47. Reid IR, Miller PD, Brown JP, et al. Effects of denosumab on bone histomorphometry: The FREEDOM and STAND studies. *J Bone Miner Res* 2010;25:2256–2265.

48. Effects of hormone therapy on bone mineral density: Results from the postmenopausal estrogen/progestin interventions (PEPI) trial. The Writing Group for the PEPI. *JAMA* 1996;276:1389–1396.

49. Cauley JA, Robbins J, Chen Z, et al. Effects of estrogen plus progestin on risk of fracture and bone mineral density: The Women's Health Initiative randomized trial. *JAMA* 2003;290:1729–1738.

50. Rossouw JE, Anderson GL, Prentice RL, et al. Risks and benefits of estrogen plus progestin in healthy postmenopausal women: Principal results from the Women's Health Initiative randomized controlled trial. *JAMA* 2002;288:321–333.

51. Lufkin EG, Wahner HW, O'Fallon WM, et al. Treatment of postmenopausal osteoporosis with transdermal estrogen. *Ann Intern Med* 1992;117:1–9.

52. Chesnut CH 3rd, Silverman S, Andriano K, et al. A randomized trial of nasal spray salmon calcitonin in postmenopausal women with established osteoporosis: The prevent recurrence of osteoporotic fractures study. PROOF Study Group. *Am J Med* 2000;109:267–276.

53. Knopp JA, Diner BM, Blitz M, et al. Calcitonin for treating acute pain of osteoporotic vertebral compression fractures: A systematic review of randomized, controlled trials. *Osteoporos Int* 2005;16:1281–1290.

54. Meunier PJ, Roux C, Seeman E, et al. The effects of strontium ranelate on the risk of vertebral fracture in women with postmenopausal osteoporosis. *N Engl J Med* 2004;350: 459–468.

55. Schoofs MW, van der Klift M, Hofman A, et al. Thiazide diuretics and the risk for hip fracture. *Ann Intern Med* 2003;139:476–482.

56. Dvorak MM, De Joussineau C, Carter DH, et al. Thiazide diuretics directly induce osteoblast differentiation and mineralized nodule formation by interacting with a sodium chloride co-transporter in bone. *J Am Soc Nephrol* 2007;18:2509–2516.

57. Binkley N, Krueger D. Combination therapy for osteoporosis: Considerations and controversy. *Curr Osteoporos Rep* 2005;3:150–154.

58. Finkelstein JS, Hayes A, Hunzelman JL, et al. The effects of parathyroid hormone, alendronate, or both in men with osteoporosis. *N Engl J Med* 2003;349:1216–1226.

59. Black DM, Greenspan SL, Ensrud KE, et al. The effects of parathyroid hormone and alendronate alone or in combination in postmenopausal osteoporosis. *N Engl J Med* 2003; 349:1207–1215.

60. Black DM, Bilezikian JP, Ensrud KE, et al. One year of alendronate after one year of parathyroid hormone (1-84) for osteoporosis. *N Engl J Med* 2005;353:555–565.

61. Heaney RP. Calcium, dairy products and osteoporosis. *J Am Coll Nutr* 2000;19:83S–99S.

62. Holick MF. Vitamin D deficiency. *N Engl J Med* 2007;357:266-281.

63. Chapuy MC, Arlot ME, Delmas PD, et al. Effect of calcium and cholecalciferol treatment for three years on hip fractures in elderly women. *BMJ* 1994;308:1081–1082.

64. Bischoff-Ferrari HA, Willett WC, Wong JB, et al. Fracture prevention with vitamin D supplementation: A meta-analysis of randomized controlled trials. *JAMA* 2005;293: 2257–2264.

65. Bolland MJ, Avenell A, Baron JA, et al. Effect of calcium supplements on risk of myocardial infarction and cardiovascular events: Meta-analysis. *BMJ* 2010;341:c3691.

66. Todd JA, Robinson RJ. Osteoporosis and exercise. *Postgrad Med J* 2003;79:320–323.

67. Feskanich D, Willett W, Colditz G. Walking and leisure-time activity and risk of hip fracture in postmenopausal women. *JAMA* 2002;288:2300–2306.

68. Kannus P, Parkkari J, Niemi S, et al. Prevention of hip fracture in elderly people with use of a hip protector. *N Engl J Med* 2000;343:1506–1513.

69. Van Staa TP, Leufkens HG, Abenhaim L, et al. Use of oral corticosteroids and risk of fractures. *J Bone Miner Res* 2000;15:993–1000.

70. Saag KG, Zanchetta JR, Devogelaer JP, et al. Effects of teriparatide versus alendronate for treating glucocorticoid-induced osteoporosis: Thirty-six-month results of a randomized, double-blind, controlled trial. *Arthritis Rheum* 2009;60:3346–3355.

Paget's Disease of Bone

26

Scott Goodwin and Michael P. Whyte

GENERAL PRINCIPLES

Definition

Paget's disease of bone (PDB) is characterized by acquired, focal acceleration of bone turnover (remodeling and expansion) and compromised structure that lead to weak bone predisposed to fracture. It is also referred to as **osteitis deformans** and was first described in 1877 by Sir James Paget.[1,2]

Classification

PDB can be localized to one skeletal area (**monostotic**) or affect multiple parts of the skeleton (**polyostotic**).

Epidemiology

- PDB is the second most common metabolic bone disorder in older adults (after osteoporosis). The prevalence is slightly greater in men than women.[3]
- PDB shows a distinctive geographic distribution globally. It occurs most commonly in Western Europe, North America, Australia, and New Zealand. It is uncommon in Asia, Africa, and the Middle East. Interestingly, however, the prevalence of PDB is similar in both white and black Americans.[3]
- PDB typically manifests in middle age or later and is considered uncommon in adults younger than 40 years of age. Population studies using radiographs and autopsy have found prevalence of 1% in adults older than age 40 years in the United States.[2]

Etiology

The etiology of PDB has been debated for decades and remains unsolved today. Evidence suggests there are both genetic and environmental factors that influence the changes associated with Pagetic bone.

- **Genetic factors:** 5% to 40% of patients with PDB have a first-degree relative also with this bone disorder.[4,5] Two gene mutations have been described. However, these mutations do not account for all cases. One mutation disrupts sequestosome 1/p62. The other mutation consists of defects within a valosin-containing protein.[2]
- **Environmental influences:** PDB due to a viral infection of osteoclasts has been postulated since the 1970s. Evidence to support this began with the visualization using electron microscopy of viral-like inclusion bodies in osetoclasts and viral-like antigens using immunohistochemical techniques.[6] However, these observations have not always been replicated and actual viruses have not been isolated from Pagetic bone.

Pathophysiology

The pathogenic abnormality in PDB is enhanced osteoclast activity. The osteoclasts in patients with Pagetic bone are excessively multinucleated, increased in number, and size with up to 100 nuclei (5 to 10 normal). The increased osteoclast activity results in three distinct clinical phases of the disease. Different parts of the skeleton may simultaneously be in different stages[7,8]:

- The **initial osteolytic phase** features intense bone resorption by the Pagetic osteoclasts, usually in the long bones, pelvis, and/or the skull.
- In the **mixed osteolytic/osteoblastic phase,** active bone resorption by osteoclasts leads to increased and uncooridinated bone formation by reactive osteoblasts.
- The **late sclerotic phase** is characterized by continued bone formation, resulting in thickened disorganized bone of poor quality.

DIAGNOSIS

Clinical Presentation

- The majority of patients with PDB are **asymptomatic,** and the disease is diagnosed incidentally on radiographs or for the investigation of an elevated serum alkaline phosphatase.
- If there are symptoms, the two most common are **bone pain** and **joint pain.**[9]
  - ○ The bone pain is typically constant, is deep-seated, may be worse at night, and frequently increases with weight bearing. The severity of pain does not always correlate with radiographic findings and tends to be more prominent with advanced lytic lesions.
  - ○ Secondary osteoarthritis and corresponding joint pain frequently develop, particularly in weight-bearing joints, especially the hip and the knee. Several mechanisms are responsible including uneven bony expansion resulting in a deformed base for articular cartilage, compromised space due to bony overgrowth, and altered joint mechanics secondary to bony deformities.
- Physical signs of PDB can include bony deformities such as bowing of the limbs, kyphosis or scoliosis, and enlargement of the skull (which can lead to cranial nerve compromise and/or deafness). Local skin warmth over pagetic lesions may also develop secondary to increased bony vascularity.
- The prevalence of skeletal involvement of PDB by location are shown in Table 26-1.

TABLE 26-1	FREQUENCY OF SKELETAL SITES INVOLVED IN PAGET'S DISEASE (%)
Skeletal site	**Frequency of involvement**
Pelvis	72
Lumbosacral spine (esp. L3–4)	58
Femur	55
Thoracic spine	45
Sacrum	43
Skull	42
Tibia	35
Humerus	31
Scapula	23
Cervical spine	14

Diagnostic Testing

- Evaluation of patients with PDB can include radiographs, a bone scan, and laboratory assessment including markers of bone turnover. The order in which the tests are obtained typically depends on whether PDB is suspected from symptoms or diagnosed incidentally.
- A **bone scan** is the best test for defining the extent of this disease. Bone scans are more sensitive, but less specific than traditional radiographs. They can detect 15% to 30% of lesions not detected by plain films.[7] Radiographs can be obtained of painful areas or areas that are abnormal on the bone scan to confirm the diagnosis and to assess the degree of abnormalities.[2]
- An **elevated serum alkaline phosphatase level** is the most useful biochemical marker to assess the degree of osteoblast activity. Alkaline phosphatase levels **correlate to the extent of disease on bone scan.**[10] However, investigators must remember that sources for an elevated alkaline phosphatase level include the liver and bone. Differentiation of these two sources can be made by either fractionating the alkaline phosphatase level or by assaying serum gama-glutamyltransferase (GTT). A normal GTT will effectively rule out hepatic source and then imaging studies could be pursued, as described, to search for bony lesions.
- At the time of initial diagnosis, markers of both bone formation and bone resorption can be useful.
  ○ Alkaline phosphatase (total or bone specific) is a good marker to assess bone formation.
  ○ **Other bone markers**, such as urinary hydroxyproline, serum osteocalcin, procollagen type I N-terminal peptide (NTX), and/or procollagen type 1 C-terminal peptide (CTX) usually require the use of referral laboratories and are therefore not routinely measured[10,11]
- **Additional optional testing**
  ○ If the traditional tests above are inconclusive, some additional laboratory and imaging tests may be useful.
  ○ Serum calcium and phosphorous concentrations are usually normal in PDB. Hypercalcemia in ambulatory patients suggests presence of a second disorder such as primary hyperparathyroidism.
  ○ Additional radiologic testing is generally unnecessary except to evaluate for complications. Computed tomography (CT) or magnetic resonance imaging (MRI) help to evaluate for malignant degeneration or neurologic complications, such as spinal stenosis.
  ○ Bone biopsy is usually not required to make a diagnosis of PDB but is obtained primarily when concern arises for malignant degeneration.

TREATMENT

- The primary goals of treatment are to decrease pain and to hopefully decrease the rate of bone turnover to prevent progression of disease and the development of complications.
- The following are generally accepted **indications for treatment**[12]:
  ○ Symptomatic disease: bone pain, deformities, or neurologic symptoms
  ○ Patients preparing for elective orthopedic surgery on involved joints (in an effort to decrease bony vascularity)

TABLE 26-2	PHARMACOLOGIC TREATMENT OPTIONS
Agent	**Dose**
First-line agents	
Alendronate	40 mg p.o. daily for 6 months
Risedronate	30 mg p.o. daily for 2 months
Pamidronate	30–60 mg i.v. daily for 3 days or 30 mg i.v. q week for 6 weeks or 30 mg i.v. q month for 6 months
Zoledronate	5 mg i.v. infused over 15 minutes × 1 dose
Second-line agents	
Tiludronate	400 mg p.o. daily for 3 months
Etidronate	200–400 mg p.o. daily for 6 months
Calcitonin	50–100 IU i.m. daily or 3×/week for 6–12 months

○ Asymptomatic patients with evidence of increased bone turnover are at risk for complications based on the areas involved:
   ■ Lytic lesions in long bones with a high risk for developing fractures
   ■ Disease in proximity to joints with risk of developing secondary osteoarthritis
   ■ Disease in the spine because of the risk of developing spinal stenosis
   ■ Disease in the skull because of the risk of deafness and cranial nerve palsy

Medications

- The newer generation, **nitrogen-containing bisphosphonates** are the perferred treatment for those PDB patients requiring therapy. These agents are now available in oral (aldendronate and risedronate) or intravenous (pamidronate and zolendronate) formulations (Table 26-2). These agents have shown to decrease bone turnover (as measured by the decline in serum alkaline phosphatase levels) as well as improve/relieve symptoms.[12,13]
- **Supplemental calcium and vitamin D** can be given to prevent defective bone mineralization, although this complication is much less common with the newer bisphosphonates.
- Older generation bisphosphonates, etidronate, and tiludronate are less effective in improving symptoms and decreasing markers of bone turnover. They are generally not given as first-line treatment.[2,12]
- Calcitonin is another older agent that can be considered for patients who are unable to tolerate bisphosphonates. Calcitonin is somewhat more effective in PDB when given as an injection (subcutaneous or intramuscular) than when given nasally. Unfortunately, symptoms and increases in bone turnover usually recur soon after stopping this therapy.[12]

Surgical Management

- Surgical therapy may be **helpful for some complications of PDB**. The most common indication is a joint replacement, usually of a hip or a knee, for secondary osteoarthritis.[14]

- Other reasons to consider surgical intervention are for a complicated nonhealing fracture, bowing deformities of long bones, spinal stenosis, and focal nerve root compression syndromes.
- Bisphosphonate therapy can be initiated prior to elective surgery to decrease bone vascularity and the risk of intraoperative bleeding.[12]

COMPLICATIONS

- Multiple complications can occur in patients with PDB (Table 26-3), although most are infrequent.
- **Fractures** are one of the most common complications and occur in 6% to 7% of patients.[14] Fractures occur most commonly in the femur, tibia, and humerus and are often associated with poor healing and nonunion.
- **Neurologic complications** can occur because of either direct nerve root compression by pagetic bone or diversion of blood flow to bone. Spinal stenosis is an important neurologic complications. Deafness occurs in 10% to 30% of patients with disease affecting the skull.[7]
- **Cardiovascular complications** are much less common than previously thought, particularly high-output heart failure.

TABLE 26-3	POSSIBLE COMPLICATIONS IN PAGET'S DISEASE
Organ system	**Possible complications**
Long bones	Fractures, deformities, arthritis
Neurologic	Spinal stenosis
	Chronic headaches
	Cranial neuropathies (especially II, V, VII, VIII)
	Noncommunicative hydrocephalus
	Dementia
	Seizure disorder
Dental	Loss of teeth/malocclusion
ENT	Deafness
	Tinnitus
	Vertigo
Rheumatologic	Hyperuricemia/gout
	Increased susceptibility to seronegative spondyloarthropathies, psoriatic arthritis
Cardiovascular	Increased vascular disease
	High-output heart failure
	Valvular heart disease (aortic > mitral)
Metabolic	Hypercalcemia (usually with immobility)
	Primary hyperparathyroidism
Tumors	Benign giant cell tumors
	Malignant sarcoma

ENT, ear, nose, and throat.

- **Malignant sarcomatous degeneration** is an uncommon but severe and usually life-threatening complication of PDB, occurring in <1% of patients and most commonly in those with severe polyostotic disease.[15]
  - The most commonly involved bones, in descending order, are the femur, humerus, pelvis, skull, and facial bones.
  - Malignant transformation may lead to a sudden or severe increase in pain, a palpable mass, a rise in the alkaline phosphatase, and/or a pathologic fracture.
  - The prognosis is poor, with a 50% mortality rate at 6 months and a 5-year survival rate of only 5% to 15%.[15] A small percentage of patients with limb-bone sarcomas without evidence of metastatic disease can be treated with wide surgical excision/amputation and aggressive chemotherapy and/or radiation therapy.

MONITORING/FOLLOW-UP

- Follow-up of patients with PDB includes monitoring their **symptoms** as well as sometimes following markers of bone turnover occasionally supplemented with radiologic studies.
- Symptoms are usually initially monitored every 3 months in those on therapy and every 6 to 12 months in those not on treatment. The markers of bone resorption typically improve quickly within days, whereas the markers of bone formation take longer to improve, often up to 1 month.[2,7,12]
- The **alkaline phosphatase** is the easiest of the markers of bone turnover to follow and is usually the only one needed in follow-up. The alkaline phosphatase could be checked every 3 to 4 months during therapy until it normalizes. It is usually followed annually in those not on treatment. Retreatment with another course of a bisphosphonate should be considered if the alkaline phosphatase increases by >20% to 25% above the posttreatment nadir.[2,10,11]
- Serial measurements of other markers of bone turnover could be useful in those with highly active lytic disease, especially if the alkaline phosphatase is relatively normal.[10,11]
- Indications for subsequent X-rays are new symptoms or worsening of stable symptoms, trauma, concern for a fracture, and concern for sarcomatous degeneration.

REFERENCES

1. Seton M. Paget's disease: Epidemiology and pathophysiology. *Curr Osteoporos Res* 2008; 6:125–129.
2. Whyte MP. Clinical practice. Paget's disease of bone. *N Engl J Med* 2006;355:593–600.
3. Altman RD, Bloch DA, Hochberg MC, et al. Prevalence of pelvic Paget's disease of bone in the United States. *J Bone Miner Res* 2000;15:461–465.
4. Siris ES, Ottman R, Flaster E, et al. Familial aggregation of Paget's disease of bone. *J Bone Miner Res* 1991;6:495–500.
5. Takata S, Yasui N, Nakatsuka K, et al. Evolution of understanding of genetics of Paget's disease of bone and related diseases. *J Bone Miner Res* 2004;22:519–523.
6. Roodman GD, Windle JJ. Paget disease of bone. *J Clin Invest* 2005;115:200–208.
7. Shoback D, Sellmeyer D, Bikle D. Metabolic Bone Disease. In: Gardner DG, Shoback D, eds. Greenspan's basic & clinical endocrinology, 8th ed. New York, NY: McGraw-Hill Companies; 2007;337–341.
8. Ralston SH. Pathogenesis of Paget's disease of bone. *Bone* 2008;43:819–825.

9. Tiegs RD. Paget's disease of bone: Indications for treatment and goals of therapy. *Clin Ther* 1997;19:1309–1329.

10. Delmas PD. Biochemical markers of bone turnover in Paget's disease of bone. *J Bone Miner Res* 1999;14(Suppl 2):66–69.

11. Alvarez L, Guanabens N, Peris P, et al. Discriminative value of biochemical markers of bone turnover when assessing the activity of Paget's disease. *J Bone Miner Res* 1995;10:458–465.

12. Siris ES, Lyes KW, Singer FR, et al. Medical management of Paget's disease of bone: Indications for treatment and review of current therapies. *J Bone Miner Res* 2006;2:94–98.

13. Merlotti D, Luigi G, Martini G, et al. Comparison of different intravenous bisphosphonate regimens for Paget's disease of bone. *J Bone Miner Res* 2007;22(10):1510–1517.

14. Parvizi J, Klein GR, Sim FH. Surgical management of Pagets disease of bone. *J Bone Miner Res* 2006;21:75–82.

15. Mirabello L, Troisi RJ, Savage SA. Osteosarcoma incidence and survival rates from 1973 to 2004: Data from the surveillance, epidemiology, and end results program. *Cancer.* 2009; 115:1531–1543.

Standards of Care for Diabetes Mellitus

27

Prajesh M. Joshi and Janet B. McGill

GENERAL PRINCIPLES

- Standards of care for patients with diabetes are developed by consensus committees both in the United States and abroad to facilitate the application of evidence-based medicine to all patients with diabetes.
- The stated goals of these committees are to provide practical guidelines for health-care providers that will reduce the risk of morbidity and mortality from acute and chronic complications of diabetes.
- Health-care providers are expected to know the health risks associated with diabetes, and to be able to develop treatment strategies for individual patients to attain the stated targets. Although individual patients may require modification of treatment targets, providers should strive to achieve the stated goal in the majority of patients with diabetes.
- Third party payers are beginning to utilize these treatment targets as benchmarks for evaluation of services and for payment.
- Standards of care for patients with diabetes have been established by the American Diabetes Association (ADA), the American Association of Clinical Endocrinologists (AACE), and the European Association for the Study of Diabetes (EASD) in conjunction with the European Society of Cardiology (ESC). Other groups such as the Joint National Committee for the Study of Hypertension (JNC VII) and the Adult Treatment Panel (ATP) have addressed specific comorbid conditions.
- Most of the recommendations from these consensus groups are similar; however, there are key differences that will be pointed out in this chapter.
- Original studies and grade of evidence supporting the recommendations discussed in this chapter are referenced in the consensus documents. And the diagnostic and treatment strategies have been discussed in Chapter 28 and Chapter 29.

SCREENING FOR DIABETES MELLITUS

Type 1 Diabetes Mellitus
- Type 1–prevention trials suggest that **measurement of autoantibodies** identifies individuals at risk for developing the disease. Testing may be appropriate in high-risk individuals with prior history of transient hyperglycemia, those who have close relatives with type 1 diabetes (T1DM), or in the context of clinical research studies. However, widespread screening is generally not recommended for low-risk populations.[1]
- Counseling regarding the risk of developing T1DM should be provided to those who have positive antibody titers.

TABLE 27-1	CRITERIA FOR TESTING FOR DIABETES IN ASYMPTOMATIC ADULTS

1. Testing should be considered in all adults who are overweight (BMI ≥25 kg/m$^{2\,a}$) and have additional risk factors:
   - Physical inactivity
   - First-degree relative with diabetes
   - Members of a high-risk ethnic population (e.g., African American, Latino, Native American, Asian American, Pacific Islander)
   - Women who delivered a baby weighting >9 lb or diagnosed with gestational diabetes mellitus
   - Hypertension (≥140/90 mm Hg or on therapy for hypertension)
   - HDL cholesterol <35 mg/dL (0.90 mmol/L) and/or a triglyceride level >250 mg/dL (2.82 mmol/L)
   - Women with polycystic ovary syndrome
   - A1c ≥5.7%, IGT, or IFG on previous testing
   - Other clinical conditions associated with insulin resistance (e.g., severe obesity, acanthosis nigricans)
   - History of CVD
2. In the absence of the above criteria, testing for diabetes should begin at age 45.
3. If the results are normal, testing should be repeated at least at 3-year intervals, with consideration of more frequent testing depending on initial results and risk status.

Adapted from Standards of Medical Care in Diabetes—2012 a Position Statement—ADA[1]

^{a}At risk BMI may be lower for some ethnic groups.

Type 2 Diabetes Mellitus

- The **ADA recommends** screening for type 2 diabetes mellitus (T2DM) at **age 45 OR in adults who are overweight (BMI ≥25 kg/m^2) with additional risk factors** (Table 27-1 for screening recommendations).
- **AACE recommends annual screening of all individuals who are risk for developing T2DM.** The risk factors include family history of T2DM; cardiovascular disease; overweight or obese; sedentary lifestyle; nonwhite ethnicity; previously identified impaired glucose tolerance (IGT) or impaired fasting glucose (IFG) and/or metabolic syndrome (see Chapter 29); hypertension; increased levels of triglycerides, low concentrations of high-density lipoprotein (HDL) cholesterol, or both; history of gestational diabetes mellitus, history of delivery of an infant with a birth weight >9 pounds (4 kg); polycystic ovary syndrome (PCOS); and antipsychotic therapy for schizophrenia and/or severe bipolar disease.[2]
- **The EASD and ECS recommend using a risk-assessment tool** such as the Finnish Diabetes Risk Score (FINDRISC) to assess the 10-year risk of T2DM, and performing laboratory testing that includes a diagnostic oral glucose tolerance test (OGTT) on persons at high risk.[3]
- The **same tests are used for screening and diagnosis of diabetes.** Diagnostic criteria are covered in Table 29-2 in Chapter 29.
- **Hemoglobin A1c** (HbA1c) performed in a laboratory using a method that is National Glycohemoglobin Standardization Program (NGSP) certified and standardized to the Diabetes Control and Complication Trial (DCCT) assay, has

TABLE 27-2	CORRELATION BETWEEN HBA1c AND MEAN PLASMA GLUCOSE[1]	
HbA1c	**Mean plasma glucose**	
%	**mg/dL**	**mmol/L**
6	126	7.0
7	154	8.6
8	183	10.2
9	212	11.8
10	240	13.4
11	269	14.9
12	298	16.5

HbA1c, Hemoglobin A1c.

recently been added as one of the tests for screening and diagnostic test for diabetes (Table 27-2).[4]

Gestational Diabetes Mellitus

Gestational diabetes mellitus (GDM) is defined as **any degree of glucose intolerance with onset or first recognition during pregnancy.**

- Screening for diabetes in pregnancy is important to ensure optimal maternal and fetal outcomes.
- Because the number of pregnant women with undiagnosed type 2 diabetes has increased with the ongoing epidemic of obesity, patients with preconception T2DM may be wrongly classified as gestational. Hence **ADA recommends screening women with risk factors for diabetes (see Table 27-1) using standard diagnostic testing at the first prenatal visit.** Women who satisfy diagnostic criteria should receive a diagnosis of overt diabetes.[1]
- All pregnant women previously undiagnosed with diabetes should undergo GDM testing with a **75 gm OGTT at 24 to 28 weeks of gestation.** The OGTT should be performed in the morning after an overnight fast of at least 8 hours. The **diagnosis of GDM is made if any of the following criteria are met**[1,5]:
  ○ Fasting plasma glucose ≥92 mg/dL (5.1 mmol/L)
  ○ 1-hour plasma glucose ≥180 mg/dL (10 mmol/L)
  ○ 2-hour plasma glucose ≥153 mg/dL (8.5 mmol/L)
- **Women with GDM should also be tested at 6 to 12 weeks postpartum** to detect persistence of diabetes and followed more closely in subsequent years.

PREVENTION OF DIABETES

- Several randomized controlled studies have shown that diabetes can be prevented in individuals at high risk with either lifestyle modification or with medication.[6,7]
- All three-consensus groups recommend **counseling in lifestyle management to reduce weight in those who are overweight and to increase physical activity.**[1–3]

- Studies of lifestyle management that have resulted in weight loss of ≥5% through diet and exercise (150 minute/week) have demonstrated up to 58% reduction in risk of progression to diabetes.[6,7]
- Based on these clinical trials, lifestyle changes with a goal weight loss of at least 7% and moderate physical activity ~150 minutes/week are recommended for prevention of progression from IFG or IGT to diabetes.[1–3]
- **Medications that have proved effective in preventing diabetes** include metformin, α-glucosidase inhibitors (e.g., acarbose), orlistat, and thiazolidinediones. None of these drugs have been approved by the FDA in the United States for use in prediabetes/prevention of progression of diabetes. After consideration of cost, side effects, and lack of persistence of their effect in clinical trials, ADA recommends against the use of these drugs in prediabetes/prevention of progression of diabetes. However, if lifestyle management fails, metformin therapy could be considered.[1,2]

GLYCEMIC CONTROL

- Targets for glycemic control in diabetes reflect evidence from randomized controlled trials that have demonstrated protection from long-term microvascular complications. Reduction in macrovascular events has not been demonstrated in clinical trials comparing tight versus less tight glycemic control. However, long-term follow-up of the DCCT and UKPDS cohorts has demonstrated risk reduction of macrovascular disease in tight control group. It is, therefore, important to individualize the goal HbA1c according to the risk of hypoglycemia, presence of comorbidities, and life expectancy.[1]
- In pregnancy, glycemic targets are lower than in nonpregnant adults to mimic nondiabetic pregnant women, and to ensure optimal fetal outcomes.
- The **two primary ways to monitor glycemic control are** self-monitored blood glucose (SMBG) and HbA1c.[4]
- Continuous glucose monitoring (CGM) using a real-time sensor that measures glucose concentration in the interstitial fluid has become an ancillary method for glucose monitoring and management.[4]

Self-monitoring of Blood Glucose

- The **frequency of SMBG** should range from 1 to 4 or more readings per day, depending on the intensity of therapy and risk of hypoglycemia. In patients with T1DM and T2DM on multiple insulin injections or insulin pump as well as pregnant women taking insulin, more frequent testing (three or more times a day) is necessary to reach HbA1c targets.[1] The optimal frequency, timing, and overall utility of SMBG for noninsulin treated patients with T2DM is a matter of debate.
- SMBG is **generally checked before meals and at bedtime**, with periodic checks of glucose during the postprandial period and during sleep.
- The capillary blood glucose levels are 10% to 15% lower than plasma glucose levels. Newer blood glucose meters are calibrated to report plasma glucose values, so each patient should be informed whether his/her meter reports plasma values.[4]
- If there is a discrepancy between SMBG values reported by the patient or depicted in meter readings and the HbA1c, it may be useful to measure postprandial glucose 1 to 2 hours after meals. Persistently high HbA1c despite lower than expected blood

TABLE 27-3   GLYCEMIC TARGETS FOR ADULTS WITH DIABETES

Glycemic parameter	ADA[1]	AACE[2]	EASD[3]	GDM[8]	Pregnancy[9]
Hemoglobin A1c	<7.0%[a]	≤6.5%	≤6.5%	N/A	<6.0%
Fasting and preprandial blood glucose	90–130 mg/dL	<110 mg/dL	≤108 mg/dL	≤95 mg/dL	60–99 mg/dL
Postprandial blood glucose	<180 mg/dL	<140 mg/dL	≤135 mg/dL	1 hour post meal ≤140 mg/dL 2 hour post meal ≤120 mg/dL	100–129 mg/dL

---

[a]Using a DCCT-referenced assay.

AACE, American Association of Clinical Endocrinologists; ADA, American Diabetes Association; EASD, European Association for the Study of Diabetes.

---

glucose readings, or wide fluctuations in blood glucose, should prompt further investigation, which is often done best by a certified diabetes educator (CDE).

- The HbA1c **reflects blood glucose levels over the previous 2 to 3 months**. The HbA1c **should be monitored every 3 months until a patient reaches goal, and then every 6 months if the patient is at target and stable.** Use of point-of-care HbA1c test enables timely decisions on therapeutic changes during office visits. Table 27-2 lists correlation between HbA1c and mean plasma glucose levels. A calculator for converting HbA1c results into estimated average glucose (eAG) is available at **http://professional.diabetes.org/eAG**.[1,4]

- Guidelines for glycemic goals established by consensus groups are listed in Table 27-3.[1–3]

- The **goals for glycemic control should be individualized**. HbA1c goal may be near normal (<6%) for individuals with short duration of diabetes, long life expectancy, and no significant cardiovascular disease if possible to achieve it without hypoglycemia; and less stringent targets may be appropriate for those with a history of severe hypoglycemia, limited life expectancy, extensive comorbid conditions, advanced microvascular or macrovascular complications, and difficult to manage long-standing diabetes. Targets for children are adjusted to permit scrupulous avoidance of serious hypoglycemia.[1,2]

- **HbA1c can be misleading in patients with certain forms of anemia and hemoglobinopathies.** HbA1c assay without interference from abnormal hemoglobins (list of assays and impact of abnormal hemoglobin on them is available at **http://www.ngsp.org/factors.asp**) should be used for hemoglobinopathies with normal red cell turnover (e.g., sickle cell trait). HbA1c is unreliable for diagnosis and management in conditions of abnormal cell turnover as in pregnancy or anemia from hemolysis and iron deficiency.[4]

TREATMENT RECOMMENDATIONS

The ADA and EASD have developed a consensus statement on the management of hyperglycemia in diabetes. The basic tenets are early intervention with metformin and lifestyle therapy, which include medical nutrition therapy (MNT) and exercise with frequent adjustment to achieve the glycemic goal. Diabetes Self-Management Education (DSME) is an integral part of management strategy.

Diabetes Self-Management Education

Patients with newly diagnosed as well as established diabetes should receive comprehensive DSME by a CDE. This approach should be patient centered and done in collaboration with health-care professionals.

Lifestyle Therapy

- Nutrition recommendations need to be individualized with consideration to the patient's level of overweight, ethnicity, diabetes therapy, and food choices.
- **Carbohydrate intake monitoring** with carbohydrate counting, exchanges, or experience-based estimation have been shown to improve glycemic control.
- **Aerobic exercise** of at least 150 minutes (50% to 70% of maximum heart rate) per week and supplemental **repetitive resistance training** are recommended for all adults with diabetes in the absence of contraindications.
- Studies have shown that high levels of physical activity, either as part of a daily work routine or for pleasure, are associated with reduced cardiovascular risk in both primary and secondary prevention that is equivalent to first-line pharmacologic therapy. Health-care providers should assess the level of physical activity in patients with diabetes and provide encouragement to reach the target of 150 minutes of aerobic exercise weekly or 10,000 steps daily. Physical limitations should be addressed and alternative exercise programs developed as needed.
- Nutrition advice specific to cardiovascular risk reduction includes avoidance of trans and saturated fats, increased intake of fiber, and intake of five or more servings of fruits and vegetables daily. Reduction of salt intake is advised in persons who are hypertensive. This advice should be provided to all patients as part of routine health-care visits and included in MNT instructions.
- **Smoking cessation** is critically important for persons with diabetes, and counseling regarding smoking cessation should be documented in medical records.

Drug Therapy

- Medication intervention **should normally begin with metformin,** with other agents added sequentially to achieve glycemic targets.
- **Earlier treatment with insulin is recommended to correct blood glucose level >250 to 300 mg/dL at presentation** or any time in the course of treatment.
- **Hypoglycemia** is a limiting factor in the glycemic management of diabetes. **Glucose values <70 mg/dL should be treated with 15 to 20 g of glucose (preferred) or other carbohydrate, and rechecked in 15 minutes.** Persons at risk for severe hypoglycemia should have a prescription for **glucagon** and instructions for use by a companion.

Bariatric Surgery

- Gastric banding or bypass surgery should be considered in morbidly obese T2DM individuals (BMI >35 kg/m^2), especially when lifestyle and pharmacologic therapies have failed to achieve the goals of therapy.

- Bariatric surgery has resulted in near or complete normalization of glycemia in ~55% to 95% of patients with T2DM in various studies.[10]

PREVENTION OF COMPLICATIONS DUE TO DIABETES

Cardiovascular Disease

- Cardiovascular disease is the **leading cause of mortality in patients with diabetes**. Diabetes confers an increased risk of acute coronary syndrome, myocardial infarction, heart failure, atrial fibrillation, stroke, peripheral vascular disease, and sudden death that is 2 to 5 times the risk in nondiabetic comparator groups.
- Persons with diabetes also experience greater morbidity after vascular events, and interventions such as coronary angioplasty may not be as effective at reducing morbidity and mortality in diabetic patients compared to nondiabetic comparison groups. Although the increased risk is not entirely explained by usual risk factors, studies have shown that aggressive management of hypertension and lipids and the use of antiplatelet agents in patients with diabetes can reduce the risk of cardiovascular events, and that the benefits of treatment of each risk factor in diabetes may exceed the benefits in lower risk cohorts.
- Consequently, health-care providers are expected to address cardiovascular risk in a comprehensive manner, and achieve targets that are more stringent for blood pressure, lipids, and healthy lifestyles than in nondiabetic patients.

Hypertension

- Hypertension is present in more than 75% of persons with T2DM, and more than 50% of persons with T1DM.[1–3,11,12]
- Blood pressure reduction has been shown to reduce the frequency of myocardial infarction, cerebrovascular disease, and diabetes-related deaths. In addition, blood pressure reduction slows the progression of nephropathy, retinopathy, and vision loss.
- Blood pressure should be checked at every visit in patients with diabetes.
- Lifestyle therapy and medical treatment should be considered if the blood pressure is ≥130/80 mm Hg. Lifestyle therapy for hypertension includes weight loss, DASH (dietary approaches to stop hypertension)-style diet, moderation of alcohol intake, and increased physical activity. DASH-style diet consists of decrease in sodium and increase in potassium intake.
- **All of the consensus guidelines suggest using angiotensin-converting enzyme (ACE) inhibitors (ACEIs) or angiotensin receptor blockers (ARBs) as initial therapy** because of proven benefit in lowering cardiovascular mortality and progression of both retinopathy and nephropathy in individual with diabetes.
- Second- and third-line treatment with diuretics, β-blockers, or calcium channel blockers should be tailored to the individual patient. β-blockers are indicated in patients who have had a myocardial infarction, heart failure, or for rate control in atrial fibrillation. Vasodilating agents such as carvedilol or nebivolol may be particularly useful in patients with diabetes, since they do not worsen insulin resistance or symptomatic peripheral vascular disease.
- Use of ACEIs in diabetic patients with blood pressure below the stated target of 130/80 mm Hg and with retinopathy or microalbuminuria may provide protection

from progression of these complications. ACEIs and ARBs have been associated with birth defects, so caution is advised in premenopausal women, especially those women who indicate a desire to become pregnant or who are not using adequate birth control.

Hyperlipidemia

- Diabetic patients should have a fasting lipid profile (total cholesterol, low-density lipoprotein [LDL] cholesterol, HDL cholesterol, and triglycerides) checked yearly. Lipid targets for patients with diabetes are listed in Table 27-4.[1–3,13,14]
- Therapy is initially directed toward meeting the LDL cholesterol goal. A secondary goal is to raise HDL cholesterol above the gender-specific target. For

TABLE 27-4	**LIPID TARGETS FOR PERSONS WITH DIABETES**	
	ADA, AACE, ATP III[1,2,13]	**EASD/ESC**[3,a]
Total cholesterol		<4.5 mmol/L (174 mg/dL)
LDL cholesterol	<100 mg/dL	<2.5 mmol/L (97 mg/dL)[b]
• DM + CVD	≤70 mg/dL, or ↓ by 30%–40% regardless of baseline	<1.8 mmol/L (70 mg/dL)
• DM older than age 40	↓ by 30%–40% regardless of baseline using a statin	
HDL	>40 mg/dL in men	>1 mmol/L (39 mg/dL) in men
	50 mg/dL in women	>1.2 mmol/L (46 mg/dL) in women
Triglycerides	<150 mg/dL If >500 mg/dL, lowering TG becomes a priority	>1.7 mmol/L (151 mg/dL) is a marker for increased vascular risk; begin treatment when >2.3 mmol/L (189 mg/dL) and LDL is at target
Non-HDL (TC-HDL)	<130 mg/dL (especially for those with TG >200 mg/dL)	0.8 mmol/L (31 mg/dL) above stated LDL goal

[a]With the Third Joint European Societies Task Force on Cardiovascular Disease Prevention in Clinical Practice.

[b]Includes patients with type 1 diabetes.

AACE, American Association of Clinical Endocrinologists; ADA, American Diabetes Association; ATP, Adult Treatment Panel; CVD, cardiovascular disease; DM, diabetes mellitus; EASD, European Association for the Study of Diabetes; ESC, European Society of Cardiology; HDL, high-density lipoprotein; LDL, low-density lipoprotein; TC, total cholesterol; TG, triglycerides.

those with triglycerides ≥200 mg/dL, current National Cholesterol Education Program/Adult Treatment Panel III guidelines have established a non-HDL cholesterol (total HDL cholesterol) target of <130 mg/dL as the secondary goal.
- If the triglyceride level is >500 mg/dL, therapy should first be directed at lowering triglycerides to prevent pancreatitis.
- HMG-CoA reductase inhibitors (statins) have provided the greatest benefit in patients with diabetes, and should be considered first-line therapy. Combination therapy with fibrates, fish oil, or niacin may be needed in selected patients to achieve HDL and triglyceride targets. Additional LDL lowering with ezetimibe or a bile acid sequestrant may be required to reach LDL targets. For specific recommendations on treatment of hyperlipidemia, please refer to Chapter 33.

Retinopathy
- Patients with diabetes are at risk for retinopathy. Diabetic retinopathy poses a serious threat to vision and is the leading cause of blindness in middle-aged Americans.[1,2]
- Annual dilated ophthalmologic evaluations are recommended to monitor retinopathy.
- Newly diagnosed T1DM patients should have an initial dilated eye examination within 3 to 5 years after onset of their disease. Persons with T2DM should have a comprehensive eye examination at the time of diagnosis and yearly thereafter.[15]
- Women who are planning a pregnancy, or who present early in pregnancy, should have a comprehensive eye examination due to the risk of development or progression of retinopathy during pregnancy. An eye examination should be performed in the first trimester with close follow-up throughout the pregnancy and for 1 year postpartum.
- Eye examinations more frequently than once a year should be done in patients with active retinopathy and in patients receiving active treatment for retinopathy.
- Laser photocoagulation therapy has been the mainstay treatment for preservation of vision in diabetic retinopathy, but it does not restore lost vision. Close ophthalmologic follow-up is recommended to determine the timing and extent of laser or other therapies.

Nephropathy
- Diabetic nephropathy accounts for nearly 50% of end-stage renal disease in the United States and is a leading cause of diabetes-related morbidity and mortality.[1,2]
- The earliest sign of diabetic nephropathy is microalbuminuria, which can be measured by albumin-to-creatinine ratio in a spot urine sample or by the more cumbersome method of 24-hour or timed collections of urine, which do not lead to improved accuracy.
- Microalbuminuria is defined as a **albumin:creatinine ratio of 30 to 300 mcg/mg**, and macroalbuminuria is defined as **albumin:creatinine ratio of ≥300 mcg/mg.**
- Macroalbuminuria carries a worse prognosis with regard to progression of kidney disease and need for renal replacement therapy.
- In patients with T1DM, testing for albuminuria should be performed within 5 years of diagnosis and repeated annually. Testing should be done at the time of diagnosis and annually in persons with T2DM.

- Microalbuminuria should be confirmed in two of three tests within 3 to 6 months to eliminate positive tests due to transient conditions such as exercise, urinary tract infections, hematuria, viral illness, and hyperglycemia. **Once microalbuminuria is diagnosed, treatment should begin with either an ACEI or an ARB** (even if normotensive), hypertension should be treated to goal, and glycemic control should be optimized. These treatments can slow the progression of diabetic nephropathy. If the patient develops clinical macroalbuminuria (>300 mcg/mg or 300 mg/24 hours) modest dietary protein restriction to 0.8 g/kg/day may help slow progression of this renal complication.
- **Serum creatinine should be measured annually** in patients with both T1DM and T2DM. Calculation of estimated glomerular filtration rate (eGFR) should be done using the Modification of Diet in Renal Disease (MDRD) equation. The MDRD eGFR formula can be found at: www.kidney.org/professionals/kdoqi/gfr_calculator.cfm.
- Recent studies have shown that kidney function can decline in the absence of albuminuria and retain pathologic features of diabetic nephropathy. Careful attention to blood pressure and glycemic control, along with the use of ACEIs or ARBs, can slow the progression of kidney disease.
- When the eGFR is <60 mL/minute/1.73 m^2 by the modified MDRD formula, testing for anemia, vitamin D, and parathyroid hormone should be undertaken and abnormal values treated. A referral to a nephrologist is recommended in all patients with eGFR <60 mL/minute/1.73 m^2, regardless of etiology.

Neuropathy

- Neuropathy is considered a microvascular complication of diabetes, which can present in several forms, generally categorized as focal or diffuse and involving peripheral sensory, autonomic, or sensory plus motor pathways.[1,2]
- The **most common forms are distal symmetric sensorimotor diabetic polyneuropathy (DPN) and autonomic neuropathy** involving gastrointestinal, genitourinary, and cardiovascular systems, as well as contributing to hypoglycemic unawareness. Focal neuropathy is less common and typically presents acutely.

Diagnosis of Neuropathy

- Evaluation of possible neuropathy should begin with a thorough history of symptoms such as pain, numbness, paresthesias, weakness in the feet or hands, early satiety, or erectile dysfunction. A neurologic examination should be performed annually and should evaluate deep tendon reflexes and various sensory modalities (pain/temperature, vibration, light touch, and joint position sense).
- Individuals with diabetes should undergo annual screening for DPN using tests such as pinprick sensation, vibration perception (using a 128-Hz tuning fork), and 10 g monofilament sensory testing. Sensitivity of detecting DPN increases to >87% with combination of these tests.
- Sensory testing with a 10 g monofilament detects the presence or absence of "protective sensation." Loss of monofilament sensation and vibration is predictive of foot ulcers.

Treatment of Neuropathy

- Although there is no specific therapy that alters the course of DPN, **strict control of blood glucose**, with attention to reducing glucose fluctuation, may prevent progression.
- **Symptomatic pain relief** can be attained, through the use of some anticonvulsant medications, tricyclic antidepressants, and serotonin/norepinephrine reuptake

inhibitors. Large-fiber neuropathies are managed with strength, gait, and balance training; pain management; orthotics to treat and prevent foot deformities; and surgical reconstruction in some cases. Small-fiber neuropathies are managed by foot protection, supportive shoes with orthotics, regular foot and shoe inspection, prevention of heat injury, and use of emollient creams.

- **Gastroparesis symptoms** respond to dietary changes and prokinetics like metoclopramide or erythromycin. Erectile dysfunction is treated with phosphodiesterase type 5 inhibitors, intracorporeal or intraurethral prostaglandins, vacuum devices, or penile prosthesis.
- A multidisciplinary approach should be adopted to manage patients with foot ulcers or at high risk for foot ulcers due to conditions such as Charcot deformity.

Lower Extremity Complications

- Patients with diabetes develop foot problems owing to a combination of vascular and neurologic compromise and poor wound healing.[1,2]
- Diabetes is the leading cause of nontraumatic lower extremity amputation in the United States.
- Annual foot examinations should include evaluation of touch and vibration sense (Semmes-Weinstein 10 g monofilament and 128 mHz tuning fork), deep tendon reflexes, and pedal pulses. At every visit, the feet should be visually inspected for skin breakdown, callus, discoloration, or signs of vascular or neurologic disease.
- Individuals with foot ulcers or at high risk for foot ulcers should be managed by a multidisciplinary team to ensure healing and prevent recurrence.

ANTIPLATELET THERAPY

- Treatment with **low-dose (75 to 162 mg/day) aspirin** has been shown to reduce recurrence of cardiovascular events, including myocardial infarction (~30%) and stroke (~20%) in persons with diabetes.
- Low-dose aspirin is recommended as primary prevention measure for individuals with T1DM and T2DM at increased cardiovascular risk (10-year risk >10%). The evidence is, however, insufficient to recommend aspirin in lower risk individuals. Aspirin should be used as a secondary prevention strategy in those patients with CVD with diabetes.
- Other antiplatelet agents such as clopidogrel are a reasonable alternative to aspirin when the patient is intolerant to aspirin.

Screening for Cardiovascular Disease

Routine screening of asymptomatic patients for coronary artery disease is not recommended by the ADA due to evidence that shows no difference in outcome measures with screening stress electrocardiograms and no difference in intensive medical therapy versus invasive revascularization. However, individuals with typical or atypical cardiac symptoms and an abnormal resting ECG should undergo exercise stress cardiac testing.[1]

IMMUNIZATIONS

- **Influenza vaccine should be administered annually** to all diabetic patients ≥6 months of age, beginning each October.

- The **pneumococcal vaccine** should be administered once the diagnosis of diabetes is established to all patients ≥2 years of age. Other specific vaccines are left to clinical judgment.

INPATIENT MANAGEMENT

- Hyperglycemia in hospitalized patients is recognized as an important modifiable contributor to increased morbidity and mortality. Persons with diabetes (whether previously diagnosed or not) are admitted to the hospital more often than individuals without diabetes, and the stress of acute illness and surgery can cause hyperglycemia in previously nondiabetic individuals. Therefore, more than half of patients in some intensive care units (ICUs) and 25% of ward patients will require management of hyperglycemia.[16]
- In a joint consensus statement, the ADA and AACE made the following recommendations:
  - Identify all patients with a known diagnosis of diabetes clearly in the medical record.
  - Measure blood glucose on admission and institute point-of-care glucose testing in all patients with a prior diagnosis of diabetes, in those with hyperglycemia identified in the hospital, and in those with high-risk medical or surgical illnesses or procedures.
  - Target blood glucose for non-ICU, nonpregnant patients should be premeal of <140 mg/dL, with random blood glucose values <180 mg/dL. To avoid hypoglycemia, the insulin regimen should be reassessed if blood glucose declines below 100 mg/dL.
  - Target blood glucose for ICU patients should be maintained between 140 and 180 mg/dL.
  - Use of continuous insulin infusion has been shown to be the most effective method to achieve glycemic control in ICU settings, to treat diabetes hyperglycemic emergencies, and in labor and delivery.
  - Scheduled subcutaneous insulin for medical and surgical ward patients should include the following components:
    - Basal insulin using an intermediate (NPH) or long-acting (glargine or detemir) insulin preparation, which should be marked "Do not hold."
    - Prandial insulin using a rapid-acting preparation (lispro, aspart, glulisine), with orders to give immediately with the meal and held if the meal is missed or not eaten.
    - Correction factor using a rapid-acting preparation (lispro, aspart, glulisine), to be given at prespecified times and at intervals at least 4 hours apart to avoid stacking doses.
  - Orders for treatment of hypoglycemia with oral carbohydrate source if mild and the patient is able to take oral nutrients (intravenous if unable to handle oral intake) should be prespecified, along with retest intervals and physician notification.
  - Safety is of paramount importance in the management of inpatient hyperglycemia, so a systems approach with appropriate training, boundaries, and monitoring is needed to ensure success.
  - Follow-up of patients who were hyperglycemic during their hospital stay is appropriate, either to adjust newly instituted therapy or to perform diagnostic testing for diabetes.

OUTCOMES

Optimum care of patients with diabetes prevents acute complications and reduces the risk of development of long-term complications of this disease. This can be accomplished through patient education, regular health screening, medical care, laboratory evaluation, and timely referral to specialists.

REFERENCES

1. American Diabetes Association-Position Statement. Standards of medical care in diabetes–2012. *Diabetes Care* 2012;35(Suppl 1):S11–S63.
2. Handelsman Y, Mechanick JI, Blonde L, et al. American Association of Clinical Endocrinologists Medical Guidelines for Clinical Practice for Developing a diabetes mellitus comprehensive care plan. *Endocr Pract* 2011;17(Suppl 2):1–53.
3. Rydén L, Standl E, Bartnik M, et al. The Task Force on Diabetes and Cardiovascular Diseases of the European Society of Cardiology (ESC) and of the European Association for the Study of Diabetes (EASD). Guidelines on diabetes, pre-diabetes, and cardiovascular diseases: executive summary. *Eur Heart J* 2007;28:88–136.
4. Sacks DB, Arnold M, Bakris GL, et al. Position Statement Executive Summary: Guidelines and Recommendations for Laboratory Analysis in the Diagnosis and Management of Diabetes Mellitus. *Diabetes Care* 2011;34:1419–1423.
5. International Association of Diabetes and Pregnancy Study Groups Consensus Panel, Metzger BE, Gabbe SG, et al. International association of diabetes and pregnancy study groups recommendations on the diagnosis and classification of hyperglycemia in pregnancy. *Diabetes Care* 2010;33:676–682.
6. Diabetes Prevention Program Research Group. Reduction in the incidence of type 2 diabetes with lifestyle intervention or metformin. *N Engl J Med* 2002;346:393–403.
7. Tuomilehto et al. Prevention of type 2 diabetes mellitus by changes in lifestyle among subjects with impaired glucose tolerance. *N Engl J Med* 2001;344:1343–1350.
8. Metzer BE, Buchanan TA, Coustan DR et al. Summary and recommendations of the Fifth International Workshop-Conference on Gestational Diabetes Mellitus. *Diabetes Care* 2007; 30(Suppl. 2):S251–S260.
9. Kitzmiller JL, Block JM, Brown FM, et al. Managing preexisting diabetes for pregnancy: Summary of evidence and consensus recommendations for care. *Diabetes Care* 2008;31; 1060–1079.
10. Buchwald H, Estok R, Fahrbach K, et al. Weight and type 2 diabetes after bariatric surgery: Systematic review and meta-analysis. *Am J Med* 2009;122:248–256.
11. AACE Hypertension Task Force. American association of clinical endocrinologists medical guidelines for clinical practice for the diagnosis and treatment of hypertension. *Endocr Pract* 2006;12:196–222.
12. Chobanian AV, et al. The seventh report of the Joint National Committee on prevention, detection, evaluation, and treatment of high blood pressure (the JNC 7 report). *JAMA* 2003; 289:2560–2572.
13. Expert Panel on Detection, Evaluation, and Treatment of High Blood Cholesterol in Adults. Executive summary of the third report of the National Cholesterol Education Program (NCEP) expert panel on detection, evaluation, and treatment of high blood cholesterol in adults (Adult Treatment Panel III). *JAMA* 2001;285:2486–2497.
14. Grundy SM, Cleeman JI, Merz NB, et al. Implications of recent clinical trials for the national cholesterol education program adult treatment panel III guidelines. *Circulation* 2004;110:227–239.
15. Harris MI, Klein R, Welborn TA, et al. Onset of NIDDM occurs at least 4–7 years before clinical diagnosis. *Diabetes Care* 1992;15:815–819.
16. The AACE/ADA Task Force on Inpatient Diabetes. American College of Endocrinology and American Diabetes Association consensus statement on inpatient glycemic control. *Endocrine Practice* 2009;15:1–17

Diabetes Mellitus Type 1

28

Judit Dunai and Janet B. McGill

GENERAL PRINCIPLES

- Type 1 diabetes mellitus (T1DM) is an illness in which autoimmune destruction of pancreatic beta cells causes **insulin deficiency** and **hyperglycemia**.
- Insulin deficiency can lead to acute metabolic decompensation known as **diabetic ketoacidosis (DKA)**; however, exogenous insulin taken in excess can produce life-threatening hypoglycemia.
- Chronic hyperglycemia is the root cause of disabling microvascular complications and contributes to macrovascular disease.
- The treatment goal of T1DM is normalization of blood glucose (BG) by physiologically based insulin replacement therapy.

Epidemiology

- The overall prevalence of the disease is 0.25% to 0.5% of the population, or 1 in 400 children and 1 in 200 adults in the United States.
- The incidence of T1DM is increasing in developed countries, and it is appearing at younger ages.[1,2]
- The peak onset occurs at age 10 to 12 years, but it can be diagnosed from a few months of age into the ninth decade of life.
- Males and females are equally affected.
- T1DM accounts for 5% to 10% of all cases of diabetes and needs to be accurately diagnosed so that insulin therapy is not delayed or withheld inappropriately.

Etiology and Pathogenesis

- The **autoimmune process that selectively destroys pancreatic beta cells** is T-cell mediated with an unknown antigenic stimulus, in genetically susceptible individuals.[3,4]
  - Environmental factors, including coxsackie and rubella viruses, and dietary factors, such as early exposure to cow's milk, have been implicated.
  - Insulitis (lymphocytic infiltration of pancreatic islets) is an early finding, followed by apoptosis of beta cells, which leads to their virtual absence later in the disease course.
  - Antibodies to beta-cell antigens can be found in the majority of patients before diagnosis, and for some time after the onset of clinical diabetes.
  - These disease markers are antibodies to **glutamic acid decarboxylase (GAD65)**, to **tyrosine phosphatases IA-2** and **IA-2 beta**, and to **insulin (IAA)**.
    - Of these markers, GAD65 is positive in 80% of children and adults near the time of diagnosis, whereas IA-2 and IAA are positive in ~50% of children and are less likely to be present in adults.
    - The presence of two antibodies has high sensitivity and specificity for rapid progression to insulin dependency and may help clarify the diagnosis in some patients.

- In cases of T1DM in which no evidence of autoimmunity can be detected, the classification used is *idiopathic T1DM*.
- Several organ-specific **autoimmune diseases occur with increased frequency in patients with T1DM**, including autoimmune thyroiditis (Hashimoto's and Graves' diseases), Addison's disease, pernicious anemia, celiac sprue, vitiligo, alopecia, and chronic active hepatitis.[5,6]
  - In a study of 265 adults with T1DM, the risk of thyroid disease was 32% for the proband, 25% for siblings, and 42% for parents, with females more commonly affected than males.
  - The risk of developing autoimmune thyroid disease increases with age, so periodic screening should continue throughout adulthood in patients with T1DM and their family members.
- The **genetic susceptibility** to T1DM is manifested by linkage with several gene loci and association with HLA-DR and DQ.[7]
  - Genome-wide association studies identified additional risk loci BACH2, C1QTNF6, CTSH, and PRKCQ.[7]
  - The *IDDM1* gene located in the HLA region of chromosome 6p21.3, and the *IDDM2* gene in the region 5' upstream of the insulin gene on chromosome 11p15.5 contribute 42% and 10%, respectively, to the observed familial clustering.
  - In the family of a patient with T1DM, the risk of an identical twin developing T1DM is 50%, an offspring is 6%, and a sibling is 5%.
- The striking familial discordance supports the importance of environmental factors.

Pathogenesis of Complications

- Patients with both T1DM and type 2 diabetes mellitus (T2DM) are susceptible to organ dysfunction that is caused by long-term exposure to hyperglycemia and which leads to devastating morbidity and mortality.[8]
- The **microvascular complications** of diabetes are retinopathy, nephropathy, and neuropathy.
- Although they share some pathogenic features, they may not appear at the same time or with the same severity in all individuals with diabetes. The pathogenesis of each of these complications includes increased oxidative stress or the generation of reactive oxygen species with inadequate scavenger activity.
  - **Advanced glycation end-products** are formed by processes of glycation and/or oxidation of proteins, nucleotides, and lipids, and have intrinsic cellular toxicity.
  - High levels of glucose and reactive oxygen species have been shown to increase diacylglycerol and stimulate protein kinase C activity, causing alterations in intracellular signal transduction and production of cytokines and growth factors.[9]
- Glucose enters peripheral nerves by mass action, is converted first to sorbitol by aldose reductase, and is then converted to fructose by sorbitol dehydrogenase. These saccharides produce osmotic stress, increase glycation, and cause alterations in the NADH/NAD ratio, which collectively contributes to nerve fiber damage and loss leading to the symptoms of **peripheral neuropathy**.
- **Diabetic retinopathy** is associated with the adverse effects of hyperglycemia on the vascular endothelium and upregulation of cytokines such as vascular endothelial growth factor.
- In **diabetic nephropathy**, hyperglycemia induces transforming growth factor β, which stimulates matrix synthesis and inhibits matrix degradation in renal mesangial cells. Investigational agents that target these processes are currently in clinical development.

DIAGNOSIS

Clinical Presentation

- T1DM develops most commonly in childhood but can present at any age.
- Because 80% of cases occur without a positive family history, symptoms may be overlooked until hyperglycemia reaches critical levels.
- The **prodromal symptoms are related to hyperglycemia** and include weight loss, polyuria, polydipsia, polyphagia, and blurred vision. If **diabetic ketoacidosis** (DKA) is present, the patient might complain of abdominal pain, nausea, vomiting, myalgias, and shortness of breath and exhibit changes in mental and hemodynamic status.

History

- In previously diagnosed patients, the **history of present illness** should document the duration of the illness, frequency of hyper- and hypoglycemia, results of self-monitored BG (SMBG) testing, dietary habits, and the status of any microvascular or macrovascular complications.
- The history of present illness or medication history should **record the insulin regimen in detail** and should provide an assessment of adequacy of, or problems with, the regimen.
- In female adolescents and adult women, menstrual, sexual, and gestational histories should be elicited and the method of birth control should be documented.
- Smoking behavior, alcohol and drug use, and socioeconomic status and social support are all important factors in the care of a patient with T1DM.

Physical Examination

- If the patient presents in **DKA**, signs of dehydration and acidosis, such as tachycardia, orthostatic hypotension, and dry mucus membranes, might be evident.
- Fruity odor to the breath reflects the presence of ketones.
- Routine follow-up physical examinations should document height, weight, and Tanner staging in children to determine that growth and development are advancing normally.
- Blood pressure and heart rate are important measures for all patients with T1DM.
- At least annually, the physical examination should include skin, funduscopic, oral, thyroid, and cardiovascular examinations, as well as sensory testing and foot screening.
- Dilated eye examination by an ophthalmologist is recommended at 3 to 5 years of T1DM duration, with scheduling of repeat examinations based on clinical findings.

Diagnostic Testing

- The diagnosis of diabetes mellitus, based upon the guidelines of the American Diabetes Association (ADA) is one of four abnormalities of glucose metabolism[10]:
  - Hyperglycemia symptoms and a random venous plasma glucose ≥200 mg/dL.
  - Fasting plasma glucose ≥126 mg/dL, confirmed on a second sample if <200 mg/dL.
  - Glycated hemoglobin (A1C) ≥6.5 percent (using an assay that is certified by the National Glycohemoglobin Standardization Program).
  - Abnormal oral glucose tolerance test (OGTT). Two-hour plasma glucose level of ≥200 mg/dL after ingestion of a 1.75 g/kg glucose drink. However, OGTT is rarely needed to diagnose T1DM.

○ Typically, people with T1DM present with symptoms of hyperglycemia, possibly DKA), and markedly elevated blood glucose, **random plasma glucose ≥200 mg/dL.**

• After the diagnosis of diabetes mellitus is made, T1DM must be differentiated from other types of diabetes.
  ○ This is based upon clinical presentation (body habitus, age, signs of insulin resistance, history (family history), and if necessary, laboratory studies.
  ○ If patient has not had DKA and the diagnosis of T1DM is unclear, testing for islet-specific pancreatic autoantibodies, GAD65, or the 40K fragment of tyrosine phosphatase IA-2B (also known as *ICA*), or IAA or C-peptide level can be useful.[10]
    ▪ C-Peptide levels are typically low or undetectable in patients with T1DM.
    ▪ Of note, the absence of pancreatic autoantibodies does not rule out T1DM. Also, antibodies may be present in up to 30 percent of individuals with other forms of diabetes.

• **Hemoglobin A1c** (HbA1c) should be measured 2 to 4 times per year, and a lipid profile, serum creatinine and electrolytes, and urine microalbumin-to-creatinine ratio should be checked at least annually in adolescents and adults. Screening for thyroid antibodies is recommended, and thyroid-stimulating hormone (TSH) should be checked annually if the patient is antibody positive or has a goiter.[10]

TREATMENT

Goals of Treatment

• The goal of diabetes treatment is to **maintain the BG as close to normal as possible** and to **avoid hypoglycemia**.
• All patients with T1DM require insulin therapy, and early achievement of a near-normal HbA1c has been shown to preserve residual beta-cell function and to reduce long-term complications.[11]
  ○ The Diabetes Control and Complications Trial (DCCT) and its follow-up study have shown that every 1% reduction in HbA1c reduces retinopathy by 33%,[11,12] microalbuminuria by 22%,[13] and neuropathy by 38%.[14]
  ○ Tight control early on, during the first 5 to 10 years of diabetes before the manifestation of complications, confers long-term risk reduction, supporting the hypothesis that hyperglycemia induces organ toxicity that can be self-perpetuating (glycemic memory).
• In children, the therapeutic goals include ensuring normal growth and development and the scrupulous avoidance of severe hypoglycemia at young ages.
• In the postpubertal adolescent and adult patient, maintenance of normal blood pressure, achievement of target lipid levels, smoking cessation, aspirin use in patients older than age 40, and preconception counseling are important treatment goals. (Please refer to Chapter 27 for detailed recommendations.)

Glucose Monitoring

• Patients with T1DM should be encouraged to do **SMBG** at least 4 times daily so that appropriate insulin adjustments can be made based on ambient glucose levels.
• These recommendations may be modified for children with school considerations.

- Increased monitoring is required during acute illnesses, for intense exercise, and before and during pregnancy.
  - ○ Alternate site testing; rapid readings; and meters with averaging, graphing, and download functions have helped patients with the challenging task of SMBG.
  - ○ Periodic monitoring during the nighttime is recommended for all patients to check for nocturnal hypoglycemia.
  - ○ **Continuous glucose monitoring systems** (CGM) are now available to assist with diabetes management. This is a supplemental tool especially useful for those with hypoglycemia unawareness.
    - ■ CGM devices measure glucose level in the interstitial fluid on a near-continuous basis, providing information about the direction, magnitude and duration of glycemic fluctuations.
    - ■ The use of CGM-directed therapy has been shown to decrease the frequency of hypoglycemia and improve HbA1c.[15,16]

Diet

- Patients should receive Medical Nutrition Thereapy (MNT), which is an **individualized assessment and instruction** on diet and is most effectively provided by a registered dietitian.
- The caloric requirement for people with moderate physical activity is approximately 35 kcal/kg/day, but there is significant variation from person-to-person and day-to-day.[10]
  - ○ Individualized instruction should consider the patient's caloric needs, ethnicity, habits, constraints, and prescribed insulin regimen.
  - ○ The diet for patients with diabetes should aim to achieve an ideal HbA1c, blood pressure, and lipid profile.
  - ○ Attention should be payed to balancing energy intake and expenditure to avoid excess weight gain.
  - ○ Patients on fixed-dose insulin regimens need to have a consistent day-to-day carbohydrate intake.
  - ○ Mastery of either an exchange system or carbohydrate-counting allows for flexibility in meal planning, and helps avoid postprandial hypo- or hyperglycemia.[5]
  - ○ Review of dietary principles is a cost-effective way to help the patient achieve treatment targets.

Medications

Insulin Therapy

- Insulin regimens must be individualized to cater to a given patient's lifestyle and comorbidities.
- Insulin types and pharmacokinetics are shown in Table 28-1.
- Flexible insulin regimens with **multiple daily injections (MDI)** or use of an insulin pump can best approximate the physiologic insulin response (Table 28-2).
- Insulin prescriptions consisting of a long-acting basal, and rapid-acting preprandial insulin formulations (given based on carbohydrate intake), are best suited for reaching HbA1c goals while minimizing the risk of hypoglycemia.
- **Continuous subcutaneous insulin infusion (CSII)** via an insulin pump has the added benefit of allowing for variable basal rates and flexibility in delivering bolus insulin doses.

TABLE 28-1	INSULIN TYPES AND PHARMACOKINETICS[a]		
Insulin	Onset	Peak	Duration
Rapid acting[b]			
Insulin aspart (NovoLog)	10–20 minutes	1–3 hours	3–5 hours
Insulin lispro (Humalog)	10–15 minutes	1–2 hours	3–4 hours
Insulin glulisine (Apidra)	10–20 minutes	1 hour	3–4 hours
Short acting			
Regular ("R")	0.5–1.0 hour	2–4 hours	4–8 hours
Intermediate acting			
NPH ("N")[c]	1.5–3 hours	4–10 hours	10–18 hours
Long acting			
Insulin detemir (Levemir)	1–2 hours	None	Up to 24 hours
Insulin glargine (Lantus)[d]	2–3 hours	None	24 hours

[a]Insulin pharmacokinetics show significant inter- and intrasubject variation. The onset, peak, and duration may be influenced by the dose administered, the injection site, skin temperature, and other less well-defined factors.

[b]Rapid-acting insulin should be administered immediately before or after meals. Also suitable for insulin pump use.

[c]Cloudy, suspended formulations require resuspension by rolling and tipping (but not shaking) the vial before administration. Resuspension is a potential source of erratic pharmacokinetics.

[d]Do not mix with any other type of insulin in the same syringe due to incompatible pH. Clear preparation, no resuspension needed.

TABLE 28-2	MDI INSULIN DOSING REGIMEN	
Time	Dose	Regimen
Before breakfast, lunch, and dinner	$0.15 \times$ TDD or units determined by carbohydrate counting plus correction factor	Rapid acting insulin
Before bed (can be given in the morning or split into two doses)	$0.55 \times$ TDD	Insulin glargine or detemir. If NPH is used, give one-half in the morning and one-half in the evening.

- The DCCT and other studies have clearly demonstrated that patients are more likely to achieve glycemic targets using **intensified insulin therapy with basal and bolus components** than with conventional therapy with one or two injections.[11]
  - Decisions about the appropriate insulin regimen should be made with the patient's abilities and scheduling constraints in mind.
  - In general, patients need an **intermediate- or long-acting insulin to cover basal needs** and a **rapid- or short-acting insulin to provide meal coverage.**
  - When initiating or changing an insulin regimen, an estimation of the **total daily dose (TDD)** should be made. Individual requirements vary, but usually range from 0.5 to 0.8 U/kg/day, higher if insulin resistance is present.
- Historically, the most widely prescribed regimen was "split-mixed," which used NPH as the basal insulin and a short- or rapid-acting analog before breakfast and dinner.
  - Use of this regimen presumed that the patient would eat lunch at a standard time, because the morning NPH is likely to peak at about midday. Patient scheduling problems and the erratic pharmacokinetics of NPH have made this regimen less popular.
  - If NPH is used, the dose will be about 0.2 U/kg, twice a day.
- The most commonly prescribed regimens for patients with T1DM by endocrinologists today are **MDI** or **CSII**. These regimens use the concepts of basal and bolus (premeal) dosing.

Multiple Daily Injections

- The **basal dose** is generally 45% to 55% of the total daily dose (TDD), ~0.4 U/kg/day, and is often given in one injection of insulin, glargine or detemir, at bedtime. Many patients take their basal insulin in the morning, or about 0.2 U/kg twice daily.
  - The basal insulin dose is adjusted so that the fasting BG is routinely within the target of 80 to 120 mg/dL, and there is <30 mg/dL variation between evening and morning values.
  - Changes in weight, exercise, persistent hyperglycemia, or frequent hypoglycemia should prompt reconsideration of the basal insulin dose.
- **Bolus doses** are administered to cover carbohydrate intake and to correct high BG readings. Premeal bolus doses are determined by one or more of the following methods:
  - Fixed amount before each meal, ~0.13 U/kg or one-sixth of the TDD.
  - Fixed dose before each meal as above plus a sliding scale "correction factor" (see subsequent text) based on the premeal SMBG.
  - Carbohydrate counting plus "correction factor" uses variable amounts depending on the anticipated carbohydrate intake and the premeal SMBG.
  - Both the patient and the physician need to learn important concepts to succeed in the use of MDI regimens. If fixed amounts of premeal insulin are to be used, the patient should have a clear idea of the prescribed meal plan and be able to follow it precisely.
  - Alternatively, the patient can adjust the premeal dose based on the anticipated carbohydrate content, which allows greater flexibility. To do this, the physician or diabetes educator must determine the **"insulin-to-carbohydrate" ratio**, which can be calculated by dividing 500 by the TDD.
    - A patient who takes 50 U of insulin daily needs 1 U of insulin for every 10 g of carbohydrate intake.

- The patient needs to learn which foods contain carbohydrate, how to estimate the grams of carbohydrate in the serving provided, and how to calculate the premeal dose.
- Additional adjustments are sometimes made for high-fat meals or for meals that have high fiber content.
- Occasional postprandial SMBG is needed to test whether the "insulin-to-carbohydrate" ratio is correct or whether the patient has been able to estimate the carbohydrate content of the meal appropriately.
  - In addition to covering calories, the patient must be able to compensate for high or low BG readings. An individualized sliding scale, known as the **correction factor** is determined, which provides the number of units to be added (or subtracted) to each premeal dose. The correction factor is estimated by dividing 1800 by the TDD.

Sample Calculations

- Example 1: a modestly overweight patient takes 60 U of insulin daily. His current BG is 178 mg/dL, and he is about to eat a meal with 90 g of carbohydrate. His physician has told him that his target SMBG is 120 mg/dL. What dose of rapid-acting insulin should he take?
  - Insulin-to-carbohydrate ratio = 500/60 = 1 U insulin/8.33 g.
  - Correction factor = 1800/60 = 30 (predicts that 1 U insulin drops the BG 30 mg/dL) 90 g carbohydrates/8.33 g/U insulin = ~10 U insulin to cover carbohydrates.
  - SMBG – target BG = 178 mg/dL – 120 = 58 mg/dL. He will take 2 U insulin as correction.
  - Thus, the patient should take 12 U of rapid-acting insulin.
- Example 2: a thin, insulin-sensitive patient takes 30 U of insulin per day. If this patient has a current BG of 178 mg/dL and is about to eat her usual meal containing 45 grams of carbohydrate, how much insulin should she use?
  - Insulin to carbohydrate ratio = 500/30 = 1 U insulin/16.66 g.
  - Correction factor = 1800/30 = 60 (predicts that 1 U insulin will drop the BG 60 mg/dL).
  - 45 g carbohydrates/16.66 g/U insulin = ~3 U insulin to cover carbohydrates.
  - SMBG – target BG = 178 – 120 = 58 mg/dL.
  - She will take 1 U insulin as correction.
  - Thus, this patient should take 4 U of rapid-acting insulin. Using an insulin pen that provides doses in half units, this patient may elect to take 3.5 units.

Continuous Subcutaneous Insulin Infusion

- **Insulin pump therapy** has become an accepted alternative to MDI and has both advantages and disadvantages.
- Technologic advances have contributed to smaller pumps with features such as multiple basal rates, dose calculators, and alternate dosing modalities.
- CSII systems now include continuous glucose monitoring, which assist with dosing adjustments. CSII offers the patient with T1DM the greatest flexibility and is more socially acceptable than needles and syringes for frequent dosing. Insulin pumps are the size of a pager and contain 180 to 300 U of insulin in a specialized syringe that is connected to a subcutaneous (SC) catheter by thin tubing.
- The SC catheter should be changed and repositioned every 3 days. The pump is preprogrammed to infuse the basal rate of insulin, but the patient must activate the pump to deliver bolus doses at the time of the meal or when a correction is needed.

- Only rapid-acting insulin is used. Diabetes education from an educator experienced in CSII is necessary to teach the patient how to use the pump, which requires several hours of instruction.
- **Insulin dose prescribing is conceptually similar to MDI;** however, the TDD is reduced 10% to 20%.
  - The **basal rate** (equal to one-half of the new TDD) is divided by 24 and programmed as an hourly rate. For example, a patient taking 48 U/day with MDI will need ~20 U for basal requirements, or ~0.8 U/hour to start. The basal rate can be adjusted to accommodate nighttime low BG, morning rise, and increased or decreased activity during the day. The basal rate can be temporarily reduced for exercise or the pump can be put in suspended mode for hypoglycemia.
  - **Bolus dosing** is handled similarly to MDI, with a key exception. Today's insulin pumps can administer doses in very small quantities, so the correction factor can be prescribed as a fraction. The opportunity to give smaller doses is helpful for children and insulin-sensitive patients.
- The **major disadvantage** of CSII is the high cost of an insulin pump and supplies. Because only rapid-acting insulin is used, if there is a pump or catheter failure, the BG can rise quickly and DKA can ensue within 12 hours of the interruption of insulin delivery.
- Another potential disadvantage is the risk of catheter-site infection, which is minimized by instruction in semi-sterile techniques.

Adjusting Insulin Doses
- Insulin dose adjustments or changes to the insulin regimen are made after evaluating SMBG values and looking for patterns.
- **The efficacy of a specific rapid-acting insulin dose is monitored by the SMBG that follows the dose in question** (e.g., postprandial or noon SMBG reflects the breakfast dose of rapid-acting insulin).
- Intermediate and long-acting insulin doses are evaluated by scrutinizing the SMBG after the injection (e.g., morning SMBG to determine adequacy of evening dose) and review of overall frequency of hyper- and hypoglycemia.
- Diabetes educators are skilled at insulin dose adjustments and provide a valuable resource for patients who are experiencing problems keeping their glucose values near the target range.
- Diabetes education is cost-effective and necessary to achieve tight glycemic control while avoiding hypoglycemic episodes.

Adjunct Therapy
- Pramlintide (Symlin), a synthetic analog of the beta-cell secretory product amylin, is approved for use as adjunctive therapy to insulin in patients with T1DM. It is given as a separate injection of 15 to 45 mcg before meals, and helps reduce postprandial glucose excursions by suppressing glucagon and enhancing satiety.
- It has a modest effect on HbA1c of about 0.5%, and may contribute to modest weight loss. Side effects are nausea, vomiting, and increased risk of hypoglycemia. Insulin adjustments are needed when pramlintide is prescribed.[17,18]

Diabetic Ketoacidosis
- DKA is the direct result of relative insulin deficiency; dehydration and excess counter-regulatory hormones (glucagon, epinephrine, and cortisol) are accelerating factors.

- Typically, an **exacerbating factor** can be identified: new diagnosis of diabetes, omission of insulin doses, infection, pregnancy, trauma, emotional stress, excessive alcohol ingestion, myocardial infarction, stroke, intercurrent illness, hyperthyroidism, Cushing's disease, or, rarely, pheochromocytoma.
- The major clinical features of DKA are hyperglycemia, dehydration, acidosis, abdominal pain, nausea, vomiting, change in hemodynamic status, and altered mental status.

Pathophysiology
- The pathophysiology of DKA begins with insulin levels that are insufficient to support peripheral glucose uptake and to suppress hepatic gluconeogenesis.
- Hyperglycemia is further driven by increases in the counterregulatory hormones glucagon, catecholamines, cortisol, and growth hormone. Activation of catabolic pathways in muscle and fat produce amino acids and free fatty acids, which fuel hepatic gluconeogenesis and ketone production.
- The osmotic diuresis imposed by hyperglycemia causes marked fluid and electrolyte losses, further stimulating catecholamine release.
- Catecholamines are antagonistic to insulin action and contribute to increased lipolysis, which pumps free fatty acids into the circulation that then undergo fatty acid oxidation to ketone bodies.
- Volume depletion decreases renal blood flow, which contributes to reduced excretion of glucose and ketones and increased serum levels of creatinine and potassium.
- Acidosis ensues when the levels of acetone, acetoacetate, and β-hydroxybutyrate exceed the buffering capacity of bicarbonate and the respiratory response.
- Low $Paco_2$ reflects the respiratory effort and the severity of the metabolic acidosis.
- The presence of an anion gap and low bicarbonate in the setting of high BG and an ill-appearing patient should prompt immediate treatment for DKA while confirmatory laboratory evaluation is under way. The differential diagnosis for anion-gap acidosis is outlined in Table 28-3.

Symptoms
- The symptoms of DKA are nonspecific and include anorexia, nausea, vomiting (coffee ground emesis in 25%), abdominal pain, and myalgias or weakness.
- Polyuria and polydipsia are characteristic of high BG, but may become blunted due to vomiting, reduced renal clearance, and altered mental status as the severity of DKA worsens.
- Hyperpnea is noted with mild acidosis, and the patient may complain of shortness of breath. Kussmaul breathing is a sign of a critically ill patient.
- The physical examination reveals tachycardia, hypotension, or orthostatic hypotension, dry mucous membranes, poor skin turgor, abdominal tenderness, and other signs of clinical events that may have prompted the DKA episode. Mental status can be normal or severely compromised. Signs of a concurrent illness or event that precipitated the DKA may be present.

Laboratory Findings
- Laboratory findings of DKA include the following: glucose >250 mg/dL, glycosuria, an elevated anion gap (normal gap is ≤12), and the presence of serum or urine ketones.
- The anion gap is calculated as follows: (Anion gap = Na^+ – [Cl + HCO_3]). The serum bicarbonate is typically <15 mEq/L, the Pco_2 <40 mm Hg, and the arterial pH <7.3.
- Creatinine and K^+ are generally increased above baseline.
  ○ If hypokalemia is present at the time of diagnosis, the patient has severe K^+ depletion and requires careful monitoring.

TABLE 28-3	DIFFERENTIAL DIAGNOSIS OF ANION-GAP ACIDOSIS (THE MUDPILES MNEMONIC)

Conditions	Clinical associations
M: Methanol ingestion	Visual impairment/blindness; osmol gap between the calculated and measured osmolality (seen with any alcohol ingestion)
U: Uremia	History of renal failure; increased serum urea and creatinine
D: Diabetic ketoacidosis	History of diabetes, hyperglycemia
P: Paraldehyde	Formaldehyde-like breath odor; increased paraldehyde level
I: Iron; isoniazid	Increased serum iron level; patient may have elevated hepatic transaminases with isoniazid toxicity
L: Lactic acidosis	May be due to hypovolemia/sepsis, infarction, metformin, cyanide, hydrogen sulfide, CO, methemoglobin; lactate levels are elevated
E: EtOH; Ethylene glycol	Osmol gap between the calculated and measured osmolality (seen with any alcohol ingestion); increased EtOH level seen with EtOH intoxication; calcium oxalate crystals seen in the urine with ethylene glycol
S: Salicylates	Tinnitus, increased salicylate level, may have a concurrent respiratory alkalosis

EtOH, ethanol.

○ Often the initial potassium level is high, and the ECG should be checked for signs of hyperkalemia, which include peaked T waves, shortened QT intervals, widened QRS complexes, and flattened or absent P waves.
○ Later in the course of treatment, if hypokalemia occurs, a repeat ECG might show ST-segment depression, flattened or inverted T waves, a prolonged QT interval, and appearance of U waves.
• Hyponatremia may be present, but the measured serum sodium should be corrected for the high glucose (add 1.6 to the reported sodium for every 100 mg/dL that the glucose is >100 mg/dL), and may be further depressed by high triglycerides.
• Amylase and lipase may be elevated via unclear mechanisms, do not necessarily indicate pancreatitis, and resolve with treatment of the DKA.

Treatment of DKA
Clinical Evaluation and Triage
• Intensive care admission is required for patients with hemodynamic instability or mental status changes, for pediatric patients, or if frequent monitoring is not possible on a medical ward.
• Hemodynamic monitoring may be required for patients in shock, with possible sepsis, with DKA complicated by myocardial infarction, or in patients with end-stage renal disease or chronic heart failure.

- Nasogastric tube placement may be needed for patients with hematemesis or for comatose patients.

Fluids and Electrolytes

- Fluid resuscitation in adults should begin with normal saline at 1 L/hour unless there is a contraindication (chronic heart failure, end-stage renal disease).
  - The typical total body water deficit is 4 to 6 L, sodium deficit is 7 to 10 mEq/kg, K^+ deficit is 3 to 5 mEq/kg, and PO_4 deficit is 5 to 7 mmol/kg. If the corrected sodium is normal or high on repeat testing, change the intravenous fluids to 0.45% NaCl; continue 0.9% saline if it is low.
  - When the K^+ drops to <5.0 mEq/L and the patient has adequate urine output, add 20 to 30 mEq K^+ to each liter of intravenous fluid.
  - Plan to correct the water and salt deficits over 24 hours, slower in children. The starting fluid administration rate for children should be 10 to 20 mL/kg/hour and should not exceed 50 mL/kg over the first 4 hours of therapy.
- Patients presenting with DKA have a total body PO_4 depletion due to osmotic diuresis, although this may not be apparent on presentation because insulin deficiency and acidosis cause PO_4 to shift out of cells. Serum PO_4 levels decrease with insulin therapy. Except in very severe cases of hypophosphatemia (serum PO_4 <1.0 mg/dL) or concomitant cardiorespiratory compromise, routine administration of PO_4 has not been shown to be beneficial and may, in fact, be harmful because excess replacement can cause hypocalcemia.
- Bicarbonate therapy in DKA is controversial and it should not be routinely administered, unless the serum pH is <7.0 or the patient has life-threatening hyperkalemia.

Insulin and Glucose

Initial intravenous loading bolus 0.1 to 0.15 U/kg of regular (R) insulin followed by continuous infusion 0.1 U/kg/hour (100 units R insulin/100 mL normal saline solution). Children should not receive intravenous bolus doses of insulin; infusion should be started.[14]

- Monitor serum glucose every hour and expect the BG to decline by 50 to 75 mg/dL/hour. A slower response could indicate insulin resistance, inadequate fluid resuscitation, or improper insulin delivery.
- As the acidosis clears, the glucose is likely to fall more rapidly. When the serum glucose is <250 mg/dL, add 5% dextrose to the intravenous fluids, and decrease the insulin infusion rate by up to one-half.
- If the glucose infusion rate is kept stable, the insulin infusion requirements will be more predictable.
- Continue intensive insulin therapy and monitoring until the patient is tolerating oral intake and the anion-gap acidosis has resolved. As the acidosis resolves, the anion gap closes, arterial and venous pH rise, and serum bicarbonate rises.
- The ADA position paper regarding the treatment of DKA states that criteria for the resolution of DKA include a glucose <200 mg/dL, a serum bicarbonate ≥18 mEq/L, and a venous pH >7.3.[19,20]
- Patients recovering from DKA may develop a transient non–anion gap hyperchloremic metabolic acidosis that occurs because of urinary loss of "potential bicarbonate" in the form of ketoanions and their replacement by chloride ions from intravenous fluids. This non–anion-gap acidosis is transient and has not been shown to be clinically significant, except in renal failure.

○ **Common error:** the hyperglycemia will respond to treatment faster than the acidosis will resolve. **Do not decrease or discontinue the insulin infusion when
glucose levels approach the normal range.** This can lead to worsening of the
ketoacidosis. Instead, continue the intravenous insulin infusion, but adjust the
dose and/or add 5% dextrose. If 5% dextrose is infused at excessively rapid rates,
the BG will increase, and the transition to SC insulin will be delayed.

Monitoring
• Fingerstick BG every hour during insulin infusion.
• Electrolytes, blood urea nitrogen (BUN), and creatinine levels every 2 to 4 hours
until the K^+ has stabilized and the anion gap acidosis is resolved.
• Serum ketones or β-hydroxybutyrate level by fingerstick on admission only. Use of
the fingerstick β-hydroxybutyrate test to follow DKA treatment is under review.
• Intake and output, weight.

Transition to Subcutaneous Insulin
• Continue the intravenous insulin infusion and intravenous fluids until the acidosis
has cleared, the glucose is <250 mg/dL, and the patient is able to eat.
  ○ Note: it is possible for the patient to attempt a small or clear liquid meal while on
  an insulin drip, but the drip rate may need to be increased for the meal hour and
  then returned to the usual rate.
  ○ Make the transition to subcutaneous insulin before a meal or at bedtime, but not
  during the middle of the night or between meals.
  ○ If the patient has been previously diagnosed, give the usual premeal insulin dose plus
  any correction factor, and cover basal needs with intermediate- or long-acting insulin.
    ▪ For example, if the drip can be stopped at noon, give a premeal dose of short-
    acting insulin according to the patient's usual schedule and add a partial dose
    of NPH to cover until dinner or bedtime.
    ▪ Start basal insulin (NPH, detemir [Levemir], or glargine [Lantus]) and short-
    acting insulin 1 to 2 hours before stopping the insulin drip.
    ▪ Reduce the rate of intravenous dextrose to ≤100 mL/hour or discontinue it if
    the patient is able to eat.
    ▪ Note that intravenous fluids may need to be continued until the serum creati-
    nine has returned to baseline.

Problem Solving
Recurring DKA should prompt additional history to search for precipitating causes.
• Insulin pump malfunction, noncompliance with insulin doses, social distress, medication problems, or concomitant illness should warrant attention of an experienced
diabetes care provider.
• Newly diagnosed patients require additional time in the hospital for the institution
of an insulin regimen and diabetes education.

CHRONIC COMPLICATIONS

• Care of the patient with T1DM includes screening for microvascular and macrovascu-
lar complications, and the application of proven therapies to reduce morbidity and
mortality.
• Tight glycemic control prevents against macrovascular disease, as established by the
DCCT and the Epidemiology of Diabetes Interventions and Complications
(EDIC) study.[11,12,13]

- Maintaining strict glycemic control in type 1 diabetics has beneficial effects on primary and secondary prevention of microvascular complications; this was demonstrated by the DCCT.[11]
- The best-studied intervention in T1DM is the use of angiotensin-converting enzyme (ACE) inhibitors (ACEIs) to prevent progression of microalbuminuria to macroalbuminuria and slow the progression of diabetic nephropathy.[21]
  - ACEIs may also slow the progression of retinopathy.
  - ACEIs should be started if blood pressure increases above the normal range for the patient's age or even at or below goal blood pressure (130/80) when persistent microalbuminuria is identified.[10]
  - ACEIs should be avoided in premenopausal women who are not using effective birth control, are planning a pregnancy, or who are pregnant, due to the risk of birth defects.
- Blood pressure control, lipid parameters, and other prevention measures are covered in Chapter 27 and Chapter 29.
- Preconception counseling is mandatory for young women with T1DM, and very tight glucose control with near-normalization of glucoses is recommended before conception and during pregnancy for optimal maternal and fetal outcomes.

REFERENCES

1. Patterson CC, Dahlquist GG, Gyurus E, et al. Incidence trends for childhood type 1 diabetes in Europe during 1989-2003 and predicted new cases 2005-20: A multicentre prospective registration study. *Lancet* 2009;373:2027.
2. Dabelea D, Bell RA, D'Agostino RB Jr, et al. Incidence of diabetes in youth in the United States. *JAMA* 2007;297:2716.
3. Cook A. Etiology/pathogenesis of type 1 diabetes. In: Gill RG, Harmon JT, Maclaren NK, eds. *Immunologically Mediated Endocrine Diseases.* Philadelphia, PA: Lippincott Williams & Wilkins; 2002:287–301.
4. Concannon P, Rich SS, Nepom GT. Genetics of type 1A diabetes. *N Engl J Med* 2009; 360:1646.
5. Furmaniak J, Rees SB. Addison's disease. In: Gill RG, ed. *Immunologically Mediated Endocrine Diseases.* Philadelphia, PA: Lippincott Williams & Wilkins; 2002:167–187.
6. Barker JM. Type 1 diabetes-associated autoimmunity: Natural history, genetics, associations, and screening. *J Clin Endocrinol Metab* 2006;91:1210–1217.
7. Cooper JD, Smyth DJ, Smiles AM, et al. Meta-analysis of genome-wide association study data identifies additional type 1 diabetes risk loci. *Nat Genet* 2008;40:1399.
8. Brownlee M. Biochemistry and molecular cell biology of diabetic complications. *Nature* 2001;414:813–820.
9. Sheetz MJ, King GL. Molecular understanding of hyperglycemia's adverse effects for diabetic complications. *JAMA* 2002;288:2579.
10. American Diabetes Association. Standards of medical care in diabetes–2012. *Diabetes Care* 2012;35(Suppl 1):S11–S63.
11. The Diabetes Control and Complications Trial Research Group. The effect of intensive treatment of diabetes on the development and progression of long-term complications in insulin-dependent diabetes mellitus. *N Engl J Med* 1993;329(14):977–986.
12. White NH, Sun W, Cleary PA, et al. Prolonged effect of intensive therapy on the risk of retinopathy complications in patients with type 1 diabetes mellitus: 10 years after the Diabetes Control and Complications Trial. *Arch Ophthalmol* 2008;126(12):1707–1715.
13. Diabetes Control and Complications Trial/Epidemiology of Diabetes Interventions and Complications Research Group. Sustained effect of intensive treatment of type 1 diabetes mellitus

on development and progression of diabetic nephropathy: The Epidemiology of Diabetes Interventions and Complications (EDIC) study. *JAMA* 2003;22;290(16):2159–2167.

14. Albers JW, Herman WH, Pop-Busui R, et al. Effect of prior intensive insulin treatment during the Diabetes Control and Complications Trial (DCCT) on peripheral neuropathy in type 1 diabetes during the Epidemiology of Diabetes Interventions and Complications (EDIC) Study. *Diabetes Care* 2010;33(5):1090–1096.

15. Juvenile Diabetes Research Foundation Continuous Glucose Monitoring Study Group, Bode B, et al. Sustained benefit of continuous glucose monitoring on A1C, glucose profiles, and hypoglycemia in adults with type 1 diabetes. *Diabetes Care* 2009;32(11):2047–2049.

16. Block CD, et al. A review of current evidence with continuous glucose monitoring in patients with diabetes. *J Diabetes Sci Technol* 2008;2(4):718-727.

17. Edelman S, Garg S, Frias J, et al. A double-blind, placebo-controlled trial assessing pramlintide treatment in the setting of intensive insulin therapy in type 1 diabertes. *Diabetes Care* 2006;29:189–195.

18. Ryan G, Briscoe TA, Jobe L. Review of pramlintide as adjunctive therapy in treatment of type 1 and type 2 diabetes. *Drug Des Devel Ther* 2009;2:203–214.

19. Kitabchi AE, Umpierrez GE, Miles JM, et al. Hyperglycemic crises in adult patients with diabetes. *Diabetes Care* 2009;32:1335.

20. Kitabchi AE, Umpierrez GE, Murphy MB, et al. For the American Diabetes Association. Hyperglycemic crises in diabetes. *Diabetes Care* 2004;27(Suppl 1):S94–S102.

21. Lewis EJ, Hunsicker LG, Bain RP, et al. For the Collaborative Study Group. The effect of angiotensin-converting enzyme inhibition on diabetic nephropathy. *N Engl J Med* 1993; 329:1456–1462.

Diabetes Mellitus Type 2

29

Zhiyu Wang and Janet B. McGill

GENERAL PRINCIPLES

Definition
- Type 2 diabetes mellitus (T2DM) results from a combination of resistance to insulin action and an inadequate compensatory insulin secretory response.[1]
- It is a metabolic disorder with carbohydrate intolerance as the cardinal feature.

Epidemiology
- Diabetes has an estimated total prevalence of 23.5 million among people ≥20 years of age, or 10.7% of the adult population.[2] T2DM accounts for about 95% of all cases of diabetes in the United States and is a growing public health concern.
- Diabetes is the sixth leading cause of death in the United States and a leading cause of morbidity and mortality in other countries.
- Diabetes is the leading cause of end-stage renal disease, blindness in individuals age 20 to 74 years, and nontraumatic limb amputation.
- The major cause of mortality in diabetes is cardiovascular, and the diagnosis of diabetes confers a two- to four-fold increase in cardiovascular risk.

Etiology
The etiology of T2DM is multifactorial. It is complex and involves the interaction of genetic and environmental factors.
- Patients often have a family history of T2DM, supporting the role of genetic predisposition in the pathogenesis.
- Genome-wide association studies have contributed to our understanding of the genetic architecture of T2DM. While many genetic loci have been associated with T2DM, these new discoveries represent but a small proportion of the genetic variation underlying the susceptibility to this disorder.[3]
- A number of environmental factors have been shown to play a critical role in the development of T2DM.
  - Sex, age, and ethnic background are important factors in determining risk of developing T2DM.
  - Excessive caloric intake leading to obesity, especially visceral adiposity, and physical inactivity contribute significantly to insulin resistance and, in epidemiologic studies, are the factors associated with the increasing incidence of T2DM.
  - Lifestyle modification that includes weight loss and exercise improves insulin resistance and prevents diabetes in high-risk cohorts.[4]

Pathophysiology
- **Insulin resistance**, the inability of cells to respond to stimulation by insulin, is present in most individuals with T2DM.[5]

- ○ Insulin resistance precedes the onset of T2DM by years.
- ○ The cellular features of insulin resistance include reduction of nonoxidative glucose storage as glycogen, impaired fatty acid oxidation and reduced ability to switch between fatty acid and glucose oxidation during hyperinsulinemia. Mitochondrial content and oxidative capacity may be reduced in insulin-responsive tissues of persons with insulin resistance.[6]
- ○ Inflammation also plays a role in insulin resistance, and elevated levels of free fatty acids and inflammatory markers are present. Insulin sensitivity declines with age, but this may be due to the changes in body composition that occur with aging.[7]
- • **Insulin deficiency,** on the other hand, typically follows a period of hyperinsulinemia, which compensates for insulin resistance.[8]
- ○ The initial defects in insulin secretion are loss of first-phase insulin release and loss of the oscillatory secretion pattern. The clinical correlate of this early defect is postprandial hyperglycemia. Further decline in insulin secretion leads to inadequate suppression of hepatic glucose output and presents clinically as fasting hyperglycemia.
- ○ Hyperglycemia and T2DM develop when insulin secretion by pancreatic beta cells is inadequate to meet the metabolic demand.
- ○ Hyperglycemia contributes to impaired beta-cell function and worsening insulin deficiency, a phenomenon known as glucose toxicity.
- ○ Chronic elevation of free fatty acids, another characteristic of T2DM, may contribute to reduced insulin secretion and islet cell apoptosis.
- • There are no definitive histopathologic findings of insulin resistance; however, increased cellular triglyceride and reduced numbers of mitochondria may be seen.
- • Histopathologic changes in the islets of Langerhans in long-standing T2DM include amyloid accumulation and a reduction in the number of insulin-producing beta cells.
- • Longitudinal data from the UK Prospective Diabetes Study (UKPDS) suggest progressive beta-cell failure occurs during the lifespan of individuals with T2DM. Early in the course of diabetes, improvement in insulin secretion can be achieved by reducing insulin resistance and improving hyperglycemia, thereby reducing the functional defects imposed by hyperglycemia and elevated free fatty acids.[9]
- • The definitive tests for insulin resistance measure insulin-mediated glucose uptake and/or hepatic glucose output and are available in research settings.
- • In the clinical settings, insulin resistance is often inferred when features of the metabolic syndrome are present, with or without a diagnosis of diabetes.

Classification

In addition to type 1 diabetes (**T1DM**), **T2DM,** and **gestational DM,** the American Diabetes Association (ADA) classifies a heterogeneous group of hyperglycemic disorders as "**other specific types of diabetes.**"[1]

- • The most common of this group of disorders are the **drug- or chemical-induced forms of diabetes.** Typical offending agents include glucocorticoids, nicotinic acid, thiazides, β-adrenergic agonists, atypical antipsychotic agents, and some antiretroviral agents. Hyperglycemia can be relatively mild or quite severe with the institution of these therapies.
- • **Pancreatic disease** can result in partial or complete insulin deficiency. Patients with hemochromatosis or advanced cystic fibrosis may present with nonketotic hyperglycemia. Pancreatitis, pancreatectomy, pancreatic neoplasia, or fibrocalculous pancreatopathy may cause insulin deficiency, and insulin therapy may be needed early in the course of the illness.

TABLE 29-1 MONOGENIC FORMS OF DIABETES

Associated with insulin resistance
Mutations in the insulin receptor gene
- Type A insulin resistance
- Leprechaunism
- Rabson–Mendenhall syndrome

Lipoatrophic diabetes
Mutations in the PPARγ gene

Associated with defective insulin secretion
Mutations in the insulin or proinsulin genes
Mitochondrial gene mutations

Maturity-onset diabetes of the young (MODY)
HNF-4α (MODY 1)
Glucokinase (MODY 2)
HNF-1α (MODY 3)
IPF-1 (MODY 4)
HNF-1β (MODY 5)
NeuroD1/Beta2 (MODY 6)

HNF, hepatocyte nuclear factor; IPF, insulin promoter factor; NeuroD1/Beta2, neurogenic differentiation 1/beta cell E-box *trans*-activator 2; PPAR, peroxisome proliferator-activated receptor.

This table was published in *Type 2 Diabetes Mellitus,* Buse JB, Polonsky KS, Burant CF. In: Kronenberg HM, Melmed S. Polonsky KS, et al., eds., *Williams Textbook of Endocrinology,* 11th ed., Philadelphia, PA: Saunders/Elsevier 1329–1389, Copyright Saunders/Elsevier, 2008.

- Diabetes can occur with **critical illness** and other endocrine diseases such as **Cushing's syndrome** and **acromegaly.** Resolution of the diabetes often occurs when the hormone excess is corrected.
- Diabetes can be due to genetic defects of the beta-cell and/or insulin action. It consists of monogenic and polygenic forms.
  ○ The monogenic forms of diabetes generally occur in young patients, often in the first two to three decades of life, although if only mild asymptomatic elevations in blood glucose (BG) occur the diagnosis may be missed until later in life (Table 29-1).[10]
    ■ **Maturity-onset diabetes in the young (MODY)** is one of the common monogenetic forms of diabetes. It is a genetically and clinically heterogeneous group of disorders resulting from mutations in any one of at least six different genes, which cause a primary defect in pancreatic beta cell function. MODY often presents with mild to moderate nonketotic hyperglycemia in young adults with a family history. Obesity and insulin resistance are not characteristic features of MODY. Most of the T2DM that is diagnosed in children and teenagers is not MODY, but is rather early onset classic T2DM.[11]
    ■ There are other rare monogenetic forms of diabetes, including mitochondrial gene defects and defects in the insulin molecule or insulin receptor (type A insulin resistance).

TABLE 29-2	METABOLIC SYNDROME	
Metabolic syndrome characteristics	**Men**	**Women**
Waist circumference	>40 inches	>35 inches
	>102 cm	>88 cm
Triglycerides	≥150 mg/dL	≥150 mg/dL
High-density lipoprotein	<40 mg/dL	<50 mg/dL
Blood pressure	≥130/85 mm Hg	≥130/85 mm Hg
Fasting glucose	≥100 mg/dL	≥100 mg/dL

- Patients with Down's syndrome, patients with Prader–Willi syndrome, and others may develop diabetes as a consequence of obesity.
- **Latent autoimmune diabetes in adults (LADA)** is an insulin-deficient form of diabetes that develops more slowly than classic T1DM and is associated with other autoimmune diseases.[12] The majority of patients with LADA require exogenous insulin within 5 years of diagnosis. Later in the course of the illness, patients with LADA may become C-peptide negative and are at risk for ketoacidosis. When LADA is suspected, testing for anti-GAD antibodies and C-peptide may help rule in or rule out the diagnosis.

Risk Factors

Individuals at high risk for the development of T2DM can often be identified before the onset of clinical diabetes.[13] Risk factors for the development of T2DM include

- Older age
- Overweight or obesity (body mass index [BMI] ≥25 kg/m^2)
- Physical inactivity
- First-degree relative with diabetes
- Members of high-risk ethnic population (e.g., African American, Latino, Native American, Asian American, Pacific Islander)
- Women who delivered a baby weighing >9 lb or were diagnosed with gestational diabetes mellitus (GDM)
- Women with polycystic ovary syndrome
- A1C ≥5.7%, impaired glucose tolerance (IGT) or impaired fasting glucose (IFG)
- Other conditions associated with insulin resistance (e.g., metabolic syndrome,[14] defined as three or more of the characteristics listed in Table 29-2, acanthosis nigricans)

DIAGNOSIS

Clinical Presentation

- Mild hyperglycemia is asymptomatic. Patients presenting with symptoms of polyuria, nocturia, polydipsia, polyphagia, fatigue, weight changes, or blurred vision are likely to have significant BG elevation and may have been undiagnosed for some time.
- Patients who present with complaints of extremity pain, sexual dysfunction, or visual changes from diabetic retinopathy are likely to have been hyperglycemic for years before being diagnosed with diabetes.

History

Medical history of a patient with diabetes should include documentation of:

- The onset and progression of diabetes, with information about episodes of diabetic ketoacidosis (DKA), prior response to medications, and level of glycemic control.
- Health behaviors, such as frequency of self-monitoring of BG, use of medical nutrition therapy (MNT), and exercise frequency and intensity, should be recorded.
- Usual BG values and problems with both hyperglycemia and hypoglycemia require assessment to plan changes in therapy.
- Symptoms of hyperglycemia and hypoglycemia should be elicited to augment a careful review of glucose records or meter readings.
- The past medical history (PMH) should record history of diabetes-related complications.
  - Macrovascular: coronary heart disease, cerebrovascular disease, peripheral vascular disease.
  - Microvascular: retinopathy, nephropathy, and neuropathy including history of foot ulceration or joint problems.
  - Other: psychosocial problems, dental disease.
  - The vaccine status should be recorded. Menstrual history, pregnancy history, and use of contraception need to be addressed in the PMH of adolescent and adult women.

Physical Examination

- Physical examination may be completely normal or may include hypertension, obesity, or acanthosis nigricans.
- Funduscopic examination may be normal or abnormal (dot hemorrhages, exudates, neovascularization, or laser scars).
- The cardiovascular examination for patients with diabetes should include carotid and peripheral pulses.
- Examination of the feet, including skin, nails, joints, and sensation with a 10 g Semmes-Weinstein monofilament, should be done at regular intervals.
- The diagnosis of neuropathy is based on a combination of symptoms and physical findings, with documented decrease in more than one sensory modality (e.g., absent reflexes plus loss of vibratory sensation).

Diagnostic Criteria

- Classically, diabetes has been diagnosed on the basis of prospective epidemiologic data associating circulating glucose levels with the future development of diabetes retinopathy. The diagnostic criteria for diabetes and prediabetic conditions are listed in Table 29-3.
- **ADA current criteria for the diagnosis of diabetes**[1]
  - Hemoglobin A1c (HbA1c) ≥6.5%;
  - Fasting plasma glucose (FPG) ≥126 mg/dL and confirmed on a second sample;
  - 2-hour plasma glucose is ≥200 mg/dL after a 75 g oral glucose tolerance test (OGTT);
  - Or a random BG of ≥200 mg/dL accompanied by classic symptoms of hyperglycemia or hyperglycemic crisis.
  - In the absence of unequivocal hyperglycemia, tests should be confirmed by repeat testing.
- **Categories of increased risk for diabetes**
  - This is an intermediate group of individuals whose glucose levels do not meet criteria for diabetes, yet are higher than those considered normal.[1]

TABLE 29-3 DIAGNOSIS OF DIABETES

Stage	HbA1c	FPG	OGTT	Random blood glucose
Normal	≤5.6%	<100 mg/dL	2-hour PG <140 mg/dL	—
Prediabetes	5.7%–6.4%			
IFG		≥100 mg/dL and <126 mg/dL	—	—
IGT	—		2-hour PG ≥140 mg/dL and <200 mg/dL	—
Diabetes	≥6.5%	FPG ≥126 mg/dL	2-hour PG ≥200 mg/dL	≥200 mg/dL with symptoms

FPG, fasting plasma glucose; OGTT, oral glucose tolerance test; PG, plasma glucose; IFG, impaired fasting glucose; IGT, impaired glucose tolerance.

In the absence of unequivocal hyperglycemia, diagnosis should be confirmed by repeat testing.

○ They have been referred to as having **prediabetes,** indicating the relative high risk for the future development of diabetes. They may be at higher risk for cardiovascular events even in the absence of T2DM.
○ These patients are defined as having:
  ▪ IFG (FPG 100 mg/dL to 125 mg/dL);
  ▪ IGT (2-hour values on the 75 g OGTT of 140 mg/dL to 199 mg/dL);
  ▪ Or HbA1c of 5.7% to 6.4%.
• Testing for T2DM in asymptomatic patients
○ Although the effectiveness of early identification of prediabetes and diabetes through mass testing of asymptomatic individuals has not been proven definitively, prediabetes and diabetes meet established criteria for conditions in which early detection is appropriate.
○ ADA recommends testing for diabetes in asymptomatic patients based on their risks.[13]
  ▪ Testing to detect T2DM in asymptomatic people is recommended in adults of any age who are overweight or obese (BMI ≥25 kg/m^2) and who have ≥1 risk factors for diabetes.
  ▪ In those without risk factors, testing should begin at age 45.
  ▪ HbA1c, FPG, or 2-hour 75 g OGTT are appropriate tests.
  ▪ If tests are normal, repeat testing is recommended at least at 3-year intervals.

Diagnostic Testing

• **Routine laboratory testing** of a patient with T2DM should include the following:
○ HbA1c, chemistry panel, fasting lipid profile, urine microalbumin (usually done as microalbumin-to-creatinine ratio on a random spot urine sample), and liver function panel.

- HbA1c should be done at diagnosis and at least semiannually. If the HbA1c is significantly above the target of 7% and therapy is being changed, it should be checked every 1 to 3 months.
- Liver function testing is required for monitoring of statin and thiazolidinedione (TZD) therapies and should be considered for all patients with insulin resistance due to the increased risk of nonalcoholic fatty liver disease (NAFLD).
- Patients with T2DM and proteinuria or renal insufficiency require increased surveillance of renal parameters.
- A **baseline electrocardiogram** (ECG)

TREATMENT

- T2DM is best managed with a multidisciplinary team, including doctors, diabetes educators, pharmacists, dietitians, and support groups.[13]
- Diabetes is a lifelong disease, and health care providers have almost no control over the extent to which patients adhere to the day-to-day treatment regimen. Therefore, it is critical for the health care professional to understand the context in which patients are taking care of their disease, and carefully engage patients in the therapeutic process. Any plan should recognize diabetes self-management education (DSME) and on-going diabetes support as an integral component of care.
- Diabetes therapy should be individually designed to achieve glycemic, blood pressure, lipid, and prevention targets while accommodating the patient's age and socioeconomic and cultural status and presence of complications of diabetes and other medical conditions (see Chapter 27 for further details).

LIFESTYLE MODIFICATION

- Lifestyle modification incorporating both MNT and physical activity is the first-line therapy for the prevention of diabetes and treatment of new-onset T2DM.
  - Weight loss has been shown to reduce insulin resistance. Moderate weight loss (7% body weight) and regular physical activity (150 minutes/week) with dietary strategies are effective in reducing the progression from prediabetes to diabetes.[4]
  - Weight loss is recommended for all overweight or obese individuals who have or are at risk for diabetes.[14]
  - Individuals who have prediabetes or diabetes should receive individualized MNT as needed to achieve treatment goals.
    - Low-carbohydrate or low-fat calorie-restricted diets are effective for short-term weight loss. Several randomized controlled trials suggested low-carbohydrate diets (<130 g/day) achieved more weight loss than low-fat diets and a greater decrease of Hb1Ac in T2DM patients.[15]
    - Monitoring carbohydrate intake remains a key strategy in achieving glycemic control.
    - Structured exercise interventions have been shown to lower Hb1Ac in T2DM patients.[16] In the absence of contraindications, T2DM patients should be encouraged to perform resistance training 3 times/week and at least 150 minute/week of moderate-intensity aerobic physical activity (50% to 70% of maximum heart rate).[17]

- However, the UKPDS study showed that only 8% of patients treated with dietary therapy alone were able to achieve and maintain glycemic control over a 9-year period.[18]

Medications

- **Oral hypoglycemic agents** (Tables 29-4 and 29-5)
  - **Metformin**
    - Metformin is the only biguanide available in the United States.[19]
    - It decreases hepatic glucose output and lowers fasting glycemia.
    - Metformin monotherapy decreases HbA1c by 1% to 2%.
    - Metformin is related to either weight stability or modest weight loss.
    - The most common adverse effect is gastrointestinal intolerance. Metformin may interfere with Vitamin B12 absorption. Renal dysfunction is considered a contraindication to metformin use.
  - **Sulfonylureas**
    - Sulfonylureas enhance insulin secretion.
    - They can lower HbA1c by 1% to 2%.
    - The major adverse effect is hypoglycemia, especially in the elderly. Weight gain is common following sulfonylurea therapy.
  - **Glinides**
    - Glinides are short-acting insulin secretagogues. They bind to a different site within the sulfonylurea receptor. They have a shorter half-life than the sulfonylureas and must be administered more frequently.
    - Glinides decrease HbA1c by 1% to 1.5%
    - They have similar adverse effects to sulfonylureas.
  - **TZDs**
    - TZDs are peroxisome proliferator-activated receptor γ modulators.
    - They decrease the sensitivity of muscle, fat, and liver to insulin.
    - Monotherapy with TZDs has demonstrated a 0.8% to 1.8% decrease in HbA1c.
    - The most common adverse effects are weight gain, fluid retention, and an increased incidence of fractures in women.
    - Several meta-analyses have suggested a 30% to 40% relative increase in risk for MI with rosiglitazone, which is no longer available for use. Pioglitazone has been associated with an increased risk of bladder cancer.
  - **α-Glucosidase inhibitors**
    - α-Glucosidase inhibitors reduce the rate of digestion of polysaccharide in the proximal small intestine, lowering postprandial glucose without causing hypoglycemia.
    - They decrease HbA1c by 0.6% to 1.2%.
    - Increased gas production and gastrointestinal symptoms are the most common side effects.
  - **Dipeptidyl peptidase 4 inhibitors (DPP-4 inhibitors)**
    - DPP-4 inhibitors are small molecules inhibiting the enzyme that breaks down endogenous glucagon-like peptide-1 (GLP1) and glucose-dependent insulinotropic polypeptide (GIP). Therefore, they enhance the effects of GLP1 and GIP, increase glucose-mediated insulin secretion, and suppress glucagon secretion and gastric emptying.
    - DPP-4 inhibitors lower Hb1Ac by 0.6% to 1.8% and are weight neutral.
    - The potential side effect is to interfere with immune function. Dosage needs adjustment for impaired renal function except for linagliptin.

TABLE 29-4 NON-INSULIN ANTIDIABETIC DRUGS

Drug	Daily dose	Mode of action	Efficacy	Advantages	Disadvantages
Biguanide					
Metformin (Glucophage, Glucophage XR, Glumetza) (Riomet, liquid formulation)	500–2000 mg daily, divided doses	Reduces hepatic glucose output	↓ A1c by 1%–2%	No weight gain, may ↓ triglycerides; inexpensive	GI side effects (nausea, diarrhea); risk of lactic acidosis. Avoid if creatinine is >1.4 in women; >1.5 in men; chronic heart failure, age >80 years, liver impairment.
Sulfonylureas (SFUs, second generation)					
Glyburide (DiaBeta, Micronase)	2.5–20 mg divided doses	Stimulate insulin release by receptor mediated, glucose independent mechanism	↓ A1c by 1%–2%	Well tolerated, inexpensive	Hypoglycemia, weight gain, allergy. Use with caution in the elderly or in patients with liver or renal insufficiency.
Glipizide (Glucotrol)	2.5–20 mg, divided doses				
Glimepiride (Amaryl)	2–8 mg q.d.				
Meglitinides					
Repaglinide (Prandin)	0.5–2 mg t.i.d. a.c.	Short-acting insulin secretagogue	↓ A1c by 1%–1.5%	Well tolerated, may have less risk of hypoglycemia compared to sulfonylureas	Hypoglycemia, t.i.d. dosing, more expensive than sulfonylureas
Nateglinide (Starlix)	60–120 mg t.i.d. a.c.				

Thiazolidinediones (TZDs)

Pioglitazone (Actos)	15, 30, 45 mg q.d.	Insulin sensitizer; reduces insulin resistance peripherally	↓ A1c by 0.8%–1.8%	Neutral to positive effect on CV outcomes, carotid IMT	Weight gain, fluid retention, congestive heart failure, anemia; fracture in women; variable lipid effects, expensive; rare liver toxicity. Increased risk of bladder cancer.

Alpha-glucosidase inhibitors (AGIs)

Acarbose (Precose), Miglitol (Glyset)	Both agents: 50–100 mg t.i.d. before meals, start with lower doses	Inhibit gut enzymes that break down carbohydrates	↓ A1c by 0.6%–1.2%	No weight gain	GI side effects, including flatulence, diarrhea, and cramping; rare liver toxicity.

Dipeptidyl peptidase IV inhibitor (DPP-4 inhibitor)

Sitagliptin (Januvia)	100 mg q.d., 50 mg q.d. in stage 3 CKD, 25 mg q.d. in stage 4 CKD	Increases endogenous GLP-1 by inhibiting the enzyme that breaks down GIP and GLP-1	↓ A1c by 0.6%–1.2%	Weight neutral, well tolerated	Dose adjustment in CKD; risk of interfering immune function; hypersensitivity: expensive
Saxagliptin (Onglyza)	5 mg q.d., 2.5 mg q.d. in CKD stage 3, 4, 5				
Linagliptin (Tradjenta)	5 mg q.d., no dose adjustment in CKD				

(continued)

TABLE 29-4	NON-INSULIN ANTIDIABETIC DRUGS (Continued)				
Drug	Daily dose	Mode of action	Efficacy	Advantages	Disadvantages
Bile acid sequestrant (BAS)					
Colesevelam (WelChol)	3.75 g/day (6 tablets)	Reduction or delay in glucose absorption, or modulation of FXR mediated pathways	↓ A1c by 0.6%–1.0%	Weight neutral, lowers LDL cholesterol	Constipation, increased pill count, possible interaction with absorption of other drugs
Dopamine receptor agonist					
Bromocriptine mesylate (Cycloset)	0.8 mg to 4.8 mg q.d.	Glucose lowering mechanism of action is unknown	↓ A1c by 0.4%–0.6%	Weight neutral	Can cause orthostatic hypotension and syncope; may exacerbate psychosis or limit the effectiveness of anti-psychotics
GLP-1 Mimetic					
Exenatide (Byetta, Bydureon) Liraglutide (Victoza)	5–10 mcg b.i.d. a.c. 2 mg once weekly 0.6–1.8 mg q.d. by subcutaneous injection	Stimulates insulin secretion, decreases appetite	↓ A1c by 0.5%–2%	Satiety effect, promotes weight loss	GI: Nausea, vomiting, diarrhea in one-third. Must be given by injection; risk of pancreatitis; warning regarding thyroid C-cell tumors in rodents; expensive
Amylin Analog					
Pramlintide (Symlin)	30–120 mcg t.i.d. a.c. by subcutaneous injection	Decreases postprandial BG by slowing gastric emptying, inducing satiety, enhancing GLP	↓ A1c by 0.5%	Satiety effect, flattens postprandial BG	GI: Nausea and vomiting. Indicated for use with MDI. Can contribute to hypoglycemia

TABLE 29-5	ORAL COMBINATION PILLS
Trade names	**Generic names and doses**
Glucovance	Glyburide/metformin: 1.25 mg/250 mg; 2.5 mg/500 mg; 5 mg/500 mg
Metaglip	Glipizide/metformin: 2.5 mg/250 mg; 2.5 mg/500 mg; 5 mg/500 mg
Actoplus Met	Pioglitazone/metformin: 15 mg/500 mg and 15 mg/850 mg
Duetact	Pioglitazone/glimepiride: 2 mg/30 mg and 4 mg/30 mg
Janumet	Sitagliptin/metformin: 50 mg/500 mg and 50 mg/1000 mg
Kombiglyze	Saxagliptin/metformin extended release: 5/500, 5/1000 and 2.5/1000 mg
Jentadueto	Tradjenta/metformin: 2.5/500, 2.5/850 and 2.5/1000 mg

- ○ **Colesevelam hydrochloride (WelChol)**
  - ■ WelChol is a resin originally developed for the treatment of high LDL. It also lowers HbA1c in patients with T2DM by 0.4% to 0.6%.[20]
- ○ **Bromocriptine mesylate (Cycloset)**
  - ■ Cycloset lowers HbA1c by 0.4% to 0.6%.
  - ■ The major side effect is orthostatic hypotension and syncope.
- ○ Because the agents have different mechanisms of action, most have been tested for use in combination with the other classes. Appropriate patient-specific prescribing can often provide excellent glycemic control with low risk of hypoglycemia, weight gain, and adverse effects.
- • **Non-insulin injectable hypoglycemic agents**
  - ○ **GLP-1 agonists**
    - ■ **Exenatide (Byetta, Bydureon)** and **liraglutide (Victoza)** are GLP-1 mimetics. They bind to the GLP-1 receptors on the pancreatic beta cells and augment glucose-mediated insulin secretion. They also suppress glucagon secretion and slow gastric motility.
    - ■ GLP-1 agonists decrease HbA1c by 0.5% to 2%, mainly by lowering postprandial glucose.
    - ■ They have a high incidence of gastrointestinal side effects, but have an ancillary benefit of contributing to weight loss while lowering blood glucose.
    - ■ Acute pancreatitis has been reported in patients taking exenatide, although the actual incidence is not known.
    - ■ GLP-1 agonists are administered subcutaneously once or twice daily. A once weekly formulation of exenatide is in phase 3 clinical development.
  - ○ **Pramlintide (Symlin)**
    - ■ Symlin is a synthetic analogue of the beta cell hormone amylin. It slows stomach emptying, improves satiety, and inhibits glucose-dependent glucagon production, which is reflected in reduced postprandial glucose and modest weight loss.
    - ■ Symlin decreases HbA1c by 0.5% to 0.7%.
    - ■ The major side effects are gastrointestinal in nature.
    - ■ It is given in doses of 30 to 120 mcg subcutaneously before each meal.
    - ■ Symlin is approved for use in patients with T2DM who are also taking insulin.

- **Insulin** (see Chapter 28 for an overview of insulin types and pharmacokinetics.)
  - When adding insulin in the management of inadequately controlled T2DM, generally the oral antidiabetic agents can be continued. (Table 29-6)
  - Initially, a basal insulin can be added at bedtime. The long-acting insulins glargine (Lantus) and detemir (Levemir) have been shown to cause less nighttime hypoglycemia when used with oral agents in an evening dosing regimen.
  - If the response to one or more oral agents has been poor, or a contraindication develops, a more complex insulin regimen might be required. Multiple daily dosing regimens have been used to achieve tight glucose control and reduce the risk of hypoglycemia by carefully adjusting the premeal doses according to ambient BG, anticipated carbohydrate intake, and activity level.
  - Insulin requirements vary with changes in weight, diet, activity, concomitant medication use, acute illnesses, and infections.
  - The regimen should be tailored to the patient's needs and abilities.
  - Diabetes education is highly recommended when insulin is started or when the regimen is changed.
    - Instruction in signs and symptoms of hypoglycemia and in methods of treatment is required.
    - Instruction in the use of glucagon should be provided to the patient's household members.
- **Concentrated insulin**
  - **U500** (500 U/mL) is available only as Humulin R, or regular.
  - It is an option for patients who require exceptionally large doses of insulin.
  - An endocrinology consultation should be sought if U500 insulin use is contemplated.

Bariatric Surgery

- Bariatric surgery that involves either gastric banding or bypassing sections of the small intestine can be an effective weight loss treatment, particularly for severe obesity.
- Bariatric surgery has been shown to lead to near or complete normalization of glycemia in 50% to 90% of T2DM patients.[21]
- The mechanisms of glycemic improvement, long-term benefits and risks, and cost-effectiveness of bariatric surgery in T2DM need further investigation.
- Bariatric surgery should be considered for T2DM adults with BMI ≥35 kg/m^2, especially if their diseases are difficult to control with lifestyle and medications.[11]
- Currently, there is insufficient evidence to support general recommendation for bariatric surgery in T2DM patients with BMI <35, however some patients may benefit from the procedure.
- Patients who have undergone bariatric surgery need lifelong lifestyle support and medical monitoring.

Prevention of T2DM

Randomized controlled trials have shown that early interventions significantly decrease the rate of onset of diabetes in high-risk individuals. The ADA recommends prevention of T2DM.[13]

- Prediabetic patients are recommended to have an effective ongoing support program for weight loss of 5% to 10% of body weight and increase in physical activity to at least 150 minute/week of moderate activity.

TABLE 29-6 INSULIN REGIMENS FOR DIABETES MELLITUS TYPE 2

Regimen	Oral agents	Insulin types	Glucose monitoring	Starting Doses
Oral agents + basal insulin—*Usual starting regimen*	Continue all types of oral agents. Use submaximal doses of TZDs.	Intermediate (NPH) or long-acting (glargine, detemir).	Fasting and as needed during the day	0.1–0.2 U/kg given at bedtime; increase until FPG is at target.
Premixed insulin, generally bid.—*OK for patients with regular meal schedules*	Continue insulin sensitizers. TZDs: Use up to 30 mg pioglitazone.	70/30 NPH/regular; Humalog mix 75/25; NovoLog mix 70/30.	2–4 × daily and as needed to avoid hypoglycemia	0.1 U/kg a.m. and p.m.; increase doses equally until blood glucose near the target range; evaluate with q.i.d. self-monitored blood glucose.
MDI regimens—*Helpful for patients with irregular meal schedules; may be necessary to achieve tight control*	Continue sensitizers at doses above if the patient is insulin resistant and there are no contraindications. Discontinue secretagogues.	Basal insulin: Insulin glargine given at bedtime or detemir/NPH/Lente given q.d. or b.i.d.; premeal insulin: Lispro (Humalog), aspart (NovoLog), glulisine (Apidra) or regular.	4 × daily is required: Before meals and at bedtime	In general, a total dose of 0.5–2 U/kg will be required. Give 50% as basal; divide the remaining 50% into premeal doses. Use adjustable scales ± carbohydrate counting for premeal dosing.
Continuous SC insulin infusion—*Many attractive features for patients*	Sensitizers may still be useful for insulin-resistant patients.	Lispro (Humalog) Aspart (NovoLog) and glulisine (Apidra)	4 × daily and as needed	Conceptually similar to MDI regimens. Intensive diabetes education is needed.

FPG, fasting plasma glucose; MDI, multiple daily injection; TZD, thiazolidinedione.

- In addition to lifestyle counseling, metformin can be considered in those who are at very high risk for developing diabetes (combined IFG and IGT plus other risk factors) and who are obese and <60 years of age.
- Follow-up counseling and monitoring for development of diabetes should be performed annually.

SPECIAL CONSIDERATIONS

Nonketotic Hyperosmolar Coma

- Nonketotic Hyperosmolar Coma (NKHC) evolves over a period of time but presents emergently when neurologic deterioration occurs in the setting of high glucose levels and dehydration.
- Elderly or disabled patients with significant hyperglycemia who are unable to compensate for the free water loss with oral intake are predisposed to develop this syndrome.[22]
- Patients with NKHC present with a plasma glucose that is generally >600 mg/dL, normal or slightly elevated anion gap, increased BUN and creatinine, increased serum osmolality, and a free water deficit of 2 to 6 L.
- The initial goal of therapy is to replace volume and correct the free water deficit with the infusion of appropriate intravenous fluids.
  - The nature of the fluids (isotonic vs. hypotonic) administered and the rate of infusion are determined by the clinical circumstances.
  - As in DKA, patients in NKHC also present with total body K^+ deficit.
  - Intravenous insulin should be given as repeated intravenous bolus doses (0.1 U/kg/1 to 2 hours) or via insulin drip (see Chapter 28 for further details).
  - The glucose may decline more rapidly in NKHC than in DKA. Electrolytes and the clinical status of the patient should be checked closely and intravenous fluids adjusted accordingly.
  - Neurologic changes should be evaluated to rule out stroke or other central nervous system (CNS) conditions.
  - Mortality is high in patients who present with NKHC due to age and underlying conditions.

REFERENCES

1. American Diabetes Association. Diagnosis and Classification of Diabetes Mellitus. *Diabetes Care* 2010;33:S62-S69.
2. Center for Disease Control and Prevention. *National Diabetes Fact Sheet: General Information and National Estimates on Diabetes in the United States, 2007*. Atlanta, GA:: Department of Health and Human Services, Centers for Disease Control and Prevention; 2008.
3. Frayling TM. Genome-wide association studies provide new insights into type 2 diabetes aetiology. *Nat Rev Genet* 2007;8:657–662.
4. Diabetes Prevention Program Research Group. Reduction in the incidence of type 2 diabetes with lifestyle intervention or metformin. *N Engl J Med* 2002;346:393–403.
5. Diabetes Prevention Program Research Group. Role of insulin secretion and sensitivity in the evolution of type 2 diabetes in the Diabetes Prevention Program. Effects of lifestyle intervention and metformin. *Diabetes* 2005;54;2404–2414.

6. Szendroedi J, Phielix E, Roden M. The role of mitochondria in insulin resistance and type 2 diabetes mellitus. *Nature Reviews/Endocrinology* 2011;8(2):92–103.

7. Donath MY, Shoelson SE. Type 2 diabetes as an inflammatory disease. *Nature Reviews/Immunology* 2011;11;98–107.

8. Weyer C, Bogardus C, Mott DM, et al. The natural history of insulin secretory dysfunction and insulin resistance in the pathogenesis of type 2 diabetes mellitus. *J Clin Invest* 1999; 104:787–794.

9. Statton IM, Adler AI, Neil HA, et al. Association of glycaemia with macrovascular and microvascular complications of type 2 diabetes (UKPDS 35): Prospective observational study. *BMJ* 2000;321:405–412.

10. Buse JB, Polonsky KS, Burant CF. Type 2 Diabetes Mellitus. In: Kronenberg HM, Melmed S, Polonsky KS, et. al., *Williams Textbook of Endocrinology,* 11th ed. Philadelphia, PA: Saunders/Elsevier, 2008:1329–1389.

11. Fajans SS, Bell GI, Polonsky KS. Molecular mechanisms and clinical pathophysiology of maturity-onset diabetes of the young. *N Engl J Med* 2001;345:971–980.

12. Naik RG, Brooks-Worrell BM, Palmer JP. Latent autoimmune diabetes in adults. *J Clin Endocrinol Metab* 2009;94:4635–4644.

13. American Diabetes Association. Standards of medical care in diabetes–2010. *Diabetes Care* 2010;33(Suppl 1):S11–S61.

14. Park Y, Zhu S, Palaniappan L, et al. The metabolic syndrome: Prevalence and associated risk factor findings in the U.S. population from the third national health and nutrition exam survey, 1988–1994. *Arch Intern Med* 2003;163:427–436.

15. Stern L, Iqbal N, Seshadri P, et al. The effects of low-carbohydrate versus conventional weight loss diets in severely obese adults: One-year follow-up of a randomized trial. *Ann Intern Med* 2004;140:778–785.

16. Boulé NG, Haddad E, Kenny GP, et al. Effects of exercise on glycemic control and body mass in type 2 diabetes mellitus: A meta-analysis of controlled clinical trials. *JAMA* 2001; 286:1218–1227.

17. U.S. Department of Health and Human Services. *2008 Physical Activity Guidelines for Americans.* Atlanta, GA: Center for Disease Control and Prevention, 2008.

18. Turner RC, Cull CA, Frighi V, et al. Glycemic control with diet, sulfonylurea, metformin, or insulin in patients with type 2 diabetes mellitus: Progressive requirement for multiple therapies (UKPDS 49). UK Prospective Diabetes Study (UKPDS) Group. *JAMA* 1999; 281:2005–2012.

19. Nathan DM, Buse JB, Davidson MB, et al. Medical management of hyperglycemia in type 2 diabetes: a consensus algorithm for the initiation and adjustment of therapy: A consensus statement of the American Diabetes Association and the European Association for the Study of Diabetes. *Diabetes Care* 2009;32:193–203.

20. Handelsman Y, Goldberg RB, Garvey WT, et al. Colesevelam hydrochloride to treat hyper-cholesterolemia and improve glycemia in prediabetes: A randomized, prospective study. *Endocr Pract* 2010;16:617–628.

21. Buchwald H, Estok R, Fahrbach K, et al. Weight and type 2 diabetes after bariatric surgery: Systematic review and meta-analysis. *Am J Med* 2009;122:248–256.

22. Ennis ED, Stahl EJVB, Kreisberg RA. The hyperosmolar hyperglycemic syndrome. *Diabetes Rev* 1994;2:115–126.

Inpatient Management of Diabetes

30

David A. Rometo and Garry Tobin

GENERAL PRINCIPLES

- Hyperglycemia is a common occurrence in hospitalized patients, including those with previously diagnosed diabetes, those diagnosed with diabetes during the admission, and those with acute illness, stress, or intervention-induced hyperglycemia.
- Hypoglycemia is less common, and is most often caused by therapy to treat or prevent hyperglycemia.
- Guidelines defining appropriate glucose targets and how to achieve them in hospitalized patients have been published by several organizations. They are specific to either a critically ill or non-critically ill patient population (Table 30-1).[1]
- The use of insulin to treat hyperglycemia is almost universally favored over oral hypoglycemic therapy in the hospital setting.
- Diabetes care is more complex than ordering the correct dose of medication. Coordination of care between physicians, nurses, nurse assistants, dietary staff, diabetes educators, and social workers is important to allow for appropriate timing of glucose measurement, insulin administration, meal/nutrition delivery, treatment of hypoglycemia, patient self-management education, and discharge planning.

Epidemiology

- It is estimated that 22% of all inpatient (IP) hospital days are incurred by patients with diabetes.[1]
- Hyperglycemia (>180 mg/dL) is found on 46% of all blood glucose (BG) readings in intensive care units (ICUs), and 31.7% of all non-ICU readings (from a 2007 survey of over 12 million point-of-care (POC) glucose readings from 126 US hospitals).[2]

Outcomes

- **BG <60 or >110 mg/dL are associated with higher inpatient mortality.**[3]
- Non-critically ill patients with previously diagnosed diabetes who are hyperglycemic while hospitalized have increased in-hospital mortality compared to euglycemic patients. Those without a prior diagnosis of diabetes but with new hyperglycemia while hospitalized have an even greater increase in mortality compared to euglycemic patients. Critically ill patients with newly diagnosed hyperglycemia also have higher inpatient mortality rates than patients with known diabetes or with euglycemia.[4]
- Patients who are hyperglycemic at admission and are placed on TPN have increased mortality compared to those on TPN who were euglycemic at admission.[5]
- Patients who have had an episode of hypoglycemia (<50 mg/dL) in the hospital have increased in-hospital mortality, longer hospital stays, increased hospital charges, and increased rates of discharge to skilled nursing facilities.[6]

TABLE 30-1	RECOMMENDED GLUCOSE TARGETS FOR INPATIENTS	
Recommended blood glucose targets for inpatients		
	Critically ill	**Non-critically ill**
AACE/ADA	140 mg/dL to 180 mg/dL using IV insulin protocol	Premeal glucose <140 mg/dL Random glucose <180 mg/dL Using basal/prandial regimen with correction dose

- Intensive insulin therapy administered by a variable dose IV infusion improves many clinical outcomes in ICU settings, including reductions in wound infections and in organ failure after cardiothoracic surgery. However, the risk of hypoglycemia is increased and may contribute to increased mortality in medical ICU settings.[1]
- Only small-scale clinical trials of insulin therapy in non-critically ill inpatients have been conducted.

DIAGNOSIS

For diagnostic criteria for diabetes, see Chapter 29.

Acute or Chronic Hyperglycemia?

- **Inpatient hyperglycemia** can be defined as **any blood glucose value >140 mg/dL.**
- Checking a hemoglobin A1c (HbA1c) can distinguish acute hyperglycemia from undiagnosed diabetes, the latter likely having an HbA1c > 6.5%.[1] Hemoglobin A1c values are affected by hemoglobinopathies, acute blood loss, and blood transfusion. These issues must be taken into consideration when ordering a HbA1c in the hospital.

Glucose Monitoring

- "Fingerstick" or capillary BG testing using point-of-care (POC) glucose meters is an integral part of diabetes management in hospitalized patients. **The timing of glucose checks should be adjusted to the patient's clinical condition.** Glucose testing is performed hourly in patients receiving insulin by IV infusion, every 4 to 6 hours in patients who are NPO, or who are receiving enteral nutrition or TPN. Monitoring of blood glucose should be performed 30 to 60 minutes before meals in patients who are eating meals so that prandial and correction factor insulin can be administered before the meal. In general, inpatients receiving insulin should have their blood glucose checked ≥4X daily.
- Attention should be paid to the limitations of the glucose analyzer and the source of the specimen. Measurement of glucose with standardized lab measurements, including blood gas analyzers and the clinical chemistry laboratory, are more accurate than POC technology.
- The source of the patient's sample (arterial, capillary, central venous), the patient's clinical conditions (anemia, hypoxia, poor peripheral perfusion) and current medications (acetaminophen, ascorbic acid, IVIG, peritoneal dialysis) can all affect the POC glucose results.

- Anemia (Hct <34%) has been shown to cause significant error, overestimating glucose with POC glucose meters. Dosing insulin based on falsely elevated glucose values may contribute to hypoglycemia in intensively treated patients in ICU settings. The use of formulas to correct BG for the level of anemia has been shown to reduce hypoglycemic events in ICU patients.[7]
- Meters using glucose dehydrogenase enzymatic strips are affected by maltose in IVIG and Icodextrin peritoneal dialysis solution, and therefore should be used with caution in healthcare facilities.[7]
- In the absence of an interfering substance, the current FDA standard for POC glucose meters is +/− 20% accuracy above 75 mg/dL, and +/− 15% for <75 mg/dL, 95% of the time. This standard may be lowered to +/− 10% in the future.
- Arterial blood measured by POC glucose meters is more accurate than capillary glucose, and should be used when available in ICU patients on IV insulin.[8]

MANAGEMENT OF THE NON-CRITICALLY ILL

Assessment

- A history of diabetes should include the age of onset, duration, type of diabetes, and history of DKA or other diabetes-related hospitalizations.
- Ability to monitor blood glucose at home, frequency of home monitoring and availability of supplies is an important part of the history that will be useful for discharge planning.
- The home anti-diabetes medications, including insulin doses and regimen, should be documented in detail. "Sliding scale" does not describe a specific regimen, and provides insufficient information. When the patient adjusts their insulin dose at home, recording either the adjustment scale (e.g., 1 unit/10 g of carbohydrate plus correction of 1 unit/30 mg/dL over 150 mg/dL) or typical doses (e.g., 5 to 10 units before meals) is necessary to discern insulin needs in the hospital. Calculation of the typical total daily dose (TDD) taken at home is very helpful for medication reconciliation.
- Appropriateness of the home regimen can be assessed by obtaining a history of prior HbA1c values, frequency of hypoglycemia, injection site problems, and reported adherence to the regimen.
- **Risk factors for inpatient hypoglycemia** include low weight, advanced age, chronic kidney disease or renal impairment, liver dysfunction, autonomic instability, hypoglycemia unawareness, and malnutrition.
- Ongoing assessment of nutritional intake, including dextrose containing IV fluids, is necessary when prescribing insulin or other anti-diabetes therapies.
- Note corticosteroid use as this will affect the planned dosage regimen.

Oral Hypoglycemics

- **Oral and non-insulin injectable hypoglycemic agents are generally discontinued in the hospital setting,** although selected anti-diabetic agents may be used in inpatients with stable kidney function and nutritional intake.
- Sulfonylureas may contribute to hypoglycemia, particularly during periods of poor intake or NPO status.
- Metformin is contraindicated in patients with renal impairment, and in situations of possible fluctuation in kidney function, such as during IV contrast studies or surgery.

- Dipeptidyl-peptidase IV inhibitors may be options for those with mild hyperglycemia (see Chapter 29).
- Other agents such as thiazolidinediones and GLP analogs have contraindications that may apply to hospitalized patients.[1]

Insulin Therapy

- Insulin is the most accepted anti-hyperglycemic medication in the IP setting since it can be used in patients with varying severities of illness and titrated to the individual patient needs. The major adverse effects of insulin relate to the difficulty with individualized dosing, causing some patients to have persistent hyperglycemia and/or episodes of hypoglycemia.
- Target glucose levels set by the ADA/AACE guidelines are based on clinical experience and judgment, as no large clinical trial has been conducted to determine the best target range in non-critically ill patients. These guidelines recommend a fasting blood glucose <140 mg/dL, and random BG <180 mg/dL.[1]
- Glucose levels <100 mg/dL should prompt reconsideration of insulin doses, and levels below 70 necessitate a dose change (unless the event is easily explained by another factor).[1]
- DKA and hyperosmolar hyperglycemic non-ketotic coma are considered "never events" by CMS and may result in loss of Medicare/Medicaid reimbursement for the hospitalization if the cause is due to inappropriate treatment of patients with diabetes while hospitalized. Discontinuation of insulin or providing inadequate doses of insulin can result in these events during hospitalization.

Patients Taking Oral Nutrition

- **For patients eating meals, a subcutaneous basal-bolus regimen consisting of basal, prandial, and correction doses of insulin is recommended.** AACE/ADA guidelines recommend the use of insulin analogs in the hospital setting. Basal insulin is provided by NPH, glargine or detemir in single or divided daily doses. Use of a rapid acting analogue (aspart, lispro, glulisine) is recommended for prandial and correction doses of insulin. Correction doses, previously known as "sliding scale", are added to the prandial insulin to correct glucose values above a specified target.
- The efficacy and safety of a basal-bolus regimen was tested against "sliding scale" regular insulin alone in a RCT trial of non-critically ill insulin-naïve patients with type 2 diabetes on medicine wards in the RABBIT 2 trial. Patients were placed on a basal-bolus regimen based on weight and level of hyperglycemia, and the dose was titrated based on a treatment algorithm. More patients on basal-bolus therapy reached target BG <140 than the sliding scale group, and there was no difference in hypoglycemia.[9]
- The starting doses for an inpatient basal-bolus regimen could be determined by either 1) a logical adjustment of home insulin therapy, based on the medication history and patient's condition, or 2) the "start from scratch" approach, often a weight-based method of dosing, taking additional patient-specific risk factors into consideration.
- Table 30-2 shows a basal-bolus insulin dosing algorithm. Determination of the TDD of insulin needed by the patient is the first step in planning an insulin regimen.
- Some hospitals offer a "diabetic," "carb-consistent," or "carb-restricted" diets. The dose of prandial insulin may need to be reduced if the diet contains <60 g of

TABLE 30-2 SUBCUTANEOUS INSULIN DOSING ALGORITHM

	Patients not previously on insulin:	**Patients previously insulin treated:**
Estimate TDD	• If Type 1 or pancreatectomy 0.3–0.45 U/kg/day • If Type 2 ≥ 0.5 U/kg/day (less if thin)	Obtain TDD in U/day
Calculate Doses	• Basal dose = TDD/2 • Bolus (prandial) doses = TDD/6 (assuming three isocaloric meals daily)	
Administer Basal Prandial	• Give the total basal dose once daily (glargine or detemir) or one-half of the basal dose every 12 hours (NPH, detemir) • If eating, give prandial plus correction (bolus) doses 15 minutes before meal, or when tray arrives • Meal should contain 60–90 g carbohydrate • If NPO, withhold prandial insulin dose	
Monitoring	• If eating, check BG before meals and at bedtime • If NPO, check BG every 6 hours	

Correction doses	BG (mg/dL)	Insulin sensitive	Usual	Insulin resistant	TDD recalculation
Before meal: Add indicated number of units	<70	Withhold bolus dose; call physician; administer PO or IV carbohydrate as per hypoglycemia orders			Reduce by 20%
At bedtime: Add HALF of indicated number of units	70–100	Delay bolus dose until after meal			Reduce by 10%
	101–139	No change	No change	No change	No change
	140–175	1	2	3	
	176–200	1	3	5	Add 75% of correction dose
	201–250	2	4	7	
	251–300	3	6	9	
	301–350	4	8	11	Add 100% of correction dose
	>350	Call MD			

carbohydrate per meal (check with dietary services about the carbohydrate content of regularly ordered diets).

• The choice of correction dose scale is determined by the patient's sensitivity to insulin. This can be inferred by their TDD of insulin. Those using >100 units/day would require the "insulin resistant" scale, while those using <50 units/day would apply the "insulin sensitive" scale on this algorithm.

- Mixed insulins (such as NPH 70/regular 30 and analog mixes) increase the risk of hypoglycemia in the hospital. Mixed insulin regimens should be converted to basal-bolus regimens during the IP stay.

NPO

- **In general, basal insulin doses should be continued during short periods of NPO status**, such as for tests. The prandial insulin should be held and sliding scale doses reconsidered, possibly only administered if the BG is >200 mg/dL.
- **During prolonged periods of NPO status, low-dose dextrose may be required in addition to basal insulin or an insulin drip** for insulin-deficient patients to avoid the development of ketones or iatrogenic diabetic ketoacidosis (DKA).
- The following scenario is a relatively common occurrence and can be prevented: hypoglycemia (BG <70 mg/dL) is discovered prior to the scheduled basal insulin dose in a patient with T1DM and the dose is held. Twelve to 16 hours later (longer if the patient is receiving correction doses), the patient is found to have DKA. Adjustment of the basal insulin dose is the recommended approach depending on the proximal cause of the hypoglycemia. The risk for DKA is much less in type 2 diabetes (T2DM), but inappropriate holding of a basal insulin dose will likely result in poor glycemic control for the following day.
- Blood glucose should be monitored every 4 to 6 hours while NPO on insulin.

Enteral Tube Feeding

- When possible, tube feedings in hyperglycemic IP should be continuous for 24 hours. This may help simplify the dosing schedule of insulin and prevent errors and hypoglycemia.
- Products containing a lower concentration of simple carbohydrate may be appropriate choices for persons with hyperglycemia.
- A recent RCT in 50 hospitalized patients with hyperglycemia on tube feeds showed basal glargine with correction dose regular insulin was equivalent to regular sliding scale with NPH added only for persistent hyperglycemia. However, 48% of the patients in the sliding-scale group needed added NPH. These patients had higher glucose at randomization and tended to have diabetes prior to admission.[10]
- Basal insulin can be provided as glargine or detemir given once or twice daily, or human NPH in divided doses every 6, 8, or 12 hours. Dividing the basal insulin into 2 to 4 doses offers opportunities for dose adjustment if there are problems with the tube feeds.
- Orders should include instructions for starting dextrose containing IV fluids if insulin has been administered and the tube feed is interrupted.
- Bolus tube feeds are handled similar to the patient taking PO with regularly scheduled doses of short-acting insulin based on the carbohydrate content of the feeding.

Total Parenteral Nutrition (TPN)

- Intravenous nutrition containing a mix of macro- and micronutrients has a profound effect on glucose and insulin requirements. Failure to control blood glucose in patients receiving TPN has been associated with poor patient outcomes.
- To determine a starting dose of insulin, the total daily carbohydrate intake should be calculated, and the initial insulin dose is based on this value. A common starting ratio is 1 unit: 10 g carbohydrate.

- Insulin can be mixed in the TPN infusate. This ensures that when the TPN stops, the insulin also stops, reducing the risk of hypoglycemia. Small doses of basal insulin should be given subcutaneously in patients with T1DM to reduce the risk of DKA during periods between TPN infusions.

Special Circumstances

Corticosteroids

- The use of oral, IV, and IM corticosteroids can cause or exacerbate hyperglycemia. The effect is most pronounced in the postprandial state.
- Hyperglycemia secondary to once-daily prednisone can be managed with a dose of NPH at the time of the steroid administration, or with higher meal doses of rapid acting insulin. Multiple daily doses of dexamethasone or methylprednisolone can be offset by giving NPH at the time of each dose.
- If the patient has persistent hyperglycemia despite attempts at insulin dose adjustment, consider IV insulin with titration protocol to achieve glucose targets and to determine daily insulin requirements.[11]
- The insulin dose should be proactively, preemptively increased when high-dose corticosteroids are planned. While the exact dose adjustment is not known, it is often necessary to increase doses dramatically.

Insulin Pump Therapy

- For patients who are using an insulin pump prior to admission, inpatient diabetes management can sometimes be achieved with pump continuation and diabetes self-management. This requires that the hospital have strict policies and procedures in place, as there are issues of medical/legal liability for self-administered medications in the hospital. A patient must show the physical and mental capacity for self-management with the pump, and staff must document the timing and amount of insulin administered in the medical record.[1]
- Obtaining an **endocrinology consultation or assessment by a certified diabetes educator (CDE)** to evaluate the appropriateness of the insulin pump regimen, and to make setting adjustments when hyper- and hypoglycemia, are encountered is recommended.
- Hospitals without policies and procedures in place or experienced staff to ensure safe insulin pump use should disallow pump use and convert patients to an appropriate basal/bolus subcutaneous regimen.
- The use of an insulin pump can increase the risk of DKA due to tube or catheter occlusion or insufficient insulin in the reservoir.

U-500 Insulin

- U-500 insulin is **concentrated 5 times compared to the standard U 100 insulin**. One mL of U-500 contains 500 units of regular insulin, compared to 100 units of U-100 insulin.
- The use of U-500 insulin requires special care and is **generally discouraged in the hospital setting**.
- Patients with severe insulin resistance, often needing more than 200 units/day of U-100 insulin, may use U-500 at home prior to admission. It is generally prescribed as TID before meals or QID with a bedtime dose.
- Studies have been done regarding its use in the hospital setting. If it is available in the hospital pharmacy, precautions must be made to prevent dosing or medication substitution errors.

- When possible, the U-500 home dose should be converted to a basal/bolus regimen using U-100 insulin in the hospital.
- If U-500 insulin is needed for control of hyperglycemia, the doses should be written in volume (e.g., 0.1 cc instead of 10 units) to prevent errors. Having the dose predrawn in pharmacy might be necessary to avoid having the concentrated insulin on the floor.
- A predetermined lower dose should be given for any missed meal to ensure basal coverage, and to decrease hypoglycemic events while NPO.

MANAGEMENT OF HYPERGLYCEMIA IN THE CRITICALLY ILL

- Hyperglycemia is a common finding in patients in the ICU, occurring in both diabetic and non-diabetic patients. Numerous observational studies have shown that hyperglycemia is an independent risk factor for morbidity and mortality in patients in ICUs, including postoperative cardiac and general surgery patients, patients with acute myocardial infarction and stroke, and general medicine patients.
- Historically, a few single-center randomized trials had shown that treating hyperglycemia in critically ill patients could reduce morbidity and mortality. More recent multicenter trials have demonstrated that hypoglycemia and intensive glycemic control were associated with adverse outcomes, including increased hospital mortality.

Clinical Trials

- **Van den Berghe et al. 2001.** This randomized trial in a single surgical ICU showed that mortality was reduced in hyperglycemic patients assigned to intensive insulin treatment (goal glucose 80 to 110 mg/dL) compared with standard care (IV insulin to goal glucose 180 to 200 mg/dL).[12]
- **Van den Berghe et al. 2006.** This trial applied the intensive intervention of the earlier study to patients in a medical ICU, and showed significantly reduced morbidity, but not in-hospital mortality, in patients assigned to the intensive treatment arm. Those staying in the ICU <3 days had increased mortality, while those staying ≥3 days had decreased mortality, but this was statistically insignificant. There were more hypoglycemic events in the intensive therapy group, but no associated hemodynamic instability or seizures.[13]
- **NICE-SUGAR 2009.** Compared to the single-center Van den Berghe studies, this multinational study compared critically ill medical and surgical patients expected to remain in the ICU >3 days randomized to intensive glucose control (81 to 108 mg/dL) versus conventional glucose control (180 mg/dL or less). NICE-SUGAR demonstrated that intensive treatment increased the incidence of hypoglycemia (6.8 vs. 0.5%) and 90-day mortality (27.5 vs. 24.9%). Trauma patients and those on corticosteroids did show mortality benefit with intensive control, but did not reach statistical significance.[14]
- There were numerous methodologic differences in the studies mentioned above, including methods of measuring blood glucose and the nutritional support of the different patient populations.[1]

Therapy

Target Glucose
ADA/AACE guidelines have set a range of 140 to 180 mg/dL for critically ill patients, with recommendations to start IV insulin therapy when the BG goes above 180 mg/

dL. Greater benefit may be realized at the lower end of this range, and some patients may benefit from a lower target range. However, a target range below 110 mg/dL is not recommended (Table 30-1).[1]

Medications
- In critically ill patients admitted to the ICU, oral hypoglycemic agents and subcutaneous insulin should be stopped. Insulin in critically ill patients should be given intravenously.
- Most ICUs now have standardized glucose algorithms, generally managed by ICU nurses, which have been shown to be valid ways to manage glucose. The most effective glucose algorithms are dynamic and incorporate the rate of glucose change into the insulin dose adjustments (Table 30-3).[15]

Insulin Adjustments
- Changes in the insulin-infusion rate are predicated on the current blood glucose, rate of change from past measurements, changes in the clinical condition, and changes in carbohydrate intake.
- For example, a change in the 5% dextrose infusion rate from 150 mL/hour (180 g carbohydrates normalized during a 24-hour period) to 75 mL/hour (90 g carbohydrates normalized during a 24-hour period) will require a decrease in the insulin infusion rate in order to prevent hypoglycemia. In critically ill patients, multiple sources of carbohydrate need to be taken into consideration when calculating the insulin dose, such as parenteral nutrition, enteral tube feeds, and dextrose-containing IV fluids.
- Nutrition, whether enteral or parenteral, should be given as a continuous infusion rather than intermittent boluses to prevent significant fluctuations in blood glucose. It is often critical to reassess caloric intake every 12 to 24 hours.
- The **patients most at risk for hypoglycemia are those with kidney or liver failure**. Close attention to details and a less aggressive upward titration in patients with liver and renal failure allow insulin drips to be used safely.
- ICU patients in general are not able to perceive, much less respond, to low glucose levels. Thus, avoidance of hypoglycemia is entirely the responsibility of the physicians and staff managing the insulin and nutrition orders.

Transition from IV to Subcutaneous Insulin
- At the time of transfer from the ICU, intravenous insulin doses need to be converted to a subcutaneous insulin regimen. Using an insulin sliding scale alone results in rebound hyperglycemia, and could risk the development of severe hyperglycemia.[16]
- Subcutaneous insulin should overlap with IV insulin to prevent hyperglycemia after discontinuation of an insulin drip. The first dose of long-acting insulin should be given 2 to 3 hours prior to the end of the IV drip.[17]
- For patients with diabetes, the subcutaneous insulin regimen doses can be estimated from a TDD that is 75% to 80% of the total insulin received via IV in the prior 24 hours.[1]
- When non-diabetic patients with stress hyperglycemia are transitioned to subcutaneous insulin, using 60% to 70% of the daily IV dose is an appropriate starting place. The daily insulin requirement may fall as patients recover from stress due to illness or surgery. For example, in patients who are recovering from cardiothoracic surgery, the subcutaneous insulin dose may need to be tapered rapidly, with daily changes in the subcutaneous TDD until a stable regimen is established.

TABLE 30-3   IV INSULIN INFUSION PRINCIPLES

Initiating insulin infusion

Standard insulin infusion is 100 units of **regular human insulin** in 100 mL
0.9% normal saline.

Preferred administration is via an infusion pump.

Give initial bolus if blood glucose (BG) >150 mg/dL;

Divide initial BG by 100 and round to nearest 0.5 U (e.g., BG 255: 255/100 =
2.55, rounded to 2.5, so IV bolus 2.5 U.).

After bolus, start infusion at same hourly rate as bolus (2.5 U/hour IV in
above example).

If **BG <150 mg/dL,** divide by 100 for initial hourly rate with **NO bolus** (e.g., BG
145 would be 145/100 = 1.45, rounded to 1.5, so start at 1.5 U/hour IV).

Changes to the insulin infusion rate are made hourly, based on: blood
glucose, rate of change of glucose, change in nutrition, administration of
corticosteroids.

Blood glucose monitoring

Check BG q1h until stable (three consecutive values in target range).

Once stable, can change BG monitoring to q2h.

If stable q2h for 12–24 hours, can change to q3–4h if no significant change
in nutrition or clinical status.

Resume q1h BG monitoring for BG >70 md/dL with any of the following:

Change in insulin-infusion rate.

Initiation or cessation of corticosteroid or vasopressor therapy.

Significant change in clinical status.

Change in nutritional support (initiation, cessation, or rate change).

Initiation or cessation of hemodialysis or CVVHD.

Hypoglycemia (BG ≤70 mg/dL)

If **BG <50 mg/dL,** stop infusion and give 25 g dextrose 50% (1 amp D50) IV.
Recheck BG q10–15min.

When BG > 100 mg/dL, recheck in 1 hour. If still >100 mg/dL after 1 hour,
resume insulin infusion at **50% most recent rate.**

If **BG 50–69 mg/dL,** stop infusion.

If symptomatic or unable to assess, give 25 g dextrose 50% (1 amp D50) IV.
Recheck BG q15min.[a]

If asymptomatic, consider 12.5 g dextrose 50% (1/2 amp D50) or 8 oz. fruit
juice PO.

Recheck q15–30min.[a]

[a]When, BG >100 mg/dL, recheck in 1 hour. If still >100 mg/dL after 1 hour,
resume insulin infusion at **75% most recent rate**.

—

BG, blood glucose; CVVHD, continuous venovenous hemodialysis; IV, intravenous; PO, by
mouth.

Adapted from Goldberg PA, Siegel MD, Sherwin RS, et al. Implementation of a safe and effective
insulin-infusion protocol in a medical intensive care unit. *Diabetes Care.* 2004;27:461–467.

DISCHARGE

- Patients with prior or newly diagnosed diabetes (or missed diagnosis) who have hyperglycemia during admission have higher rates of re-hospitalization than euglycemic patients.[18]
- Discharge planning should include instruction in basic diabetes management skills, such as glucose monitoring and insulin injections, as appropriate.
- Follow-up with a healthcare provider skilled in diabetes management will help with adherence and prevent readmissions for diabetes-related problems.

Select Discharge Regimen

- The AACE bases its 2010 discharge recommendations for those with prior diabetes on the level of glucose control or severity of disease prior to admission. Those at goal (A1C < 7) should return to previous therapy, while those not at goal should intensify therapy, including continuing basal-bolus therapy at hospital doses for an A1C > 9%. Adjustments to this regimen should be made based on glycemic control in the hospital and risk of hypoglycemia.
- Though not recommended for inpatient use, mixed insulin can be beneficial for convenience, improving adherence, and reducing errors (compared to the complex basal-bolus regimen) for patients who require insulin at discharge. Lingvay et al. showed that 0.2 U/kg/day of a rapid-acting analog 70/30 mix, divided into BID equal doses administered via pen, in addition to metformin, was effective and safe in treatment-naïve persons with newly diagnosed diabetes. The average HbA1C declined from 10.8% to 5.9% in 3 months, and the hypoglycemia rate over 3 years was 0.51 mild events/person-month.[19]
- Treatment of diabetes diagnosed during the hospitalization (with elevated A1C proving preadmission hyperglycemia) should follow outpatient guidelines (see Chapter 27).
- For those requiring insulin for corticosteroid-induced hyperglycemia, a plan to taper the insulin dose during steroid taper should be included in the discharge plan.

Education and Supplies

- All patients with newly diagnosed diabetes, those with uncontrolled diabetes prior to admission, and those who will require hypoglycemic therapy after discharge would benefit from diabetes education from a CDE during the hospital stay. Early consultation of these services will allow for repeat visits and assessment of retention. Education should include:
  - Assessment of level of understanding related to the diagnosis of diabetes
  - Self-monitoring of BG and explanation of home BG goals
  - Definition, recognition, treatment, and prevention of hyper- and hypoglycemia.
  - Information on consistent eating patterns
  - Insulin administration (if appropriate)
  - Sick day management
- It is also important to ensure that the patient will have all the needed equipment and supplies at home, and be able to afford and obtain them. Supplies may include glucose meter, test strips, lancets, needles, syringes, urine ketone strips, and a Glucagon kit.[1]

Follow-up Care

- Short-term follow up with a healthcare provided skilled in diabetes management should be scheduled for patients with new or changed diabetes treatment regimens.

- The discharge summary should include the extent of inpatient hyperglycemia, the A1C on admission, and any medication changes made, and should be communicated in a timely manner to the out-patient provider.
- Patients may also need a phone contact for problems with hyperglycemia or hypoglycemia that develop after discharge.

REFERENCES

1. Moghissi ES, Korytkowski MT, DiNardo M, et al. American Association of Clinical Endocrinologists and American Diabetes Association consensus statement on inpatient glycemic control. *Diabetes Care* 2009;32(6):1119–1131.
2. Cook CB, Kongable GL, Potter DJ, et al. Inpatient glucose control: A glycemic survey of 126 U.S. hospitals. *J Hosp Med* 2009;4(9):E7–E14.
3. Bruno A, Gregori D, Caropreso A, et al. Normal glucose values are associated with a lower risk of mortality in hospitalized patients. *Diabetes Care* 2008;31(11):2209–2210.
4. Umpierrez GE, Isaacs SD, Bazargan N, et al. Hyperglycemia: An independent marker of in-hospital mortality in patients with undiagnosed diabetes. *J Clin Endocrinol Metab* 2002; 87(3):978–82.
5. Cheung NW, Napier B, Zaccaria C, et al. Hyperglycemia is associated with adverse outcomes in patients receiving total parenteral nutrition. *Diabetes Care* 2005;28(10):2367–2371.
6. Curkendall SM, Natoli JL, Alexander CM, et al. Economic and clinical impact of inpatient diabetic hypoglycemia. *Endocr Pract* 2009;15(4):302–312.
7. Pidcoke HF, Wade CE, Mann EA, et al. Anemia causes hypoglycemia in intensive care unit patients due to error in single-channel glucometers: Methods of reducing patient risk. *Crit Care Med;*38(2):471–476.
8. Scott MG, Bruns DE, Boyd JC, et al. Tight glucose control in the intensive care unit: Are glucose meters up to the task? *Clin Chem* 2009;55(1):18–20.
9. Umpierrez GE, Smiley D, Zisman A, et al. Randomized study of basal-bolus insulin therapy in the inpatient management of patients with type 2 diabetes (RABBIT 2 trial). *Diabetes Care* 2007;30(9):2181–2186.
10. Korytkowski MT, Salata RJ, Koerbel GL, et al. Insulin therapy and glycemic control in hospitalized patients with diabetes during enteral nutrition therapy: A randomized controlled clinical trial. *Diabetes Care* 2009;32(4):594–596.
11. Smiley D, Rhee M, Peng L, et al. Safety and efficacy of continuous insulin infusion in noncritical care settings. *J Hosp Med* 2010;5(4):212–217.
12. van den Berghe G, Wouters P, Weekers F, et al. Intensive insulin therapy in the critically ill patients. *N Engl J Med* 2001;345(19):1359–1367.
13. Van den Berghe G, Wilmer A, Hermans G, et al. Intensive insulin therapy in the medical ICU. *N Engl J Med* 2006;354(5):449–461.
14. Finfer S, Chittock DR, Su SY, et al. Intensive versus conventional glucose control in critically ill patients. *N Engl J Med* 2009;360(13):1283–1297.
15. Goldberg PA, Siegel MD, Sherwin RS, et al. Implementation of a safe and effective insulin infusion protocol in a medical intensive care unit. *Diabetes Care* 2004;27(2):461–467.
16. Olansky L, Sam S, Lober C, et al. Cleveland Clinic cardiovascular intensive care unit insulin conversion protocol. *J Diabetes Sci Technol* 2009;3(3):478–486.
17. Clement S, Braithwaite SS, Magee MF, et al. Management of diabetes and hyperglycemia in hospitals. *Diabetes Care* 2004;27(2):553–591.
18. Robbins JM, Webb DA. Diagnosing diabetes and preventing rehospitalizations: The urban diabetes study. *Med Care* 2006;44(3):292–296.
19. Lingvay I, Legendre JL, Kaloyanova PF, et al. Insulin-based versus triple oral therapy for newly diagnosed type 2 diabetes: Which is better? *Diabetes Care* 2009;32(10):1789–1795.

Hypoglycemia

31

Nadia Khoury and Philip E. Cryer

GENERAL PRINCIPLES

- Glucose is the principle metabolic fuel for the brain under physiologic conditions. This makes it essential for the body to protect itself against hypoglycemia and for plasma glucose to be maintained in a narrow range.
- This regulation occurs in the postprandial state due to increased insulin secretion from the beta cell and increased glucose use and energy storage by target tissues. In the postabsorptive (fasting) state, plasma glucose is maintained between approximately 70 and 100 mg/dL. It can fall further without causing symptoms in some individuals, especially young women.
- The body has multiple counter-regulatory mechanisms to prevent or correct hypoglycemia.[1] These include, in order of occurrence, decreased insulin secretion followed by increased secretion of counter-regulatory hormones (glucagon and epinephrine) that amplify release of glucose from liver stores (glycogenolysis), increase glucose production and release by the liver (gluconeogenesis), and further reduce glucose use by tissues. All of these mechanisms serve to raise plasma glucose levels. Later, other counter-regulatory hormones (cortisol and growth hormone) assist in defending against hypoglycemia.

Definition

- Hypoglycemia is **a plasma glucose concentration low enough to cause signs or symptoms**. Due to shifting thresholds of symptoms with recurrent hypoglycemia (hypoglycemic symptoms occur at lower BG) or poorly controlled diabetes (hypoglycemic symptoms occur at higher BG), it is not possible to identify a single plasma glucose value that defines hypoglycemia.
- Hypoglycemia is most convincingly documented by **Whipple's triad** of signs or symptoms consistent with hypoglycemia, a low measured plasma glucose concentration, and relief of symptoms or signs on raising the glucose levels.
  - Documentation of Whipple's triad is especially important in the non-diabetic patient because hypoglycemia is rare in this population.
  - Documentation of low blood glucose in the setting of symptoms in a diabetic patient using insulin or insulin secretagogue therapy is preferable but less critical because hypoglycemia is common.

Pathophysiology

- Hypoglycemia occurs, in general, when disappearance of glucose from the circulation is greater than the appearance of glucose in the circulation.
- Sources of circulating glucose include exogenous glucose from ingested carbohydrates and endogenous processes such as hepatic gluconeogenesis and glycogenolysis and renal gluconeogenesis.

DIAGNOSIS

- Traditional classification schemes have placed hypoglycemia occurring in non-diabetic individuals into categories of fasting or postprandial (after meals).
- Alternatively, classification of hypoglycemia may be based on patient characteristics: That occurring in those who are ill or on medication or those who are seemingly well.[2]
- Reactive hypoglycemia is a term no longer in use that described a functional disorder with postprandial hypoglycemia symptoms without demonstration of Whipple's triad.

Clinical Presentation

- Symptoms of hypoglycemia can be classified as **neurogenic symptoms** that result from activation of the sympathetic nervous system, and **neuroglycopenic symptoms** that result from inadequate delivery of glucose to the brain (Table 31-1).[3]
- Neurogenic and neuroglycopenic **symptoms normally begin to occur at a glucose level of approximately 50 to 55 mg/dL**. Lower glucose levels may be associated with cognitive and behavioral changes and may produce coma, convulsions, and even death.

History

A detailed history is essential and should include the following: The circumstances of the episode and its temporal relationship to meals or exercise, associated symptoms, weight changes, recurrence of the episode, drug/alcohol history, medication history, history of gastric surgery, personal or family history of diabetes or of multiple endocrine neoplasia 1 (MEN1) or MEN-associated conditions, comorbid conditions, and symptoms of other hormone deficiencies.

Physical Examination

- Acutely, hypoglycemia can present with changes in mental status and even focal neurologic findings that are usually transient.
- Chronic or recurrent hypoglycemia may have no obvious physical signs, but may result in weight gain or subtle neurologic deficits.
- There are no specific physical findings associated with insulinoma. A complete physical examination may reveal other causes of hypoglycemia, including signs of chronic alcohol use, other hormone deficiencies, or MEN1.

Diagnostic Criteria

Confirmation of low blood glucose by a reliable laboratory method rather than with self monitoring of blood glucose (SMBG) is essential in the work-up of hypoglycemia in the non-diabetic. If the patient's apparent hypoglycemia was asymptomatic, it is

TABLE 31-1	SYMPTOMS OF HYPOGLYCEMIA
Neurogenic (autonomic)	**Neuroglycopenic (brain glucose deprivation)**
Palpitations	Confusion
Tremor	Fatigue
Anxiety	Seizure
Sweating	Loss of consciousness
Hunger	Focal neurologic deficit
Paresthesia	

TABLE 31-2	CAUSES OF HYPOGLYCEMIA IN ADULTS

Ill or medicated individual

Drugs
- Insulin or insulin secretagogue
- Alcohol
- Others

Critical illnesses
- Hepatic, renal, or cardiac failure
- Sepsis
- Inanition

Hormone deficiency
- Cortisol
- Glucagon and epinephrine (in insulin deficient diabetes mellitus)

Nonislet cell tumor

Seemingly well individual

Endogenous hyperinsulinism
- Insulinoma
- Functional β-cell disorders (nesidioblastosis)

Noninsulinoma pancreatogenous hypoglycemia

Postgastric bypass hypoglycemia
- Insulin autoimmune hypoglycemia

Antibody to insulin

Antibody to insulin receptor
- Insulin secretagogue
- Other

—

Accidental, surreptitious, or malicious hypoglycemia

Adapted from Cryer PE et al. Evaluation and management of adult hypoglycemic disorders. *J Clin Endocrinol Metab* 2009;94:709–728.[2]

important to consider artifacts caused by improper collection, storage, or error in analytic methods. Measured plasma glucose can drop 10 to 20 mg/dL/hour after the blood sample is drawn, so it is important for samples to be processed quickly. In addition, large numbers of blood cells, as in patients with leukemia, can consume plasma glucose, thereby artifactually lowering the measured value, even in the presence of glycolytic inhibitors.[4]

Differential Diagnosis

- In the ill or medicated person without diabetes, there are **four main causes of hypoglycemia** (see Table 31-2):
  - **Drugs** are the most common cause of hypoglycemia.[5] Insulin, sulfonylureas, and alcohol account for the majority of cases. Although hypoglycemic agents used in the treatment of diabetes are the drugs most often implicated in iatrogenic hypoglycemia, it is important to remember that many other medications—some of which are commonly used—can also lower blood sugar. Included in this list are

salicylates, quinine, quinolone antibiotics (especially gatifloxacin), haloperidol, disopyramide, angiotensin-converting enzyme (ACE) inhibitors, β-blockers, pentamidine, trimethoprim-sulfamethoxazole, and propoxyphene. Ingestion of alcohol during prolonged fasting (i.e., an alcohol binge) may lead to hypoglycemia by inhibition of gluconeogenesis.

○ In **critical illness**, such as end-stage liver disease, renal failure, starvation, and sepsis, glucose utilization may exceed production, thereby causing hypoglycemia.

○ **Counter-regulatory hormone deficiencies** (adrenal insufficiency, growth hormone deficiency) rarely cause hypoglycemia.

○ **Non-islet cell tumors** can cause hypoglycemia, albeit rarely. Malignancies such as lymphoma, hepatoma, some sarcomas, and teratomas can cause hypoglycemia by secretion of insulin-like growth factor 2 (IGF-2), which can increase glucose use and suppress production.[6]

• In the seemingly well individual, hypoglycemia generally results from one of two causes:

○ Hypoglycemia can be accidental, malicious, or surreptitious.

○ Factitious hypoglycemia should be considered in any patient with a history of psychiatric illness, or access to insulin or oral hypoglycemia agents (e.g., health care workers, friends and relatives of people with diabetes).[7]

• Endogenous hyperinsulinism may be due to the following:

○ **Insulinoma** is a rare but life-threatening condition characterized by excessive insulin secretion by a pancreatic beta-cell tumor, leading to primarily fasting but occasionally postprandial hypoglycemia. The incidence of insulinoma is one to two cases per million patient-years. The median age at presentation is 47 with a slight female predominance. Malignant insulinoma, which occurs in 10% of all such tumors, is more common in older patients.[8] In younger patients, insulinoma is more frequently associated with MEN1. Insulinomas associated with MEN may be multifocal or malignant and may secrete other hormones such as gastrin or adrenocorticotropic hormone (ACTH).

○ **Noninsulinoma pancreatogenous hypoglycemia syndrome** (NIPHS) leads to neuroglycopenic spells typically after a meal. It occurs predominately in men and is due to diffuse islet hypertrophy and sometimes, hyperplasia.[9]

○ Some patients after Roux-en-Y gastric bypass surgery develop **postprandial endogenous hyperinsulinemic hypoglycemia** through a yet unknown mechanism.[10]

• Rarely, the presence of autoantibodies against insulin can cause a picture of predominantly reactive hypoglycemia, or antibodies against the insulin receptor can present as fasting hypoglycemia.

Diagnostic Testing

Evaluation of hypoglycemia involves demonstration of Whipple's triad with simultaneous laboratory evaluation. When Whipple's triad has not been documented or laboratory evaluation has not been done during symptomatic hypoglycemia, it is necessary to recreate the circumstances in which symptoms occur either through a **monitored 72-hour fast for a history of fasting hypoglycemia** or a **mixed meal challenge for a history of postprandial hypoglycemia.**

Laboratory Evaluation

• Laboratory evaluation should start with confirmation that hypoglycemia has occurred and there is a risk of recurrence. The focus should then be placed on **documentation of insulin and C-peptide levels during an episode of symptomatic hypoglycemia (plasma glucose <54 mg/dL).**

- If the C-peptide is low in the presence of high measured insulin, exogenous insulin is the probable etiology. With high insulin and high C-peptide, screening for sulfonylurea, and non-sulfonylurea (repaglinide and nateglinide) secretagogues should be performed to rule out surreptitious or inadvertent drug use. Insulin antibodies should also be considered and ordered early in the course of the work-up when there is a suspicion of exogenous insulin administration.
- During a 72-hour fast, the fast is ended once symptomatic hypoglycemia is documented and appropriate samples are collected. Diagnostic values include the following:
  ○ glucose <54 mg/dL,
  ○ insulin ≥3 µU/mL,
  ○ C-peptide ≥0.2 nmol/L,
  ○ proinsulin ≥5.0 pmol/L,
  ○ β-hydroxybutyrate ≤2.7 mmol/L, and
  ○ negative screen for insulin secretagogues.
    ■ If Whipple's triad has been previously documented, the diagnostic fast can be concluded with these measurements at an asymptomatic plasma glucose of <54 mg/dL.
    ■ If Whipple's triad has not been previously documented, the fast should be continued until symptoms occur even if this means a lower blood sugar. Once symptomatic, the patient can be treated with 1 mg intravenous glucagon. An increase in glucose of >25 mg/dL over 30 minutes is consistent with the diagnosis of endogenous hyperinsulinemia.[2]
- For postprandial hypoglycemia, a mixed meal challenge including foods recognized by the patient to cause hypoglycemia should be performed over 5 hours. An oral glucose tolerance test should never be used to diagnosis postprandial hypoglycemia. The same laboratories that are obtained in a fasting challenge are obtained in the mixed meal challenge.

Imaging and Diagnostic Procedures
- Once a diagnosis of endogenous hyperinsulinemia is made clinically and biochemically, insulinoma localization is usually performed first by **dual-phase thin-section multidetector computed tomography (CT)**. Alternative imaging procedures include **MRI** or **transabdominal ultrasonography**. These methods detect 75% of insulinomas.[1]
- **Endoscopic ultrasound** with the possibility of fine needle aspiration allows preoperative localization of the vast majority of insulinomas.[11]

TREATMENT

- Immediate treatment of hypoglycemia is necessary to prevent further decline in blood glucose, neuroglycopenia, and its associated adverse outcomes.
- To prevent recurrent hypoglycemia, identification and correction of the underlying mechanism are necessary. For insulinoma, surgical resection is preferred.

Medications
- **Immediate treatment of severe hypoglycemia** includes **oral or intravenous dextrose** [initial bolus of 1 ampule D50 (25 g) followed by infusion of glucose to maintain blood glucose >100 mg/dL] or 1 mg intramuscular or subcutaneous **glucagon**.

- Conscious patients may be given readily absorbable carbohydrates orally in the form of fruit juices or glucose tablets.
- Medical therapy with diazoxide (notable side effects include edema and hirsutism), verapamil, or octreotide is reserved for patients with endogenous hyperinsulinism who are not surgical candidates, who have recurrent disease and refuse reoperation, or who have inoperable disease.
- Alpha-glucosidase inhibitors, diazoxide, and octreotide may be helpful in NIPHS or postgastric bypass hypoglycemia.
- Oral formulations of inhibitors of mammalian target of rapamycin (mTOR), such as everolimus, have recently been used with some success for refractory hypoglycemia in malignant insulinoma.[12] Studies have shown improvement in glucose levels with and without tumor regression.

Other Nonpharmacologic Therapies

- If surgical or medical treatments fail, **frequent daytime feedings** and **provision of large amounts of uncooked cornstarch at bedtime** or even overnight gastric glucose infusion may be necessary.
- Patients should be educated about the symptoms of hypoglycemia and the appropriate corrective measures (including when to seek medical attention), and diabetic patients should be provided with a medical alert bracelet and a glucagon emergency kit.

Surgery

- The **treatment of choice for insulinoma is surgical resection**, usually via a laparoscpic procedure. For solitary adenomas, surgery is curative.
- Multiple insulinomas associated with MEN1 are treated with an 80% subtotal pancreatectomy, although the recurrence rate is still 21% at 20 years.
- Partial pancreatectomy in NIPHS and postbariatric surgery hyperinsulinemic hypoglycemia is sometimes curative.

SPECIAL CONSIDERATIONS

- Drug treatment of diabetes is, by far, the most common cause of hypoglycemia. Iatrogenic hypoglycemia from insulin and insulin secretagogues limits the glycemic management of diabetes.
- Recurrent morbidity and sometimes mortality can result from insulin or insulin secretagogue-induced hypoglycemia, and the risk or occurrence of hypoglycemia can abrogate the full realization of the vascular benefits of glycemic control.
- Persons with type 1 diabetes experience innumerable episodes of hypoglycemia each year and most experience at least one severe episode each year.
- Hypoglycemia is less common in type 2 diabetes but carries a bigger burden of morbidity and mortality due to the 20-fold greater prevalence of the disease.[1]
- The American Diabetes Association (ADA) recommends that people with diabetes become concerned about developing hypoglycemia at blood glucose <70 mg/dL (3.9 mmol/L). At this level, patients should consider actions including repeat measurement, carbohydrate ingestion, and avoiding exercise or driving until the glucose level is raised.
- In both type 1 and long-term type 2 diabetes, glucose counter-regulatory mechanisms may be reduced or lost. When hypoglycemia is caused by exogenous insulin or insulin secretagogue, reduction in ambient insulin level is not possible. Both

glucagon secretion and epinephrine responses may be attenuated. This cluster of abnormal responses leads to the clinical syndromes of **defective glucose counter-regulation** and **hypoglycemia unawareness** which are associated with 25-fold or greater and six-fold or greater risks of severe hypoglycemia respectively.

• In addition, repeated hypoglycemia shifts glycemic thresholds for epinephrine secretion and awareness of hypoglycemia. This phenomenon is known as **hypoglycemia-associated autonomic failure** (HAAF) and is a common complication of tight glycemic control in people with diabetes.[13] In most cases, avoidance of hypoglycemia for 2 to 3 weeks can restore awareness.[14]

REFERENCES

1. Cryer PE. Hypoglycemia. In: Melmed S, Polonsky KS, Larsen PR, et al., eds. *Williams Textbook of Endocrinology,* 12th ed. Philadelphia, PA: WB Saunders; 2011:1552–1577.
2. Cryer PE, Axelrod L, Grossman AB, et al. Evaluation and management of adult hypoglycemic disorders: An endocrine society clinical practice guideline. *J Clin Endocrinol Metab* 2009;94:709–728.
3. Cryer PE, Davis SN, Shamoon H. Hypoglycemia in diabetes. *Diabetes Care* 2003;26:1902–1912.
4. Field JB, Williams HE. Artifactual hypoglycemia associated with leukemia. *N Engl J Med* 1961;265:946–948.
5. Murad MH, Coto-Yglesias F, Wang AT, et al. Clinical review: Drug-induced hypoglycemia: A systematic review. *J Clin Endocrinol Metab* 2009;94:741–745.
6. Daughaday W. The pathophysiology of IGF-II hypersecretion in non-islet cell tumor hypoglycemia. *Diabetes Rev* 1995;3:62–72.
7. Marks V, Teale JD. Hypoglycemia: Factitious and felonious. *Endocrinol Metab Clin North Am* 1999;28:579–601.
8. Service FJ, McMahon MM, O'Brien PC, et al. Functioning insulinoma–incidence, recurrence, and long-term survival of patients: A 60-year study. *Mayo Clin Proc* 1991;66:711–719.
9. Won JG, Tseng HS, Yang AH, et al. Clinical features and morphological characterization of 10 patients with noninsulinoma pancreatogenous hypoglycaemia syndrome (NIPHS). *Clin Endocrinol (Oxf)* 2006;65:566–578.
10. Service GJ, Thompson GB, Service FJ, et al. Hyperinsulinemic hypoglycemia with nesidioblastosis after gastric-bypass surgery. *N Engl J Med* 2005;353:249–254.
11. Tucker ON, Crotty PL, Conlon KC. The management of insulinoma. *Br J Surg* 2006;93:264–275.
12. Kulke MH, Bergsland EK, Yao JC. Glycemic control in patients with insulinoma treated with everolimus. *N Engl J Med* 2009;360:195–197.
13. Dagogo-Jack SE, Craft S, Cryer PE. Hypoglycemia-associated autonomic failure in insulin-dependent diabetes mellitus. Recent antecedent hypoglycemia reduces autonomic responses to symptoms of, and defense against subsequent hypoglycemia. *J Clin Invest* 1993;91:819–828.
14. Dagogo-Jack S, Rattarasarn C, Cryer PE. Reversal of hypoglycemia unawareness but not defective glucose counterregulation in IDDM. *Diabetes* 1994;43:1426–1434.

Obesity

32

David A. Rometo, Dominic N. Reeds, and Richard I. Stein

GENERAL PRINCIPLES

Definition

- Obesity constitutes the condition of excessive adiposity.
- It is classified using body mass index (BMI).
  - **BMI = weight in kilograms/square of the height in meters, or kg/m^2**. Alternatively, lb/in^2 × 703.
  - For adults, obesity is defined as having a BMI ≥ 30.
  - For children, obesity is having a BMI ≥ 95th percentile for sex/age on a BMI growth chart (http://www.cdc.gov/growthcharts/clinical_charts.htm).
- Adults with significant muscle mass (athletes, bodybuilders) can have elevated BMIs without excess fat. If adiposity is minimal on physical examination, they are not obese.

Classification

- **Overweight** describes adults with BMI between 25 and 30, and children with BMI in the 85th to 95th percentile.
- **Obesity** can be classified by severity and by distribution
  - **Class 1:** BMI 30 to 34.9
  - **Class 2:** BMI 35 to 39.9
  - **Class 3:** BMI ≥40 (extreme)
  - **Central or visceral-abdominal obesity:** waist circumference >102 cm (40 in) in men, >88 cm (35 in) in women.
  - **Gluteal-femoral obesity:** adiposity distributed over the buttocks and upper legs without the above waist circumference
- The term **morbid obesity** has been used to describe patients with a BMI ≥ 35 with a comorbid condition, a BMI ≥ 40 (used interchangeably with extreme), and with weights >150 kg.

Epidemiology

- National Health and Nutrition Examination Survey (NHANES) has been tracking/estimating overweight/obesity in the US since 1960. The rates began to significantly increase between 1976 and 1994. The most recent evaluation of NHANES data showed further increases in obesity prevalence from 1999 to 2008 for men, but the trend began to plateau after 2003. There was no significant trend in obesity prevalence for women during this 10-year period.[1]
- African American (AA) and Hispanic women have the highest rates of overweight and obesity.
- Health risks associated with obesity may be lower for AAs than whites at the same BMI level.

- NHANES also tracks obesity in children and adolescents. Among all, 16.9% of children age 2 to 19 had a BMI ≥ 95th percentile in 2007 to 2008 (triple the prevalence from 1980). There has been a significant rise in the prevalence of BMI ≥ 97th percentile for boys age 6 to 19 since 1999.
  - Prevalence of BMI ≥ 95th percentile is highest among Hispanic boys and adolescent AA girls.[2]
  - The normative growth curves for children are based on historical data. Therefore, as the population increases in weight, more than 5% of children today can be ≥ 95th percentile for BMI.

Etiology/Pathophysiology

Obesity is the result of the interaction among the environment, polygenic genetic factors, and behavior of an individual. Fundamentally, these interactions result in the imbalance between energy intake and energy expenditure, or an imbalance between caloric intake/fat synthesis and fat oxidation. Excess caloric energy is stored as triacylglycerols in adipocytes.

Genetics
- Although polygenic inheritance may play a large role in susceptibility to obesity amongst close relatives, identifiable monogenic obesity, usually extreme obesity with early onset, is very rare.
- Mutations of leptin, leptin receptor, prohormone convertase 1 (PC1), pro-opiomelanocortin (POMC), and peroxisome proliferator-activated receptor (PPAR) gamma 2 result in syndromic conditions and are inherited in a recessive pattern. They are seen in consanguineous pedigrees.[3]
- Melanocortin 4-receptor (MC4-R) mutation is non-syndromic and autosomal dominant.[4]
- Prader–Willi results from the deletion of paternally derived chromosome 15q11–13, resulting in hyperphagia at a young age. Anecdotally, parents must padlock the refrigerator and pantry.[5]

Hypothalamic Obesity
Results from damage to the satiety/hunger signaling regions of the hypothalamus, leading to insatiable appetite and overeating. This is sometimes seen after craniopharyngioma resection.

Medications
- Antipsychotics: both typical and atypical
- Antidepressants: paroxitine, tricyclics
- Neuroleptics: gabapentin, valproic acid
- Beta-blockers
- Glucocorticoids
- Some hypoglycemic agents: insulin, sulfonylureas, thiazolidinediones (TZDs)

Associated Conditions
- Type 2 diabetes mellitus (T2DM)
  - Only 20% of obese people have T2DM, while 80% of those with T2DM are obese.
  - The risk for T2DM increases with weight at a BMI of 23 for women (RR1.3).[6]
  - Weight gain of >5 kg after age 18 increases risk of T2DM.[7]
- Coronary artery disease (CAD): correlation begins with increasing BMI within the normal range.[8]

- Congestive heart failure: increased risk 5% to 7% for every 1 kg/m^2 above 30[9]
- Cerebrovascular disease, hypertension, insulin resistance/hyperinsulinemia, dyslipidemia (high triglycerides, low high-density lipoprotein [HDL])
- Obstructive sleep apnea (OSA), obesity hypoventilation syndrome (OHS)
- Venous thromboembolism
- Gastroesophageal reflux disease (GERD), gallstones, non-alcoholic steatohepatitis (NASH)/non-alcoholic fatty liver disease (NAFLD)
- Polycystic ovary syndrome (PCOS)
- Osteoarthritis (OA), gout
- Increased risk of colorectal, esophageal, kidney, pancreatic, thyroid, endometrial, gallbladder, and postmenopausal breast cancers. A weaker correlation exists for leukemia, malignant melanoma, multiple myeloma, non-Hodgkin lymphoma, and premenopausal breast cancer.[10]

Mortality

- Obesity is associated with increased all-cause mortality in several large retrospective and prospective studies.
  - In the year 2000, there were 111,909 excess deaths associated with/attributed to obesity, according to conservative interpretation of NHANES data.[11]
  - Mortality rate increases 30% for every 5 kg/m^2 increase in BMI over 25.[12]
  - Men over 50 years old who have never smoked have a two- to three-fold increase in risk of death if BMI > 30.[13]
- Disease-specific mortality. Prospective studies show increase in mortality with every 5 kg/m^2 increase in BMI above 25.[12]
  - T2DM (HR 2.16)
  - CAD (HR 1.39)
  - Cancer (HR 1.1)
- Life expectancy is reduced by 7 years in those at age 40 with a BMI > 30 compared to normal weight, and reduced by 14 years if they also smoke.[14]

DIAGNOSIS

Clinical Presentation

Patients often do not present with a complaint about body weight, and thus a practitioner should be very sensitive when addressing the issue, tying the need for weight loss to medical issues and not communicating disapproval or blame. It is only rarely necessary to rule out secondary causes of obesity. Red flags that would prompt this include rapid weight gain without an attributable cause or symptoms of new onset fatigue or skin coloration changes. Otherwise, review of the medication list, history, and physical examination should be adequate to raise a clinical suspicion of Cushing's syndrome, thyroid illness, or hypothalamic obesity. Hyperthyroidism may also present with weight gain, although this is less common than weight loss. The evaluation of associated cardiovascular risk and comorbidities may prompt medical treatment and prevention, but it is also useful to determine the risks and benefits of the treatments for obesity itself.

History

- Family history should include obesity, diabetes, and early-onset CAD in parents and siblings.

- Weight history should start with childhood/adolescence and include previous weight loss attempts. A behavioral assessment for underlying eating disorders should also be obtained when a clinical suspicion arises.
- To evaluate for OSA, it is important to elicit a history of snoring and apneic episodes (ask sleeping partner), as well as excessive daytime sleepiness (can use the Eppworth Sleepiness Scale, ESS)
- Review systems for hypo-/hyperthyroidism, Cushing's, OA, gout, GERD, CAD/PAD, incontinence (weight loss and bariatric surgery may alleviate incontinence by decreasing intra-abdominal pressure).
- Discuss current lifestyle: diet, activity level, smoking, recent smoking cessation (can cause significant weight gain), alcohol, recreational drug use (indicator of poor outcomes with weight loss and bariatric surgery), life stressors.

Physical Examination
- In addition to a routine exam, the exam of the obese patient should identify comorbid conditions and secondary causes of weight gain.
- Measure height and weight after removing the shoes, coat, and any other accessories. Having the patient change into an appropriate-size gown will both provide an accurate and comparable weight for future visits and facilitate the remainder of the physical exam.
- Measure the waist circumference using a tape measure, with the patient standing after relaxed exhalation. Keep the tape parallel to the floor at the level of the right lower costal margin (see Figure 32-1). This measurement can function as a starting point to monitor the effects of intervention, though there can be significant variability when abdominal folds are present.
  - It is very important to have a gown, scale, and tape measure that accommodate the severely obese, and that clinic protocols minimize embarrassment to the patient.
- Use a size-appropriate cuff to measure the blood pressure.
- Look for a narrow/crowded oropharynx, neck circumference >17 inches, pulmonary rales, right-sided heart failure (jugular venous distension, hepatosplenomegaly, lower extremity edema), goiter, deep tendon reflexes (brisk or delayed relaxation), tremor, facial plethora, purple abdominal striae, bruising, thin skin, acanthosis nigricans, proximal weakness, supraclavicular/dorsoclavicular fat, hirsutism, acne, paniculitis, cellulitis, and candidiasis in deep skin folds.

Diagnostic Testing
Laboratories
- **Routine laboratory tests:** fasting blood glucose, fasting lipid panel, thyroid-stimulating hormone (TSH), complete metabolic panel including alanine aminotransferase (ALT), aspartate aminotransferase (AST), and alkaline phosphatase.
  - Though NAFLD is common in obesity (present in 85% of those with a BMI > 40), other causes of liver dysfunction should be ruled out (as clinically indicated) before ascribing transaminitis to obesity.[15]
- **Additional laboratory testing to diagnose *suspected* secondary causes of obesity and comorbidities:**
  - Cushing's syndrome: proximal muscle weakness, moon face, hyperpigmented stretch marks, mood change (see Chapter 14)
  - PCOS: Rotterdam criteria include two out of anovulation, physical, or biochemical evidence of hyperandrogenism, radiographic evidence of polycystic ovaries (see Chapter 20)

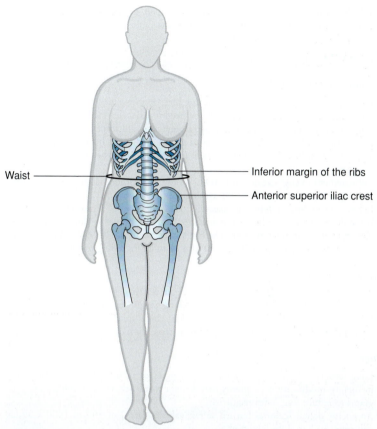

Waist — Inferior margin of the ribs

— Anterior superior iliac crest

FIGURE 32-1 Guide to measuring waist circumference

○ OHS: OSA, dyspnea on exertion, cyanosis. Check arterial blood gas on room air.[16]

○ Screening for genetic causes of obesity is not cost effective or recommended.

Imaging

Dual-energy X-ray absorptiometry (DXA), CT, and MRI do not have a clear role in clinical practice.

Diagnostic Procedures

If a patient has symptoms of sleep apnea (snoring, excessive daytime sleepiness, observed apneas), polysomnography should be obtained.[17] Among patients in whom there is a clinical suspicion of an underlying disorder contributing to obesity, appropriate lab testing should be performed.

Miscellaneous

Routine evaluation for CAD is not indicated in asymptomatic obese patients without diabetes. Evaluation of any suspected comorbidities (e.g., CAD, GERD) should be conducted according to current evidence- or expert opinion–based standards and guidelines. These are beyond the scope of this text.

TREATMENT

Benefits of Weight Loss
- Five percentage weight loss achieved using lifestyle intervention (diet and exercise) can reduce fasting glucose and reduce the need for diabetes medications.
- Those with prediabetes (impaired glucose tolerance and impaired fasting glucose) have a decreased incidence of progression to T2DM with as little as 4 kg of weight loss when combined with regular physical activity, as seen in the Diabetes Prevention Program.[18]
- Improvement in triglycerides and HDL. Weight loss without changing macronutrients rarely dramatically alters LDL cholesterol.[19]
- For every 1 kg loss, systolic and diastolic blood pressure fall 1 mm Hg.[20]
- It should be noted that the recommendations for weight loss in this chapter do not pertain to obese pregnant women. The Institute of Medicine (IOM) recommends that women with a prepregnancy BMI > 30 gain 11 to 20 lbs during pregnancy.[21]

Weight Loss Goals
- A reasonable, achievable, safe, and effective goal is 5% to 10% weight loss, at a rate of 1 to 2 lbs/week over 6 months, with lifelong weight maintenance.
- Weight loss >2% per week increases the risk of cholelithiasis and should be avoided after the first few weeks, when weight loss is typically more rapid.

Diet
- Long-term (i.e., >1 year) weight loss is challenging to achieve. Patients participating in dietary modification programs may benefit from behavioral modification programs to reduce long-term recidivism.
- An energy deficit (calories burned minus calories eaten) of 500 to 1000 kcal/day will result in 1 to 2 lbs loss/week.
- Very low-calorie diets (<800 kcal/day) can result in 20% weight loss in 4 months, but increase the risk of gallstones and do not have added benefit in long-term weight loss.[19]

Low-Fat or Low-Carbohydrate Diets
- A low-fat diet (<30% of calories from fat, >50% from carbohydrates) has been the recommended diet by the American Diabetes Association (ADA) since at least the mid-1990s. Very low-fat diets (<15% from fat), such as the Ornish diet, are quite high in carbohydrates and can exacerbate hypertriglyceridemia and hyperglycemia in patients with diabetes. The LEARN diet (lifestyle, education, attitudes, relationships, and nutrition) recommends <10% of calories from saturated fat, 55% to 60% from carbohydrates, and overall calorie restriction.[22]
- Low-carbohydrate diets are another option, with variable popularity. The USDA recommended daily allowance (RDA) for carbohydrate is 130 g. Low-carbohydrate diets have less than this amount, but can vary widely in carbohydrate, protein, and fat content. A ketogenic diet contains a level of carbohydrates so low that glycogen stores are depleted, glucose is produced from amino acids and triglycerides by gluconeogenesis, and hepatic fatty acid metabolism results in increased circulating

and urinary ketone bodies. This begins at below 50 g of carbohydrates/day. These diets, including the Atkins™ diet, often allow ad lib protein and fat ingestion to achieve satiety. Patients tend to automatically eat a calorie-restricted diet when given these parameters, due to increased satiety and/or fewer palatable food choices. The Zone® diet limits carbohydrates to 40% of a calorie-restricted diet, but is not ketogenic.[22]

- Several studies have contrasted the efficacy and metabolic effects of low-carbohydrate and low-fat diets to achieve weight loss. Initial 6-month weight loss is often greater in the low-carbohydrate diet, but several studies show that weight loss is equal to low-fat diets by 1 year.[23] Randomized control trials (RCTs) show HDL and triglycerides improve more on low-carbohydrate diets, but LDL improves more on low-fat diets.[24] An RCT comparing the Atkins™, Zone®, LEARN, and Ornish diets showed that Atkins™ resulted in more weight loss, higher HDL, lower triglycerides, better blood pressure, and same LDL at 1 year compared to the other diets.[22]

- These findings were confirmed with a 2-year-long multi-center RCT of 307 patients that compared a low-carbohydrate diet (starting at 20 g/day) and a low-fat diet. The low-carbohydrate diet resulted in improved weight loss at 3 months, lower diastolic blood pressure for most of the 24 months, lower triglycerides and VLDL up to 12 months, and higher HDL throughout the entire 2 years. The low-fat diet group had better LDL for the first 6 months. There were no serious cardiovascular events in either group.[25]

Low-Fat or Low-Carbohydrate Diets in Diabetes

- A low-carbohydrate diet would reduce average blood glucose levels in patients with T2DM by limiting postprandial glucose excursions from absorbed dietary carbohydrates, in addition to any improvement in insulin sensitivity from weight loss. The above studies either examined all patients, or excluded diabetics.

- In patients with insulin resistance/glucose intolerance, 48 hours of calorie restriction with a low-carbohydrate diet results in a greater decrease in intrahepatic triglyceride content, hepatic glucose output, fasting glucose level, and insulin resistance compared to a low-fat diet.[26]

- The ADA now recommends either a low-fat or low-carbohydrate (≤130 g/day) diet for weight loss in overweight/obese patients with T2DM.

- A meta-analysis indicated that low-carbohydrate diets showed improvement in A1c and triglycerides in diabetic patients compared to low-fat diets, but no statistically significant difference in weight or lipids.[27]

- A 4-year RCT of overweight, newly diagnosed T2DM patients assigned to a Mediterranean diet (increased unsaturated fats, <50% calories from carbohydrates) or low-fat diet showed significant reduction in the need to start oral hypoglycemics with the low-carbohydrate diet.[28]

- A low-carbohydrate Mediterranean diet (LCM: <35% calories from carbohydrates) was compared to the ADA-recommended low-fat diet in overweight T2DM patients for 1 year. LCM showed a statistically significant improvement in triglycerides, A1c, fasting glucose, HDL, and LDL compared to the low-fat diet. Improvements in weight were similar.[29]

- A ketogenic diet in obese diabetic patients for 24 weeks resulted in a lower A1c, weight, and triglycerides, a higher HDL, and reduction in diabetes medications compared to a low glycemic index diet (and a mean LDL increase of only 1.3 mg/dL) for those who completed the trial.[30]

- Authors' conclusion: for overweight or obese patients without diabetes, prediabetes, or dyslipidemia, any diet that creates an energy deficit to induce and maintain weight loss will be beneficial. For patients with these conditions, a low-carbohydrate approach may provide additional metabolic and cardiovascular risk factor benefit, and may reduce the use of diabetes medications, compared to a low-fat diet. Long-term studies of cardiovascular and microvascular outcomes have not been done to compare these two strategies.

Special Considerations for Low-Carbohydrate Diet

- Before recommending carbohydrate restriction to an individual patient, consider the potential consequences of increasing the other macronutrients, which a patient may do to replace the carbohydrates in meals. Patients with significant chronic kidney disease may benefit from protein limitation, those with CAD and elevated LDL need to restrict cholesterol and saturated fats, and those with primary hypertriglyceridemia need to strictly limit total fat intake. Specifying protein and fat quality and content, or avoiding a low-carbohydrate approach completely, may be appropriate in these individuals.
- Those with T2DM will need a medication adjustment that reflects this change in diet, specifically to prevent hypoglycemia. Sulfonylureas, prandial insulin, and basal insulin doses may need to be decreased or discontinued. These changes should be made proactively, and further adjustments made based on frequent monitoring of blood glucose levels.
- Use caution with low-carbohydrate diets among obese patients with type 1 diabetes who are prone to diabetic ketoacidosis (DKA) and/or severe hypoglycemia. A keto-genic diet is not recommended for type 1 diabetes, as it has not been adequately studied in this population and may increase the risk of DKA.

Physical Activity

- An increase in physical activity alone, without caloric restriction, does not result in significant or sustainable weight loss, but regular physical activity helps to maintain weight loss and prevent weight gain during and after successful dieting.[31]
- Before starting an obese patient with cardiovascular disease risk factors on a moderate to intense exercise program, a provider should consider evaluation with an exercise stress test based on current guidelines.[32]
- Recommended physical activity for weight loss is 30 to 45 minutes of aerobic activity at moderate intensity, 3 to 5 days per week, and gradual increase in frequency and duration from there. Those who were previously inactive should start with 10 minutes/day and gradually increase low-intensity activity. To maintain weight loss long-term, many studies show that 60 to 75 minutes of moderate-intensity activity daily is needed. This kind of exercise can be done in/around the home and be divided into several sessions/day to increase compliance.[19]
- Physical activity level and cardiorespiratory fitness are associated with decreased cardiovascular disease risk factors, independent of obesity. Patients should be encouraged to continue exercise even if weight loss goals are not met in order to achieve these potential benefits.[33]

Lifestyle Change Programs

- Just giving a list of goals to a patient regarding his/her caloric intake and exercise requirements does not result in significant weight loss or medical benefit. The use of behavior modification techniques to help the patient modify his/her diet and physical activity may improve adherence and sustained weight loss.

- Success is correlated with frequency of visits to a provider managing weight loss, which is unrealistic in a physician practice. The patient can be referred to a **dietitian, a comprehensive medical weight management program, or to a commercial weight loss program** to provide this frequency/intensity. Examples of behavioral topics addressed typically include social support for dietary/activity changes, overcoming high-risk situations (e.g., parties, restaurants, cold weather for exercise), maintaining motivation over time, and emotional eating.
- One should assess the patient's desire and willingness to make lifestyle changes, and set realistic goals to promote an energy deficit. A common first step is for the patient to keep a **food diary** (paper-and-pencil or computer/web-based), recording all foods and drinks for at least **3 days**, including a weekend day. It is helpful for the patient and practitioner to know the patient's current energy intake to make an evaluation and initiate a change, though patient self-reporting can be highly inaccurate and unreliable.
- To promote honest recording, it is essential for the practitioner to be nonjudgmental when reviewing a patient's food diary. It will be most helpful for a practitioner and patient to generate concrete changes for the patient's eating (e.g., cut fast food to one time per week, eliminate caloric soft drinks) and physical activity (e.g., walk for 30 minutes, 3 times per week), and problem-solve barriers, in order for patients to achieve success.

Medical Therapy

- Pharmacotherapy can be added to lifestyle modification if the patient was unable to achieve weight loss goals with lifestyle alone. Overall, medical therapy provides modest benefit during treatment, but needs to be continued lifelong to maintain weight loss. There is limited data on improvements in morbidity, and none on mortality, with drug-induced weight loss.
- National Heart, Lung and Blood Institute (NHLBI) recommends that medications for weight loss only be used in patients with a BMI > 30, or >27 with a comorbidity that may improve with weight loss.

FDA Approved

- **Anorexiant sympathomimetics** are Schedule IV drugs due to potential for abuse. They were FDA approved for short-term use only (12 weeks) prior to new standards set in 1996. They are not recommended for prolonged use or sustained weight loss and carry significant cardiovascular side effects.
  - **Phenteremine** (Adipex-P): 18.75 to 37.5 mg/day taken before breakfast or divided BID. Efficacy: in RCT, lost 13 kg versus 4.8 kg with placebo in 36 weeks.[34]
  - **Phendimetrazine** (Bontril): 105 mg PO daily before breakfast (slow-release capsule)
  - **Diethylpropion:** 75 mg PO daily (controlled-release capsule)
- **Orlistat** (Xenical, Alli) acts as an intestinal lumen lipase inhibitor, decreasing the absorption of ingested fats, thereby increasing the fecal fat content. It is the only medication approved for prolonged use (4 years) by the FDA.
  - 120 mg PO TID with any fat-containing meal. Each meal should contain <30% calories from fat.
  - Produced 11% versus 6% weight loss in 1 year. Reduced conversion from pre-diabetes to diabetes at 4 years. Reduction in LDL also seen.[35]
  - Less than 1% of the drug is absorbed into the blood stream, so the side effects are mostly lower GI, including fatty/oily stool, increased defecation, and fecal urgency.

These occur within the first 4 weeks in 15% to 20% of patients, then resolve spontaneously. A patient should start this medication over the weekend (with easy access to a restroom) so the initial effects do not interfere with work/school.

○ It also blocks the absorption of fat-soluble vitamins, so patients should also take a daily multivitamin 2 hours before or after orlistat.

• **Sibutramine** (Meridia) was previously the only appetite suppressant approved for long-term use (2 years) for weight loss. It was voluntarily taken **off the market** in October 2010 after the Sibutramine Cardiovascular Outcomes Trial (SCOUT) showed that there was a 16% increase in the relative risk of nonfatal MI and stroke, and about a 5% weight loss.[36]

Off-Label Use

• **Antidepressants**
  ○ **Fluoxetine** 60 mg/day showed 4.8 kg versus 2.4 kg loss with placebo at 6 months, with half regained at 1 year.[37]
  ○ **Bupropion SR** 400 mg/day showed 10.1% versus 5% weight loss at 24 weeks. Weight loss was sustained at 48 weeks.[38]
• **Antiepileptics**
  ○ **Topiramate:** 6.5% versus 2% at 6 months. Side effects include somnolence and metabolic acidosis.[39]
  ○ **Zonisamide:** 9.6 versus 1.6% at 32 weeks.[40]
• **Diabetes drugs**
  ○ **Metformin, pramlintide, exenatide, and liraglutide** have been shown to be either weight-neutral or weight loss inducing compared to insulin, sulfonylureas, and TZDs. Regarding the injectable therapies, nausea and decreased caloric intake may be the mechanism for this effect.

BARIATRIC SURGERY

Bariatric surgery encompasses any surgery on the gastrointestinal system that is meant to result in weight loss for the obese patient. These procedures cause weight loss by a combination of restriction and malabsorption. **Restrictive procedures** physically limit the amount of food that can be eaten in a short amount of time before the patient feels satiated or even nauseated, thereby significantly reducing daily caloric intake without inducing hunger. A **malabsorptive procedure** limits the exposure of fully digested food (after mixing with bile and pancreatic enzymes) to the small intestinal lumen.

Appropriate Patients
• BMI > 40
• BMI > 35 with a significant comorbid condition:
  ○ T2DM
  ○ OSA
  ○ Obesity-hypoventilation syndrome
  ○ Gastroesophaeal reflux
  ○ Non-alcoholic steatohepatitis
  ○ Hypertension
  ○ Dyslipidemia
  ○ Lifestyle-limiting joint disease
  ○ CAD

○ Pseudotumor cerebri
○ Asthma
○ Venous stasis disease
○ Severe urinary incontinence
• Attempted and failed lifestyle intervention for weight loss (though failure is generally not defined).
• Exclusion criteria:
○ Active substance abuse
○ Mental illness that may prevent safe compliance after the procedure
○ Eating disorder

Improvement in Comorbidities with Surgical Therapy

• Diabetes resolution, see Results under section on Roux-en-Y Gastric Bypass.
• Hypertension: resolved in 62%. Resolved or improved in 78.5%.
• OSA: resolved in 85.7%.[41]
• NAFLD: 84% resolution of steatosis at 2 years.[42]
• High triglycerides, low HDL: 85% remission.
• OHS: 76% remission after 2 years.[43]
• GERD: 95% resolution/significant improvement almost immediately.[44]
• Osteoarthritis: 50% of patients are able to decrease pain medication dose.[45]
• **Mortality:** 40% decrease in long-term all-cause mortality despite an increase in deaths from non-disease (accidents, suicides, etc.). There was a reduction in death rate from diabetes (92%), CAD (59%), and cancer (60%) in a matched control study of nearly 10,000 surgery patients with mean 7.1-year follow-up. This equated to preventing 136 deaths per 10,000 surgeries.[46]

Preoperative Care

• Optimize glycemic control in patients with diabetes. Determining the need for medications including insulin and their doses to achieve control prior to surgery may help predict the chances of complete remission.
• A perioperative glycemic control plan should be discussed preoperatively, including discontinuation of oral hypoglycemics at admission, and anticipating that those requiring insulin and those having diabetes for over 10 years preoperatively are likely to continue to require medication after discharge.
• Estrogen therapy should be discontinued 1 month prior to surgery to reduce risk of thromboembolic events. Some form of contraception should be used in premenopausal women before and for 1 year after surgery. Women with PCOS may have a significant and rapid improvement in fertility postoperatively.
• Smokers should stop smoking at least 8 weeks prior to surgery and have a plan to maintain cessation postoperatively.
• Evaluation for deep vein thrombosis and consideration of preoperative inferior vena cava (IVC) filter placement in high-risk patients.
• Psychiatry or psychology evaluation is mandatory, as significant mental illness and eating disorders can result in morbidity and mortality after surgery.
• Prior to malabsorptive procedures, micronutrient deficiencies including vitamin D should be assessed and treated.
• Patients at risk for cardiac disease should undergo risk stratification/evaluation for perioperative beta-blockade according to current guidelines.
• Preoperative weight loss using meal replacements (shakes or bars) is often done to attempt to reduce liver volume and to potentially improve outcomes.[43]

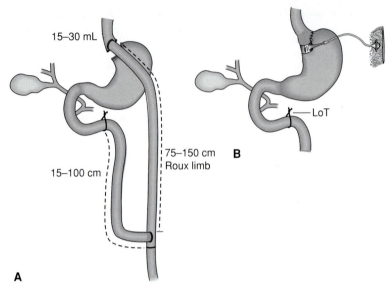

FIGURE 32-2 **A.** Roux-en-Y gastric bypass. **B.** Laparoscopic adjustable gastric banding.

Roux-en-Y Gastric Bypass (RYGB)

- Combines both restrictive and malabsorptive elements (see Figure 32-2A).
- A small proximal **gastric pouch**, 10 to 30 mL, is created. This provides the restrictive component.

Procedure

- The jejunum is transected 15 to 100 cm distal to the ligament of Treitz. The proximal end of the distal jejunum is anastomosed to the gastric pouch, creating the **Roux limb**, which will carry food away from the stomach. The free distal portion of the proximal jejunum is anastomosed to the Roux limb 75 to 150 cm from the gastric pouch, creating the **biliopancreatic limb**. This will carry bile, gastric, and pancreatic secretions to mix with ingested food at the point where the Roux and biliopancreatic limbs meet.
- Ingested food, therefore, bypasses most of the stomach, the duodenum, and the proximal jejunum, and is not broken down by digestive enzymes to enhance absorption until mixing with them in the distal jejunum. The entire ileum is still present for nutrient absorption, making malabsorption a small contributor to weight loss compared to earlier surgeries, which resulted in significant malabsorption.

Results

- **Seventy percentage excess weight loss at 1 year**. Twenty percentage weight regain between 2 and 5 years, then plateau (15 year follow-up showing 50% EWL).[47]
- **Resolution of diabetes:** >80% complete resolution (normoglycemic off medications) often within weeks. Those with diabetes > 10 years and those who require

insulin treatment prior to surgery are less likely to achieve complete resolution, but still have significant improvements in control with less need for medication. These metabolic improvements often precede clinically detectable weight loss.[41,48]

• Also reduces the conversion of impaired glucose tolerance to diabetes by 30-fold.[49]

Surgical Complications
• 30-day mortality: 0.2% laparoscopic, 2.1% open (higher BMI, more severe comorbidities).[50]
• Bowel leak, ulcer, gastro-gastric fistula, PE, MI, pneumonia, wound infection, SBO, stomal stenosis, nausea, incisional hernia, suboptimal weight loss.
• Rates of surgical complications including mortality in any bariatric procedure are variable, and associated with the experience of the performing surgeon.

Medical Complications
• Cholelithiasis, nutritional deficiencies, dumping symptoms—common
• Hyperinsulinemic hypoglycemia—rare

Laparoscopic Adjustable Gastric Banding
A purely restrictive procedure with the benefits of adjustability and reversibility (see Figure 32-2B).

Procedure
An **inflatable band** is placed around the top of the stomach, creating a **gastric pouch.** The gastric fundus is stitched to the area above the band. A **subcutaneous port** is placed in the anterior abdomen. There is no rearrangement of gastrointestinal sequence. The amount of band inflation can be adjusted by accessing the subcutaneous port with a needle, and adding or subtracting saline. The bariatric surgeon will frequently assess symptoms and rate of weight loss to determine the need for adjustment.

Results
• 35% to 45% EWL at 2 to 10 years[51].
• Resolution of diabetes in 60% at 2 years, proportional to weight loss.

Complications
• Operative mortality 0.1%.[51]
• Acute obstruction, PE, MI, band slippage, esophageal dilation, band erosion, balloon failure, port malposition, band and port infections, maladaptive eating, suboptimal weight loss.

Less Common Surgeries
• **Vertical banded gastroplasty:** 15 to 45 mL pouch, 10 to 11 mm outlet, replaced by LAGB because the latter is less invasive, adjustable, reversible, and has better outcomes.
• **Biliopancreatic diversion (BPD):** subtotal gastrectomy (200 to 500 mL pouch). Small intestines divided 250 cm from the cecum and the proximal portion of the distal segment is anastomosed to the gastric pouch, creating the alimentary limb. The biliopancreatic limb is anastomosed to the ileum 50 cm from the cecum. BPD is less restrictive but much more malabsorptive than RYGB. Protein calorie malabsorption, steatorrhea, iron and fat-soluble vitamin deficiencies, and metabolic bone disease are common. It is rarely performed in the United States anymore, but may be appropriate for some patients with a BMI > 60.

- **Sleeve gastrectomy:** resection of the greater curve of the stomach, preserving the gastric antrum. This leaves a path for food along the lesser curve, from the esophageal to the pyloric sphincter, but greatly reduces gastric volume.
- **BPD with duodenal switch:** BPD, but with a sleeve gastrectomy, and the alimentary limb is anastomosed to the gastric pylorus.

Postoperative Care

Diet

- There are minor differences in the recommendations for RYGB and LAGB, and these details are beyond the scope of this text.
- Stages I–III (at least 5 weeks): initially clear liquid (always sugar-free) slowly advanced to solid **protein (>60 g/day)**, fruits, vegetables, and salads (chewing thoroughly), avoiding rice, bread, and pasta. Multiple small meals. Greater than 1.5 L fluid daily. Do not drink until 30 minutes after meals.
- Stage IV: balanced meals including whole grains, using small plates and utensils, and vitamin/mineral supplements (1 to 2 chewable multivitamins per day, containing iron, calcium, and B-complex).[43]

Diabetes Control

- See Chapter 30.
- Avoid long-acting insulin in the immediate perioperative period. IV insulin can be used intra/postoperatively if necessary. All oral and non-insulin injectable hypoglycemic agents should be avoided during hospitalization.
- Achieving inpatient glucose control should be no different than other postoperative populations. Critically ill patients require IV insulin titrated per protocol to keep BG in the 140–180 mg/dL range. In non-critically ill patients, long-acting insulin analogues should be used to achieve target fasting glucose <140. A correction-dose of rapid-acting insulin should also be given every 4 to 6 hours for hyperglycemia.
- In the only published RCT of inpatient diabetes management after gastric bypass, those treated with 0.3 U/kg glargine once daily plus sliding scale had improved glucose control compared to those on sliding scale regular insulin only, without significant hypoglycemia.[52]
- The basal insulin requirements may fall significantly over several postoperative days as glycogen stores are depleted and insulin resistance wanes. Fixed-dose prandial insulin should not be needed, as the Stage I diet is carbohydrate-free liquids. Insulin can be discontinued if the patient has T2DM and continues to meet glycemic targets without insulin.
- There are no published guidelines regarding outpatient management of glucose control after weight loss surgery. The following is the authors'/editors' personal recommendation.
  - At discharge, some patients may still require basal insulin to maintain a fasting blood glucose <140 mg/dL. They can be placed on metformin titrated to maximum dose as tolerated if not contraindicated. They can be discharged on their hospital dose of basal insulin, and instructed to check glucose fasting daily. When fasting glucoses fall below 100, basal insulin doses can be reduced by 20%. This reduction can be repeated when fasting glucose again falls below 100 mg/dL, until insulin can be discontinued.
  - It is unknown how often a patient with T2DM will require prandial insulin on the prescribed low-carbohydrate diet (Stage I–III). Those that do should be very cautious and check 2-hour postprandial blood glucose to monitor for hypoglycemia.

A plan to titrate down this dose for postprandial lows should be provided to the patient at discharge.
  ○ Once a patient is no longer on insulin, he/she can remain on metformin until the A1c falls into the normal range.
• An A1c under 5.7 and a fasting glucose under 100 on no hypoglycemic medication are indicative of diabetes remission. The effect of continued metformin treatment on weight regain and diabetes recurrence after weight loss surgery has not been assessed.

Hyperlipidemia
There is no evidence to support empiric discontinuation of statin therapy after surgery. Routine monitoring is recommended, following National Cholesterol Education Program (NCEP) Adult Treatment Panel III (ATPIII) guidelines.[53]

Hypertension
Hypotension may develop postoperatively in the setting of poor fluid intake, leading to hypovolemia. Consider holding diuretic therapy until adequate intake is confirmed to avoid hypotension and electrolyte imbalances.

Gallbladder Disease
300 mg/day ursodiol for 6 months reduces clinically significant gallstone disease in patients who have not undergone prophylactic cholecystectomy.[54]

Skeletal/Mineral Homeostasis
• Obese patients presenting for bariatric surgery have high rates of vitamin D deficiency and secondary hyperparathyroidism. In RYGB, dietary calcium bypasses the duodenum, where vitamin D-dependent calcium absorption takes place. There is increased risk of hypocalcemia and secondary hyperparathyroidism in the absence of supplementation.[55]
• After RYGB, routine daily vitamin D and calcium supplementation (1500 mg + 800 IU) improves vitamin D levels and prevents hypocalcemia in vitamin D deficient patients, but secondary hyperparathyroidism may persist.[56]
• Urine N-telopeptides and serum osteocalcin rise while bone mineral density falls. The fall in bone density and increased bone turnover can be attributed to weight loss itself, as there is a decrease in the mechanical weight-bearing of bones when significant weight is lost. DXA may not truly reflect the change in bone density when the density of surrounding tissues drastically changes over a period of months.[57]
• In a RCT of 60 women with vitamin D insufficiency prior to surgery, 50,000 units ergocalciferol/week for 1 year after RYGB showed:
  ○ Significant improvement in vitamin D levels, fewer patients with deficiency
  ○ No difference in calcium, PTH, bone-specific alkaline phosphatase, urine N-telopeptides
  ○ Hip bone mineral density fell 0.08% versus 0.12%
  ○ Rate of hypertension resolution: 75% versus 32% ($p = 0.029$)
  ○ The authors concluded that all patients undergoing RYGB should receive daily elemental calcium 1500 mg, and cholecalciferol 2000 IU. Patients with low vitamin D levels preoperatively should also be treated with 50,000 IU ergocalciferol weekly, checking a vitamin D level every 6 to 12 months.[58]
• Calcium carbonate preparations should be chewable and taken with food to assist absorption. Calcium citrate will be better absorbed, and can be taken without food, as it does not need acidic gastric contents.

- The Endocrine Society guidelines recommend vitamin D, calcium, phosphorus, PTH, and alkaline phosphatase levels be checked every 6 months.[53]
- Osteoporosis treatment with IV bisphosphonates is preferred over orals due to concern over absorption and anastomotic ulceration, but only after correction of vitamin D deficiency and with adequate calcium supplementation.[43]

Micronutrient Deficiencies after RYGB
- **Iron deficiency** is found in 25% to 75% of patients by 5 to 10 years. Iron is absorbed predominantly in the duodenum and requires gastric acid for optimal absorption. Deficiency should be monitored for biannually with CBC and iron studies, and treated. It should be prevented in menstruating women after RYGB with twice-daily 65 mg elemental iron supplementation. Vitamin C coadministration (and taking separately from calcium supplementation) will help iron absorption. IV iron is sometimes needed if oral supplementation fails to correct deficiency.
- **B12 deficiency** (in RYGB) is found in 8% to 40% of patients by 1 year. Routine supplementation with vitamin B12 > 350 ug/day is appropriate in all RYGB patients. Biannual assessment of B12 status is recommended.
- **Folate deficiency** can be prevented with folic acid 400 mcg/day, which may be included in multivitamin preparations.
- **Thiamine deficiency**, which can lead to Wernicke encephalopathy, is seen in patients with recurrent/persistent vomiting needing IV fluids. Consider thiamine supplementation for those patients.[43]
- **Copper deficiency** is increased after gastric bypass, as copper is absorbed in the stomach, duodenum, and upper jejunum. Signs include anemia, leukopenia, and neurologic manifestations similar to B12 deficiency. Prevention strategies beyond multivitamin are unclear, but persistent illness/anemia after correcting for other deficiencies should prompt evaluation for copper deficiency. IV copper may be necessary in patients with a deficiency.

Dumping Syndrome
- Abdominal pain, cramping, nausea, diarrhea, lightheadedness, flushing, tachycardia, and syncope shortly after eating in patients who have had RYGB. It results from the consumption of carbohydrate-dense or hypertonic foods and beverages that enter the intestines quickly. It has been reported in 70% to 76% of RYGB patients, but may serve an important role in behavior adjustment, causing patients to avoid behaviors that lead to the uncomfortable symptoms.
- Behaviors that prevent or lessen these symptoms include eating small frequent meals, not drinking until 30 minutes after meals, and avoiding simple sugars, replacing them with fiber, complex carbohydrates, and protein.[53]

Postprandial Hyperinsulinemic Hypoglycemia
- Presents with neuroglycopenic symptomatic hypoglycemia after meals. Diagnosis is made by a negative 72-hour fast for hypoglycemia, but positive hyperinsulinemia with hypoglycemia within 5 hours after a mixed meal tolerance test, and negative imaging for an insulinoma. This rare syndrome presents between years 2 and 9 postoperatively from RYGB.
- Medical management includes low-carbohydrate meals, acarbose, calcium channel blockers, diazoxide, and octreotide. Refractory patients have been treated with 80% pancreatectomy with improvement, but not absolute resolution. Pathology suggests islet hyperplasia.[59]

REFERENCES

1. Flegal KM, Carroll MD, Ogden CL, et al. Prevalence and trends in obesity among US adults, 1999-2008. *JAMA* 2010;303(3):235–241.
2. Ogden CL, Carroll MD, Curtin LR, et al. Prevalence of high body mass index in US children and adolescents, 2007-2008. *JAMA* 2010;303(3):242–249.
3. Farooqi IS, Wangensteen T, Collins S, et al. Clinical and molecular genetic spectrum of congenital deficiency of the leptin receptor. *N Engl J Med* 2007;356(3):237–247.
4. Santini F, Maffei M, Pelosini C, et al. Melanocortin-4 receptor mutations in obesity. *Adv Clin Chem* 2009;48:95–109.
5. Ohta T, Gray TA, Rogan PK, et al. Imprinting-mutation mechanisms in Prader-Willi syndrome. *Am J Hum Genet* 1999;64(2):397–413.
6. Willett WC, Dietz WH, Colditz GA. Guidelines for healthy weight. *N Engl J Med* 1999; 341(6):427–434.
7. Colditz GA, Willett WC, Rotnitzky A, et al. Weight gain as a risk factor for clinical diabetes mellitus in women. *Ann Intern Med* 1995;122(7):481–486.
8. Willett WC, Manson JE, Stampfer MJ, et al. Weight, weight change, and coronary heart disease in women. Risk within the 'normal' weight range. *JAMA* 1995;273(6):461–465.
9. Kenchaiah S, Evans JC, Levy D, et al. Obesity and the risk of heart failure. *N Engl J Med* 2002;347(5):305–313.
10. Basen-Engquist K, Chang M. Obesity and cancer risk: Recent review and evidence. *Curr Oncol Rep*2011;13(1):71–76.
11. Flegal KM, Graubard BI, Williamson DF, et al. Excess deaths associated with underweight, overweight, and obesity. *JAMA* 2005;293(15):1861–1867.
12. Whitlock G, Lewington S, Sherliker P, et al. Body-mass index and cause-specific mortality in 900 000 adults: Collaborative analyses of 57 prospective studies. *Lancet* 2009; 373(9669):1083–1096.
13. Adams KF, Schatzkin A, Harris TB, et al. Overweight, obesity, and mortality in a large prospective cohort of persons 50 to 71 years old. *N Engl J Med* 2006;355(8):763–778.
14. Peeters A, Barendregt JJ, Willekens F, et al. Obesity in adulthood and its consequences for life expectancy: A life-table analysis. *Ann Intern Med* 2003;138(1):24–32.
15. Klein S, Mittendorfer B, Eagon JC, et al. Gastric bypass surgery improves metabolic and hepatic abnormalities associated with nonalcoholic fatty liver disease. *Gastroenterology* 2006;130(6): 1564–1572.
16. Nowbar S, Burkart KM, Gonzales R, et al. Obesity-associated hypoventilation in hospitalized patients: Prevalence, effects, and outcome. *Am J Med* 2004;116(1):1–7.
17. Chung F, Yegneswaran B, Liao P, et al. STOP questionnaire: A tool to screen patients for obstructive sleep apnea. *Anesthesiology* 2008;108(5):812–821.
18. Knowler WC, Barrett-Connor E, Fowler SE, et al. Reduction in the incidence of type 2 diabetes with lifestyle intervention or metformin. *N Engl J Med* 2002;346(6):393–403.
19. Klein S, Sheard NF, Pi-Sunyer X, et al. Weight management through lifestyle modification for the prevention and management of type 2 diabetes: Rationale and strategies: A statement of the American Diabetes Association, the North American Association for the Study of Obesity, and the American Society for Clinical Nutrition. *Diabetes Care* 2004;27(8):2067–2073.
20. Neter JE, Stam BE, Kok FJ, et al. Influence of weight reduction on blood pressure: A meta-analysis of randomized controlled trials. *Hypertension* 2003;42(5):878–884.
21. Rasmussen KM, Abrams B, Bodnar LM, et al. Recommendations for weight gain during pregnancy in the context of the obesity epidemic. *Obstet Gynecol* 2010;116(5):1191–1195.
22. Gardner CD, Kiazand A, Alhassan S, et al. Comparison of the Atkins, Zone, Ornish, and LEARN diets for change in weight and related risk factors among overweight premenopausal women: The A TO Z Weight Loss Study: A randomized trial. *JAMA* 2007;297(9): 969–977.
23. Sacks FM, Bray GA, Carey VJ, et al. Comparison of weight-loss diets with different compositions of fat, protein, and carbohydrates. *N Engl J Med* 2009;360(9):859–873.

24. Nordmann AJ, Nordmann A, Briel M, et al. Effects of low-carbohydrate vs low-fat diets on weight loss and cardiovascular risk factors: A meta-analysis of randomized controlled trials. *Arch Intern Med* 2006;166(3):285–293.

25. Foster GD, Wyatt HR, Hill JO, et al. Weight and metabolic outcomes after 2 years on a low-carbohydrate versus low-fat diet: A randomized trial. *Ann Intern Med* 2010;153(3): 147–157.

26. Kirk E, Reeds DN, Finck BN, et al. Dietary fat and carbohydrates differentially alter insulin sensitivity during caloric restriction. *Gastroenterology* 2009;136(5):1552–1560.

27. Kirk JK, Graves DE, Craven TE, et al. Restricted-carbohydrate diets in patients with type 2 diabetes: A meta-analysis. *J Am Diet Assoc* 2008;108(1):91–100.

28. Esposito K, Maiorino MI, Ciotola M, et al. Effects of a Mediterranean-style diet on the need for antihyperglycemic drug therapy in patients with newly diagnosed type 2 diabetes: A randomized trial. *Ann Intern Med* 2009;151(5):306–314.

29. Elhayany A, Lustman A, Abel R, et al. A low carbohydrate Mediterranean diet improves cardiovascular risk factors and diabetes control among overweight patients with type 2 diabetes mellitus: A 1-year prospective randomized intervention study. *Diabetes Obes Metab* 2010;12(3):204–209.

30. Westman EC, Yancy WS Jr, Mavropoulos JC, et al. The effect of a low-carbohydrate, ketogenic diet versus a low-glycemic index diet on glycemic control in type 2 diabetes mellitus. *Nutr Metab (Lond)* 2008;5:36.

31. Catenacci VA, Ogden LG, Stuht J, et al. Physical activity patterns in the National Weight Control Registry. *Obesity (Silver Spring)* 2008;16(1):153–161.

32. Gibbons RJ, Balady GJ, Bricker JT, et al. ACC/AHA 2002 guideline update for exercise testing: Summary article. A report of the American College of Cardiology/American Heart Association Task Force on Practice Guidelines (Committee to Update the 1997 Exercise Testing Guidelines). *J Am Coll Cardiol* 2002;40(8):1531–1540.

33. Wing RR, Jakicic J, Neiberg R, et al. Fitness, fatness, and cardiovascular risk factors in type 2 diabetes: Look ahead study. *Med Sci Sports Exerc* 2007;39(12):2107–2116.

34. Munro JF, MacCuish AC, Wilson EM, et al. Comparison of continuous and intermittent anorectic therapy in obesity. *Br Med J* 1968;1(5588):352–354.

35. Torgerson JS, Hauptman J, Boldrin MN, et al. XENical in the prevention of diabetes in obese subjects (XENDOS) study: A randomized study of orlistat as an adjunct to lifestyle changes for the prevention of type 2 diabetes in obese patients. *Diabetes Care* 2004; 27(1):155–161.

36. James WP, Caterson ID, Coutinho W, et al. Effect of sibutramine on cardiovascular outcomes in overweight and obese subjects. *N Engl J Med* 2010;363(10):905–917.

37. Goldstein DJ, Rampey AH, Jr., Enas GG, et al. Fluoxetine: A randomized clinical trial in the treatment of obesity. *Int J Obes Relat Metab Disord* 1994;18(3):129–135.

38. Anderson JW, Greenway FL, Fujioka K, et al. Bupropion SR enhances weight loss: A 48-week double-blind, placebo- controlled trial. *Obes Res* 2002;10(7):633–641.

39. Li Z, Maglione M, Tu W, et al. Meta-analysis: Pharmacologic treatment of obesity. *Ann Intern Med* 2005;142(7):532–546.

40. Gadde KM, Franciscy DM, Wagner HR 2nd, et al. Zonisamide for weight loss in obese adults: A randomized controlled trial. *JAMA* 2003;289(14):1820–1825.

41. Buchwald H, Avidor Y, Braunwald E, et al. Bariatric surgery: A systematic review and meta-analysis. *JAMA* 2004;292(14):1724–1737.

42. Furuya CK Jr, de Oliveira CP, de Mello ES, et al. Effects of bariatric surgery on nonalcoholic fatty liver disease: Preliminary findings after 2 years. *J Gastroenterol Hepatol* 2007; 22(4):510–514.

43. Mechanick JI, Kushner RF, Sugerman HJ, et al. American Association of Clinical Endocrinologists, The Obesity Society, and American Society for Metabolic & Bariatric Surgery Medical guidelines for clinical practice for the perioperative nutritional, metabolic, and nonsurgical support of the bariatric surgery patient. *Endocr Pract* 2008;14(Suppl 1):1–83.

44. Nelson LG, Gonzalez R, Haines K, et al. Amelioration of gastroesophageal reflux symptoms following Roux-en-Y gastric bypass for clinically significant obesity. *Am Surg* 2005; 71(11): 950–953; discussion 953–954.

45. Abu-Abeid S, Wishnitzer N, Szold A, et al. The influence of surgically-induced weight loss on the knee joint. *Obes Surg* 2005;15(10):1437–1442.

46. Adams TD, Gress RE, Smith SC, et al. Long-term mortality after gastric bypass surgery. *N Engl J Med* 2007;357(8):753–761.

47. Pories WJ, Swanson MS, MacDonald KG, et al. Who would have thought it? An operation proves to be the most effective therapy for adult-onset diabetes mellitus. *Ann Surg* 1995;222 (3):339–350; discussion 350–352.

48. Schauer PR, Burguera B, Ikramuddin S, et al. Effect of laparoscopic Roux-en Y gastric bypass on type 2 diabetes mellitus. *Ann Surg* 2003;238(4):467–484; discussion 84–85.

49. Long SD, O'Brien K, MacDonald KG Jr, et al. Weight loss in severely obese subjects prevents the progression of impaired glucose tolerance to type II diabetes. A longitudinal interventional study. *Diabetes Care* 1994;17(5):372–375.

50. Flum DR, Belle SH, King WC, et al. Perioperative safety in the longitudinal assessment of bariatric surgery. *N Engl J Med* 2009;361(5):445–454.

51. Favretti F, Segato G, Ashton D, et al. Laparoscopic adjustable gastric banding in 1,791 consecutive obese patients: 12-year results. *Obes Surg* 2007;17(2):168–175.

52. Datta S, Qaadir A, Villanueva G, et al. Once-daily insulin glargine versus 6-hour sliding scale regular insulin for control of hyperglycemia after a bariatric surgical procedure: A randomized clinical trial. *Endocr Pract* 2007;13(3):225–231.

53. Heber D, Greenway FL, Kaplan LM, et al. Endocrine and nutritional management of the post-bariatric surgery patient: An Endocrine Society Clinical Practice Guideline. *J Clin Endocrinol Metab* 2010;95(11):4823–4843.

54. Sugerman HJ, Brewer WH, Shiffman ML, et al. A multicenter, placebo-controlled, randomized, double-blind, prospective trial of prophylactic ursodiol for the prevention of gallstone formation following gastric-bypass-induced rapid weight loss. *Am J Surg* 1995; 169(1):91–96; discussion 96–97.

55. Carlin AM, Rao DS, Meslemani AM, et al. Prevalence of vitamin D depletion among morbidly obese patients seeking gastric bypass surgery. *Surg Obes Relat Dis* 2006;2(2):98–103; discussion 104.

56. Carlin AM, Rao DS, Yager KM, et al. Effect of gastric bypass surgery on vitamin D nutritional status. *Surg Obes Relat Dis* 2006;2(6):638–642.

57. Coates PS, Fernstrom JD, Fernstrom MH, et al. Gastric bypass surgery for morbid obesity leads to an increase in bone turnover and a decrease in bone mass. *J Clin Endocrinol Metab* 2004;89(3):1061–1065.

58. Carlin AM, Rao DS, Yager KM, et al. Treatment of vitamin D depletion after Roux-en-Y gastric bypass: A randomized prospective clinical trial. *Surg Obes Relat Dis* 2009;5(4):444–449.

59. Mathavan VK, Arregui M, Davis C, et al. Management of postgastric bypass noninsulinoma pancreatogenous hypoglycemia. *Surg Endosc* 2010;24(10):2547–2555.

Dyslipidemia

33

Mariko Johnson and Anne C. Goldberg

GENERAL PRINCIPLES

Definition

- The National Cholesterol Education Program (NCEP) has developed optimal ranges for fasting levels of all four lipid parameters for adults.[1] Dyslipidemia can be diagnosed if any of the following are present:
  - Total cholesterol >200 mg/dL
  - Low-density lipoprotein (LDL) cholesterol >100 mg/dL
  - High-density lipoprotein (HDL) cholesterol <40 mg/dL
  - Triglycerides >150 mg/dL
- Dyslipidemia usually fits one of four general patterns:
  - Isolated hypertriglyceridemia
  - Isolated elevation in LDL-cholesterol
  - Combined elevation of triglycerides and LDL-cholesterol
  - Any of the above with the addition of a low HDL-cholesterol

Epidemiology

Dyslipidemia is very common in Western society. It affects 90% of patients with coronary artery disease[2] and close to 30% of patients without clinical coronary disease.[3]

Etiology

- It is widely accepted that both genetic and environmental factors play a role in the development of dyslipidemia.
- The underlying pathophysiology of dyslipidemia in most cases is likely complex and remains obscure. However, certain cases have a clear genetic basis, and in a subset of these, a well-defined underlying mechanism exists (see Table 33-1).
- Differential diagnosis of the major lipid abnormalities is summarized in Table 33-2.

Prevention

Diet, exercise, and weight loss play a large role in the prevention and treatment of dyslipidemia.

Associated Conditions

- Dyslipidemia is a major modifiable risk factor for cardiovascular, cerebrovascular, and peripheral vascular disease. Targeted lowering of LDL-cholesterol has demonstrated a benefit in both primary and secondary prevention of coronary disease.[4] Elevated triglycerides and low HDL-cholesterol likely confer additional risk, although the benefit of lowering triglycerides and raising HDL-cholesterol is less well established.

TABLE 33-1   REVIEW OF MAJOR GENETIC DYSLIPOPROTEINEMIAS

Genetic dyslipidemia	Typical lipid profile	Inheritance pattern	Phenotypic features	Pathophysiology
Isolated LDL elevation				
Familial hypercholesterolemia (FH)	Heterozygous form: LDL > 220 mg/dL Homozygous form: LDL > 550 mg/dL	Autosomal dominant	• Premature CAD • Tendon xanthomas • Xanthelasmata • Premature arcus corneae	Caused by mutations of the LDL receptor that lead to defective uptake and degradation of LDL
Familial defective apolipoprotein B-100	Similar to familial hypercholesterolemia	Autosomal dominant	• Similar to familial hypercholesterolemia	Caused by a mutation in apo B-100 which impairs the interaction of LDL with the receptor leading to decreased LDL clearance
Isolated triglyceride elevation				
Lipoprotein lipase (LPL) OR apo C-II deficiency	TGs 1,000–25,000 mg/dL	Autosomal recessive	• Diagnosed in childhood • Eruptive xanthomas* • Lipemia retinalis* • Pancreatitis* • Hepatosplenomegaly* *Clinical manifestations occur when triglycerides exceed 1500 mg/dL	Deficiency in LPL or its cofactor apo C-II impairs uptake of triglycerides into peripheral tissues
Familial hypertriglyceridemia	TGs 150–500 mg/dL or higher in the presence of secondary factors (obesity, alcohol use, diabetes)	Autosomal dominant	• Diagnosed in adulthood • Same as for LPL if triglyceride levels are severely elevated	Caused by overproduction of VLDL triglycerides Genetic defects are not been established

(continued)

TABLE 33-1 REVIEW OF MAJOR GENETIC DYSLIPOPROTEINEMIAS (Continued)

Genetic dyslipidemia	Typical lipid profile	Inheritance pattern	Phenotypic features	Pathophysiology
Combined elevations in LDL and triglycerides				
Familial combined hyper-lipidemia (FCH)	Moderately elevated levels of LDL, triglycerides or both	Autosomal dominant	• Premature CAD • Xanthelasma only Tendon and cutaneous xanthomas are absent	Caused by overproduction of VLDL Genetic defects are not established
Type III hyperlipoproteinemia (familial dysbetalipoproteinemia)	Symmetric elevations of cholesterol and triglycerides (300–500 mg/dL) Emergence of hyperlipidemia often requires a secondary factor	Autosomal recessive	• Premature CAD • Tuberous or tuberoeruptive xanthomas • Planar xanthomas of the palmar creases are essentially pathognomonic	Caused by homozygous mutation in apo E (apo E2/E2) leading to defective clearance of chylomicron and VLDL remnants
Isolated low HDL				
Familial hypoal-phalipoproteinemia	HDL levels below the 10th percentile (<30 mg/dL for men and <40 mg/dL for premenopausal women)	Autosomal dominant	• Premature CAD • No characteristic findings on physical exam	Genetic defects are not established

CAD, coronary artery disease; LDL, low-density lipoprotein; VLDL, very low-density lipoprotein; HDL, high-density lipoprotein; TGs, triglycerides

| TABLE 33-2 | DIFFERENTIAL DIAGNOSIS OF MAJOR LIPID ABNORMALITIES |

Lipid abnormality	Primary disorders	Secondary disorders
Hypercholesterolemia	Polygenic, familial hypercholesterolemia, familial defective apo B-100	Hypothyroidism, nephrotic syndrome, obstructive liver disease, thiazide diuretics
Hypertriglyceridemia	Lipoprotein lipase deficiency, apo C-II deficiency, familial hypertriglyceridemia	Poorly controlled diabetes mellitus, hypothyroidism, renal failure, obesity, high carbohydrate diets, alcohol use, oral estrogen, beta blockers, protease inhibitors glucocorticoids, retinoids, bile acid binding resins, antipsychotics, thiazide diuretics
Combined hyperlipidemia	Familial combined hyperlipidemia, type III hyperlipopro-teinemia	Poorly controlled diabetes mellitus, hypothyroidism, glucocorticoids, immunosuppressants, protease inhibitors, nephrotic syndrome
Low HDL	Familial alpha lipoproteinemia, Tangier's disease, familial HDL deficiency, lecithin:cholesterol acyltransferase deficiency	Anabolic steroids, retinoids, tobacco use

HDL, high-density lipoprotein.

- Dyslipidemia is often associated with a constellation of additional metabolic abnormalities including obesity, hypertension, insulin resistance, and fatty liver disease.
- Severely elevated triglycerides are a risk factor for pancreatitis.

DIAGNOSIS

Screening for dyslipidemia should be performed at least once every 5 years beginning at age 20 and in high-risk patients diagnosed with vascular disease, diabetes, or pancreatitis.[1] Certain physical examination findings (see Physical Examination section) can be a clue to a lipid disorder and should prompt a screening lipid panel (see Table 33-1).

Clinical Presentation

History

The history should focus on identification of secondary causes of dyslipidemia or family history of premature coronary disease, and evaluation of cardiovascular risk factors. Consideration of secondary causes requires that the clinician pay attention to diet, medications, and alcohol consumption in addition to comorbid conditions (see Table 33-2). A detailed family history should also be sought, as a strong family history of premature coronary disease may suggest a genetic dyslipoproteinemia (see Table 33-1). Determination of risk factors is important because cardiovascular risk determines an individual patient's goal LDL-cholesterol, thereby affecting treatment (see Section Treatment).

Physical Examination

The physical examination should focus on identification of occult vascular disease (bruits) and physical findings that suggest a severe dyslipoproteinemia, such as tendon xanthomas, palmar xanthomas, eruptive xanthomas, tuberous xanthomas, xanthelasma, lipemia retinalis, or premature arcus corneae.

Diagnostic Testing

- The **fasting lipid panel** is the cornerstone of diagnosis.
- Most laboratories directly measure levels of triglycerides, total cholesterol, and HDL-cholesterol, but calculate LDL-cholesterol. If triglycerides are >400 mg/dL, calculated LDL-cholesterol measurements are not reliable and direct LDL-cholesterol should be measured.
- A new diagnosis of hypertriglyceridemia should prompt screening for diabetes, hypothyroidism, and renal failure.
- A new diagnosis of elevated LDL-cholesterol should prompt screening for hypothyroidism, obstructive liver disease, and the nephrotic syndrome.

TREATMENT

- The NCEP adult treatment panel (ATP) III guidelines define a stepwise approach to the patient with dyslipidemia.[1] An update to these guidelines was published in 2004[5] and release of revised guidelines is expected in 2012. The guidelines make optimization of LDL-cholesterol the primary target of therapy but guide clinicians in addressing abnormalities in other lipid parameters.
- *Step 1: Treat severely elevated triglycerides.*
  - If triglycerides are severely elevated (>500 mg/dL), this must be addressed before LDL-cholesterol as it predisposes to pancreatitis.
  - Treatment should include:
    - A very low fat diet (<15% of calories from fat)
    - Increased physical activity
    - Weight loss if overweight
    - Drug therapy with a fibrate or niacin (if necessary)
  - Once triglycerides are <500 mg/dL, clinicians can turn their attention to LDL-cholesterol targets.
- *Step 2: Determine coronary heart disease (CHD) risk.*
  - The ATP III guidelines provide a formal method of CHD risk assessment.

TABLE 33-3	ADULT TREATMENT PROGRAM III (ATP III) CATEGORIES OF CORONARY HEART DISEASE (CHD) RISK
Category	**Definition**
Very high risk	CHD and:
	Multiple risk factors (especially diabetes)
	Severe and poorly controlled risk factors (especially continued cigarette smoking)
	Multiple risk factors of the metabolic syndrome
	Acute coronary syndromes
High risk	CHD or CHD risk equivalent
Moderately high risk	2+ risk factors and 10-year CHD risk 10%–20%
Moderate risk	2+ risk factors and 10-year CHD risk <10%
Lower risk	0–1 risk factors

Adapted from Grundy SM, Cleeman C, Merz NB, et al. Implications of recent clinical trials for the National Cholesterol Education Program Adult Treatment Panel III Guidelines. *Circulation* 2004;110:227.

- ATP III recognizes **five categories of CHD risk**—very high, high, moderately high, moderate, and lower risk. These CHD risk categories are defined in Table 33-3 and risk can be assigned using the following algorithm:
- **Task 1: Determine whether CHD or a CHD risk equivalent is present.**
  - CHD
  - Diabetes
  - Symptomatic cerebrovascular disease
  - Peripheral artery disease
  - Abdominal aortic aneurysm
- **Task 2: Determine what CHD risk factors are present.**
  - Cigarette smoking
  - Hypertension (blood pressure ≥140/90 mm Hg or on antihypertensive medication)
  - Low HDL-cholesterol (<40 mg/dL)
    High HDL-cholesterol (≥60 mg/dL) serves as a "negative" risk factor if present, removing one risk factor from the total count
  - Family history of premature CHD (CHD in a male first degree relative < age 55 or CHD in a female first degree relative < age 65)
  - Age (Men ≥ age 45 or Women ≥ age 55)
- **Task 3: Assess risk level for patients with CHD or a CHD risk equivalent.**
  - All patients with CHD or a CHD risk equivalent fall into the high or very high-risk categories.
    - High risk: CHD or a CHD risk equivalent without additional CHD risk factors
    - Very high risk: CHD with combined with multiple, severe, or poorly controlled CHD risk factors, diabetes, acute coronary syndrome, or metabolic syndrome.
    - Once risk category is determined, clinicians can skip to *Step 3*.
- **Task 5: Assess risk level for patients without CHD or a CHD risk equivalent.**
  - Patients without CHD or a CHD risk equivalent can fall into any of the four following categories:

- □ Low risk: 0 to 1 CHD risk factors are present
- □ Moderate risk, moderately high risk, high risk: 2+ CHD risk factors are present
- □ If risk category is determined, clinicians can skip to *Step 3*. If risk category has not yet been determined, clinicians must move to *Task 6*.

- ○ Task 6: Calculate Framingham score for patients with 2+ CHD risk factors.
  - ■ A Framingham score can be calculated and translated into a 10-year CHD risk using the system outlined in Table 33-4.
  - ■ Patients with 2+ CHD risk factors can then be assigned a risk level based on 10-year CHD risk.
    - □ Moderate risk: 2+ risk factors and 10-year CHD risk <10%
    - □ Moderately high risk: 2+ risk factors and 10-year CHD risk 10% to 20%
    - □ High risk: 2+ risk factors and 10-year CHD risk >20%
    - □ Risk category for all patients should now be determined and clinicians can move to *Step 3*.

- • *Step 3: Determine LDL goal and initial treatment strategy.*
  - ○ An LDL-cholesterol goal and initial treatment strategy can be determined directly from the CHD risk (see Table 33-5).
  - ○ The NCEP guidelines recommend two basic interventions to reduce LDL-cholesterol.
    - ■ **Therapeutic lifestyle changes** are recommended for *all* patients whose LDL-cholesterol is above goal and in all very high-risk patients.
      - □ Dietary changes (saturated fat <7% of calories, cholesterol <200 mg/day, consideration of soluble fiber at doses of 10 to 25 g/day and plant phytosterols at doses of 2 g/day)
      - □ Increased physical activity
      - □ Weight management
    - ■ **Drug therapy** should be started at the thresholds recommended by the NCEP (see Table 33-5).
      - □ In low- and moderate-risk patients, a three-month trial of TLC alone prior to drug therapy is permitted.
      - □ In high-risk patients (those in the moderately high-, high-, and very high-risk categories), drug therapy should be initiated immediately and an LDL-cholesterol lowering of 30% should be targeted.

- • *Step 4: Choose appropriate drug therapy if it is indicated.*
  - ○ The NCEP guidelines defer the choice of drug to the clinician though **we recommend that a statin be the first-line agent**. The potency of available statins can be found in Table 33-6.
  - ○ Four additional classes of drugs can be used to lower LDL-cholesterol if statins are contraindicated, poorly tolerated, or if additional LDL-cholesterol lowering is needed. Efficacy and side effects of the different classes vary and are summarized in Table 33-7.
    - ■ **Bile acid sequestrants** are safe and effective if significant isolated LDL-cholesterol lowering is needed. Bile acid sequestrants may elevate triglycerides and so should be avoided in cases of combined hyperlipidemia.
    - ■ **Niacin** is an excellent choice if LDL-cholesterol lowering needs are modest, particularly if triglycerides are also elevated.
    - ■ **Fibrates** are less often used because they can increase risk of myopathy when used in combination with statins and may paradoxically increase LDL-cholesterol when triglycerides are also elevated. Fibrates lower LDL-cholesterol in the setting of normal triglycerides.

TABLE 33-4	ESTIMATE OF 10-YEAR RISK (FRAMINGHAM POINT SCORES) FOR MEN AND WOMEN

Estimate of 10-year risk for men

Age (years)	Points
20–34	–9
35–39	–4
40–44	0
45–49	3
50–54	6
55–59	8
60–64	10
65–69	11
70–74	12
75–79	13

Total Cholesterol	Points Age 20–39	Age 40–49	Age 50–59	Age 60–69	Age 70–79
<160	0	0	0	0	0
160–199	4	3	2	1	0
200–239	7	5	3	1	0
240–279	9	6	4	2	1
≥280	11	8	5	3	1

	Points Age 20–39	Age 40–49	Age 50–59	Age 60–69	Age 70–79
Nonsmoker	0	0	0	0	0
Smoker	8	5	3	1	1

HDL (mg/dL)	Points	Systolic BP (mm Hg)	If Untreated	If treated
≥60	–1	<120	0	0
50–59	0	120–129	0	1
40–49	1	130–139	1	2
<40	2	140–159	1	2
		≥160	2	3

Point total	10-year risk (%)	Point total	10-year risk (%)
<0	<1	9	5
0	1	10	6
1	1	11	8
2	1	12	10
3	1	13	12

Point total	10-year risk (%)	Point total	10-year risk (%)
4	1	14	16
5	2	15	20
6	2	16	25
7	3	≥17	≥30
8	4		

(*continued*)

Estimate of 10-year risk for women

Age (years)	Points
20–34	–7
35–39	–3
40–44	0
45–49	3
50–54	6
55–59	8
60–64	10
65–69	12
70–74	14
75–79	16

Total Cholesterol	Points Age 20–39	Age 40–49	Age 50–59	Age 60–69	Age 70–79
<160	0	0	0	0	0
160–199	4	3	2	1	1
200–239	8	6	4	2	1
240–279	11	8	5	3	2
≥280	13	10	7	4	2

	Points Age 20–39	Age 40–49	Age 50–59	Age 60–69	Age 70–79
Nonsmoker	0	0	0	0	0
Smoker	9	7	4	2	1

HDL (mg/dL)	Points	Systolic BP (mm Hg)	If untreated	If treated
≥60	–1	<120	0	0
50–59	0	120–129	1	3
40–49	1	130–139	2	4
<40	2	140–159	3	5
		≥160	4	6

Point total	10-year risk (%)	Point total	10-year risk (%)
<9	<1	17	5
9	1	18	6
10	1	19	8
11	1	20	11
12	1	21	14
13	2	22	17
		23	22
14	2	24	27
15	3	≥25	≥30
16	4		

BP, blood pressure; HDL, high-density lipoprotein.

Adapted from Third Report of the National Cholesterol Education Program (NCEP). Expert panel on detection, evaluation, and treatment of high blood cholesterol in adults (adult treatment panel III). National Heart, Lung, and Blood Institute; National Institutes of Health; U.S. Department of Health and Human Services.

TABLE 33-5	ADULT TREATMENT PROGRAM III (ATP III) LOW-DENSITY LIPOPROTEIN CHOLESTEROL (LDL-C) GOALS AND THRESHOLDS FOR THERAPEUTIC LIFESTYLE CHANGE (TLC) AND DRUG THERAPY		
Category	LDL-C goal	Start TLC	Start Drug Therapy
Very high risk	<70 mg/dL	Any LDL-C	LDL-C ≥70 mg/dL
High risk	<100 mg/dL	≥100 mg/dL	≥100 mg/dL (optional if baseline LDL-C <100 mg/dL)
Moderately high risk	<130 mg/dL (<100 mg/dL optional)	≥130 mg/dL	≥130 mg/dL (optional if baseline LDL-C 100–129 mg/dL)
Moderate risk	<130 mg/dL	≥130 mg/dL	≥160 mg/dL
Lower risk	<160 mg/dL	≥160 mg/dL	≥190 mg/dL (optional if baseline LDL-C 160–189 mg/dL)

Adapted from Grundy SM, Cleeman JI, Merz CN, et al. Implications of recent clinical trials for the National Cholesterol Education Program Adult Treatment Panel III guidelines. *Circulation* 2004;110(2):227–239.

- **Ezetimibe** is an efficacious LDL lowering agent, but data on benefit in clinical endpoint studies is limited.[6,7]
- *Step 5: Assess response to therapy and titrate drug therapy.*
  Response to therapy can be assessed every 6 weeks and drug therapy titrated until LDL-cholesterol goals are met.
- *Step 6: Manage the metabolic syndrome.*
  The metabolic syndrome is a common constellation of cardiovascular risk factors affecting around 25% of Americans.[8]

TABLE 33-6	POTENCY OF AVAILABLE STATINS	
Statin potency	Drug name	Expected LDL-C reduction
Least	Fluvastatin Pravastatin Lovastatin	~20%–40%
Mid	Simvastatin Pitavastatin	~25%–45%
High	Atorvastatin Rosuvastatin	~35%–55%

LDL-C, low-density lipoprotein cholesterol.

Adapted from Hou R, Goldberg AC. Lowering low-density lipoprotein cholesterol: Statins, ezetimibe, bile acid sequestrants, and combinations: comparative efficacy and safety. *Endocrinol Metab Clin North Am* 2009;38(1):79–97. Data on efficacy of pitavastatin from Teramoto T, Shimano H, Yokote K, et al. New evidence on pitavastatin: Efficacy and safety in clinical studies. *Expert Opin Pharmacother* 2010;11(5):817–828.

TABLE 33-7	CHARACTERISTICS OF THE LIPID-LOWERING DRUGS			
Drug class	Agents and daily doses	Lipid/lipoprotein effects	Side effects	Contraindications
HMG CoA reductase inhibitors (statins)	Lovastatin (20–80 mg) Pravastatin (20–40 mg) Simvastatin (20–40 mg) Fluvastatin (20–80 mg) Atorvastatin (10–80 mg) Pitavastatin (1–4 mg)[17] Rosuvastatin (5–40 mg)	LDL-C ↓18%–55% HDL-C ↑5%–15% TG ↓7%–30%	Myopathy Increased liver enzymes	Absolute: Active or chronic liver disease Relative: Concomitant use of certain drugs[a]
Bile acid Sequestrants	Cholestyramine (4–16 g) Colestipol (5–20 g) Colesevelam (2.6–3.8 g)	LDL-C ↓15%–30% HDL-C ↑3%–5% TG No change or increase	GI distress Constipation Decreased absorption of other drugs	Absolute: Dysbetalipoproteinemia, TG > 400 mg/dL Relative: TG > 200 mg/dL
Nicotinic acid	Immediate release (1.5–3 g) Extended release (1–2 g)	LDL-C ↓5%–25% HDL-C ↑15%–35% TG ↓20%–50%	Flushing Hyperglycemia Hyperuricemia GI distress Hepatotoxicity	Absolute: Chronic liver disease, Severe gout Relative: Poorly controlled diabetes, Hyperuricemia, Peptic ulcer disease
Fibric acids	Gemfibrozil (600 mg BID) Fenofibrate (various dose forms 135 to 200 mg)	LDL-C ↓5%–20%[b] HDL-C ↑10%–20% TG ↓20%–50%	Dyspepsia Gallstones Myopathy	Severe renal disease Severe hepatic disease

Cholesterol absorption inhibitor[16]	Ezetimibe (10 mg)	LDL-C ↓14%–25% HDL-C No change TG No change	Diarrhea Myalgias	Severe hepatic disease
Omega-3 fatty acids[16]	Lovaza (3–4 g) OTC Fish oils (1–4 g of EPA + DHA)	LDL-C No significant change HDL-C No change TG ↓20%–50%	Eructation Diarrhea Gastrointestinal distress	None

---

[a]Cyclosporine, macrolide antibiotics, various anti-fungal agents, and cytochrome P-450 inhibitors.

[b]May be increased in patients with elevated TG.

LDL-C, low-density lipoprotein cholesterol; HDL-C, high-density lipoprotein cholesterol; TG, triglycerides.

Adapted from the Third Report of the National Cholesterol Education Program (NCEP) Expert Panel on Detection, Evaluation, and Treatment of High Blood Cholesterol in Adults (Adult Treatment Panel III) At-A-Glance Quick Desk Reference available at http://www.nhlbi.nih.gov/guidelines/cholesterol/atglance.htm. Data on ezetimibe and omega-3 fatty acids from Semenkovich CF, Goldberg, Anne C., and Goldberg, Ira J. Disorders of Lipid Metabolism, in press. *Williams Textbook of Endocrinology*. 12th edition ed, 2010. Data on pitavastatin from Teramoto T, Shimano H, Yokote K, Urashima M. New evidence on pitavastatin: efficacy and safety in clinical studies. *Expert Opin Pharmacother* 2010;11(5):817–828.

TABLE 33-8	ADULT TREATMENT PROGRAM III (ATP III) DIAGNOSTIC CRITERIA FOR THE METABOLIC SYNDROME

Patients must meet 3 out of 5 criteria to qualify for the diagnosis of metabolic syndrome

Category	Criteria
Carbohydrate metabolism	Fasting glucose ≥100 mg/dL[a]
Abdominal obesity	Men, waist >40 in; women, waist >35 in[b]
Dyslipidemia	Triglycerides ≥150 mg/dL[a]
	Men, HDL <40 mg/dL; women, HDL <50 mg/dL[a]
Hypertension	BP ≥130/85 mm Hg[a]

[a]Or current use of drug treatment for these indications

[b]For Asian Americans: Men, waist >35 in; women, waist >31 in

BMI, body mass index; BP, blood pressure; HDL, high-density lipoprotein.

Adapted from Grundy SM, Cleeman JI, Daniels SR, et al. Diagnosis and management of the metabolic syndrome: an American Heart Association/National Heart, Lung, and Blood Institute Scientific Statement. *Circulation* 2005;112(17):2735–2752.

○ The defining characteristics of the metabolic syndrome[9] can be found in Table 33-8.

○ It has not yet been established whether the presence of the metabolic syndrome confers a cardiovascular risk equal to or greater than the sum of its individual components.

○ Dietary modification, increased physical activity, and management of cardiovascular risk factors are the cornerstones of therapy.

• *Step 7: Manage elevated non-HDL-cholesterol (elevated triglycerides).*

○ ATP III recommends treatment beyond LDL-cholesterol lowering when triglycerides are ≥200 mg/dL.

○ If triglycerides remain ≥200 mg/dL after LDL-cholesterol goals are achieved, a goal for non-HDL-cholesterol should be set 30 mg/dL higher than the original LDL-cholesterol goal.

○ Non-HDL-cholesterol can be calculated according to the following formula: Non-HDL-cholesterol = total cholesterol—HDL-cholesterol.

○ Non pharmacologic therapy is very important in the management of elevated triglycerides and should include:

■ Encouraging weight loss and exercise

■ Decreasing alcohol intake

■ Controlling hyperglycemia in patients with diabetes mellitus

■ Avoiding simple sugars and very high carbohydrate diets

■ Changing oral estrogen replacement to transdermal estrogen

○ If non-HDL-cholesterol remains elevated despite nonpharmacologic therapies, LDL-cholesterol lowering therapy can be intensified or triglyceride-lowering agents such as fibrates, niacin, or omega-3 fatty acids can be added.

• *Step 8: Manage low HDL-cholesterol.*

• If HDL-cholesterol remains low (<40 mg/dL), niacin or fibrate treatment can be started or intensified.

SPECIAL CONSIDERATIONS

- **Statin intolerance**
  - Adverse reactions to statins can be idiosyncratic and may not occur with a different statin or a lower dose.
  - Pravastatin and fluvastatin appear to have less intrinsic muscle toxicity than other statins and may be useful if patients experience myalgias with other statins.[10]
  - Significant LDL-cholesterol lowering can be achieved with low-dose statins using every other day or weekly dosing if the minimum dose of a daily statin is not tolerated.[11–15]
  - Musculoskeletal complaints in patients on statins are not always due to statin use. These patients should be assessed for hypothyroidism, vitamin D deficiency, depression, and rheumatologic disease.
- **Liver function test abnormalities**
  - Transaminitis with statin use may be transient and mild elevations (<3 × upper limit of normal) can simply be monitored.
  - Changing the statin, lowering the dose, or choosing an agent from a different class should be considered when serum transaminases remain persistently elevated >3 × upper limit of normal).[16]
  - Non-alcoholic steatohepatitis (fatty liver) is not a contraindication to statin use.[16]
  - Statin use can be considered in chronic well-compensated liver disease after consideration of the risk benefit ratio.
- **The elderly**
  ATP III does not place age restrictions on treatment of hypercholesterolemia in elderly adults.
- **Young adults (men ages 20 to 35 and women ages 20 to 45)**
  - ATP III recommends TLC for young adults once LDL-cholesterol level ≥130 mg/dL.
  - Drug therapy should be considered in the following high-risk groups:
    - Men who both smoke and have elevated LDL-cholesterol levels (160 to 189 mg/dL)
    - All young adults with LDL-cholesterol ≥190 mg/dL
    - All young adults with an inherited dyslipidemia
- **Diabetics and other high-risk patients**
  - ATP III recognizes the benefit of statin therapy in high-risk patients and gives clinicians the option of treating with statins even when baseline LDL-cholesterol is not elevated (<100 mg/dL).
  - Niacin can be used judiciously in well-controlled diabetic patients already on antidiabetic therapy, since therapy can be intensified to compensate if hyperglycemia develops.
- **Pregnancy**
  As a rule, lipid-lowering drugs should be avoided in pregnancy and statins, niacin, and ezetimibe are contraindicated.

REFERRAL

- Patients with hyperlipidemia are often managed very successfully by primary care providers.
- Endocrinology referral should be considered in cases of severe dyslipidemias after exclusion and treatment of secondary causes.

MONITORING/FOLLOW-UP

- Fasting lipid panels can be checked every 6 to 12 weeks during medication titration.
- Once lipid goals are achieved, fasting lipid panels should be assessed every 4 to 6 months.
- Transaminases can be monitored with addition or dose titration of statins, fibrates, or niacin and every 6 months once the regimen is stable.
- Other laboratory studies are assessed to evaluate for side effects as determined by symptoms. Creatinine kinase can be checked to distinguish myalgias (muscle pain without muscle damage) from myopathy (muscle pain due to muscle damage) in patients taking statins.

ADDITIONAL RESOURCES

- The ATP III guidelines are available in summary form at http://www.nhlbi.nih.gov/guidelines/cholesterol/atglance.htm.
- The 2004 update to the ATP III guidelines is available in summary form at http://www.nhlbi.nih.gov/guidelines/cholesterol/upd-info_prof.htm.

REFERENCES

1. Third Report of the National Cholesterol Education Program (NCEP). Expert panel on detection, evaluation, and treatment of high blood cholesterol in adults (adult treatment panel III) final report. *Circulation* 2002;106(25):3143–421.
2. Muntner P, DeSalvo KB, Wildman RP, et al. Trends in the prevalence, awareness, treatment, and control of cardiovascular disease risk factors among noninstitutionalized patients with a history of myocardial infarction and stroke. *Am J Epidemiol* 2006;163(10):913–920.
3. Goff DC Jr, Bertoni AG, Kramer H, et al. Dyslipidemia prevalence, treatment, and control in the Multi-Ethnic Study of Atherosclerosis (MESA): Gender, ethnicity, and coronary artery calcium. *Circulation* 2006;113(5):647–656.
4. Baigent C, Keech A, Kearney PM, et al. Efficacy and safety of cholesterol-lowering treatment: Prospective meta-analysis of data from 90,056 participants in 14 randomised trials of statins. *Lancet* 2005;366(9493):1267–1278.
5. Grundy SM, Cleeman JI, Merz CN, et al. Implications of recent clinical trials for the National Cholesterol Education Program Adult Treatment Panel III guidelines. *Circulation* 2004;110(2):227–239.
6. Kastelein JJ, Akdim F, Stroes ES, et al. Simvastatin with or without ezetimibe in familial hypercholesterolemia. *N Engl J Med* 2008;358(14):1431–1443.
7. Baigent C, Landray MJ, Reith C, et al. The effects of lowering LDL cholesterol with simvastatin plus ezetimibe in patients with chronic kidney disease (Study of Heart and Renal Protection): A randomised placebo-controlled trial. *Lancet* 2011;377(9784):2181–2192.
8. Ford ES, Giles WH, Dietz WH. Prevalence of the metabolic syndrome among US adults: Findings from the third National Health and Nutrition Examination Survey. *JAMA* 2002;287(3):356–359.
9. Grundy SM, Cleeman JI, Daniels SR, et al. Diagnosis and management of the metabolic syndrome: An American Heart Association/National Heart, Lung, and Blood Institute Scientific Statement. *Circulation* 2005;112(17):2735–2752.
10. Bruckert E, Hayem G, Dejager S, et al. Mild to moderate muscular symptoms with high-dosage statin therapy in hyperlipidemic patients–the PRIMO study. *Cardiovasc Drugs Ther* 2005;19(6):403–414.

11. Rindone JP, Hiller D, Arriola G. A comparison of fluvastatin 40 mg every other day versus 20 mg every day in patients with hypercholesterolemia. *Pharmacotherapy* 1998;18(4):836–839.
12. Matalka MS, Ravnan MC, Deedwania PC. Is alternate daily dose of atorvastatin effective in treating patients with hyperlipidemia? The Alternate Day Versus Daily Dosing of Atorvastatin Study (ADDAS). *Am Heart J* 2002;144(4):674–677.
13. Jafari M, Ebrahimi R, Ahmadi-Kashani M, et al. Efficacy of alternate-day dosing versus daily dosing of atorvastatin. *J Cardiovasc Pharmacol Ther* 2003;8(2):123–126.
14. Ferrer-Garcia JC, Perez-Silvestre J, Martinez-Mir I, et al. Alternate-day dosing of atorvastatin: Effects in treating type 2 diabetic patients with dyslipidaemia. *Acta Diabetol* 2006;43(3):75–78.
15. Wongwiwatthananukit S, Sansanayudh N, Dhummauppakorn R, et al. Efficacy and safety of rosuvastatin every other day compared with once daily in patients with hypercholesterolemia. *Ann Pharmacother* 2006;40(11):1917–1923.
16. Semenkovich CF, Goldberg Anne C, Goldberg Ira J. Chapter 37, Disorders of lipid metabolism. In: Melmed et al, eds. *Williams Textbook of Endocrinology.* 12th ed. Elsevier; 2011:1633–1661.
17. Teramoto T, Shimano H, Yokote K, et al. New evidence on pitavastatin: Efficacy and safety in clinical studies. *Expert Opin Pharmacother* 2010;11(5):817–828.

Multiple Endocrine Neoplasia Syndromes

34

Shunzhong Bao and Thomas J. Baranski

GENERAL PRINCIPLES

- Multiple endocrine neoplasia (MEN) syndromes are sporadic or hereditary neoplastic disorders of more than one endocrine organ. Broadly, there are two distinct syndromes: MEN1 and MEN2. Each of these syndromes is characterized by complete penetrance but variable expressivity. The main subtypes of MEN2 are MEN2A, with its variant, familial medullary thyroid cancer (FMTC), and MEN2B.
- Both MEN syndromes have an autosomal-dominant pattern of inheritance and provide examples of different genetic mechanisms of tumorigenesis. MEN1 is caused by loss of function or inactivation of a tumor suppressor gene. MEN 2, on the other hand, is caused by gain of function or activation of a proto-oncogene.

Definition

- **MEN1 is defined as presence of at least two of three main MEN1 tumor types: parathyroid, pituitary, and enteropancreatic.** Familial MEN1 is defined as one index case plus one relative with at least one of the three main MEN1 tumor types.
- **MEN2 is subclassified into three syndromes:** MEN2A, FMTC, and MEN2B.
  - **MEN2A** is an autosomal dominant disorder characterized by medullary thyroid cancer (MTC), pheochromocytoma, and parathyroid hyperplasia.
  - **FMTC** is a variant of MEN2A. There is a strong predisposition to MTC but not for the other clinical manifestations of MEN2, such as pheochromocytoma, or hyperparathyroidism.
  - **MEN2B** is an autosomal dominant disorder characterized by MTC, marfanoid habitus, medullated corneal nerve fibers, ganglioneuromatosis of the gut and oral mucosa, and pheochromocytoma; hyperparathyroidism is absent.

Epidemiology

- MEN1 is inherited as an autosomal dominant trait with an incidence of 2 to 20 per 100,000 in the general population (see Table 34-1).
- MEN2 is also a rare autosomal-dominant syndrome with an estimated incidence of 1 to 10 per 100,000 in the general population. It has been identified in 500 to 1000 kindred worldwide. MEN2A accounts for 80% of cases, FMTC for 15%, and MEN2B for 5%.

Etiology

- Multiple endocrine neoplasia 1 (see Table 34-1)
  - The gene for MEN1 has been identified and is located on the long arm of chromosome 11 (11q13). The MEN1 gene functions as a tumor suppressor gene and encodes a 610 amino acid nuclear protein called menin. The complete function

TABLE 34-1	GENERAL FEATURES OF MEN1 AND MEN2 SYNDROMES	
	MEN1	**MEN2**
Incidence	2–20 per 100,000	1–10 per 100,000
Inheritance	Autosomal dominant	Autosomal dominant
Gene	*MEN1* gene	*RET* gene
Gene product	Menin (nuclear protein)	RET (transmembrane tyrosine kinase–linked protein)
Location	Chromosome 11 (11q13)	Chromosome 10 (10q11-2)
Function	Tumor suppresser gene	Proto-oncogene
Type of mutation in tumors	Inactivation	Activation
Genotype–phenotype correlation	No	Yes
Genetic testing guides intervention to prevent and cure cancer	No	Yes

Adapted from Brandi ML, Gagel RF, Angeli A, et al. Guidelines for diagnosis and therapy of MEN type 1 and type 2. *J Clin Endocrinol Metab* 2001;86:5658–5671.

of menin is not yet fully known, although studies suggest it might have a role in transcriptional regulation. Although ~10% of MEN1 mutations arise de novo, more than 400 different germline mutations have been identified.

○ Rare germline mutations in other genes such as cyclin-dependent kinase inhibitor gene have been implicated in MEN1-like syndromes.[1,2]

○ There is no correlation between the genotype and phenotype in MEN1, making genetic screening and rational therapeutic intervention difficult.

• Multiple endocrine neoplasia 2

○ **Nearly all patients with the MEN2 syndrome will develop medullary thyroid carcinoma** (MTC), which is derived from the cells of the neural crest rather than from thyroid follicular cells. Approximately 25% of patients with MTC have one of the MEN2 variants. **Pheochromocytoma is the second most common tumor in MEN2** and is present in ~50% of patients.

○ The gene for MEN2 has been identified and its function well characterized. MEN2 is caused by specific mutations in the RET (REarranged during Transfection) proto-oncogene, located on chromosome 10 (10q11-2), containing 21 exons and encoding a membrane-bound tyrosine kinase receptor.[3]

○ In contrast to MEN1, there is a high degree of correlation between a specific RET mutation and clinical phenotype. Among all, 80% to 98% of cases of MEN2A and FMTC are caused by mutations involving exon 10 or exon 11 that lead to ligand-independent homodimerization of the receptor with constitutive activation and downstream signaling of the mitogen-activated protein (MAP) kinase pathway.

○ In most MEN2A kindreds, one of four cysteine residues (C634, C609, C618, C620) in the RET extracellular domain has been involved.[4]

○ On the other hand, more than 95% of MEN2B cases exhibit a single mutation at codon 918 met to thr mutation in exon 16, and 2% to 3% have a mutation at codon 883 in exon 15 that leads to autophosphorylation and alteration of substrate specificity. Therefore, these are the exons that are routinely screened for RET mutations, and because of the tight genotype–phenotype correlation, both genetic screening as well as curative therapeutic interventions are feasible.[3]

DIAGNOSIS

Clinical Presentation

Multiple Endocrine Neoplasia 1

• Although the presentation can be variable, the three most common features of the MEN1 syndrome are parathyroid, enteropancreatic, and pituitary tumors. Thus clinically, a patient with primary hyperparathyroidism and either a pituitary adenoma or an islet cell tumor is considered to have MEN1.[5] The incidence of MEN1 has been estimated from randomly chosen postmortem studies to be 0.25% and to be 1% to 18% among patients with primary hyperparathyroidism, 16% to 38% among patients with gastrinomas, and <3% among patients with pituitary tumors (see Table 34-2).[5]

○ **Primary hyperparathyroidism** is the most common and earliest manifestation of MEN1 and occurs in nearly 95% of patients by the age of 50 years. Hyperparathyroidism in MEN1, compared to its sporadic counterpart, typically presents around at age 20 to 25 years (vs. 55 to 60 years), with an equal male-to-female ratio (compared to 1M:3F ratio), and involves all four glands (rather than a single adenoma). Although most patients are asymptomatic, they may present with typical symptoms and signs of hypercalcemia (polyuria, myalgias, fatigue, renal stones).

○ **Enteropancreatic tumors** are the second most common tumors and occur in 30% to 80% of MEN1-affected individuals. They can be functional or nonfunctional. Symptoms of hormone excess usually occur by age 40, although with biochemical testing and imaging asymptomatic tumors in carriers can be identified much earlier.

■ **Gastrinoma** is the most common enteropancreatic tumor, presenting in ~50% of MEN1 patients. An initial diagnosis of gastrinoma should suggest MEN1, because 25% to 30% of all gastrinoma patients have MEN1. The tumor causes hypergastrinemia with increased gastric acid output (Zollinger–Ellison syndrome). It is usually multicentric and has malignant potential. More than half of the gastrinomas in MEN1 have already metastasized before diagnosis, although the metastatic tumors in MEN1 are usually less aggressive than sporadic gastrinoma tumors. These tumors account for the major morbidity and mortality associated with MEN1. They are often located in the duodenum and may be associated with pancreatic tumors. Patients may present with peptic ulcer disease, diarrhea, cachexia, and abdominal pain.

■ **Insulinoma** is the second most common enteropancreatic tumor, occurring in ~10% of patients with MEN1 syndrome. Most insulinomas arise spontaneously because <5% of patients with insulinoma have MEN1 syndrome. Patients typically present with fasting hypoglycemia. The finding of inappropriately

TABLE 34-2	CLINICAL MANIFESTATIONS OF MEN1, MEN2A, AND MEN2B

MEN1	MEN2A	MEN2B
Hyperparathyroidism (90%–95%)	**Medullary thyroid cancer (~100%)**	**Medullary thyroid cancer (~100%)**
Enteropancreatic tumors (30%–80%)	**Pheochromocytoma (~50%)**	**Pheochromocytoma (~50%)**
• Gastrinoma (50%)	**Hyperparathyroidism (~30%)**	**Other**
• Insulinoma (10%)	**Other**	• Mucosal neuroma (95%)
• Glucagonoma	• Cutaneous lichen amyloidosis	• Intestinal ganglioneuromatosis (40%)
• VIPoma	• Hirschsprung's disease	• Marfanoid habitus (75%)
• Non-hormone secreting		
Pituitary tumors (15%–90%)		
• Prolactinoma (60%)		
• GH-secreting (acromegaly) (25%)		
• ACTH-secreting (Cushing's disease) (2%–6%)		
• Non-hormone secreting		
Other tumors		
• Facial angiofibromas and collagenomas (70%–88%)		
• Multiple lipomas (30%)		
• Adrenocortical tumors (5%–40%)		
• Carcinoid tumors (3%)		

GH, growth hormone; VIP, vasoactive-intestinal polypeptide.

Adapted from Brandi ML, Gagel RF, Angeli A, et al. Guidelines for diagnosis and therapy of MEN type 1 and type 2. *J Clin Endocrinol Metab* 2001;86:5658–5671; Lakhani VT, You YN, Wells SA. The multiple endocrine neoplasia syndromes. *Ann Rev Med* 2007;58: 253–265.

elevated plasma levels of insulin, C-peptide, and proinsulin in a hypoglycemic patient is highly suggestive of insulinoma. The tumors are usually too small to be identified by computed tomography (CT) or magnetic resonance imaging (MRI), but intraoperative ultrasound usually identifies the tumor within the pancreas. For further details, see Chapter 31.

○ **Pituitary tumors.** Anterior pituitary adenomas are seen in 15% to 90% of patients with MEN1 and are the initial presenting tumors in 10% to 25% of cases. Two-thirds are microadenomas, which are usually functional and commonly secrete prolactin, resulting in the expected symptoms of prolactin excess (amenorrhea and galactorrhea in women; impotence in men). Nearly one-fourth of these pituitary tumors secrete growth hormone resulting in acromegaly, and a smaller percentage secrete adrenocorticotropic hormone (ACTH) resulting in Cushing's disease. The presentation, diagnosis, and management are similar to those of sporadic pituitary adenomas (see Chapter 1).

○ **Other tumors.** Patients with MEN1 syndrome can also present with multiple lipomas, facial angiofibromas, and collagenomas. Adrenocortical tumors, both functional and nonfunctional, occur in 5% to 40% of patients with MEN1.

○ **Hypercortisolism** can be ACTH-dependent (pituitary adenoma or ectopic ACTH syndrome) or ACTH-independent (adrenal adenoma). Although statistically most cases are caused by pituitary adenomas, it is nevertheless important to differentiate between the various causes by biochemical testing (see Chapter 14).

○ **Carcinoid tumors** are present in ~3% of MEN1 patients. Nearly all carcinoid tumors in MEN1 originate in tissues arising from the embryologic foregut. Thymic carcinoids are predominantly seen in males, can be asymptomatic until a late stage, and tend to be more aggressive than in sporadic tumors. Bronchial carcinoids, by contrast, tend to occur mainly in females, can secrete ACTH, and may present with Cushing's syndrome. Gastric enterochromaffin-like cell carcinoids have been found incidentally during gastric endoscopy for gastrinoma in MEN1. Carcinoid syndrome generally does not occur unless the tumor has metastasized to the liver (see Chapter 35).

Multiple Endocrine Neoplasia 2

• The presenting features of MEN2 are largely dependent on the subtype (see Table 34-2). However, the **common underlying feature in virtually all patients with MEN2A, MEN2B, and FMTC is the development of MTC**, which is the most common cause of morbidity and death in patients with the MEN2 syndrome.[6]

○ **MTC** is the first clinical manifestation in MEN2 kindreds because of its earlier and higher penetrance, occurring in nearly all patients with MEN2. MTC is preceded by C-cell hyperplasia (CCH), with resultant secretion of calcitonin, which serves as an excellent plasma tumor marker. CCH progresses to microscopic MTC, followed by local disease (usually multicentric), and eventually by metastatic disease (commonly to lymph nodes, lung, liver, and bones). MTC usually presents as a thyroid nodule and/or increased serum calcitonin.

▪ The severity of MTC depends on the MEN2 subtype. It tends to be more aggressive in MEN2B, usually presenting before 5 years of age and as early as infancy.[6]

▪ By contrast, MTC is the only manifestation of **FMTC** (a variant of MEN2A) and has an indolent clinical course. FMTC presents later in life, with a peak incidence in the fourth and fifth decades. It tends to be less aggressive than the other subtypes of MEN2. The criteria to characterize kindred as having FMTC include MTC in more than 10 carriers in the kindred, multiple carriers or affected members older than age 50, and an adequate history to rule out pheochromocytoma or hyperparathyroidism. Such strict diagnostic criteria are necessary because some MEN2A patients may manifest only MTC and thus be incorrectly designated as FMTC, with the resulting danger of missing a diagnosis of pheochromocytoma.

○ **Pheochromocytoma.** Almost one-half of the patients with MEN2A and MEN2B have pheochromocytoma. Compared to sporadic cases, pheochromocytoma in MEN2 is almost always benign, bilateral, and confined to the adrenal glands and presents earlier in life. If unrecognized, it can present as hypertensive crisis during surgery for MTC early in childhood. The clinical presentation, diagnosis, and management are similar to that seen in sporadic cases (see Chapter 15). The earliest reported age of diagnosis of pheochromocytomas is 12 years old in patients with 918 codon RET mutation.[7]

○ **Primary hyperparathyroidism** is seen in about one-third of the patients with MEN2A, but it is absent in MEN2B. It is usually caused by four-gland hyperplasia, although it is less aggressive than in MEN1. The clinical presentation, diagnosis, and management are similar to those in MEN1 and that seen in sporadic cases (see Chapter 22). It is important to evaluate the parathyroid glands during thyroidectomy for patients with MEN2A because they may be enlarged even though the preoperative calcium level is normal.

○ **Cutaneous lichen amyloidosis (CLA)** can occur in some MEN 2A or FMTC families. This is most often associated with mutations in the RET codon 634. It presents with intensive pruritis and is sometimes difficult to treat. The American Thyroid Association recommends that patients with lichen planus amyloidosis or pruritis in the central upper back be tested for the presence of a 634 codon mutation.[8,9]

○ **Other features associated with MEN2B.** In addition to MTC and pheochromocytoma, patients with MEN2B also manifest a characteristic marfanoid habitus, but do not have lens subluxation or aortic disease.[10]

○ **Ganglioneuromas** occur in 95% of MEN2B patients, which can present at the lips, eyelids, and tongue, giving these patients a characteristic phenotype that can be apparent at birth.

○ **Intestinal ganglioneuromatosis** can occur as early as infancy with gastrointestinal motility disorders. One study reported 90% of patients had colonic disturbances, typically chronic constipation since birth.[9]

Diagnostic Criteria

• **MEN1** is present if the patient has **two of the three main MEN1-related tumors: parathyroid, pituitary, and enteropancreatic.** Familial MEN1 is diagnosed as at least one case of MEN1 plus a first-degree relative with one of the three tumors.[5]

• **The MEN2 syndrome** is diagnosed in a patient with **personal or family history of MTC and positive germline RET gene mutation.** This is a great example of a genetic disorder in which genetic testing allows for early diagnosis and effective prophylactic surgical intervention. In patients who present with a suspicious thyroid nodule, fine-needle aspiration biopsy may establish the diagnosis of MTC.

• **The MEN 2A syndrome** is diagnosed in a patient with **personal or family history of the presence of MTC, pheochromocytoma, and primary hyperparathyroidism associated with a germline RET mutation.** Clinical diagnosis of MEN 2A can be made if at least two of the classical clinical features of MEN 2A are present in the index case or two generations, even in the absence of an autosomal dominant familial inheritance pattern or RET mutation. In the presence of a germline RET mutation and in the absence of any clinical features, that individual is said to be at risk for the clinical features of MEN 2A, and appropriate medical management should be followed.

• **Familial MTC** is a **clinical variant of MEN2A.** There is no other manifestation of MEN2. To prove that a particular kindred has FMTC, it is necessary to demonstrate the absence of a pheochromocytoma or primary hyperthyroidism in two or more generations within a family or to have a RET mutation identified only in kindreds with FMTC. It is very difficult to be sure that FMTC is the diagnosis instead of MEN 2A.

• **The MEN2B syndrome** is diagnosed in a patient with personal or family history of MTC and positive germline RET gene mutation at 918 or 883. The index patient or family member can have clinical manifestation of MTC, pheochromocytoma,

and other **features associated with MEN2B** such as **marfanoid habitus, ganglioneuromas, intestinal ganglioneuromatosis.**

Diagnostic Testing

Laboratories

- MEN1
  ○ The diagnostic tests are the same as sporadic counterparts. Laboratory tests are
    directed to gain evidence for hyperparathyroidism (PTH, total and ionized cal-
    cium), pituitary tumors (prolactin, ACTH, GH, and its glucose suppression tests,
    alpha subunit, TSH), insulinoma(Glucose, Insulin, C-peptide, Beta-hydroxybutyrate,
    Proinsulin, Sulfonylurea, and meglitinide screen), glucagonoma (CBC, a normo-
    chromic, normocytic anemia is common; hypoaminoacidemia), gastrinoma, car-
    cinoid tumors.
  ○ DNA testing in diagnosis or screening MEN1 is still very controversial.
- MEN2
  ○ **Biochemical tests are not required for diagnosis of MEN2**, but maybe useful for
    disease follow-up and diagnosis of hyperparathyroidism and pheochromocytoma.
    Most useful tests are calcitonin, CEA, calcium. The plasma free metanephrines
    and normetanephrines, or 24-hour urine metanephrines and normetanephrines
    are useful tests in diagnosis and follow-up for pheochromogyctoma. PTH can be
    obtained if hyperparathyroidism is suspected.
  ○ Once an index case is identified (any patient with MTC), the individual should
    be referred for **genetic counseling**. The counseling should include, but is not
    limited to, the scope and severity of the disease, responsibility of the competent
    patient or guardian to inform family members for testing, and option of prenatal
    or preimplantation diagnostic testing if patient in childbearing age.
  ○ Most laboratories screen for the five most commonly mutated codons in exons
    10 and 11 (C634R, C609, C611, C618, and C620) for MEN2A, and codons
    918 and 883 for MEN2B. If the initial analysis is negative, then the remaining
    exons can be sequenced.[9]
  ○ **To find a laboratory** that provides specific needs for your patient, go to http://
    www.ncbi.nlm.nih.gov/sites/GeneTests/lab?db=GeneTests. Only if the patient
    tests positive for a mutation in one of these exons should RET molecular genetic
    analysis be extended to the patient's first-degree relatives (parents and children).
    If either parent tests positive, all the at-risk family members should be tested for
    that mutation.
  ○ The main indications for molecular genetic testing include
    - Confirmation of diagnosis of MEN2A, FMTC, and MEN2B
    - Presymptomatic screening of family members at risk
    - Identification of germline mutations to distinguish sporadic from familial MTC
  ○ Given a relatively low false-negative rate (2% to 5%), if an individual tests nega-
    tive for the RET mutation, he or she is not likely to be at risk for development
    of the MEN2 syndrome. In such cases, the patient could have a sporadic MTC
    or pheochromocytoma.
  ○ Less likely is the possibility of a highly unusual or new RET mutation. Although
    entirely replaced by RET mutation analysis for carrier diagnosis, the calcitonin
    test can be used in such situations in which the MEN2 carrier ascertainment with
    DNA testing is not helpful or no RET mutation is detected.
  ○ It is important to note that RET genetic testing does not obviate the need for bio-
    chemical studies to detect pheochromocytoma or hyperparathyroidism in MEN2

patients. In addition, RET genetic testing before symptoms develop cannot identify spontaneous mutations that have not yet occurred.

Imaging
- **MEN1**
  - ○ **Neck ultrasonography** should be done in primary hyperparathyroidism. It has been reported to have a sensitivity of 72% to 89% in detecting solitary adenomas.
  - ○ **99mTc-sestamibi scan**. The sensitivity is similar to ultrasound and is reported to be 68% to 95% in detecting single adenomas. An advantage of scintigraphy is that it can detect ectopic glands outside the neck. Therefore, some favor a combined approach to preoperative evaluation, which has been shown to more accurately predict solitary adenomas than either approach alone.
  - ○ **Pituitary MRI and computed tomography (CT)** should be done if pituitary tumor is suggested. MRI is the single most specific and sensitive imaging technique in diagnosing pituitary mass.
  - ○ Somatostatin receptor imaging with 111-Indium-penetreotide (**Octreoscan**) and **SPECT** has a higher sensitivity than all other imaging modalities in localizing enteropancreatic tumors and is particularly useful in identifying liver and bone metastases.
  - ○ **Endoscopic ultrasound** is especially valuable in imaging small pancreatic endocrine tumors.
- **MEN2**
  - ○ **Neck ultrasonography** by a skilled neck ultrasonographer is mandatory to visualize superior mediastinum and central and bilateral lateral neck compartments in MEN2 patients or suspecting MTC.
  - ○ **Chest CT, neck CT, three-phase contrast-enhanced multidector liver CT, or contrast-enhanced MRI is** indicated if metastatic MTC is suspected.
  - ○ Abdominal or adrenal CT or MRI is required in localized pheochromocytoma. Pheochromocytoma is most present on adrenal glands.
  - ○ Other imaging options used in localizing pheochromocytoma are 123-I-metaiodobenzylguanidine (MIBG) scintigraphy and 111-In-pentetreotide scintigraphy (Octreoscan). For details, please refer to Chapter 15.

Diagnostic Procedures
- **MEN1**
  - ○ The diagnosis and follow-up of MEN1 components are mainly based on biochemical laboratory tests and imaging.
  - ○ Endoscopic biopsy might be useful in diagnosing certain enteropancreatic tumors. Skin biopsy may be helpful in diagnosing cutaneous tumors associated with MEN1, such as angiofibromas and collagenomas.
- **MEN2**
  - ○ Fine-needle aspiration biopsy is safe for the diagnosis of MTC and suspected lymph node metastasis.
  - ○ Several studies have suggested that measurement of calcitonin in the FNA washout fluid from suspected local recurrences and lymph node metastases may have higher sensitivity and specificity.
  - ○ Skin biopsy may be useful in establishing the diagnosis of **ganglioneuromas** in MEN2B **and CLA** in MEN2A.
  - ○ Rectal biopsy or endoscopic intestinal biopsy may be useful in establishing the diagnosis of **ganglioneuromatosis**.

TREATMENT

Multiple Endocrine Neoplasia 1

- Patients with MEN1 are not treated until there is clinical or biochemical evidence of a characteristic disease because there is no genotype–phenotype correlation, and, consequently, there is no rationale for prophylactic intervention in an attempt to prevent the disease. However, a patient with a known MEN1 mutation should be followed closely for evidence of the tumors that are characteristically associated with this syndrome.
- **Hyperparathyroidism**
  ○ The principle and modality in treating MEN1-associated hyperparathyroidism is similar to sporadic hyperthyroidism. For details, please see Chapter 22.
  ○ Parathyroid tumors. The most common surgical approach is either a four-gland parathyroidectomy with autotransplantation, or a 3.5-gland parathyroidectomy. Minimally invasive parathyroidectomy is not recommended, as the hyperparathyroidism in MEN1 patients is invariably due to hyperplasia of all four glands.
  ○ A decrease in PTH >50% from baseline indicates adequate resection of parathyroid tissue. There is a high incidence of recurrence. In one series, 10 years after parathyroidectomy, 50% of the MEN1 patients had recurrent hyperparathyroidism.
  ○ Because calcimimetics have proved effective in the treatment of patients with hypercalcemia from other causes, they also have a role in treating persistent or recurrent hypercalcemia following surgery in MEN1 patients.[11]
- **Zollinger–Ellison syndrome**
  ○ Proton pump inhibitors are the treatment of choice to effectively control hypergastrinemia, but they are administered at double the usual dose (e.g., omeprazole 40 mg orally daily; pantoprazole 80 mg orally daily).
  ○ The role of surgery in management of gastrinoma in MEN1 is still controversial. It is usually reserved for patients who (a) are refractory to or intolerant of medical therapy, (b) have gastrinomas >2 cm, (c) are at increased risk of metastasis (family history), and (d) are free of liver metastasis. Outcomes of surgery are also relatively poor in MEN1 patients (only 16% disease-free survival), compared to those with sporadic gastrinomas (45% disease-free survival).
  ○ Patients with persistent or recurrent gastrinomas after surgery could undergo repeat surgery or medical therapy with five-fluorouracil, octreotide, or interferon.
  ○ For patients with hepatic metastases, surgical debulking and/or hepatic artery chemoembolization may be employed. Chemotherapy with streptozotocin and doxorubicin can also be considered for patients with metastatic gastrinomas. However, observation is often preferable due to the indolent behavior of the metastases in many patients and the relative lack of efficacy of these agents.
- **Nonfunctioning pancreaticoduodenal tumors**
  How and when to have surgery is still very controversial. Most expert advocate surgery to cure or to prevent malignancy transformation and metastasis. If the tumor is >1 cm by imaging, surgery is generally offered. The generally applied operative procedure has consisted of enucleation of tumors in the pancreatic head and concomitant distal 80% subtotal pancreatic resection.[12]
- **Insulinoma**
  ○ Surgery is the treatment of choice for insulinoma and is usually curative. For other islet cell tumors, surgery is still a first-line indication, since medical therapy alone is unsatisfactory.

○ Tumor recurrence is treated symptomatically with agents such as octreotide.
* Other functional tumors, VIPoma, glucagonoma, and somatostatinoma.
  ○ These tumors are very rare, but have a high risk of malignancy. When clinically evident, 30% to 50% patients have metastatic lesions already.
  ○ Radical surgery **is generally** offered. For liver metastases, liver resection, or radio-frequency ablation should be considered to alleviate severe hormonal symptoms.[13]
* Intrathoracic neoplasia
  Benign and malignant intrathoracic neuroendocrine tumors occur in approximately 5% of MEN1 patients. Malignant thymic carcinoid present at an advance stage and are incurable. Prophylactic thymectomy at the time of parathyroidectomy is not totally preventive.[14]
* **Pituitary and other tumors**
  The treatment for MEN1 patients with these tumors, as well as those with carcinoid or adrenocortical tumors, is similar to that for patients who develop these tumors sporadically. After medical or surgical treatment, patients should be followed for recurrence or persistent disease, as is usually done.

Multiple Endocrine Neoplasia 2

* **Medullary thyroid carcinoma**
  ○ The decision to perform **prophylactic thyroidectomy** in MEN2 patients should be based on the results of RET mutation testing, rather than on biochemical (calcitonin) testing. This recommendation is derived from the fact that there is not only a clear relationship between the particular RET codon mutation and aggressiveness of the MTC, but that early detection and intervention can significantly alter the clinical course of MTC. Therefore, the timing of prophylactic thyroidectomy is dependent on the risk-group stratification based on the RET codon mutation.
  ○ In patients >5 years old with MEN2A or FMTC with thyroid nodules <5 mm on neck ultrasound and serum calcitonin <40 pg/mL, a total thyroidectomy without prophylactic lymph node dissection is recommended.[9]
  ○ In MEN2B patients >1 year with thyroid nodules <5 mm on ultrasound and serum calcitonin level <40 pg/mL, a total thyroidectomy with a prophylactic central neck dissection without lateral compartment neck dissection is recommended.
  ○ **For clinically apparent diseases**, the preoperative evaluation should include basal calcitonin, CEA, and calcium (albumin corrected or ionized) and RET proto-oncogene mutation analysis. Preoperative screening for pheochromocytoma should begin by age 8 for MEN2B and mutated RET codon of 634 and 630, and by age 20 for other RET mutations.[9]
  ○ For patients with local lymph node metastases, or calcitonin >400 pg/dL, further imaging tests such as preoperative chest CT, neck CT, and three-phase contrast-enhanced multidetector liver CT or contrast-enhanced MRI can be considered.
  ○ For limited local metastatic disease to regional lymph nodes in the central compartment, a total thyroidectomy coupled with level VI compartmental dissection is appropriate.
  ○ For presence of extended metastatic disease, less aggressive neck surgery may be appropriate to preserve speech, swallowing, and parathyroid function while maintaining regional disease control to prevent central neck morbidity. These patients should be referred to a well-designed clinical trial.

○ After thyroidectomy, patients are followed with serial calcitonin measurements, as it is often the first index of persistent or recurrent MTC. Local disease can be surgically resected, whereas widespread metastases are difficult to cure since conventional chemotherapy or radiotherapy is not very effective.[15]

• **Pheochromocytoma**

Treatment of pheochromocytoma in MEN2 is similar to that in sporadic cases (see Chapter 15). If a pheochromocytoma is detected at the same time as MTC, adrenalectomy should be performed before thyroidectomy with appropriate adrenergic blockade to avoid intraoperative catecholamine crisis. Laparoscopic adrenalectomy is the recommended surgical approach.

• **Hyperparathyroidism**

○ Those at risk for hyperparathyroidism (with mutations in codons 611, 618, 620, and 634) should be screened annually with ionized calcium and intact PTH, starting at age 15.

○ Hyperparathyroidism is managed with subtotal parathyroidectomy or total parathyroidectomy with autotransplantation. If parathyroid hyperplasia is found at the time of thyroidectomy, this should be considered as hyperparathyroidism even in the absence of biochemical evidence of disease.[15]

PATIENT EDUCATION

Counseling of patients and family members is an important part of disease management. A genetic counseling referral should be obtained. Useful websites include http://ghr.nlm.nih.gov/condition/multiple-endocrine-neoplasia, and http://www.amend.org.uk/.

MONITORING/FOLLOW-UP

Multiple Endocrine Neoplasia 1

• Once an index case of MEN1 is identified, genetic counseling and testing should be considered but not absolutely required for all family members. The age to start screening is still controversial. Direct DNA analysis for mutations in the MEN1 gene identifies patients who have inherited a mutated allele and are destined to develop MEN1.[14]

• Once an individual is identified as high risk for MEN1 (positive gene test or family history), periodic biochemical screening to detect symptoms related to hormone excess associated with the tumors characteristic of MEN1 should be carried out. However, as mentioned previously, because of a lack of genotype–phenotype correlation, prophylactic treatments have no beneficial role in patients with MEN1.

• On the basis of current consensus guidelines, a proposed screening scheme for tumor expression in a carrier of MEN1 mutation is as follows[16,17]:

○ **Hyperparathyroidism.** Serum ionized calcium and PTH annually, starting at age 8. A neck ultrasonography or sestamibi scan should be considered if biochemical tests are positive.

■ For patients diagnosed with hyperparathyroidism with or without surgery management, measurement of calcium (albumin corrected total calcium or ionized calcium) and creatinine annually may be sufficient. Bone density at vertebra, hip, and forearm every 1 or 2 years is recommended.

○ **Enteropancreatic tumors.** Fasting gastrin and secretin-stimulated gastrin annually starting at age 20. An octreotide scan should be considered if biochemical tests are positive.

○ **Insulinoma.** Fasting glucose with or without insulin annually, starting at age 5 to 20. Selective measurement of pancreas vein insulin during arterial calcium infusion may also be considered based on the clinical picture.

○ **Glucagonoma.** Chromogranin A and glucagon annually, starting at age 20 for other enteropancreatic tumors as indicated, followed up with octreotide scan, CT, or MRI if biochemical tests are positive.

○ **Pituitary tumors.** Prolactin and insulin-like growth factor 1 (IGF-1) annually starting at age 5. MRI if biochemical tests are positive.

• Imaging studies to detect or follow enteropancreatic tumors should be performed every 1 to 3 years depending on the risk and rate of growth. CT/MRI or endoscopic ultrasound are the usual imaging modalities.[5]

Multiple Endocrine Neoplasia 2

• **Medullary thyroid carcinoma**

○ A key issue is to distinguish individuals who have MEN2 from those with sporadic MTC. This is particularly relevant for individuals who present with multifocal MTC with a negative family history. Because MTC is the first clinical manifestation and is the major cause of morbidity and mortality in patients with MEN2A, MEN2B, and FMTC, total thyroidectomy with regional lymphadenectomy is the treatment of choice for MTC whether patients have hereditary or sporadic disease.[18,19]

○ All patients thought to have sporadic MTC should undergo RET mutation analysis as ~40% to 50% of putative sporadic cases have been shown to harbor germline RET mutations.

○ For patients with RET mutation who elect to wait for prophylaxis thyroidectomy, calcitonin, neck ultrasonography should be obtained every 6 to 12 months.

○ For patients who achieve a complete biochemical cure, long-term biochemical monitoring of annual measurement of serum calcitonin is required.

○ For patients with detectable basal serum calcitonin levels postoperatively, basal calcitonin and CEA levels should be obtained approximately every 6 months to determine their doubling time (DT). Ongoing follow-up of these tumor markers and physical examination should occur at one-fourth the shortest DT or annually, whichever is more frequent. The timing of follow-up anatomic imaging may be based on the relative stability of these tests, presence or absence of symptoms, and the location of known or likely sites of metastasis.

○ For patients in a family that meets clinical criteria for MEN 2A or 2B, or FMTC but no RET gene mutation has been found, periodically screening for MTC (neck US, calcitonin measurement) and associated primary hyperparathyroidism (albumin-corrected calcium or ionized calcium) and pheochromocytoma (plasma free metanephrines and normetanephrines, or 24-hour urine metanephrines and normetanephrines) should be done as indicated by the family phenotype. Screening should continue at 1- to 3-year intervals at least until age 50 or 20 years beyond the oldest age of initial diagnosis in the family, whichever is latest.

• **Pheochromocytoma**

○ Screening for pheochromocytoma with annual plasma and/or urinary fractionated metanephrine measurements is done in all MEN2 patients. The age at which to begin the screening also depends on specific codon mutations. Screening should start between age 5 and 8 in families with high-risk mutations (codons 611, 618, 634, and 918), and between age 10 and 15 in those with mutations in less high-risk codons (codon 768). An abnormal biochemical test should be followed by CT or MRI to localize tumors. Some advocate routine imaging every 3 to 5 years, even in the presence of normal biochemical tests.

○ Women with a RET mutation associated with MEN 2 who are pregnant or planning to become pregnant should be screened biochemically for pheochromocytoma.

○ For patients status-post pheochromocytoma resection, biochemical testing should be obtained 4 to 6 weeks postsurgery, then yearly if blood pressure is under control. If bilateral adrenalectomy has been done, the screening interval can be lengthened since extra-adrenal pheochromocytoma in MEN syndrome is very rare.

○ Approximately one-fourth of patients with no known family history of pheochromocytoma may have an inherited disease caused by a mutation other than RET, including mutations in the genes for von Hippel–Lindau (VHL), neurofibromatosis type 1 (NF1), and genes encoding the B and D subunits of mitochondrial succinate dehydrogenase (SDHB and SDHD). Therefore, any patient with presumably sporadic pheochromocytoma in the following clinical settings should be screened for mutations in these genes using a stepwise approach:

- Bilateral adrenal pheochromocytoma without MTC: First screen for mutations in VHL; if negative, then screen for mutations in RET.
- Age <20 with sporadic unilateral adrenal pheochromocytoma: First screen for mutations in VHL; if negative, then screen for mutations in RET; if negative, then screen for mutations in SDHB.
- Age >20 with sporadic unilateral adrenal pheochromocytoma: First screen for mutations in SDHB; if negative, then screen for mutations in SDHD.

• **Hyperparathyroidism**
○ The screening and follow-up is as in MEN1. Hyperparathyroidism is absent in MEN2B patients.

OUTCOME/PROGNOSIS

Multiple Endocrine Neoplasia 1

• The mortality of MEN1 is not well documented. Pancreatic malignancy and malignant thymic carcinoids are the principal causes of disease-related death in MEN1.[20] Our institution reported that nearly half of patients (46%) died of causes related to MEN1 at a mean age of 50. The most common causes of mortality are malignant islet cell tumors (24%) at average age of 46, followed by malignant carcinoid (10%) at age 53 and ulcer disease (10%) at age 56.[20] A report from Mayo Clinic showed 28% patients died of MEN1-related causes, the most common being metastatic islet malignancy (58.8%). The overall 20-year survival of MEN1 patients was 64%, compared to 81% for age- and gender-matched controls.[21]

• Rarely patients died of hyperparathyroidism. Parathyroid malignancy is very rare but is reported.[22] The major problem with hyperparathyroidism is postsurgical recurrence. The recurrence rate for subtotal parathyroidectomy or total parathyroidectomy in MEN1 is as high as 55% in 10 years.[23]

• Malignant insulinoma is the major cause of disease-related death. Malignancy rate is higher with MEN1-associated insulinoma compared to sporadic insulinoma. At diagnosis, more than 50% of patients were found to have metastatic disease.

- Gastrinoma also has high tendency for malignancy in MEN1. The cure rate by surgery is very low (0% to 10%). The majority (50% to 70%) of patients with tumor >2 cm on imaging had lymph node involvement. However, these patients have excellent long-term survival rate without surgery, and even with apparent metastatic disease they have a 15-year survival of 52%.[24]
- Nonfunctioning pancreatic tumor is currently the most common entity requiring surgery.[25] Nonfunctioning tumors account for 35% to 55% of all pancreatic endocrine tumors and most commonly present in the fourth or fifth decade of life. Approximately two-thirds of nonfunctioning pancreatic endocrine tumors are malignant.

Multiple Endocrine Neoplasia 2

- Eventually all patients develop medullary thyroid carcinoma, which is the major cause of MEN2-related death. Using a prior TNM classification system, 10-year survival rates for stages I, II, III, and IV are 100%, 93%, 71%, and 21%, respectively.[26]
- Prophylactic thyroidectomy can potentially cure individuals who test positive for the RET mutation.
- Medullary thyroid carcinoma in patients with MEN2B is more aggressive than in MEN2A or FMTC, and surgery is often not curative.[9] In one large study, death from MTC occurred in 50% of those with MEN2B but only 9.7% of those with MEN2A.[27]
- Pheochromocytoma occurs in approximately 40% of patients with MEN2A and probably a similar percentage in MEN2B. Malignant cases are very rare. No cases of death secondary to catecholamine crisis have been reported.[28]
- Primary hyperparathyroidism occurs in 10% to 25% of patients with MEN2A and is almost always multiglandular. In expert parathyroid surgical centers, the recurrence rate after apparently successful subtotal parathyroidectomy is very low.[29]

REFERENCES

1. Stock JL, Warth MR, Teh BT, et al. A kindred with a variant of multiple endocrine neoplasia type 1 demonstrating frequent expression of pituitary tumors but not linked to the multiple endocrine neoplasia type 1 locus at chromosome region 11q13. *J Clin Endocrinol Metab* 1997;82(2): 486–492.
2. Pellegata NS, Quintanilla-Martinez L, Siggelkow H, et al. Germ-line mutations in p27Kip1 cause a multiple endocrine neoplasia syndrome in rats and humans. *Proc Natl Acad Sci U S A* 2006;103(42):15558–15563.
3. Murakumo Y, Jijiwa M, Asai N, et al. RET and neuroendocrine tumors. *Pituitary* 2006;9(3):179–192.
4. Quayle FJ, Fialkowski EA, Benveniste R, et al. Pheochromocytoma penetrance varies by RET mutation in MEN2A. *Surgery* 2007;142(6):800–805.
5. Thakker RV. Multiple endocrine neoplasia type 1 (MEN1). *Best Pract Res Clin Endocrinol Metab* 2010;24(3):355–370.
6. Wohllk N, Schweizer H, Erlic Z, et al. Multiple endocrine neoplasia type 2. *Best Pract Res Clin Endocrinol Metab* 2010;24(3):371–387.
7. Machens A, Brauckhoff M, Holzhausen HJ, et al. Codon-specific development of pheochromocytoma in multiple endocrine neoplasia type 2. *J Clin Endocrinol Metab* 2005; 90(7):3999–4003.
8. Verga U, Fugazzola L, Cambiaghi S, et al. Frequent association between MEN 2A and cutaneous lichen amyloidosis. *Clin Endocrinol (Oxf)* 2003;59(2):156–161.

9. Kloos RT, Eng C, Evans DB, et al. Medullary thyroid cancer: Management guidelines of the American Thyroid Association. *Thyroid* 2009;19(6):565–612.

10. Eng CE, Clayton D, Schuffenecker I, et al. The relationship between specific RET proto-oncogene mutations and disease phenotype in multiple endocrine neoplasia type 2. *Jama* 1996;276(19):1575–1579.

11. Moyes VJ, Monson JP, Chew SL, et al. Clinical Use of Cinacalcet in MEN1 Hyper-parathyroidism. *Int J Endocrinol* 2010;2010: 906163.

12. Akerstrom G, Hessman O, Hellman P, et al. Pancreatic tumours as part of the MEN-1 syndrome. *Best Pract Res Clin Gastroenterol* 2005;19(5):819–830.

13. Wiedenmann B, Jensen RT, Mignon M, et al. Preoperative diagnosis and surgical management of neuroendocrine gastroenteropancreatic tumors: General recommendations by a consensus workshop. *World J Surg* 1998;22(3): 309–318.

14. Burgess JR, Greenaway TM, Shepherd JJ. Expression of the MEN-1 gene in a large kindred with multiple endocrine neoplasia type 1. *J Intern Med* 1998;243(6): 465–470.

15. Brandi ML, Gagel RF, Angeli A, et al. Guidelines for diagnosis and therapy of MEN type 1 and type 2. *J Clin Endocrinol Metab* 2001;86(12):5658–5671.

16. Falchetti A. Genetic screening for multiple endocrine neoplasia syndrome type 1 (MEN-1): When and how. *F1000 Med Rep* 2010;2(14):M2–M14.

17. Waldmann J, Fendrich V, Habbe N, et al. Screening of patients with multiple endocrine neoplasia type 1 (MEN-1): A critical analysis of its value. *World J Surg* 2009;33(6):1208–1218.

18. Wells SA Jr, Skinner MA. Prophylactic thyroidectomy, based on direct genetic testing, in patients at risk for the multiple endocrine neoplasia type 2 syndromes. *Exp Clin Endocrinol Diabetes* 1998;106(1):29–34.

19. Wiench M, Wygoda Z, Gubala E, et al. Estimation of risk of inherited medullary thyroid carcinoma in apparent sporadic patients. *J Clin Oncol* 2001;19(5):1374–1380.

20. Doherty GM, Olson JA, Frisella MM, et al. Lethality of multiple endocrine neoplasia type I. *World J Surg* 1998;22(6):581–586; discussion 586–587.

21. Dean PG, van Heerden JA, Farley DR, et al. Are patients with multiple endocrine neoplasia type I prone to premature death? *World J Surg* 2000;24(11):1437–1441.

22. Shih RY, Fackler S, Maturo S, et al. Parathyroid carcinoma in multiple endocrine neoplasia type 1 with a classic germline mutation. *Endocr Pract* 2009;15(6):567–572.

23. Tonelli F, Marcucci T, Giudici F, et al. Surgical approach in hereditary hyperparathyroidism. *Endocr J* 2009;56(7):827–841.

24. Norton JA. Surgical treatment and prognosis of gastrinoma. *Best Pract Res Clin Gastroenterol* 2005;19(5):799–805.

25. Lairmore TC, Chen VY, DeBenedetti MK, et al. Duodenopancreatic resections in patients with multiple endocrine neoplasia type 1. *Ann Surg* 2000;231(6):909–918.

26. Cupisti K, Wolf A, Raffel A, et al. Long-term clinical and biochemical follow-up in medullary thyroid carcinoma: A single institution's experience over 20 years. *Ann Surg* 2007; 246(5):815–821.

27. Wells SA Jr, Dilley WG, Farndon JA, et al. Early diagnosis and treatment of medullary thyroid carcinoma. *Arch Intern Med* 1985;145(7):1248–1252.

28. Evans DB, Lee JE, Merrell RC, et al. Adrenal medullary disease in multiple endocrine neoplasia type 2. Appropriate management. *Endocrinol Metab Clin North Am* 1994; 23(1):167–176.

29. O'Riordain DS, O'Brien T, Grant CS, et al. Surgical management of primary hyperparathyroidism in multiple endocrine neoplasia types 1 and 2. *Surgery* 1993;114(6): 1031–1037; discussion 1037–1039.

Carcinoid Syndrome

35

Judit Dunai and Thomas J. Baranski

GENERAL PRINCIPLES

- **Carcinoid syndrome** refers to the **cluster of symptoms mediated by the systemic release of vasoactive compounds and hormones produced by carcinoid tumors**.
- Carcinoid tumors are rare, slow-growing neuroendocrine tumors (NETs), arising from enterochromaffin cells. They have been reported in a wide range of organs, but most commonly involve the gastrointestinal and bronchopulmonary tracts.[1–3]
- Carcinoid tumors contain neurosecretory granules that synthesize, store, and release substances, such as serotonin, histamine, prostaglandin, kallikrein, bradykinin, substance P, gastrin, corticotropin as well as many others.[3,4] The most prominent of these substances is serotonin (5-hydroxytryptamine), the degradation of which results in 5-hydroxyindoleacetic acid (5-HIAA), which is excreted in the urine.
- The liver inactivates the bioactive products of carcinoid tumors and hence the carcinoid syndrome is not seen in most cases until hepatic metastases has occurred.[1]
- Most carcinoid tumors are discovered incidentally. Carcinoid tumors commonly present with nonspecific findings due to local mass effect and their diagnosis is challenging. The **classic carcinoid syndrome (flushing, diarrhea, wheezing, right-sided heart disease) is only seen in about 10% of the cases**.
- Most carcinoid tumors have metastasized at the time of presentation. Therefore, management requires a multidisciplinary approach that focuses on symptom management and surgical removal of tumor burden.
- Although originally named for their presumed indolent nature as "carcinoid", meaning carcinoma-like, these tumors are no longer thought to be benign.
- Patients with NETs have an increased incidence of synchronous nonendocrine malignancy.[2]

Epidemiology

- The overall prevalence of carcinoid tumors in the United States is estimated to be 1 to 2 cases per 100,000 persons. However, considering their indolent nature, the true incidence and prevalence is difficult to assess and it is likely to be higher.
- According to the Surveillance Epidemiology and End Results (SEER) database, the incidence of these tumors has increased over the last 30 years. Whether this is a reflection of advanced imaging techniques and better reporting or a true increase is unclear.[4]
- Risk factors include female sex, African American ancestry, smoking and family history of MEN1 or neurofibromatosis.[2]

Historical Aspects

- The term *karzinoide* was first introduced by Oberndorffer in 1907 to describe intestinal tumors that histologically resembled carcinomas but did not behave in their aggressive manner. Recognition of the endocrine-related properties of these tumors occurred several years later.

- In 1948, Rapport isolated serotonin and, a year later, Lembeck confirmed that this substance was responsible for carcinoid syndrome in a patient with ileal carcinoid tumor.

CLASSIFICATION

- Historically, carcinoid tumors were classified according to their embryologic site of origin into carcinoids of the **foregut** (15%; bronchi, stomach, thymus and duodenum), **midgut** (75%; small intestine, appendix, proximal large bowel), and **hindgut** (15%; distal colon, rectum). This classification emphasized the clinicopathologic differences between tumors of various locations, but has proven to be too imprecise in predicting the tumor's behavior and prognosis and is no longer used.
- In 2000, the World Health Organization (WHO) presented new classifications based on site of origin and differentiation.[4] This classification is clinically and prognostically more useful, providing information about tumor behavior and therapeutic consequences.
  - *Well-differentiated endocrine tumor*—Ki67 < 2% (a proliferation grade), absent cytologic atypia, and angioinvasion
  - *Well-differentiated endocrine carcinoma*—Ki67 > 2%, evidence of lymphovascular invasion, presence of metastasis
  - *Poorly differentiated endocrine carcinoma*—Ki67 > 15%, cellular atypia, necrosis
  - *Mixed exocrine—endocrine tumors* and *tumor-like lesions*—previously termed adenocarcinoid.
- More than 55% of carcinoid tumors are located in the gastrointestinal tract and ~30% are in the bronchopulmonary system.
- Within the gastrointestinal tract, carcinoids of the small intestine (ileum) are the most common (45%), followed by tumors of the rectum (20%), appendix (17%), colon (11%), and stomach (7%).[1]

Histology

- "*Typical*" carcinoids have a characteristic histologic appearance of monotonous sheets of small round cells with uniform nuclei and cytoplasm without pleomorphism or mitoses. "*Atypical*" carcinoids have features associated with more aggressive behavior, such as greater nuclear atypia, higher mitotic rates, and/or necrosis.[5]
- On electron microscopy, the cells in most tumors have membrane bound secretory granules which contain a variety of biogenic amines and hormones characteristic of NETs.[1]
- They are positive for immunohistochemical staining for one or more neuroendocrine markers such as **chromogranin A** and **synaptophysin**; this **confirms the diagnosis**.[1]
- The proliferation potential is evaluated with staining for the proliferation marker Ki67 which is expressed as a percentage.

Pathology
Molecular Pathogenesis

- The molecular pathogenesis of carcinoid tumors is incompletely understood.
- Most gastrointestinal (GI) carcinoids are sporadic and may exhibit a loss of heterozygosity of chromosome 18.[4]

- Sporadic foregut carcinoids, as well as those associated with multiple endocrine neoplasia 1 (MEN1) (primary hypergastrinemia [Zollinger–Ellison syndrome]), display allelic losses at chromosome 11q13.[2,6] Somatic *MEN1* gene mutations have also been reported in one-third of sporadic foregut tumors.
- Duodenal carcinoid tumors (localized in or close to the ampulla of Vater) produce somatostatin and are associated with neurofibromatosis-1. The NF_1 gene is located on chromosome 17q11.2.[2]
- For midgut carcinoids, the major areas of chromosomal loss are 18q (54%), 9p (15%), 11q (13%), and 16q (12%).
- Bronchial carcinoids are associated with mutations of the *p53* tumor suppressor gene and abnormal expression of proteins involved in apoptosis, including Bcl-2 and Bax.
- The expression of various growth factors (basic fibroblast growth factor, vascular endothelial growth factor, transforming growth factor α and β, trefoil peptides, and platelet-derived growth factor) and some of their receptors has also been reported in carcinoid tumors.

Biochemistry
- Midgut carcinoids contain the enzyme dopa decarboxylase, which converts 5-hydroxytryptophan (5-HTP) into serotonin (5-HT).[7]
- Foregut and hindgut carcinoids lack dopa decarboxylase and cannot synthesize serotonin. Foregut carcinoids often secrete histamine, while hindgut tumors tend to be hormonally silent.
  - Serotonin is largely responsible for the classic symptoms of carcinoid syndrome, including diarrhea, bronchospasm. The cause of flushing is uncertain, but has been attributed to prostaglandins, kinins and serotonin.[8]

DIAGNOSIS

- Symptoms of the carcinoid syndrome vary in intensity and timing and are usually vague, nonspecific, and organ-related, causing relatively long delays in diagnosis. The average time from symptom onset to diagnosis is more than 9 years.
- The differential diagnosis for carcinoid syndrome is listed in Table 35-1.
- **Many carcinoid tumors are found incidentally** during surgery for other reasons, usually at appendectomy (1 of 300 appendectomies) or surgery for acute pancreatitis, or surgery for bowel obstruction or diseases of the female reproductive tract.
- Small bowel carcinoids commonly metastasize to mesenteric lymph nodes, causing fibrosis, and contraction of the mesentery, which in turn leads to kinking of the bowel resulting in intermittent bowel obstruction. Also mesenteric vessels can become occluded leading to intermittent ischemia, causing abdominal pain, nausea, and vomiting.[1]
- Occasionally, a carcinoid tumor can be the lead point for an intermittent intestinal intussusception.
- The lungs and liver metabolize many of the substances secreted by carcinoid tumors, thereby preventing their release into the systemic circulation until metastases develop. This may explain why patients who have carcinoid tumors typically have the syndrome only if they have hepatic metastases. However, extraintestinal carcinoids can cause carcinoid syndrome in the absence of hepatic metastasis.[4]

TABLE 35-1 DIFFERENTIAL DIAGNOSIS OF CARCINOID SYNDROME

Flushing

Physiologic
- Menopause, hot drinks, anxiety disorder, benign cutaneous flushing

Medications
- Diltiazem, amyl nitrate, nicotinic acid, levodopa, bromocriptine, alcohol plus disulfiram

Diseases
- Systemic mastocytosis, basophilic chronic granulocytic leukemia, VIPoma, pheochromocytoma, medullary carcinoma of the thyroid, renal cell carcinoma, diencephalic seizures

Diarrhea
- Gastroenteritis, inflammatory bowel disease, infectious colitis, VIPoma, laxative abuse

Bronchospasm
- Asthma, anaphylaxis, pulmonary edema, bronchial foreign body

Valvular heart disease
- Rheumatic heart disease, subacute bacterial endocarditis, dilated cardiomyopathy, ischemic heart disease with papillary muscle dysfunction

Adapted from Robertson RG, et al. Carcinoid tumors. *Am Fam Physician* 2006;74:429–434; Sitaraman SV, Goldfinger SE. The carcinoid syndrome. In: Rose BD, ed. *UpToDate*, Waltham, MA: UpToDate; 2007.

- Carcinoid syndrome occurs in only 10% of all patients with carcinoid tumor, and it is most often associated with midgut tumors, whereas bronchial and other extraintestinal carcinoids rarely cause the syndrome.

Signs and Symptoms

- **Flushing** is usually dry without diaphoresis and occurs in 85% of patients with carcinoid syndrome, usually of faint pink to red color and involves the face and upper trunk down to the nipples.
  - Flushing is initially provoked by alcohol and food containing tyramines (blue cheese, chocolate, red wine). With time, flushing may occur spontaneously.
  - It typically lasts for 1 to 5 minutes and may occur many times per day.
  - Flushing associated with foregut tumors is more intense, lasts for hours, is frequently followed by telangiectasias, and involves the upper trunk and the limbs.
- **Diarrhea** is usually secretory (watery, nonbloody) and persists with fasting.
  - Stools may vary from a few to >30/day and can be explosive. If accompanied by severe abdominal cramping, diarrhea could be due to mesenteric fibrosis.
  - Diarrhea is usually not temporally related to flushing episodes.
- **Bronchospasm**—Among all, 10% to 20% of patients with carcinoid syndrome have wheezing and dyspnea, often during flushing episodes.
- **Carcinoid heart disease**—carcinoid heart disease can be seen in 60% to 70% of patients with metastatic carcinoid tumors.
  - It is characterized by fibrous thickening of the endocardium, valve leaflets, atria, and ventricles.

- ○ Valvular heart disease is the most common pathologic feature, with tricuspid valve regurgitation and pulmonary valve stenosis seen in 97% and 88% of patients, respectively.
- ○ Clinical manifestations are those of right-sided valvular heart disease and include peripheral edema, ascites, and pulsatile hepatomegaly.
- **Carcinoid crisis**—carcinoid crisis is a life-threatening form of carcinoid syndrome that is triggered by specific events such as anesthesia, surgery, or chemotherapy, which presumably stimulates the release of an overwhelming amount of vasoactive compounds.
  - ○ Symptoms include flushing with extreme changes in blood pressure, and may also include arrhythmias, bronchospasm, and altered mental status.
- **Other manifestations**—pellagra dermatisis (hyperkeratosis and pigmentation), Peyronie's disease of the penis, occlusion of the mesenteric arteries and veins, and intraabdominal/retroperitoneal fibrosis leading to intestinal and/or urethral obstruction may also be present.
- Rarely, carcinoid tumors of foregut or of hindgut origin can cause bone metastases. These tumors can secrete corticotropin-releasing hormone (CRH) and adrenocorticotropic hormone (ACTH) resulting in ectopic Cushing's syndrome, or growth hormone resulting in acromegaly.

Biochemical Testing

- Given the various other conditions apart from the carcinoid syndrome that result in diarrhea or flushing, one must verify that the presenting symptoms are due to an actively secreting carcinoid tumor.
- The most useful initial screening test for carcinoid syndrome is a measure of **24-hour urinary excretion of 5-HIAA**. The 5-HT released by functional tumors is metabolized by monoamine oxidase to 5-HIAA, which can be measured in the urine. This test has a sensitivity of 73% and specificity of nearly 100%.[1]
  - ○ The low sensitivity is not surprising, given that many carcinoid tumors, do not secrete 5-HT. The normal range of 5-HIAA excretion is <6 mg/day.
  - ○ **Most patients with the carcinoid syndrome have urinary 5-HIAA levels >100 mg/day;** in one study the range was from 99 to 2070 mg/day.[9] However, in other patients with the carcinoid syndrome, only modest elevations (up to 30 mg/day) are seen, comparable to that observed in patients with celiac sprue, Whipple's disease, or after the ingestion of high tryptophan-containing foods.
  - ○ Before ordering the measurement of urinary 5-HIAA, it is critical to note factors that can lead to false-positive test results (Table 35-2).
- 5-HIAA levels appear to correlate well with tumor mass, and can be used as a marker for the extent of disease and to follow response to treatment.
- Although urinary 5-HIAA excretion is useful in patients with midgut carcinoid tumors, this test may not be useful in patients with suspected foregut carcinoids that lack the enzyme needed to convert 5-hydroxytryptophan (5-HPT) to 5-HT.[5] Consequently, foregut carcinoids will have high levels of 5-HPT. This metabolite, however, cannot be accurately measured in clinical laboratories within the United States currently, and, therefore, other studies need to be performed to directly localize the tumor.
- Another commonly used biomarker is **chromogranin A (CgA)**. It is a glycoprotein secreted by NETs along with other hormones. Unlike 5-HIAA, plasma CgA testing does not rely on serotonin secretion and can detect nonsecreting tumors.[10]
  - ○ It is a sensitive marker of carcinoid tumors but has poor specificity.

TABLE 35-2 SOURCES OF ERROR IN URINARY 5-HIAA TESTING

False-positive

Foods
- Avocados, pineapples, bananas, kiwi fruit, plums, eggplant, walnuts, pecans

Drugs
- Nicotine, caffeine, acetaminophen, guafenesin, phenobarbital, reserpine, ephedrine, phentolamine, fluorouracil, melphalan

False-negative

Drugs
- Ethanol, aspirin, isoniazid, heparin, monoamine oxidase inhibitors, corticotropin, imipramine, levodopa, methyldopa, phenothiazines

- False-positive results may be seen in renal and liver failure, inflammatory bowel disease, physical stress and trauma, and hypergastrinemia caused by achlorhydria (e.g., chronic use of proton pump inhibitors, atrophic gastritis, or retained gastric antrum).
- A false-positive rate of 40% is also seen in patients with multiple myeloma.
  - Due to its poor specificity and possibility of false-positive results, CgA measurements are not generally used for the diagnosis of the carcinoid syndrome. Nevertheless, it is a good marker of tumor progression and can be used to monitor treatment. An increased CgA level has been shown to be an independent predictor of poor overall survival and correlates with tumor burden (except in gastrinoma).
- According to recent reports, **whole blood serotonin** concentration can be used when urinary 5-HIAA yields equivocal results, although the specificity of this test is undetermined. In addition, several factors can affect total blood serotonin levels. Selective serotonin reuptake inhibitors (SSRI) reduce blood serotonin concentrations, whereas paragangliomas, such as extra-adrenal pheochromocytomas, can increase serotonin levels.
- If the preceding biochemical tests are normal or only marginally elevated in a patient who describes obvious flushing and other features of the carcinoid syndrome, **provocative testing with epinephrine** (starting at 2 mcg intravenous boluses up to a maximum of 10 mcg) **or intravenous pentagastrin** (0.06 mg/kg body weight) might be considered, both of which have nearly 100% sensitivity.[11]
  - The test is considered positive if the patient has flushing, hypotension, and tachycardia that appear between 45 and 120 seconds after an injection and lasts for at least 1 minute. The test is stopped after the first positive response.
  - The advantage of the pentagastrin provocation test over the epinephrine test is that it induces flushing in patients with either foregut or midgut tumors.[12]

Imaging
- Once the biochemical diagnosis of carcinoid syndrome is confirmed, the tumor must be localized. Using a combination of imaging modalities is often the most helpful.[1]
- **Abdominal CT scanning is the diagnostic procedure of choice for tumor staging**, as it identifies the primary tumor and mesenteric lymph node enlargement.
  - Triphasic CT of the liver should be considered because the liver is the most common site for metastasis.

○ Carcinoids that have infiltrated have a characteristic CT appearance that is spiculated with a stellate pattern.

○ The combination of single photon emission CT (SPECT) and CT allows hybrid imaging and has 100% sensitivity compared to 80% sensitivity with CT alone.[4]

• The presence of somatostatin receptors in carcinoid tumors has allowed the use of **indium-111 octreotide scintigraphy** for tumor imaging. This test has >90% sensitivity in patients with carcinoid syndrome and 80% to 90% sensitivity in asymptomatic patients.

○ Specificity is lower because scintigraphy is positive in many other tumors, granulomas, and autoimmune diseases. Also, a smaller number (approximately 60%) of atypical carcinoids express somatostatin receptors. Therefore, abdominal CT and scintigraphy have complementary roles in localization procedures, with the added advantage of octreoscan in predicting responses to octreotide therapy.[1]

• Other modalities such as MRI (sensitive for detecting extrahepatic disease), endoscopic ultrasound/intraoperative ultrasound, and video capsule endoscopy are usually reserved for those patients with suspected carcinoid tumors that have not been localized by CT or the octreoscan.

• Chest CT scan can be used to localize bronchial carcinoid tumors, and echocardiography can help in establishing the severity of carcinoid heart disease.

• Imaging by PET is not routinely recommended, but as neuroendocrine markers become available, it has the potential to become a highly sensitive technique.[13]

TREATMENT

The key management issues in patients with carcinoid tumors include symptom control, biochemical control (lowering or normalizing 5-HIAA levels), objective tumor control, and improvement of quality of life.

Surgical Management

• Surgery plays an important role in the management of patients with small bowel carcinoids even for those with metastatic disease.[4,14]

• Resection of the primary tumor and nodal metastasis can help relieve symptoms of gastrointestinal obstruction and ischemia.[13]

• For **appendiceal carcinoid tumors**, size has been shown to be the best predictor of prognosis.[1]

○ According to current guidelines tumors <1 cm can be treated with appendectomy alone.

○ Tumors larger than 2 cm or those with lymphatic invasion, high proliferative index, and positive tumor margins require right hemicolectomy.[15]

○ Management of tumors between 1 and 2 cm is controversial. More aggressive management is usually employed for the young and for those with mesoappendiceal involvement.

• **Carcinoid tumors of the small intestine** can metastasize irrespective of size.

○ They are generally removed by small bowel resection with removal of involved mesentery and mesenteric lymph nodes.

○ Resection of the primary tumor should be accompanied by careful evaluation for synchronous tumors or metastasis, which is seen in up to 40% of patients with midgut carcinoids.[13]

- Radical excision of the rectum is recommended for **rectal carcinoids** and radical colectomy for **colonic carcinoids**.
- **Bronchial carcinoids** are usually removed surgically.

Metastatic Disease
- More than 90% of patients with the carcinoid syndrome have metastatic disease (except bronchial and ovarian tumors, which may cause symptoms without metastasis).
  - Potentially curative surgery can be offered to the rare patient with resectable hepatic or isolated brain metastasis, or to patients with bronchial and ovarian carcinoids. For others, cytoreductive resection should be considered.[14,16]
  - The goals of palliative surgery in patients with metastatic disease include stabilization of symptoms and lowering of 5-HIAA levels. Hepatic arterial embolization represents an alternate cytoreductive option for those who are not surgical candidates.
- Intraoperative **carcinoid crisis** is a rare but serious potential complication that can be precipitated by surgery or anesthesia. Therefore, pre- and intraoperative somatostatin analogue administration is required in patients with functional carcinoids.[13]

Medical Management

- **Somatostatin analogues** (SSA) are the mainstay of symptomatic therapy in patients with carcinoid syndrome.[17] Sandostatin and Lanreotide have demonstrated symptomatic relief in 50% to 70% of patients and biochemical response in 40% to 60% of patients.[1]
  - A depot form of octreotide LAR can be administered more conveniently on a monthly basis. Studies have shown equal efficacy with both lanreotide SR and octreotide.
  - Tachyphylaxis is commonly seen after about 12 months and can be overcome with a higher dose or with the addition of interferon-α.
  - Side effects include nausea, abdominal pain, vomiting, and diarrhea but usually resolve within a few days.
  - Cholelithiasis and biliary sludge can develop as a long-term complication in up to 50% of patients because octreotide reduces postprandial gallbladder contractility and emptying. Prophylactic treatment with ursodeoxycholic acid may help reduce this complication.
  - SSA treatment of asymptomatic patients with elevated 5-HIAA may stabilize the progression of carcinoid heart disease.
- The role of SSA in nonfunctional tumors is controversial. Recent evidence from the placebo-controlled, double-blind, prospective randomized study of the effect of octreotide LAR in the control of tumor growth in patients with metastatic neuroendocrine midgut tumors (PROMID) trial demonstrated evidence for ocreotide LAR's utility in tumor stabilization of both functional and nonfunctional tumors.[18]
- Cytotoxic chemotherapy (streptozocin, cyclophosphamide, fluorouracil, doxorubicin) has had limited success in the treatment of metastatic carcinoid tumors.
- Novel agents targeting vascular endothelial growth factor and mammalian target of rapamycin have been demonstrated to have beneficial effects in patients with advanced NETs and are under investigation.
- Specific treatments for the various symptoms of the carcinoid syndrome in addition to SSA are often helpful. Drugs such as prednisone, phenoxybenzamine, and chlorpromazine have shown efficacy for patients with flushing and severe diarrhea. Histamine blockers are useful for gastric carcinoids that secrete histamine.[19]

MONITORING/FOLLOW-UP

- The efficacy of various therapies may be evaluated by the magnitude of their biochemical response (e.g., >50% reduction in urinary 5-HIAA levels) or tumor response rate (e.g., reduction in tumor size on imaging studies).
- There is limited evidence for recommendation for follow-up after resection of a carcinoid tumor. Guidelines from the National Comprehensive Cancer Network include physical examination and history with tumor markers every 6 months for 1 to 3 years and imaging as clinically indicated.[13]
- Routine cardiac evaluation to detect early carcinoid heart disease might improve prognosis.

PROGNOSIS

- Carcinoid tumors are slow-growing, and even with metastases survival is measured in terms of years rather than months.
- Prognosis is based on the location, size, invasiveness, and histology of the primary tumor.
  - The best 5-year survival rates are for appendiceal tumors (~71% to 100%), similar to rectal tumors (~75% to 100%), followed by bronchopulmonary tumors (~75%), stomach (51% to 91%), small intestine (52% to 77%), and colon (33% to 75%).[20]
  - The presence of functional abnormalities of the tricuspid valve and the carcinoid syndrome portends a poorer median survival.
  - Data from the U.S. National Carcinoid Register showed an overall median 5-year survival for all patients of 82%. Median survival in patients with localized tumors was 94%, in those with regional lymph node metastases was 64%, and in those with metastatic tumors was 0% to 27%.[20]

REFERENCES

1. Pinchot SN, Holen K, Sippel RS, et al. Carcinoid tumors. *Oncologist* 2008;13:1255–1269.
2. Arnold R. Endocrine tumours of the gastrointestinal tract. Introduction: Definition, historical aspects, classification, stagingprognosis and therapeutic options. *Best Pract Res Clin Gastroenterol* 2005;19:491–505.
3. Kulke M, Mayer R. Carcinoid tumors. *N Engl J Med* 1999;340:858–868.
4. Pasieka J. Carcinoid tumors. *Surg Clin N Am* 2009;89:1123–1137.
5. Ghevariya V, Malieckal A, Ghevariya N. Carcinoid tumors of the gastrointestinal tract. *South Med J* 2009;102(10):1032–1040.
6. Debelenko LV, Zhuang Z, Emmert-Buck MR, et al. Allelic deletions on chromosome 11q13 in multiple endocrine neopasia-1 associated and sporadic gastrinomas and pancreatic endocrine tumors. *Cancer Res* 1997;57:2238–2243.
7. Richter G, Stöckmann F, Conlon JM, et al. Serotonin release into blood after food and pentagastrin. Studies in healthy subjects and in patients with metastatic carcinoid tumors. *Gastroenterology* 1986;91:912–918.
8. Arai T, Kino I. Histochemical and ultrastructural analyses of glandular differentiation in typical carcinoid tumor of the hindgut. *Pathol Int* 1994;44:49–56.
9. Sjöblom SM. Clinical presentation and prognosis of gastrointestinal carcinoid tumours. *Scand J Gastroenterol* 1988;23:779.
10. Vinik AI, Silva MP, Woltering G, et al. Biochemical testing for neuroendocrine tumors. *Pancreas* 2009;38(8):876–889.

11. Levine RJ, Sjoerdsma A. Pressor amines and the carcinoid flush. *Ann Intern Med* 1963; 58:818.

12. Richter G, Stöckmann F, Conlon JM, et al. Serotonin release into blood after food and pentagastrin. Studies in healthy subjects and in patients with metastatic carcinoid tumors. *Gastroenterology* 1986;91:912–918.

13. Kocha W, Maroun J, Kennecke H, et al. Consensus recommendations for the diagnosis and management of well-differentiated gastroenterohepatic neuroendocrine tumours: A revised statement from a Canadian National Expert Group. *Curr Oncol* 2010;17(3):49–64.

14. Chambers AJ, Pasieka JL, Dixon E, et al. The palliative benefits of aggressive surgical intervention for both hepatic and mesenteric metastases from neuroendocrine tumors. *Surgery* 2008;144:645–651.

15. National Comprehensive Cancer Network (NCCN). Clinical practive guidelines in oncology: Neuroendocrine tumours. 2006 *J Natl Compr Canc Netw* 2006;4:102.

16. Elias D, Lasser P, Ducreux M, et al. Liver resection (and associated extrahepatic resections) for metastatic well-differentiated endocrine tumors: A 15-year single center prospective study. *Surgery* 2003;133:375–382.

17. Oreg K, Kvols L, Caplin M, et al. Consensus report on the use of somatostatin analogs for the management of neuroendocrine tumors of the gastroenteropancreatic system. *Ann Oncol* 2004;15:966–973.

18. Rinke A, Müller HH, Schade-Brittinger C, et al. Placebo-controlled, double-blind, prospective, randomized study on the effect of octreotide LAR in the control of tumor growth in patients with metastatic neuroendocrine midgut tumors: A report from the PROMID study group. *J Clin Oncol* 2009;27(28):4656–4663.

19. Ramage JK, Davies AH, Ardill J, et al. Guidelines for the management of gastroenteropancreatic neuroendocrine (including carcinoid) tumours. *Gut* 2005;54(Suppl 4):iv1–iv16.

20. Rorstad O. Prognostic indicators for carcinoid neuroendocrine tumors of the gastrointestinal tract. *J Surg Oncol* 2005;89(3):151–160.

Polyendocrine Syndromes

36

Prajesh M. Joshi, Kavita Juneja, and Janet B. McGill

GENERAL PRINCIPLES

- Polyendocrinopathy is a heterogeneous group of disorders leading to destruction or dysfunction of multiple endocrine glands and possibly involving other tissues. The pathogenesis may be immune mediated, infiltrative, cellular destruction due to various genetic defects or a combination of these.
- The autoimmune polyendocrine syndromes (APS) are the most commonly encountered of the polyendocrinopathies, and are characterized by loss of immune tolerance to self-antigens leading to autoimmune destruction of endocrine glands and other tissues.
- Thomas Addison was the first to describe the clinical and pathologic features of adrenocortical failure in patients with pernicious anemia in 1849.[1] Later, Schmidt described the occurrence of lymphocytic infiltrates of thyroid and adrenal glands in autopsy specimens of two patients dying from Addisonian crisis (Schmidt syndrome).[2]
- APS (previously autoimmune polyglandular syndrome) can be classified into types 1 (APS1) and types 2–4 (APS2, APS3, APS4). Their features are summarized in the Table 36-1.

AUTOIMMUNE POLYENDOCRINE SYNDROME 1

GENERAL PRINCIPLES

Definition

- Autoimmune polyendocrine syndrome type 1 (APS1)—also called autoimmune polyendocrinopathy-candidiasis-ectodermal dystrophy (APECED)—is a rare monogenic autosomal recessive autoimmune disorder (GenomeNet classification OMIM 240300) consisting of the **classical triad of chronic mucocutaneous candidiasis, hypoparathyroidism, and adrenal insufficiency (Addison's disease)**. APECED develops in childhood and results in tissue-specific autoimmunity, leading to loss of function in multiple organs.
- Apart from the major clinical manifestations, primary hypogonadism, type 1 diabetes mellitus, autoimmune thyroid disease, lymphocytic hypophysitis, chronic atrophic gastritis with pernicious anemia, celiac disease, alopecia, vitiligo, and autoimmune hepatitis have also been reported in APS1. Type 1 diabetes mellitus and autoimmune thyroid disease are seen less commonly than in other APS types.

Epidemiology

APS1 is a rare condition, most commonly prevalent in the Sardinians (1:14,000), Finns (1:25,000), and Iranian Jews (1:9000).[3]

TABLE 36-1	AUTOIMMUNE POLYENDOCRINE SYNDROMES	
	APS-1	**APS-2 (type 2–4)**
Prevalence	Rare	Common
Onset	Infancy/early childhood	Late childhood, adulthood
Genetics	*AIRE* (chromosome21), autosomal recessive	Polygenic, HLA association
Gender	Male = Female	Female > Male
Common phenotype	Mucocutaneous candidiasis Hypoparathyroidism Adrenal insufficiency Ungual dystrophy, enamel hypoplasia	Adrenal insufficiency Type 1 diabetes Thyroiditis
Associated conditions	Hypogonadism Alopecia Vitiligo Celiac disease Type 1 diabetes Pernicious anemia Thyroiditis Chronic active hepatitis	Hypogonadism Alopecia Vitiligo Pernicious anemia Myasthenia gravis Celiac disease Rheumatoid arthritis Sjögren's syndrome

APS, autoimmune polyglandular syndrome; AIRE, autoimmune regulator gene, chromosome 21.

Etiology

• APS1 is caused by mutations in AIRE gene (21.q22.3),[6] which encodes the AIRE protein, a transcription factor exclusively expressed in the medullary thymic epithelial cells. The AIRE protein mediates the expression of peripheral tissue antigens, a function that is required for the deletion of auto reactive T-cells and the establishment of self-tolerance. Mutations in this gene presumably lead to incomplete negative selection and escape to the periphery of self-reactive T-cells, which in turn, initiate the destruction of self-tissues.[7] Approximately 60 types of mutations in AIRE gene have been reported thus far.[8]

• The presence of a mutation in the AIRE gene leads to proliferation of self reactive T-cells and formation of autoantibodies with destruction of affected organs.

DIAGNOSIS

Clinical Presentation

History

• A complete and thorough history including family history is essential for the proper evaluation and management of patients with the APSs.

- Chronic infection of the skin and mucous membranes with *candida albicans* usually occurs as the first major manifestation of APS1, typically presenting in infancy. It is present in 97% of cases by 30 years of age.[8]
- Clinical symptoms of oral candidiasis include soreness, redness, oral ulceration, and white-gray plaques in the mouth. Esophageal inflammation causes odynophagia and substernal pain. Involvement of intestines causes abdominal pain, flatulence, and diarrhea. Infection of skin manifests with rash, chronic onychomycosis of fingernails and toenails and genital discharge. Transformation to squamous cell carcinoma has been reported when oral and esophageal candidiasis is not strictly controlled.[11]
- Hypoparathyroidism is the second most common major component of APS-1 and presents with symptoms of hypocalcaemia including muscle cramps, circumoral paraesthesia, and seizures, as well as airway obstruction when severe.
- Adrenal insufficiency is typically the last major component of the syndrome to develop and presents with symptoms of fatigue, salt craving, weight loss, increased pigmentation of the skin, and mucous membranes and hypotension.
- In some cases, these major components may be preceded by symptoms of chronic diarrhea, keratitis, periodic rash with fever, severe constipation, autoimmune hepatitis, alopecia, and vitiligo.[11]

Physical Examination
- Evidence of mucocutaneous candidiasis, dental enamel hypoplasia, and nail dystrophy are seen in APS1.
- Presence of Chvostek's and Trousseau's signs, muscle twitching and cramping suggest hypoparathyroidism.
- Orthostatic hypotension, fatigue, hyponatremia and hyperkalemia are signs of adrenal insufficiency. Adrenal insufficiency that is not diagnosed for a lengthy period of time may lead to Nelson's syndrome, characterized by high ACTH and hyperpigmentation with characteristic darkening of the palmar creases.

Diagnostic Criteria

APS1: Classic diagnostic criterion consists of presence of at least two of the major components: Chronic mucocutaneous candidiasis, hypoparathyroidism, and primary adrenocortical insufficiency. Confirmation by genetic testing is recommended.

AUTOIMMUNE POLYENDOCRINE SYNDROME 2

GENERAL PRINCIPLES

Definition
- Autoimmune Polyendocrine Syndrome Type 2 (APS2) is characterized by the co-existence of autoimmune adrenal insufficiency with autoimmune thyroid disease and/or type 1 diabetes mellitus. It is more common than APS1. The components may not be diagnosed concurrently; consequently, the entire syndrome may not be manifest until adulthood. The presence of autoimmune adrenal insufficiency and autoimmune thyroiditis was previously termed Schmidt's syndrome. The combination of type 1 diabetes mellitus with autoimmune adrenal insufficiency and/or autoimmune thyroiditis and was called the Carpenter syndrome.[12]

- Patients with the more common organ-specific autoimmune disorders, type 1 diabetes, and autoimmune thyroid disease commonly have co-existing endocrinopathies without the presence of Addison's disease. Hence, some experts have proposed to classify them into APS types 3 and 4.[13]
- **APS type 3** includes thyroid autoimmune disease with other autoimmune diseases excluding autoimmune adrenal insufficiency, hypoparathyroidism, and chronic candiasis.
- **APS type 4** is defined as two or more organ-specific autoimmune diseases that do not fall into either of the above types.
- As in APS1, autoimmune involvement of other organs is not uncommon, and may include primary hypogonadism, type 1 diabetes mellitus, chronic thyroiditis, lymphocytic hypophysitis, chronic atrophic gastritis with pernicious anemia, celiac disease, alopecia, vitiligo, and autoimmune hepatitis.

Epidemiology

- APS2 is has an estimated prevalence in the general population of 1.4 to 2.0 per 100,000.[13] This syndrome occurs in approximately half of the cases of autoimmune Addison's disease.[4] It is three times more common in females. Adrenal failure is the initial endocrine abnormality in approximately half the cases.[5]
- APS3 and 4 are the most common, with prevalence of up to 1% of the population.

Etiology

Familial clustering of APS2 and its component disorders suggest a strong genetic component. Pedigree analyses of most APS2 families suggest polygenic inheritance. The association with HLA alleles in chromosome 6p21 has been recognized with autoimmune diseases for several decades. The class II HLA haplotypes DR3 and DR4 are strongly linked with component disorders of this syndrome. The highest risk of development of both Addison's disease and type 1 diabetes mellitus is associated with a heterozygous HLA-DR4-DQ8/HLA-DR3-DQ2 genotype.[9] Potentially complex interaction between non-HLA loci {cytotoxic T lymphocyte antigen 4 (CTLA-4)} and the environment has also been proposed in pathogenesis of the syndrome.

Risk Factors

- Apart from genetic factors, environmental factors have been associated with APS2. Administration of interferon-α has been associated with development of 21-hydroxylase autoantibodies, islet autoantibodies, and thyroid autoantibodies along with their respective autoimmune diseases.[10]
- Pregnancy is generally associated with decreased immune function; however, postpartum thyroiditis has been observed in approximately one-third of patients with type 1 diabetes.
- Prolamins, or proteins rich in proline and glutamine that resist intestinal peptidases, are known triggers for celiac disease. Gliadin (from wheat), and related proteins in barley, rye, corn, and some oats are implicated in the pathogenesis of celiac disease.
- The hygiene hypothesis proposes that a decline in communicable diseases, especially helminthic infestation, contributes to an increase in the incidence of allergy, asthma and autoimmune diseases.[19]

DIAGNOSIS

Clinical Presentation

History

- Family history and knowledge of increased risks for other endocrine disorders is key to the diagnosis of a polyendocrinopathy syndrome.

- Adrenal involvement is the initial manifestation of APS2 in half the cases. Other components may precede the diagnosis of adrenal insufficiency or follow it by years to decades.

- History of polyuria and polydipsia suggests presence of type 1 diabetes mellitus and weight gain/weight loss, heat/cold intolerance, and constipation/hyper-defection suggests autoimmune thyroid disease.

- Amenorrhea and hot flashes in a young woman should prompt a work-up for ovarian failure, whereas decreased libido and sexual function may suggest testicular failure in males. In both cases, gonadotropins LH and FSH will be elevated, while estrogen and testosterone are low. Specific antibodies have not been identified, so these diagnoses are based on physiologic diagnosis in susceptible individuals.

- Patchy depigmentation of skin, loss of hair, papulovesicular rash, unexplained anemia, chronic diarrhea, or jaundice are typical manifestations of the secondary associated autoimmune diseases including vitiligo, alopecia areata/totalis, pernicious anemia, celiac disease, or autoimmune hepatitis.

- Development of additional endocrine disorders may complicate the clinical picture of the preexisting disease. For example, symptomatic hypotension or hypoglycemia leading to a decrease in insulin dosing in a patient with type 1 diabetes may be manifestations of adrenal insufficiency. In a patient with autoimmune hypothyroidism and APS, an increase in requirement for thyroid hormone replacement to maintain euthyroidism may reflect malabsorption of drug due to the onset of celiac disease.

Physical Examination

- The signs of primary adrenal insufficiency include hypotension, hyponatremia, and hyperpigmentation (see APS1 section).

- Patients with type 1 diabetes mellitus will present with hyperglycemia, generally developing more rapidly in younger patients but more slowly in older patients. (See Chapter 28).

- Slow relaxation phases of deep tendon reflexes and periorbital edema are signs of hypothyroidism, while proptosis, presence of lid lag, and fine tremors suggest hyperthyroidism (see Chapter 8 and Chapter 9)

- Pernicious anemia (PA) may present with anemia or symptoms of peripheral neuropathy. Undiagnosed, PA can cause profound anemia and neurologic symptoms including cerebellar signs and ataxia.

- Vitiligo and alopecia areata are less common components of all of the autoimmune polyglandular syndromes. Vitiligo associated with these conditions is progressive, with a nonsegmental distribution and often occurs at sites of friction and trauma.[14] Alopecia areata presents as patchy non-scarring alopecia and may progress to total loss of scalp hair (alopecia totalis) or total loss of body hair (alopecia universalis).[15]

- Itchy papulovesicular lesions on extensor surfaces suggest dermatitis herpetiformis, which is associated with celiac disease.

Diagnostic Criteria

- **APS2:** Diagnosis requires presence of autoimmune Addison's disease with autoimmune thyroid disorder and/or type 1 diabetes. Autoimmune adrenal insufficiency is the defining component of this syndrome.
- **APS3–4:** The diagnosis rests on the presence of multiple autoimmune diseases in the same individual, diagnosed in any order and at any age.

Differential Diagnosis of Autoimmune Polyendocrine Syndromes

- Several genetic and acquired syndromes include multiple endocrine organ failure or dysfunction. These polyendocrinopathy syndromes are listed in Table 36-2.
- Other syndromes associated with specific autoimmune glandular dysfunction are noted to occur in conjunction with systemic lupus erythematosis, rheumatoid arthritis or other collagen vascular diseases. These include Type B insulin resistance, immune thrombocytopenia, autoimmune neutropenia, and hemolytic anemia.

Diagnostic Testing

Many of the autoimmune disorders that make up the APS have long prodromal phases during which time tissue-specific autoantibodies appear in the serum. The repertoire of autoantibodies present in a given individual serves as a guide to diseases that may develop, as the risk for a given disease tends to increase as the number and quantity of autoantibodies targeting that tissue increases. For example, the 5-year risk of developing type 1 diabetes in first-degree relatives of affected individuals is >50% if multiple anti-beta cell autoantibodies are present.

Laboratory Testing
- The major laboratory approaches to the diagnosis of the APS are serologic tests for autoantibodies against involved glands and tissues, and evaluation of end-organ function and hormone secretion.
- IgG-neutralizing autoantibodies against type 1 interferons, including interferon-α subtypes and interferon-ω, virtually confirm the diagnosis of APS1 when clinical presentation does not fulfill the classic diagnostic criterion and when thymoma and myasthenia gravis have been excluded. Genetic testing to look for mutations in the AIRE gene is now available. A good laboratory can detect mutations in the AIRE gene in >95% of cases.[8]
- Evaluation for the presence of adrenal (21-hydroxylase), thyroid (peroxidase and thyroglobulin), islet cell (insulin, glutamic acid decarboxylase, and IA-2A), and parietal cell (H+/K+-ATPase) autoantibodies (Table 36-3) may assist in confirming clinical suspicion of tissue autoimmunity or in assessing risk for future endocrine disorders, although serologic testing should not replace careful clinical assessment of organ-specific diseases.
- Endocrine organ function should be evaluated by laboratory measurement of appropriate hormones: Adrenal (cosyntropin-stimulation testing, serum electrolytes, aldosterone, and renin), thyroid (thyroid-stimulating hormone and free thyroxine), pancreatic islet (fasting glucose or glucose tolerance testing), parathyroid (ionized serum calcium and intact parathyroid hormone), and gonads (estrogen or testosterone, follicle-stimulating hormone, and luteinizing hormone).
- In a patient with anemia, a low serum vitamin B_{12} level suggests pernicious anemia which can be further evaluated with anti-parietal cell antibodies, anti-intrinsic factor antibodies and serum gastrin level.

TABLE 36-2 POLYENDOCRINOPATHY SYNDROMES

Polyendocrinopathy syndrome	Etiology	Clinical features
Chromosomal abnormalities (Down's syndrome and Turner syndrome)	Unknown	Autoimmune thyroid disease, type 1 diabetes mellitus, celiac disease, autoimmune hepatitis, alopecia areata, vitiligo
DiGeorge Syndrome, Velocardiofacial syndromes OMIM 188400	Microdeletion of chromosome 22q11.2	Craniofacial, pharyngeal, cardiac dysmorphism, mental retardation. Endocrine: hypoparathyroidism, thyroid agenesis and/or autoimmune hypo or hyperthyroidism, type 1 diabetes, ITP, GH deficiency
Hereditary hemochromatosis[22]	Mutation in *HFE* gene	Classical triad of hepatomegaly, diabetes mellitus, and hyperpigmented skin along with congestive heart failure. Other endocrinopathies: hypopituitarism, hypogonadism, hypothyroidism
Hirata's disease, also insulin autoimmune syndrome (IAS)[20]	HLA association with HLA DR4 + drug induction	Spontaneous hyperinsulinemic hypoglycemia. Has been associated with Grave's disease, particularly if treated with methimazole
IPEX (Immune dysregulation, polyendocrinopathy, Enteropathy, X-linked)[16] **OMIM 304930**	Mutation in FoxP3 gene leads to autoimmunity	Clinical triad of enteropathy (severe diarrhea), endocrinopathy (type 1 diabetes or thyroiditis) and dermatitis. Usually develops in neonates. Others: alopecia universalis, autoimmune hemolytic anemia/thrombocytopenia/neutropenia, interstitial nephritis, autoimmune hepatitis
Kearns–Sayre syndrome[21]	Deletion of mitochondrial DNA	Triad of progressive external ophthalmoplegia, atypical pigmentary retinopathy and cardiac conduction defects. Onset before 20 years of age. Endocrinopathy: Short stature, hypogonadism, diabetes mellitus, thyroid disease, hyperaldosteronism, hypoparathyroidism

(continued)

372 PART VII NEOPLASMS

TABLE 36-2 **POLYENDOCRINOPATHY SYNDROMES (*Continued*)**

Polyendocrinopathy syndrome	Etiology	Clinical features
McCune–Albright syndrome[24] **OMIM 174800**	Activating mutation in α-subunit of G-protein-coupled receptor	Characterized by triad of café-au-lait spots, polyostotic fibrous dysplasia, and multiple endocrine dysfunction Endocrinopathy: precocious puberty, acromegaly, prolactinoma, hyperthyroidism, Cushing's syndrome, hypophosphatemic osteomalacia, testitoxocosis
POEMS syndrome[18]	Unclear; monoclonal gammopathy suggests plasma cell disorder, elevated cytokines, and VEGF are common	Polyneuropathy, organomegaly, endocrinopathy, M protein (monoclonal plasma proliferative disorder), skin changes (POEMS) Others: osteosclerotic bone lesions, Castleman's disease, papilledema, edema, pleural effusion/ascites Endocrinopathy: hyogonadism, T2DM, hypothyroidism, adrenal insufficiency, increased PTH
Type B insulin resistance syndrome[23]	Antibody to insulin receptors (not commercially available)	Hyperglycemia, hyperandrogenism, systemic lupus erythematosus (SLE), Hashimoto's thyroiditis, primary biliary cirrhosis, hypoglycemia (rarely)
Wolfram syndrome[17] **OMIM 222300**	Mutation of WFS1 gene	Diabetes insipidus, diabetes mellitus, optic atrophy, and deafness (DIDMOAD) Others: hearing loss, neurogenic bladder, ataxia, dysarthria, dementia, psychiatric disease, other endocrine dysfunction (hypogonadism, hypothyroidism, and growth retardation) occur in this progressive syndrome

OMIM = the GenomeNet classification number.

TABLE 36-3 ORGAN-SPECIFIC AUTOANTIBODIES

Autoimmune disease	Antibodies associated	Diagnostic test
Type 1 diabetes mellitus	Antibody to Glutamic acid decarboxylase (GAD65), antibody to protein tyrosine phosphatase (IA-2A & IA-2β)^a, Insulin autoantibody (IAA), antibody to zinc transporter 8 (znt8)	Fasting glucose, oral glucose tolerance test, hemoglobin A1c
Insulin autoimmune syndrome (Hirata's disease)	Insulin autoantibodies (IAA), either monoclonal or polyclonal	Fasting and postprandial glucose for evidence of hypoglycemia, insulin and C-peptide levels, antibodies
Thyroiditis	Anti-thyroid peroxidase antibody (Anti-TPO), TSI (thyroid-stimulating immunoglobulin), anti-thyroglobulin antibody	Thyroid-stimulating hormone (TSH), free thyroxine (T4), total triiodothyronine (T3)
Primary adrenal insufficiency	Antibody to 21-hydroxylase (ACA), anti-17α-hydroxylase Ab, anti-P450scc Ab (SCA)	Adrenocorticotrophic (ACTH) stimulation test
Autoimmune gastritis Pernicious anemia	Anti-parietal cell antibody Anti-intrinsic factor antibody	Vitamin B12, measurement of antibodies, gastrin
Celiac disease	Antibody to tissue transglutaminase (tTG), anti-endomysial IgA Ab, Anti-gliadin antibody	Measurement of antibodies (in addition to serum IgA), small bowel biopsy
Hypoparathyroidism	Antibody to calcium-sensing receptor	PTH, serum calcium and phosphorus, 24 hour urinary calcium
Autoimmune hepatitis	Anti-nuclear antibody (ANA), anti-smooth muscle antibody, anti-mitochondrial antibody, anti-LKM1 antibody, anti-LC1 antibody	Liver function test, measurement of antibodies, liver biopsy
Hypogonadism	Antibodies to 17α-hydroxylase, P450 side-chain-cleavage enzyme, 3β hydroxyl steroid dehydrogenase, anti-spermAb	Follicle-stimulating hormone (FSH), luteinizing hormone (LH), testosterone, estradiol, progesterone
Vitiligo	Anti-tyrosinase antibody	Wood's lamp examination

^{a}Antibody to transmembrane protein of protein tyrosine phosphatase family is also known as insulinoma associated antigen (IA-2A & IA-2β), IA-2A is also known as ICA512.

- Patients with iron deficiency without a history of blood loss should be evaluated for celiac disease with tissue transglutaminase **IgA** autoantibodies and total IgA level. Endoscopy with small bowel biopsy is necessary for confirmation of celiac disease.

TREATMENT

- At the present time, there are no safe and effective therapies targeting the generalized autoimmunity that underlies the pathogenesis of the APSs. Patients with APS require close monitoring, and the clinician should maintain a high index of suspicion for the development of additional autoimmune diseases in these individuals.
- Therapies for the individual components of the syndromes are discussed in other chapters and the management of each disease is essentially the same for the patient with APS. A few points deserve special consideration:
  - Patients with APS1 and chronic oral candidiasis should be treated aggressively with antifungal medication (fluconazole) and closely monitored given the elevated risk of oral cancers in these individuals. In addition, good oral hygiene and abstinence from smoking and alcohol is helpful to prevent candidiasis.
  - Thyroid hormone replacement in a patient with hypothyroidism may precipitate life-threatening adrenal crisis if concomitant adrenal insufficiency is present. It is wise to evaluate adrenal function by dynamic testing in patients with multiple autoimmune endocrinopathies prior to starting levothyroxine therapy.
  - Pernicious anemia is treated by oral vitamin B12 in high doses or intramuscular injections of cyanocobalamin.
  - Celiac disease generally responds to a gluten-free diet; however, mineral and vitamin supplementation may be required if significant malabsorption persists.

MONITORING/FOLLOW-UP

- A high index of suspicion is required whenever one autoimmune disease is diagnosed in order to prevent morbidity and mortality from other associated diseases.
- Follow up with a specialist, particularly an endocrinologist, is advised.
- Proper psychological and social support is important for these patients.
- Patients should be educated about symptoms of potential new serious components.
- Patients should be provided with appropriate written instructions or should be advised to wear medical alert bracelets in case of emergent situations.

REFERENCES

1. Addison T. Anemia: Disease of the suprarenal capsules. *Lond Med Gaz* 1849;12:535–546.
2. Schmidt MB. Eine biglandulare Erkrankung (Nebennieren und Schilddrusee) bei Morbus Addisonii. *Verh Dtsch Ges Pathol Ges* 1926;21:212–221.
3. Betterle C, Greggio NA, Volpato M. Clinical review 93: Autoimmune polyglandular syndrome type 1. *J Clin Endocrinol Metab* 1998;83:1049–1055.
4. Falorni A, Lareti S, Santeusanio F. Autoantibodies in autoimmune polyendocrine syndrome type II. *Endocrinol Metab Clin North Am* 2002;31:369–389.
5. Schatz DA, Winter WE. Autoimmune polyglandular syndrome II: Clinical syndrome and treatment. *Endocrinol Metab Clin North Am* 2002;31:339–352.

6. The Finnish-German APECED Consortium. An autoimmune disease, APECED, caused by mutations in a novel gene featuring two PHD-type zince-finger domains. *Nat Genet* 1997;17:399–403.

7. Waterfield M, Anderson MS. Clues to immune tolerance: The monogenic autoimmune syndromes. *Ann N Y Acad Sci* 2010:1–18.

8. Husebye ES, Perheentupa J, Rautemaa R, et al. Clinical manifestation and management of patients with autoimmune polyendocrine syndrome type I. *J Intern Med* 2009;265:514–529.

9. Robles DT, Fain PR, Gotttlieb PA, et al. The genetics of autoimmune polyendocrine syndrome type II. 2002;31:353–368.

10. Eisenbarth G, Gottlieb P. Autoimmune polyendocrine syndromes. *N Engl J Med* 2004; 350:2068–2079.

11. Perheentupa J. Autoimmune polyendocrinopathy-candidiasis-ectodermal dystrophy. *J Clin Endocrinol Metab* 2006;91:2843–2850.

12. Kriegel MA, Lohmann T, Gabler C, et al. Defective suppressor function of human CD4+CD25+regulatory T cells in autoimmune polyglandular syndrome type II. *J Exp Med* 2004;199:1285–1291.

13. Betterle C, Dal Pra C, Mantero F, et al. Autoimmune adrenal insufficiency and autoimmune polyendocrine syndromes: Autoantibodies, autoantigens, and their applicability in diagnosis and disease prediction. *Endocr Rev* 2002;23:327–364.

14. Taieb A, Picardo M. Vitiligo. *N Engl J Med* 2009;360:160–169.

15. Shapiro J. Hair loss in women. *N Engl J Med* 2007;357:1620–1630.

16. Torgerson TR, Ochs HD. Immune dysregulation, polyendocrinopathy, enteropathy, X-linked: Forhead box protein 3 mutations and lack of regulatory T cells. *J Allergy Clin Immunol* 2007;120:744–750.

17. Rohayem J, Ehlers C, Wiedemann B, et al. Diabetes and neurodegeneration in Wolfram syndrome: A multicenter study of phenotype and genotype. *Diabetes Care* 2011;34:1503–1510.

18. Gandhi GY, Basu R, Dispenzieri A, et al. Endocrinopathy in POEMS syndrome: The Mayo clinic experience. *Mayo Clin Proc* 2007;82:836–842.

19. Gale EAM. A missing link in the hygiene hypothesis? *Diabetologia* 2002;45:588–594.

20. Uchigata Y, Eguchi Y, Takayama-Hasumi S, et al. Insulin autoimmune syndrome (Hirata disease): Clinical features and epidemiology in Japan. *Diabetes Res Clin Pract* 1994;22:89–94.

21. Harvey JN, Barnett D. Endocrinie dysfunction in Kearns-Sayre syndrome. *Clin Endocrinol (Oxf)* 1992;37:97–103.

22. Utzschneider KM, Kowdley KV. Hereditary hemochromatosis and diabetes mellitus: Implications for clinical practice. *Nat Rev Endocrinol* 2010;6:26–33.

23. Arioglu E, Andewelt A, Diabo C, et al. Clinical course of the syndrome of autoantibodies to the insulin receptor (type b insulin resistance)—A 28 year perspective. *Medicine (Baltimore)* 2002;81:87–100.

24. Dumitrescu CE, Collins MT. McCune-Albright syndrome. *Orphanet J Rare Dis* 2000;3:12.

Endocrine Disorders in HIV/AIDS

37

Scott Goodwin, Paul Hruz, and Kevin Yarasheski

GENERAL PRINCIPLES

- Acquired immunodeficiency syndrome (AIDS) is caused by the human immunodeficiency virus (HIV), which is transmitted by exchange of infected blood, semen, or vaginal secretions through mucosal membranes. HIV targets $CD4^+$ T lymphocytes, where it integrates into the host DNA, replicates, and produces new virions that infect and reduce T-cell numbers. This weakens host immunity and renders the host susceptible to common pathogens.[1]
- Currently, there is no vaccine or cure for HIV. However, since the mid-1990s the use of highly active antiretroviral therapy (HAART) has reduced HIV-related morbidity and mortality so effectively that HIV infection is now considered a chronic manageable infection.[1]
- HIV infection and HAART are associated with several endocrine, metabolic, anthropomorphic, and cardiovascular complications.
- All patients with HIV infection are at risk for endocrine disorders. Reasons include increased inflammation (HIV replication, obesity), AIDS wasting, presence of opportunistic infections, HAART toxicities, immune reconstitution syndrome, genetic risk, and traditional environmental factors.[2]
- In general, the signs and symptoms of endocrine disorders in patients with HIV infection do not differ from those observed in immunocompetent individuals. Please refer to the previous chapters for specific examples of presentations for each given disorder.

DIAGNOSIS

- A full health history should include: Personal or family history of cardiovascular risk factors, autoimmune disorders, duration of HIV infection, history of viral resistance, previous and current antiretroviral therapies, physical activity level and current diet.
- General examination of each organ system (detailed in previous chapters), and query for changes in body composition and fat redistribution (peripheral lipoatrophy, visceral lipohypertrophy, lipomas, "buffalo hump"). **Lipoatrophy** (specifically loss of fat in the face and extremities) and **lipohypertrophy** (visceral adiposity, dorsocervical fat pad, breast enlargement) are common. Skinfold thickness, limb, abdomen, and chest circumference, and the waist-to-hip ratio can quantify/document these changes. Consider **visceral adiposity** when: Waist-to-hip ratio >0.90 in men and >0.80 in women; or abdominal circumference >102 cm in men and >88 cm in women.[3]
- In general, the diagnostic criteria, differential diagnosis, and laboratory testing for specific endocrine disorders in patients with HIV infection do not differ from those observed in immunocompetent individuals. Please refer to the previous chapters for specific examples of the diagnostic procedures for each given disorder.

TREATMENT OF SPECIFIC DISORDERS

The successful management of HIV-infected patients with or at-risk for endocrinopathies requires an integrated approach that addresses predisposing factors, optimal antiretroviral therapies, management of comorbidities, and selective use of pharmacologic agents with awareness of potential drug–drug interactions.

Glucose Intolerance, Insulin Resistance, and Type 2 Diabetes

- In people with HIV, disorders of glucose metabolism are multifactorial: HAART toxicity (especially protease inhibitors), restoration of health with HAART, immune reconstitution syndrome, family history, and body composition changes (including lipoatrophy and visceral adiposity) are all contributing factors.[1]
- Protease inhibitors, especially Indinavir, Lopinavir, and Ritonavir, are associated with increased insulin resistance via blockade of the peripheral glucose transporter GLUT4, as well as increasing hepatic gluconeogenesis and glycogenolysis.[4–6]
- Hypoadiponectinemia is common and contributes to insulin resistance.[2]
- Screen for abnormal glucose metabolism in HIV-infected patients as described in Chapter 29. A fasting blood sugar measurement is simple and cost effective. Oral glucose tolerance testing should be performed for those with risk factors for diabetes. Monitor glycemic control before and after changes in HAART.
- The mainstay of treatment in people with HIV with insulin resistance is metformin with or without a sulfonylurea or insulin. The newer incretin class of diabetic medications have not yet been thoroughly investigated for safety and efficacy in this specific patient population.

Lipid Disorders

- Fasting hypertriglyceridemia and low high-density lipoprotein (HDL) cholesterol levels are the most common lipid changes in HIV-infected patients.[7]
- Obtain a fasting lipid profile in all HIV-infected patients. Monitor lipid/lipoprotein levels before and after changes in HAART. If abnormalities are not detected, annual repeat testing is adequate.[7]
- Mild to moderate elevations in low-density lipoprotein (LDL) cholesterol levels are also common. For markedly elevated LDL cholesterol levels, consider dietary counseling to reduce saturated fat intake and efforts to increase physical activity. The presence of an underlying genetic dyslipidemia should also be considered.
- The Infectious Diseases Society of America (IDSA) has issued comprehensive guidelines for the treatment of dyslipidemia in HIV-infected persons, and adherence to National Cholesterol Education Program (NCEP) recommendations with the stratification of goals according to coronary heart disease (CHD) risk categories is advisable (see Chapter 33).
- Lipid-lowering agents should be specific for the type of dyslipidemia: Fibrates and/or omega-3-fatty acids for fasting hypertriglyceridemia, HMG-CoA reductase inhibitors for high LDL-cholesterol level. Simvastatin and lovastatin should be avoided in patients receiving protease inhibitor-based HAART (CYP3A4 inducers and inhibitors).[7]

Thyroid Function

- The management of HIV-infected patients diagnosed with either hyper- or hypothyroidism is similar to that for non-HIV-infected individuals (see Chapter 8 and Chapter 9).

- The prevalence of thyroid dysfunction in HIV-infected patients is low and rarely caused by the direct manifestations of active disease (such as *Pneumocystis carinii*–induced thyroiditis). Therefore, routine screening in asymptomatic patients is not generally necessary.[2]
- Patients with a clinical history suggestive of hyper- or hypothyroidism can be screened with standard thyroid studies (i.e., serum thyroid-stimulating hormone [TSH] alone or together with total or free thyroxine [T_4] levels). Interpret these with caution, recognizing that changes indicative of nonthyroidal illness (normal or low TSH with low T_4 levels) may be present in seriously ill patients or patients with advanced HIV. In early HIV infection, thyroid-binding globulin levels can be elevated, resulting in high total T_4 levels and normal TSH levels. In such patients, free T_4 levels are generally normal.[8] A tender thyroid gland in a patient with advanced HIV disease requires a fine needle aspiration biopsy with culture to exclude an opportunistic infection.

Adrenal Function

- Although adrenal insufficiency is frequently considered in patients with HIV-infection, the signs and symptoms of glucocorticoid deficiency are relatively nonspecific and often overlap with the manifestations of AIDS. True adrenal insufficiency is uncommon with HIV infection.[9]
- In HIV infection, changes in the adrenal function are adaptive, and for the most part do not require treatment. Subclinical changes include: Diminished responsiveness to ACTH, a higher morning cortisol, and lower dihydroepiandrosterone levels.[10]
- Cushing's syndrome is often suspected based on lipoatrophy and lipohypertrophy noted in HIV patients treated with HAART. However, HIV patients have normal suppression of cortisol levels following dexamethasone administration.
- Routine screening for adrenal disease is not necessary. In symptomatic patients (see Chapter 11) a standard ACTH stimulation test can be performed. If hypercortisolemia is suspected, a 24-hour urinary free cortisol measurement or a dexamethasone suppression test can be performed (see Chapter 14).
- In patients with advanced disease, opportunistic infection of the adrenal gland is a rare, but reported phenomenon. Tissue is required for definitive diagnosis and a fine needle aspiration biopsy is preferred when technically feasible.

Gonadal Function

- Male hypogonadism is a common finding, particularly with advanced HIV disease. It can affect up to 40% of HIV-infected men and the cause is likely multifactorial.[2]
- Hypogonadism can contribute to the AIDS wasting syndrome; low testosterone levels are associated with loss of lean muscle tissue.
- Testosterone levels vary during the day, so it is advisable to screen for hypogonadism with an early morning serum collection. Sex-hormone binding globulin levels are often elevated in HIV-infected men; therefore, total testosterone levels may be normal despite low free testosterone levels. If testosterone levels are low, measurement of gonadotropin levels (luteinizing hormone [LH], follicle-stimulating hormone [FSH]) can distinguish between primary and secondary disease.[11]
- Testosterone replacement therapy in hypogonadal men with HIV results in improved sexual functioning, mood, energy, and an increase in lean body mass.[11]

Bone and Mineral Metabolism

- HIV-infected people have an increased risk for low bone mineral density. This appears to be multifactorial due to malnutrition, vitamin D deficiency, hypogonadism, as well as traditional risk factors.[12] Screening for osteopenia/osteoporosis should follow standard guidelines (see Chapter 25). Dual energy x-ray absorptiometry (DEXA) of the hip and lumbar spine is the most reliable and quantifiable. Assessment of calcium and vitamin D status (25-OH vitamin D level) can also be helpful.[13]

- Published reports of safe and effective treatments for low bone mineral density in HIV-patients are lacking. HIV-infected patients with a fragility fracture, or post-menopausal HIV-infected women with osteoporosis may be candidates for treatment with a bisphosphonate, unless other contraindications exist.

Fat Redistribution

- Fat redistribution in HIV patients includes peripheral lipoatrophy, visceral lipohypertrophy, and a combined phenotype (lipoatrophy plus lipohypertrophy). These changes are often associated with insulin resistance and dyslipidemia.[2]
- Several etiologies have been proposed, but to date no simple mechanism has been identified.
- Increased physical activity and dietary modifications can reduce visceral adiposity and lipohypertrophy, but do not improve lipoatrophy.
- Tesamorelin (Egrifta) is a growth hormone secretagogue that has recently been approved by the FDA for treatment of HIV-associated lipodystrophy. It is generally not recommended for use in individuals with insulin resistance or recent history of malignancies.[14]
- Lipoatrophy is stigmatizing and only minor improvements occur with changes in antiretroviral therapy (e.g., switch from stavudine or zidovudine to tenofovir or abacavir). In HIV, pioglitazone (Actos) does not appreciably increase limb adiposity, but improves insulin sensitivity. Infusion of biodegradable or permanent synthetic fillers has been used to treat facial lipoatrophy.[14]

REFERENCES

1. Kamps BS, Hoffman C, Mulkaby F. Introduction and ART 2007. *HIV Medicine 2007.* 1;23–29. 5;89–108. Last accessed: 10/23/2010 http://hivmedicine.com/hivmedicine2007.pdf

2. Lee G, Grunfeld C. AIDS endocrinopathies. In: Gardner D, Shoback D, eds. *Greenspan's Basic & Clinical Endocrinology.* 8th ed. New York, NY: McGraw-Hill Companies Inc; 2007:894–908.

3. Grinspoon S, Carr A. Cardiovascular risk and body-fat abnormalities in HIV-infected adults. *N Engl J Med* 2005;352:48–62.

4. Hertel J, Struthers H, Jorj CB, et al. A structural basis for the acute effects of HIV protease inhibitors on GLUT4 intrinsic activity. *J Biol Chem* 2004;279:55147–55152.

5. Woerle HJ, Mariuz PR, Meyer C, et al. Mechanisms for deterioration in glucose tolerance associated with HIV protease inhibitor regimens. *Diabetes* 2003;52:918–925.

6. Schwarz JM, Lee GA, Park S, et al. Indinavir increases glucose production in healthy HIV-negative men. *AIDS* 2004;18:1852–1854.

7. Dube MP, Stein JH, Aberg JA, et al. Guidelines for the evaluation and management of dyslipidemia in human immunodeficiency virus (HIV)-infected adults receiving antiretroviral therapy: Recommendations of the HIV Medical Association of the Infectious Diseases Society of America and the Adult AIDS Clinical Trials Group. *Clin Infect Dis* 2003;37:613–627.

8. Koutkia P, Mylonakis E, Levin RM. Human immunodeficiency virus infection and the thyroid. *Thyroid* 2002;12:577–582.

9. Mayo J, Collazos J, Martinez E, et al. Adrenal function in the human immunodeficiency virus-infected patient. *Arch Intern Med* 2002;162:1095–1098.

10. Findling JW, Buggy BP, Gilson JH, et al. Longitudinal evaluation of adrenocortical function in patients infected with the human immunodeficiency virus. *J Clin Endocrinol Metab* 1994;79:1091–1096.

11. Crum NF, Furtek KJ, Olson PE, et al. A review of hypogonadism and erectile dysfunction among HIV-infected men during the pre- and post-HAART eras: Diagnosis, pathogenesis, and management. *AIDS Patient Care STDS* 2005;19:655–671.

12. Borderi M, Gibelini D, Vescini F, et al. Metabolic bone disease in HIV infection. *AIDS* 2009;23:1297–1310.

13. Schambelan M, Benson CA, Carr A, et al. Management of metabolic complications associated with antiretroviral therapy for HIV-1 infection: Recommendations for an international AIDS society-USA panel. *J Acquir Immune Defic Syndr* 2002;31:257–275.

14. Carr A. Treatment strategies for HIV lipodystrophy. *Curr ophin HIV AIDS* 2007;2:332–338.

Index

Note: Page numbers followed by f and t indicates figure and table respectively.

71% of the large testes subjects (testis volume >4 mL), but only in 36% of the small testes subjects (testis volume <4 mL).[26]

REFERENCES

1. Synder P. Clinical features, diagnosis and treatment of male hypogonadism in adults. In: Basow D, eds. *UpToDate.* Waltham, MA: Uptodate; 2010.
2. Bhasin S, Cunningham GR, Hayes FJ, et al. Testosterone therapy in men with androgen deficiency syndromes: An Endocrine Society clinical practice guideline. *J Clin Endocrinol Metab* 2010;95(6): 2536–2559.
3. Bhasin S, Storer TW, Berman N, et al. Testosterone replacement increases fat-free mass and muscle size in hypogonadal men. *J Clin Endocrinol Metab* 1997;82(2):407–413.
4. Morales A, Schulman CC, Tostain J, et al. Testosterone deficiency syndrome (TDS) needs to be named appropriately–the importance of accurate terminology. *Eur Urol* 2006; 50(3): 407–409.
5. Feldman HA, Longcope C, Derby CA, et al. Age trends in the level of serum testosterone and other hormones in middle-aged men: Longitudinal results from the Massachusetts male aging study. *J Clin Endocrinol Metab* 2002;87(2):589–598.
6. Harman SM, Metter EJ, Tobin JD, et al. Longitudinal effects of aging on serum total and free testosterone levels in healthy men. Baltimore Longitudinal Study of Aging. *J Clin Endocrinol Metab* 2001;86(2):724–731.
7. Giltay JC, Maiburg MC. Klinefelter syndrome: Clinical and molecular aspects. *Expert Rev Mol Diagn* 2010;10(6):765–776.
8. Telvi L, Lebbar A, Del Pino O, et al. 45,X/46,XY Mosaicism: Report of 27 Cases. *Pediatrics* 1999;104(2):304–308.
9. Bianco B, Lipay M, Guedes A, et al. SRY gene increases the risk of developing gonadoblastoma and/or nontumoral gonadal lesions in Turner syndrome. *Int J Gynecol Pathol* 2009; 28(2):197–202 110.1097/PGP.1090b1013e318186a318825.
10. Howell S, Shalet S. Gonadal damage from chemotherapy and radiotherapy. *Endocrinol Metab Clin North Am* 1998;27(4):927–943.
11. Eckman A, Dobs A. Drug-induced gynecomastia. *Expert Opin Drug Saf* 2008;7(6):691–702.
12. Davis SW, Castinetti F, Carvalho LR, et al. Molecular mechanisms of pituitary organogenesis: In search of novel regulatory genes. *Mol Cell Endocrinol* 2010;323(1):4–19.
13. Hohl A, Mazzuco TL, Coral MH, et al. Hypogonadism after traumatic brain injury. *Arq Bras Endocrinol Metabol* 2009;53(8):908–914.
14. Agha A, Thompson CJ. Anterior pituitary dysfunction following traumatic brain injury (TBI). *Clin Endocrinol (Oxf)* 2006;64(5):481–488.
15. Kelly DF, Gonzalo IT, Cohan P, et al. Hypopituitarism following traumatic brain injury and aneurysmal subarachnoid hemorrhage: A preliminary report. *J Neurosurg* 2000; 93(5):743–752.
16. Carruthers M, Trinick TR, Wheeler MJ. The validity of androgen assays. *Aging Male* 2007;10(3):165–172.
17. Dobs AS, Few WL 3rd, Blackman MR, et al. Serum hormones in men with human immunodeficiency virus-associated wasting. *J Clin Endocrinol Metab* 1996;81(11):4108–4112.
18. Yeap BB. Testosterone and ill-health in aging men. *Nat Clin Pract Endocrinol Metab* 2009; 5(2):113–121.
19. Isojarvi JI, Tauboll E, Herzog AG. Effect of antiepileptic drugs on reproductive endocrine function in individuals with epilepsy. *CNS Drugs* 2005;19(3):207–223.
20. MacAdams MR, White RH, Chipps BE. Reduction of serum testosterone levels during chronic glucocorticoid therapy. *Ann Intern Med* 1986;104(5):648–651.
21. Brambilla DJ, Matsumoto AM, Araujo AB, et al. The effect of diurnal variation on clinical measurement of serum testosterone and other sex hormone levels in men. *J Clin Endocrinol Metab* 2009;94(3):907–913.

22. Wang C, Nieschlag E, Swerdloff R, et al. Investigation, treatment and monitoring of late-onset hypogonadism in males: ISA, ISSAM, EAU, EAA and ASA recommendations. *Eur J Endocrinol* 2008;159(5):507–514.

23. Finkel DM, Phillips JL, Snyder PJ. Stimulation of spermatogenesis by gonadotropins in men with hypogonadotropic hypogonadism. *N Engl J Med* 1985;313(11):651–655.

24. Spratt DI, Finkelstein JS, O'Dea LS, et al. Long-term administration of gonadotropin-releasing hormone in men with idiopathic hypogonadotropic hypogonadism. A model for studies of the hormone's physiologic effects. *Ann Intern Med* 1986;105(6):848–855.

25. Raivio T, Falardeau J, Dwyer A, et al. Reversal of idiopathic hypogonadotropic hypogonadism. *N Engl J Med* 2007;357(9):863–873.

26. Miyagawa Y, Tsujimura A, Matsumiya K, et al. Outcome of gonadotropin therapy for male hypogonadotropic hypogonadism at university affiliated male infertility centers: A 30-year retrospective study. *J Urol* 2005;173(6):2072–2075.

Polycystic Ovary Syndrome

20

Nadia Khoury and Janet B. McGill

GENERAL PRINCIPLES

- Polycystic ovary syndrome (PCOS) was first described in 1935 by Stein and Leventhal as a syndrome of signs and symptoms including amenorrhea, hirsutism, enlarged ovaries, and obesity.[1] It is also commonly associated with hyperinsulinemia, glucose intolerance, and dyslipidemia.
- PCOS is a heterogeneous disorder with manifestations that vary from person to person. It has a large impact on fertility, morbidity, and mortality. Its pathogenesis has not been clearly established.

Epidemiology

PCOS is the most common endocrine disorder in women of reproductive age, affecting between 4% and 12% of women.[2] In women with type 2 diabetes, the prevalence is higher, up to 27%.[3]

Pathophysiology

- The etiology of PCOS remains unknown. A prominent feature of the syndrome is that reproductive (hyperandrogenism, anovulation) and metabolic (insulin resistance, obesity) disorders coexist in varying degrees.
- Women with PCOS have increased lutenizing hormone (LH) pulse frequency and amplitude, which is likely due to accelerated GnRH pulse frequency from the hypothalamus. Increased LH pulse frequency favors earlier differentiation of granulosa cells, disordered follicular development, and increased androgen production by theca cells in the ovary, leading to persistence of hyperandrogenemia, normal to low estradiol levels but elevated estrone levels.
- Elevated androgens in combination with low progestin levels due to multiple anovulatory cycles feed back to the hypothalamus to further accelerate GnRH pulse frequency, creating a vicious cycle.[4]
- Androgen synthesis in the theca cells is augmented by upregulation of enzymes involved in the androgenic pathway, in particular cytochrome P-450c17 and 17β-hydroxysteroid dehydrogenase.[4]
- Increased steroidogenesis may involve the adrenal gland as well, though the contribution of the adrenal gland in most cases is difficult to determine and is controversial.
- Hyperinsulinemia further fuels this cycle by priming theca cells for LH-stimulated androgen synthesis. Insulin also decreases the synthesis of sex hormone binding globulin (SHBG), the effect of which is increased androgen bioavailability.
- PCOS is a complex polygenic disease. It is currently the subject of multiple linkage and case-control studies to identify possible candidate genes.

DIAGNOSIS

PCOS is a disorder with multiple manifestations that vary between individuals and may also vary over time in the same individual.

Clinical Presentation

Most of the features of the syndrome develop at the onset of puberty, and severity varies from mild hirsutism to amenorrhea and infertility. Infertility may be the presenting complaint. Most patients are overweight, but the degree of weight gain is variable and influenced by ethnicity.

History

- **Menstrual history** is a critical part of the evaluation for PCOS. Onset of menarche, menstrual interval and regularity, missed periods, and history of irregular bleeding should be documented. Patients should be asked about contraception, unprotected sex, and prior pregnancies.
- Irregular menses are commonly associated with chronic oligo- or anovulation. This can result in endometrial hyperplasia, manifesting as dysfunctional uterine bleeding.
- Less commonly, women with PCOS present with secondary amenorrhea (~24%). These women respond less favorably to treatment.
- Women with PCOS may take longer to conceive. A subset of women has persistent anovulation and infertility.
- The onset and severity of **hirsutism and acne** should be recorded. Androgen excess can result in hirsutism, acne, seborrhea, and androgenic alopecia (male pattern baldness) that often starts at menarche but may occur or progress with weight gain. Frank alopecia is rare in PCOS.
- **Central visceral obesity** (android type) affects 40% to 50% of women with PCOS. Interestingly, the mean body mass index (BMI) of women with PCOS in the United States is 35 to 40 kg/m², but in Europe and other countries it is 25 to 28 kg/m² or less.[5]
- **Hyperinsulinemia and insulin resistance** can be present even in the absence of obesity, but these conditions are exacerbated by the presence of it.
- **Sleep apnea or sleep-disordered breathing** may be present.
- Family history may reveal relatives with other manifestations of insulin resistance, including diabetes and hypertension.

Physical Examination

- **Hirsutism** is characterized by excess terminal pigmented hair in a male pattern of distribution and commonly occurs on the chin, upper lip, periareolar area, and the lower abdomen. It can be scored by the Ferriman–Gallwey system, discussed in Chapter 18.
- Assess the degree of **acne** and **male-pattern baldness**.
- **Acanthosis nigricans**, a marker of insulin resistance and hyperinsulinemia, can be appreciated as velvety, symmetric hyperpigmented plaques that commonly occur on the posterior neck, axilla, elbows, face, knuckles, and groin.
- To assess cardiovascular risk, accurate **blood pressure measurement** is important. **Waist and hip circumferences** may also be helpful as a waist-to-hip ratio >0.85 and waist circumference >100 cm are associated with cardiovascular morbidity.[6]

Diagnostic Criteria

- The criteria used to diagnose PCOS have evolved over 20+ years. The first guidelines were published by a NIH working group in 1990. The Rotterdam PCOS

TABLE 20-1	DIAGNOSTIC CRITERIA FOR PCOS[a,b]		
Criteria	NIH 1990 "Classic"	Rotterdam 2003	AE-PCOS
Oligomenorrhea[c]	+	+/−	+/−
Clinical or biochemical hyperandrogenism[d]	+	+/−	+
Polycystic ovaries on ultrasound[e]	+/−	+/−	+/−

[a]NIH: presence of both oligomenorrhea and clinical/biochemical hyperandrogenism; Rotterdam: any two of the above criteria; AE-PCOS: presence of clinical/biochemical hyperandrogenism and one other criterion.

[b]All guidelines require exclusion of other causes of androgen excess or ovulatory disorders (Cushing's syndrome, non-classical CAH, virilizing tumors).

[c]Eight or fewer menses per year.

[d]Acne or hirsutism or androgenic alopecia.

[e]Ovarian volume >10 mL and/or >12 follicles <9 mm in size in at least one ovary.

From Wild RA, Carmina E, Diamanti-Kandarakis E, et al. Assessment of cardiovascular risk and prevention of cardiovascular disease in women with the polycystic ovary syndrome: A consensus statement by the Androgen Excess and Polycystic Ovary Syndrome (AE-PCOS) Society. *J Clin Endocrinol Metab* 2010;95:2038–2049. Reprinted with permission.

Consensus Working Group then published guidelines in 2003, adding pelvic ultrasound criteria. The Androgen Excess Society favors a hybrid system identifying hyperandrogenism as the primary defect, indicating that lack of hyperandrogenism, regardless of the presence of menstrual irregularities, makes the diagnosis of PCOS less certain.[7] These guidelines are compared in Table 20-1.

• Exclusion of other etiologies of female hyperandrogenism is essential for the diagnosis of PCOS with all of the guidelines.

Differential Diagnosis

• Conditions to consider in the differential diagnosis of PCOS include late-onset congenital adrenal hyperplasia (CAH), androgen-secreting adrenal or ovarian tumors, Cushing's syndrome, hyperprolactinemia, pregnancy, hypothyroidism, acromegaly, and drug-induced disorders.
  ○ **Late-onset CAH** is more common in the Ashkenazi Jewish population, and patients may appear more virilized than a typical patient with PCOS and have a family history of infertility, hirsutism, or both.
  ○ With **androgen-secreting neoplasms**, symptoms start later and are more severe and progressive.
  ○ **Cushing's syndrome** may present at any time, be slowly progressive, and when mild, look similar to PCOS.
  ○ In **hyperprolactinemia** and **hypothyroidism**, symptoms of androgen excess are less prominent.
  ○ Other phenotypic features of **acromegaly** should help with this diagnosis.
  ○ **Drugs** such as topical and oral androgens, valproate, and cyclosporine can cause hyperandrogenism and variable degrees of menstrual irregularities.

Diagnostic Testing

The laboratory workup is initially aimed at excluding other disorders. There is no universally accepted definition for PCOS based on hormonal criteria.

Laboratory Studies

- To rule out other disorders, start with measurement of **testosterone** and **dehydroepi-androsterone sulfate** (DHEA-S) levels, which will both be markedly elevated in virilizing adrenal or ovarian tumors, >200 ng/dL and >600 mcg/dL respectively. **Serum LH** is usually normal or slightly elevated. A **random 17-hydroxyprogesterone level** of <200 ng/dL excludes non-classical CAH. An **overnight 1 mg dexamethasone suppression** of morning cortisol to <1.2 ng/mL or normal **24-hour urine for free cortisol** rules out Cushing's syndrome. Hyperprolactinemia and hypothyroidism are not usually associated with hyperandrogenemia, but a **serum prolactin** and **TSH** level should be checked in any woman with menstrual irregularity.
- The following hormonal abnormalities can be seen in women with PCOS:
  - Roughly 80% have total and free testosterone levels in the upper normal to two-fold or higher range. Because of decreased production of hepatic SHBG, the total testosterone may be in the normal range while the free testosterone is elevated. DHEA-S levels are sometimes mildly elevated.
  - Elevated LH and normal FSH, resulting in an elevated LH/FSH ratio may be observed, but due to the pulsatile nature of gonadotropin secretion and day-to-day variability, gonadotropin levels are too insensitive to confirm the diagnosis. LH levels could be useful as a secondary parameter, especially in lean women with amenorrhea.
  - Serum estrone may be increased, while serum estradiol is usually normal to low normal.
  - Prolactin can be mildly elevated.
  - Impaired glucose tolerance (and even frank diabetes) may be diagnosed in 30% to 40% of women when tested with a 75 g, 2-hour oral glucose tolerance test (OGTT).[8] Fasting blood glucose levels may be normal. The 2003 guidelines suggest screening all women with a BMI > 27 kg/m^2 with an OGTT.
  - Atherogenic lipid profiles are observed with increased prevalence in women with PCOS, even after adjusting for BMI. The characteristics of an atherogenic profile include high very-low-density lipoprotein (VLDL), high low-density lipoprotein (LDL), and low high-density lipoprotein (HDL). Low HDL levels are associated with obesity and high LDL levels with hyperandrogenemia.

Imaging

The specific **ultrasound characteristics** proposed by the 2003 consensus are (a) presence of 12 or more follicles in each ovary measuring 2 to 9 mm in diameter and (b) increased ovarian volume (>10 mL) and stroma. Only one ovary meeting these criteria is sufficient. The subjective appearance of polycystic ovaries should not be substituted for this definition. These ultrasound criteria do not apply to women on oral contraceptive pills (OCPs). If there is evidence of a dominant follicle (>10 mm), the scan should be repeated.[9]

T R E A T M E N T

- Treatment of PCOS should be individualized to the patient, including her goals of care.

- Several treatment options exist for each of the manifestations of PCOS. Most manifestations can be reversed by improving insulin resistance, either by weight loss or with medication.
- Typically, response to therapy is slow, with clinical changes lagging behind biochemical improvement by several months.
- **Pregnancy should be excluded before initiation of pharmacologic therapy with oral contraceptives or antiandrogens.**

Medications

Oral Contraceptives

- OCPs are standard therapy for those who do not desire pregnancy. OCPs interrupt the cycle of hyperandrogenemia and oligomenorrhea. They allow the resumption of normal menses and prevent the chronic, unopposed, estrogenic stimulation of the endometrium.
- OCPs lower androgen levels by 50% to 60%.[10] Hirsutism and acne respond well.
- Typically, treatment should be initiated by a combination preparation that contains ethinyl estradiol in conjunction with a progestin with low androgenic activity such as norgestimate or desogestrel.[11]
- Drospirenone is a progestin with antimineralocorticoid and antiandrogenic activity that is approved for use in combination with ethinyl estradiol.
- Cyproterone acetate is a unique progestin/antiandrogen that inhibits the binding of testosterone and 5-α-dihydrotestosterone to the androgen receptor. It is marketed outside the Unites States in combination with ethinyl estradiol for use as an OCP.
- Recent studies have raised concerns about increased risk of thromboembolism with the antiandrogenic progestins.[12]
- The choice of an OCP, and indeed the use of any OCP, should be individualized based on the degree of insulin resistance, degree of androgenicity, anthropometric characteristics, and presence of other risk factors for metabolic, cardiovascular, and thromboembolic complications. Insulin resistance can potentially be worsened by OCP use.[11]
- Contraindications for OCP therapy must be considered, including age, smoking, and prior thromboembolic disease.
- In women who do not desire (or cannot take) oral contraceptive therapy, intermittent oral progestin therapy with a 7- to 10-day course of medroxyprogesterone acetate (Provera) every 1 to 3 months can be considered. Although this therapy can offer endometrial protection, it does not reduce the effects of hyperandrogenism such as hirsutism and acne.

Insulin Sensitizers

- The use of medications that improve insulin sensitivity was initially based on the observation that interventions that improve insulin resistance, such as weight loss, reduce androgen levels and induce ovulation. The clinical response to insulin-lowering therapy does not seem to be related to the magnitude of insulin resistance.
- Although not approved by the Food and Drug Administration (FDA) for the treatment of PCOS, **metformin** effectively decreases testosterone levels and fasting insulin and glucose levels. It improves ovulation in multiple studies, but there is no overall increase in live births as compared to placebo across multiple studies.[13] Metformin can be used in pregnancy (category B). Effective doses of metformin are between 1500 and 2000 mg/day, although randomized studies have not been done.

- **Thiazolidinediones** may be effective. The initial studies were done with troglitazone, which has since been removed from the market. Newer agents (rosiglitazone, pioglitazone) have shown similar effects in increasing insulin sensitivity, decreasing testosterone levels, and inducing ovulation.[14] Rosiglitazone has been associated with increased risk of cardiovascular events and is not recommended. These agents should not be used in women who desire pregnancy (category C).

Antiandrogens
- Antiandrogens can be used in conjunction with oral contraceptives to derive further benefit when hirsutism is the primary complaint. Because of the teratogenic potential of antiandrogens, they must be used only when women are treated with effective contraception.
- **Spironolactone** (50 to 100 mg twice daily) inhibits androgen biosynthesis in the adrenal and ovary, inhibits 5-α-reductase, and decreases the effect of androgens by blocking the androgen receptor. When used alone, it has minimal effects on free testosterone levels. When used in combination with an oral contraceptive, both androgen levels and androgen action are decreased due to synergistic actions.
- **Finasteride** (5 mg daily) and **flutamide** (250 mg bid) can also be used to treat hirsutism. Flutamide may cause hepatotoxicity.
- **Enflornithine hydrochloride 13.9% cream,** which slows hair growth, can be used to treat facial hirsutism. It is usually not covered by insurance. **Topical minoxidil** can be used for male pattern hair loss.

Other Pharmacologic Interventions
- More recently, studies in women with PCOS have used agents like Orlistat to achieve weight loss and have shown reduction of testosterone levels in addition to weight loss.[15]
- Simvastatin, used in combination with an OCP, and atorvastatin, tested without concomitant OCP use, improved testosterone levels, hirsutism (simvastatin plus OCP), and lipid profiles.[16,17]

Other Nonpharmacologic Therapies

Weight reduction should be a central feature to any treatment plan of PCOS. This is generally done with caloric restriction and increased aerobic exercise. Studies have shown no benefit to restricting carbohydrates as opposed to fat.[18]

COMPLICATIONS

- **Infertility** is one of the biggest concerns for women with PCOS.
  - ○ It is important to complete a basic infertility evaluation of the couple, including a semen analysis of the man, to rule out other contributing factors.
  - ○ Weight loss and insulin sensitizers, such as metformin, may induce ovulatory cycles and permit conception. Clomiphene citrate is a triphenylethylene-derived nonsteroidal agent that is theorized to function at the level of the hypothalamus as an antiandrogen to restore gonadotropin secretion. It is superior to metformin in achieving conception, but there is a relatively high rate of multiple pregnancies. Combination of clomiphene with metformin may increase pregnancy rates. If pregnancy is not achieved after 6 to 9 months of clomiphene with or without metformin, the patient should be referred to a fertility specialist for use of injectable gonadotropins or in vitro fertilization.

○ An increased incidence of spontaneous miscarriage is associated with PCOS. Treatment with metformin may reduce the rate of miscarriage.

○ If pregnancy does occur, there is an increased risk for pregnancy-induced hypertension, preeclampsia, gestational diabetes, pregnancy loss, and preterm labor.

- The prevalence of **impaired glucose tolerance** and **type 2 diabetes** is increased in women with PCOS, who have a 3 to 7 times greater risk of developing diabetes. This association is present in both obese and lean women with PCOS.[19] Women with a family history of type 2 diabetes are at even greater risk for development of diabetes.

- **Hypertension** is not common in young women with PCOS, but studies have shown that a longer or irregular menstrual cycle length can lead to a two-fold increase in risk for hypertension. The prevalence of hypertension increases dramatically by the time of perimenopause.

- Women with PCOS also have an increased risk for **dyslipidemia** and have been shown to have abnormal vascular function, higher rates of coagulopathy, and increased markers of inflammation. There is likely an increased cardiovascular risk, but this research is still on-going.[20]

- Unopposed estrogenic stimulation of the uterus may increase the likelihood of **endometrial hyperplasia and endometrial carcinoma**.

MONITORING/FOLLOW-UP

- The long-term metabolic and cardiovascular disease risks associated with PCOS heighten the importance of proper diagnosis and follow-up.

- BMI, waist circumference, and blood pressure determinations are recommended for all women with PCOS.

- Oral glucose tolerance testing (75 g, 2 hour) is recommended for those with obesity, advanced age, personal history of gestational diabetes, or family history of type 2 diabetes mellitus.[21] This should be repeated every 2 years or annually if impaired glucose tolerance is found.[22]

- Other risk factors for cardiovascular disease, including tobacco abuse, sleep apnea, and hyperlipidemia, should be assessed annually.

- In women with PCOS, relative hyperandrogenemia and increased risk for glucose intolerance and dyslipidemia persist after menopause, so ongoing screening is warranted.[23]

REFERENCES

1. Stein IF, Leventhal ML. Amenorrhea associated with bilateral polycystic ovaries. *Am J Obstet Gynecol* 1935;29:181–191.
2. Azziz R, Woods KS, Reyna R, et al. The prevalence and features of the polycystic ovary syndrome in an unselected population. *J Clin Endocrinol Metab* 2004;89:2745–2749.
3. Peppard HR, Marfori J, Iuorno MJ, et al. Prevalence of polycystic ovary syndrome among premenopausal women with type 2 diabetes. *Diabetes Care* 2001;24:1050–1052.
4. Ehrmann DA. Medical progress: Polycystic ovary syndrome. *N Engl J Med* 2005;352:1223–1236.
5. Carmina E, Legro R, Stamets K, et al. Differences in body weight between American and Italian women with the polycystic ovary syndrome: Influence of the diet. *Hum Reprod* 2003;11:2289–2293.
6. Talbott E, Guzick D, Clerici A, et al. Coronary heart disease risk factors in women with polycystic ovary syndrome. *Arterioscler Thromb Vasc Biol* 1995;15:821–826.

- One must first **identify true hypercalcemia**. Hypercalcemia without elevated ionized calcium can occur in hyperalbuminemia, severe dehydration, or multiple myeloma with a calcium-binding paraprotein. Elevated ionized calcium with normal serum calcium may be seen in hypoalbuminema due to malnutrition or chronic liver disease.

Laboratory Studies

- **Serum calcium** needs to be adjusted for changes in albumin and pH. Acidosis decreases and alkalosis increases ionized calcium. Calcium should be changed by 0.8 mg/dL for every 1 g/dL change in albumin outside of the normal range.
- Start with measurement of **intact PTH**. If this elevated, it is most likely PHP. To differentiate PHP from FHH, measure spot urinary calcium and creatinine and calculate a fractional excretion of calcium—if this is <1%, it favors FHH. An elevated calcium and PTH can also be seen in lithium use.
- **If PTH is suppressed, look for other causes of hypercalcemia.**
  - ○ Malignancy leading to hypercalcemia is usually readily evident and therefore measurement of PTHrP is not needed.
  - ○ Measure **1,25-OH-Vitamin D** next. If this is elevated, consider chest x-ray and CBC to evaluate for lymphoma or other granulomatous disease such as sarcoidosis.
  - ○ If 25-OH-Vitamin D but not 1,25-OH-Vitamin D is elevated, consider exogenous vitamin D intoxication.
- Other laboratory work-up of hypercalcemia should be guided by history and could include thyroid-stimulating hormone (there may be a concominant elevated chloride) or cortisol (in the setting of weakness, hypotension, and hyponatremia). Other tests include vitamin A levels, urinary catecholamines for pheochromocytoma, and evaluation for multiple myeloma.

Electrocardiogram

Electrocardiographic findings may include a shortened QT interval and mild prolongations of the PR and QRS intervals. With severe hypercalcemia, there may be alterations in the T-wave configuration, as well.[15]

TREATMENT

- Determining when to treat hypercalcemia depends on its chronicity and the degree of elevation.
- Most patients with PHP have mild elevations in calcium (<12 mg/dL) and do not require active treatment. They need to be educated and modify their lifestyle as outlined in the Lifestyle/Risk Modification section.
- Even those with serum calcium above 12 mg/dL may not require treatment if this level is chronic. Usually, if the rise to this level is acute, patients are symptomatic and require active treatment.

Medications

The **primary focus of treating acute hypercalcemia is to increase urinary calcium excretion.** Patients should be **aggressively hydrated** with normal saline over 24 to 48 hours to lower the serum calcium concentration by as much as 3 to 9 mg/dL, depending on the initial degree of hypercalcemia. Close monitoring is needed, as fluid overload can develop, especially if there is underlying cardiac or renal insufficiency. The traditional use of loop diuresis with saline hydration has recently been questioned.[16] **Loop diuresis should be reserved for the setting of fluid overload.**

Aggressive diuresis in a volume-depleted patient may worsen the hypercalcemia by exacerbating the volume loss. In addition, precautions should be taken to prevent potassium and magnesium depletion.

Bisphosphonates

- **Intravenous bisphosphonate** treatment provides a longer term solution to hypercalemia when a cause has been identified and reversible causes have been fixed. Bisphosphonates are analogs of pyrophosphate that are concentrated in areas of high bone turnover and inhibit both calcification and osteoclastic bone resorption.
- These agents have maximum effect at 2 to 4 days and last 3 to 4 weeks. Two agents are FDA approved—**pamidronate** and **zoledronic acid**. While zoledronic acid has been found to be slightly more potent in head-to-head studies and has a shorter infusion time, pamidronate is less expensive and nearly as efficacious.[17]
- Both agents are well tolerated, and side effects are usually mild and transient. Fever is the most common reaction to intravenous administration. Renal toxicity is the most common serious side effect—doses should be given over a longer period of time or possibly reduced if renal insufficiency is present. Osteonecrosis of the jaw is a rare complication of bisphosphonate therapy, but should be considered when treating patients who have had a recent dental procedure or who are planning for major dental surgery.

Calcitonin

Until the time when bisphosphonates reach potency, salmon calcitonin administered subcutaneously or intramuscularly (4 U/kg every 12 hours, increased up to 6 to 8 U/kg every 6 hours) can be **used as a temporizing measure**. It acts quickly—within 6 to 8 hours—and has few side effects. Unfortunately, it is a relatively weak agent, only lowering serum calcium concentrations by 1 to 2 mg/dL, and acquired resistance often develops within the first 48 hours, limiting its use.

Other Treatments

- **Dialysis** against a no- or low-calcium bath may be needed in the setting of acute symptomatic hypercalcemia and renal or cardiac insufficiency leading to volume overload.
- **Gallium nitrate** inhibits osteoclastic bone resorption, takes several days to work, and lasts 1 week. Its use is limited by need for a 5-day-long infusion and severe side effects including renal failure, hypophosphatemia, and anemia.
- **Mithramycin** inhibits osteoclast RNA synthesis. It is rarely used because of its severe side effects including renal and liver toxicity, nausea, thrombocytopenia, and extravasation reactions.
- Hypercalcemia in hematologic malignancies and granulomatous diseases associated with increased production of $1,25(OH)_2D$ may be treated effectively with moderately high-dose **glucocorticoids** (e.g., prednisone 40 to 60 mg daily). Glucocorticoids increase urinary calcium excretion and decrease intestinal calcium absorption, but may also have direct antitumor effects. Calcium levels usually fall within 48 hours, with a peak response in 7 to 10 days.[2] Corticosteroids are also effective therapy for hypercalcemia related to adrenal insufficiency and excessive vitamin A or D ingestion.
- **Ketoconazole** acts as an inhibitor of the cytochrome P-450 hydroxylation of $25(OH)D$ to $1,25(OH)_2D$, and may also be effective in treating hypercalcemia caused by vitamin D intoxication.
- **Cinacalcet** is a calcimemetic that increases the sensitivity of the calcium sensing receptor, leading to reduced PTH levels. It is currently approved for treatment of

secondary hyperparathyroidism in chronic kidney disease where it reduces adverse outcomes from hypercalcemia. It is not yet approved for PHP but can be used in parathyroid carcinoma or PHP that persists after surgery or when surgery is no longer feasible.[18]

- A monoclonal antibody against RANK ligand, **denosumab**, was recently approved for treatment of postmenopausal osteoporosis. Studies of its use in MAH are ongoing.[17]

Surgical Management

Parathyroidectomy by an experienced surgeon is the mainstay of therapy for symptomatic PHP and asymptomatic disease in the presence of renal dysfunction, osteoporosis, or calcium >1 mg/dL of the upper limit of normal.[19] This is discussed in more detail in Chapter 22.

Lifestyle/Risk Modification

- Patients with mild and moderate hypercalcemia should be instructed to avoid factors that exacerbate hypercalcemia. These include lithium, thiazide diuretics, volume depletion, prolonged bed rest, and a diet high in calcium (>1 g/day).
- Patients should be instructed to maintain adequate hydration (about 3 L/day) to prevent nephrolithiasis.

REFERENCES

1. Dent DM, Miller JL, Klaff L, et al. The incidence and causes of hypercalcaemia. *Postgrad Med J* 1987;63:745–750.
2. Lafferty FW. Differential diagnosis of hypercalcemia. *J Bone Miner Res* 1991;6(Suppl 2): S51–S59; discussion S61.
3. Makras P, Papapoulus SE. Medical treatment of hypercalcemia. *Hormones* 2009;8(2):83–95.
4. Stewart AF. Clinical practice. Hypercalcemia associated with cancer. *N Engl J Med* 2005; 352(4):373–379.
5. Tian E, Zhan F, Walker R, et al. The role of the Wnt-signaling antagonist DKK1 in the development of osteolytic lesions in multiple myeloma. *N Engl J Med* 2003;349(26):2483–2494.
6. Iqbal AA, Burgess EH, Gallina DL, et al. Hypercalcemia in hyperthyroidism: Patterns of serum calcium, parathyroid hormone, and 1,25-dihydroxyvitamin D3 levels during management of thyrotoxicosis. *Endocr Pract* 2003;9:517–521.
7. Niesvizky R, Siegel DS, Busquets X, et al. Hypercalcaemia and increased serum interleukin-6 levels induced by all-trans retinoic acid in patients with multiple myeloma. *Br J Haematol* 1995;89(1):217–218.
8. Sam R, Vaseemuddin M, Siddique A, et al. Hypercalcemia in patients in the burn intensive care unit. *J Burn Care Res* 2007;28(5):742–746.
9. Nordt SP, Williams SR, Clark RF. Pharmacologic misadventure resulting in hypercalcemia from vitamin D intoxication. *J Emerg Med* 2002;22:302–303.
10. Jacobs TP, Bilezikian JP. Clinical review: Rare causes of hypercalcemia. *J Clin Endocrinol Metab* 2005;90:6316–6322.
11. Abreo K, Adlakha A, Kilpatrick S, et al. The milk-alkali syndrome. A reversible form of acute renal failure. *Arch Intern Med* 1993;153(8):1005–1010.
12. Khandwala HM, Van Uum S. Reversible hypercalcemia and hyperparathyroidism associated with lithium therapy: Case report and review of literature. *Endocr Pract* 2006;12: 54–58.
13. Mao C, Carter P, Schaefer P, et al. Malignant islet cell tumor associated with hypercalcemia. *Surgery* 1995;117:37–40.
14. Ziegler R. Hypercalcemic crisis. *J Am Soc Nephrol* 2001;12(Suppl 17):S3–S9.

15. Douglas PS, Carmichael KA, Palevsky PM. Extreme hypercalcemia and electrocardiographic changes. *Am J Cardiol* 1984;54:674–675.

16. LeGrand SB, Leskuski D, Zama I. Narrative review: Furosemide for hypercalcemia: An unproven yet common practice. *Ann Intern Med* 2008;149(4):259–263.

17. Lumachi F, Brunello A, Roma A, et al. Cancer-induced hypercalcemia. *Anticancer Res* 2009; 29(5):1551–1555.

18. Peacock M, Bilezikian JP, Klassen PS, et al. Cinacalcet hydrochloride maintains long-term normocalcemia in patients with primary hyperparathyroidism. *J Clin Endocrinol Metab* 2005;90(1):135–141.

19. Bilezikian JP, Khan AA, Potts JT Jr. Guidelines for the management of asymptomatic primary hyperparathyroidism: Summary statement from the third international workshop. *J Clin Endocrinol Metab* 2009;94(2):335–339.

Hyperparathyroidism

22

Shunzhong Bao and Dwight A. Towler

GENERAL PRINCIPLES

Definition

Hyperparathyroidism is defined as the elevated production of parathyroid hormone (PTH) by the parathyroid glands.

Classification

- **Primary hyperparathyroidism** (pHPT) occurs when one or more of the parathyroid glands produce an excessive amount of PTH for the amount of calcium present in the blood.
- **Secondary hyperparathyroidism** (sHPT) is a normal elevation in the production of PTH that occurs in response to a derangement in calcium homeostasis that causes, or would otherwise lead to, frank hypocalcemia (e.g., renal failure, hyperphosphatemia, or vitamin D deficiency).
- **Tertiary hyperparathyroidism** develops in the setting of long-standing severe sHPT with parathyroid hyperplasia. The increased mass of parathyroid gland produces a constitutive excess of PTH, even after correcting underlying derangement in calcium phosphate homeostasis. This is most commonly seen in the setting of renal transplantation for chronic kidney disease (CKD).

Epidemiology

- pHPT is one of the most common causes of hypercalcemia, especially in the outpatient setting. pHPT is a relatively common disease that affects about 1:1000 of the adult population. Women with the disease outnumber men by as much as 3:1, and the disease most commonly presents after age 45.
- A small increase in the incidence of non-endocrine malignancies (breast cancer, squamous cell skin cancer, colon cancer, renal parenchymal cancer) has been reported in patients with pHPT, but the reason for the association is not known. An association with thyroid cancer has also been reported; however, it is not clear if the reported incidence is higher simply because of increased detection during the evaluation and management of pHPT. The genetic association with multiple endocrine neoplasia (MEN) is detailed below.
- Overall, the effect of mild pHPT on mortality is still being evaluated and debated. However, recent data from PEARS (the Parathyroid Epidemiology and Audit Research Study) suggest that mild pHPT (i.e., calcium never over 12 mg/dL, no parathyroid surgery or renal complications) may increase morbidity and mortality. The association between moderate to severe pHPT and all-cause mortality—particularly from cardiovascular disease and malignancy—is more firmly established. Increasing calcium levels have also been shown to be an independent risk factor for death.[1]

Etiology

- PTH is typically secreted by the parathyroid gland as an 84 amino acid polypeptide often referred to as "intact PTH." The single most important regulator of PTH secretion is the level of serum ionized calcium, which acts through the calcium-sensing receptor (CaSR) to produce rapid (within seconds) and relatively large responses in PTH secretion to small changes in calcium.[2]
- The synthesis and processing of PTH within the parathyroid gland also adapt quickly to changes in calcium levels, and parathyroid hyperplasia may develop in response to more chronic hypocalcemia. Phosphate and vitamin D levels are also important in the regulation of PTH, with higher levels of phosphate and lower levels of vitamin D increasing synthesis and secretion of PTH. Long-standing phosphate excess and vitamin D insufficiency in CKD cause parathyroid gland proliferation and hyperplasia via paracrine TGF-alpha signals, culminating in tertiary HPT.[3]
- The effects of PTH are mediated primarily through the PTH/ PTHRP receptor (PTHR1), a transmembrane G protein–coupled receptor found in the kidneys, intestine, vascular smooth muscle, and bone.[4]
- **PTH causes an increase in serum calcium through three mechanisms**[5].
  - In the kidney, PTH acts to increase calcium and decrease phosphate reabsorption. PTH-dependent reabsorption of calcium occurs in the distal convoluted tubule via activation of the TRPV5 calcium channel. Phosphate reabsorption is reduced by PTH in the proximal tubule via inhibition of NaPi-IIc and NaPi-IIa sodium-phosphate co-transporters.
  - PTH acts to increase the activity of 1α-hydroxylase in proximal tubular cells, increasing the level of $1,25(OH)_2D$ over several hours, and ultimately leading to increased absorption of calcium and phosphate by the small intestine.
  - Prolonged secretion of PTH also increases bone resorption and decreases bone mass—although this is more variable than the response elicited by PTHrP, the PTHR1 ligand causing humoral hypercalcemia of malignancy. When given inter-mittently, PTH increases bone mass. This anabolic response occurs in part via PTH downregulation of osteocyte sclerostin, a negative regulator bone-forming Wnt-LRP5/6 signals.[6] This may explain why bone mass is often preserved to within normal limits in patients with mild pHPT. Nevertheless, total bone mass most frequently improves in patients following parathyroidectomy for pHPT.

Pathophysiology

Primary Hyperparathyroidism

- pHPT is the inappropriate secretion of PTH from one or more of the parathyroid glands that leads to hypercalcemia.
- A **single benign parathyroid adenoma** is found in 80% to 90% of cases. Over-expression of cyclin D1, encoded by the PRAD1 oncogene, is observed in ~30% of adenomas. There are several genetic abnormalities that may contribute to the development of parathyroid hyperplasia, including sporadic mutations in the multiple endocrine neoplasia 1 (MEN1) gene that occur in 12% to 16% of single adenomas.[7,8] Recent data suggest that the common CaSR 986S allele may also increase the risk of pHPT.
- **Four-gland hyperplasia** is seen in approximately 6% of cases. Parathyroid carcinoma is reported to occur in 0.5% to 1% of cases, but is probably in the lower half of this range. Carcinomas may have characteristic pathologic findings, but are often only distinguished from adenomas by the degree of vascular/local invasion or the presence of lymph node metastases.[7-9]

- Familial hyperparathyroidism is rare and is most commonly associated with MEN1 and MEN2A.
- **MEN1** is caused by a defect in gene encoding the tumor suppressor menin and is inherited in an autosomal-dominant fashion. It is most commonly associated with parathyroid hyperplasia, pancreatic tumors, and pituitary adenomas, although it may also be associated with other tumors. Hypercalcemia can be found in approximately 95% of those with MEN1, typically developing around age 25 years as the earliest manifestation of the syndrome. Although it may be associated with a single parathyroid adenoma at presentation, it almost always involves multiglandular hyperplasia.
- **MEN2** is inherited in an autosomal-dominant fashion and is associated with defects in the RET proto-oncogene. It is characterized chiefly by medullary thyroid cancer, which occurs with complete penetrance, and with pheochromocytoma. Approximately 25% to 35% of patients develop asymmetric parathyroid hyperplasia in MEN2A.[9]
- Less commonly pHPT may be caused by familial isolated hyperparathyroidism or is part of the hyperparathyroidism–jaw tumor syndrome. These are associated with mutations in the HPRT2 gene encoding parafibromin, a transcriptional suppressor of the PRAD1 oncogene. It is important to consider since the risk for developing parathyroid carcinoma is greatly increased to approximately 10%.
- **Familial hypocalciuric hypercalcemia** (FHH) is an autosomal-dominant disorder that is caused by a heterogeneous spectrum of mutations of the CaSR that shift the set point for serum calcium to a higher level. FHH is typically asymptomatic and is thought to be a rare disorder with estimates of prevalence as low as 1 in 78,000, and as high as 1 in 15,625 in Scotland and 1 in 31,250 in Australia. Nevertheless, since the biochemical abnormalities in FHH overlap with those of pHPT, the diagnosis must be considered; otherwise, a patient may undergo an unnecessary parathyroidectomy that is rarely curative in this disorder.[10,11]
- **Lithium therapy** can produce alterations in calcium metabolism that mimic the changes in FHH and resolve when lithium is withdrawn (see Chapter 21).

Secondary and Tertiary Hyperparathyroidism

- sHPT is a physiologic response in the production of PTH by the parathyroid glands, most often in response to hypocalcemia, vitamin D insufficiency, or hyperphosphatemia. It occurs commonly in CKD, but can occur in other settings including chronic hepatobiliary disease. **Vitamin D deficiency** is an often-overlooked cause of sHPT that may be misdiagnosed as "incipient" pHPT or normocalcemic hyperparathyroidism (normal calcium, elevated PTH).[12] Concurrent measurement and consideration of serum 25-hydroxyvitamin D and urinary 24-hour calcium helps to avoid this mistake, since both are reduced with sHPT due to vitamin D deficiency.
- sHPT develops in virtually all patients with CKD. Both decreased production of $1,25(OH)_2D$ and phosphate retention are involved. Even in the early stages of renal impairment, production of $1,25(OH)_2D$ may be decreased, leading to a decline in calcium absorption in the gut. Diminished phosphate clearance by the kidneys leads to hyperphosphatemia, with excess phosphate forming complexes with free ionized calcium ions. This decreases activation of the parathyroid gland CaSR, thus increasing PTH release. In addition, hyperphosphatemia impairs renal 1α-hydroxylase (CYP27B1), lowering $1,25(OH)_2D$ production and directly stimulating PTH synthesis and secretion by the parathyroid gland. Hyperphosphatemia-induced

FGF23 elevation also suppresses renal CYP27B1. Uremia may also produce changes associated with PTH-resistance in bone.[13]

- Tertiary hyperparathyroidism is said to be present when autonomously elevated PTH levels are associated with hypercalcemia following long-standing sHPT. Under chronic stimulation to produce PTH, the parathyroid glands hypertrophy over time and, in some patients, become resistant to normal feedback mechanisms and therefore autonomously produce PTH. This is commonly seen in end-stage renal disease requiring hemodialysis and after prolonged periods of sHPT, and can first become clinically significant following renal transplantation with cessation of dialysis.

DIAGNOSIS

Clinical Presentation

History

- pHPT is now most often diagnosed incidentally following the evaluation of an asymptomatic elevation of serum calcium. Eighty percent of cases are asymptomatic.
- It is important to elicit any history of previous hypercalcemia, hypophosphatemia, history of recurrent nephrolithiasis, history of low bone mass, bone pain, fracture (especially vertebral fracture or loss in height of ≥ 2"), history of hyperuricemia, gout, or pseudogout.
- The classic symptoms and findings of hyperparathyroidism are summarized in the mnemonic "bones, stones, abdominal moans, psychic groans, and hypertones."
- Many patients are asymptomatic at diagnosis, but many have non-specific symptoms such as weakness, fatigue, nocturia or polyuria, constipation, neuromuscular dysfunction, and neuropsychiatric disturbances that may improve after parathyroidectomy. Nephrolithiasis is the most common renal manifestation of pHPT and occurs in approximately 15% to 20% of patients. Other renal manifestations include hypercalciuria, nephrocalcinosis, renal tubular dysfunction, and chronic renal insufficiency.[14]
- The skeletal manifestation of classic, severe HPT is osteitis fibrosa cystica, which presents with typical radiographic features, including a "salt-and-pepper" appearance of the skull, bone cysts, and brown tumors of the long bones. However, this condition is now seen in <1% of patients with pHPT.
- The most characteristic skeletal finding is decreased bone mass with redistribution reflecting PTH's catabolic effects on periosteal cortical bone and anabolic effects on endosteal and cancellous bone (greatest loss at the distal one-third radius >hip> spine). Bone mass is often globally preserved in patients with mild pHPT.
- In severe sHPT, a "rugger jersey" spine appearance can be seen on lateral CXR due to sclerosing of vertebral endplates with rarified vertebral bone body. The distal clavicles can also be eroded.
- sHPT due to severe vitamin D deficiency may present with osteomalacia because of abnormal mineralization of bone. Uremic bone disease, also termed renal osteodystrophy, is a multifactorial and mixed bone disorder that arises in part due to sHPT in CKD.

Physical Examination

- Typically, there are no physical findings in patients with hyperparathyroidism.
- Some nonspecific findings may be present: confusion, mental status changes, possible findings of nephrolithiasis, possible findings of arthritis, slow pulse, proximal

An advantage of ultrasonography is the ability to fully image the thyroid gland and help characterize any thyroid nodules that also may require surgical management.

- **99mTc-sestamibi scanning** exhibits sensitivity similar to ultrasound and is reported to be 68% to 95% in detecting single adenomas, but like ultrasound has poor sensitivity for detecting multigland disease. Because 99mTc-sestamibi is also taken up by thyroid tissue, false positives may occur. An advantage of scintigraphy, however, is that it can detect ectopic glands outside the neck, identifying adenomas missed by ultrasound.

- Therefore, some favor a combined approach to preoperative evaluation. High-resolution neck ultrasonography (US) and 99mTc-sestamibi scanning—planar, single photon emission computed tomography (SPECT), or SPECT coupled with anatomic X-ray CT overlay (SPECT/CT)—have emerged as the two most useful imaging techniques for locating a single parathyroid adenoma versus multigland disease prior to surgery in patients with pHPT.[7] The combination of preoperative US followed by SPECT/CT as needed localizes 95% of solitary adenomas, and prospectively guides the selection of patients as candidates for minimally invasive surgery.

- Bone mineral density measurement by **dual electron X-ray absorptiometry** (DXA) is important in hyperparathyroidism patients. It is one indicator of disease severity. Multiple sites should be measured including distal one-third radius, spine, and hip.

- Magnetic resonance imaging (MRI) should not be commonly used for localization of parathyroid adenomas and are usually reserved for possible parathyroid carcinoma, failed parathyroidectomy or recurrent disease.

TREATMENT

Primary Hyperparathyroidism

- The only curative treatment for pHPT is parathyroid surgery and is recommended for all patients with symptomatic disease.

- However, in asymptomatic patients, the difficulty is in determining which patients are most appropriate for surgery versus watchful waiting. The recent data from PEARS (The Parathyroid Epidemiology and Audit Research Study) suggests that mild pHPT (i.e., calcium never over 12 mg/dL, no parathyroid surgery or renal complications) may increase morbidity and mortality. Moreover, cortical bone loss is progressive in the absence of surgery, and over a 15-year period, one-third of pHPT patients progress to meet surgical criteria. Thus, consensus guidelines concerning surgery in mild pHPT may change in the foreseeable future.

- The calcium level, phosphate, and PTH should be followed at least semiannually, and renal function and DXA bone density (distal radius, hip, and spine) should be monitored annually in patients who do not undergo surgery.

Surgical Management

Consensus guidelines formulated in 2009 recommend parathyroid surgery under the following conditions[18]:

- Age <50 years
- Albumin corrected serum calcium >1 mg/dL above the upper limit of normal, or any prior hypercalcemic crisis.
- Reduction in bone mineral density at any site to a T score < −2.5 or prior fragility fracture (also consider clinical fracture equivalents, e.g., >2" loss in height or morphometric vertebral fracture).
- GFR <60 mL/minute, or 70% of the age-adjusted norm.
- Patients for whom close medical follow-up is either not possible (e.g., risk of dehydration and hypercalcemic crisis is significant) or is not desirable.

- While symptomatic nephrolithiasis is an indication for surgery, hypercalciuria alone (>400 mg daily) is no longer considered as a guideline criteria for surgery. However, hypercalciuria decreases renal salt and water retention, and the individual pHPT patient's risk for dehydration and hypercalcemic crisis should be considered.
- The appropriate surgical procedure depends on the underlying cause of the disease. If a single adenoma (80% to 85%) is suspected by history or preoperative localization, the diseased gland can be removed by a minimally invasive approach. Because the half-life of immunoreactive parathyroid hormone (iPTH) is very short, intraoperative measurements can be very helpful in determining the success of the operation as each abnormal gland is removed. If imaging demonstrates a likely single adenoma, the surgeon can resect the suspected gland and monitor iPTH levels to ensure that the adenoma was appropriately removed. A drop of 50% from baseline is good evidence of a successful parathyroidectomy.
- In those suspected to have multigland disease, a more traditional bilateral approach is often used. If hyperplasia of all four glands is found, all parathyroid tissue is removed except for a small remnant that is left *in situ* or transplanted to the nondominant forearm musculature. A small amount of tissue may also be cryopreserved in the event that the transplanted tissue fails to engraft in the muscle.
- Several surgical approaches, radio-guided mini-invasive approach, unilateral mini-invasive approach, bilateral exploration, and conversion to bilateral exploration have very comparative probability of cure (95.5% to 99%) and morbidity (0.5% to 3%).[19]
- Complications of parathyroid surgery include the so-called **"hungry bone syndrome,"** in which profound hypocalcemia develops, requiring parenteral calcium supplementation. Rates of postsurgical hypocalcemia may be higher in those with hyperplasia than in those with a single adenoma, and in younger patients. Persistent hypoparathyroidism may also occur, mainly in those who have had surgery for parathyroid hyperplasia. Recurrent laryngeal nerve injury occurs in 1% to 2% of surgeries. In general, improved outcomes correlate directly with the experience of the surgeon.

Medications

- In those patients who do not meet the recommended guidelines for surgical intervention, and in those who either refuse surgery or are poor surgical candidates, medical management may be appropriate.
- General management: **adequate hydration** should be ensured, as should a **moderate calcium intake** (~1000 mg/day).
- **Thiazide diuretics** and other drugs (e.g., excessive over the counter anti-acid use) that can exacerbate hypercalcemia **should be avoided**.
- **Bisphosphonates** are effective treatments for osteoporosis and have shown promise in preventing loss of bone mass associated with pHPT. Alendronate has been best-studied, implementing osteoporosis treatment regimens of 10 mg/day or 70 mg/week. While bone mass is preserved, hypercalcemia and hypercalciuria are generally not controlled long-term.[20]
- **Estrogens** have been shown to lower serum and urinary calcium levels, decrease bone resorption and preserve bone mass in postmenopausal women with mild pHPT. However, use of estrogens for pHPT is not preferred due to adverse effects of hormone replacement therapy and the need for high doses of estrogen for maximal effect. **Raloxifene** has potential for decreasing serum calcium and has fewer adverse effects associated with hormone replacement; however, further studies are required before it can be recommended for use in pHPT.

- The calcimimetic **cinacalcet hydrochloride** represents a highly useful and promising new class of medications. Cinacalcet hydrochloride is a type II calcimimetic that increases the parathyroid gland CaSR to serum calcium levels, thus decreasing PTH production and release. Cinacalcet is currently FDA approved for treatment of sHPT and parathyroid carcinoma. However, cinacalcet also controls PTH and calcium levels in patients with pHPT, and can be used to control serum calcium in patients with symptomatic hypercalcemia who are unable to undergo surgery. Cinacalcet is usually initiated at 30 mg PO twice daily and then increased with titration to serum calcium responses. Note that cinacalcet does not improve bone mineral density, and only surgery has been shown to reduce fracture risk in pHPT. Cinacalcet is also a useful therapy for bridging severely hypercalcemic/hypercalciuric patients until surgery. The drug has a very short half-life, and can be stopped the day prior to surgery.
- **Percutaneous ethanol ablation** of parathyroid adenomas has been recently advocated as a therapeutic alternative for patients with pHPT.
- To date, in the setting of pHPT only parathyroid surgery has been demonstrated to decrease risk of hip fracture and reverse bone loss as a clinically relevant primary endpoint. Since parathyroid surgery is curative in the vast majority of patients, it should be viewed as the preferred definitive therapy for pHPT.

Secondary Hyperparathyroidism

Treatment should be directed to the correction of the causes leading to hyperparathyroidism. Surgery should not be pursued in most patients.

Medications

- **Vitamin D** deficiency is relatively easy to correct. In general, vitamin D stores should be repleted until the 25(OH)D level is >30 ng/mL. Vitamin D deficiency is common, and thus a frequent concomitant of pHPT. An established replacement regimen in the setting of pHPT when surgery is not indicated is ergocalciferol (vitamin D2) 50,000 IU PO per week for 4 weeks, then 50,000 IU per month. Even prior to surgery for pHPT, the initiation of this vitamin D replacement regimen is appropriate. In total, approximately 600,000 IU to 750,000 IU of vitamin D is required to replete a severely deficient patient, assessed by monitoring serum 25(OH)D levels after 3 months of therapy. Oral cholecalciferol (vitamin D_3) at 1000 to 2000 IU daily can be used for maintenance, and may possess more favorable pharmacodynamic properties and bioactivity.
- **Managing CKD** causing sHPT can be far more challenging. The goal of therapy is to maintain PTH levels in the acceptable range based on the stage of CKD in order to prevent both renal osteodystrophy (high-turnover bone disease) due to hyperparathyroidism and adynamic (low turnover) bone disease due to overly suppressed PTH levels.
  - The initial goal is to decrease the calcium-phosphorus product to <55 mg^2/dL^2, primarily by decreasing dietary uptake of phosphorus from the gut. In patients with CKD, the goal for daily intake of phosphorus is <800 to 1000 mg/day, and consultation with a dietitian is necessary to help patients achieve this goal.
  - Ultimately, most patients will require therapy with **phosphorus-binding agents**. The aluminum-containing agents that were once used have been linked to osteomalacia and encephalopathy and are now avoided. Currently, the mainstays of therapy are inexpensive calcium-based binders such as **calcium carbonate** and **calcium acetate**. Calcium acetate has the benefit of binding more phosphorus with less calcium being absorbed per milligram of elemental calcium than calcium carbonate. To minimize calcium absorption, the dose should be limited to

<2000 mg/day and titrated to the lowest dose needed to maintain a PO4 level between 2.7 and 5.5 mg/dL (depending on the stage of CKD).

○ However, recent data have now significantly called into question whether calcium-based phosphate binders should be used. **Sevelamer** is a copolymer that binds to dietary phosphate and prevents absorption. As compared to sevelamer, calcium-based binders significantly reduce bone mass (over suppression of PTH) and increase vascular calcification in CKD. Because of the severe cardiovascular mortality associated with vascular calcification in ESRD, non-calcium based phosphate binders such as sevelamer are seen as preferable by many nephrologists.[21,22]

○ Once the levels of calcium and phosphorus are in an acceptable range, vitamin D therapy may be necessary to lower PTH levels into the target range. **Calcitriol** or one of its analogs can be used to stabilize or reduce PTH levels to an acceptable range (the National Kidney Foundation Disease Outcomes Quality Initiative guidelines for iPTH are currently 150 to 300 pg/mL).

○ Newer analogs of vitamin D (doxercalciferol and paricalcitol) have less calcemic and phosphatemic effects, but to date have not been proven to be more effective or safer than calcitriol. Over suppression of PTH and attendant negative impact on bone and vascular calcium accrual should be avoided.

• **Calcimimetics** are a useful new therapy for hyperparathyroidism and have recently been approved by the FDA for the treatment of sHPT in patients on dialysis. **Cinacalcet** is the first available calcimimetic and has been shown to produce a dose-dependent reduction in PTH as well as a decrease in the calcium–phosphate product. The initial dose of cincalcet is 30 mg/day, and incremental BID dosing increases can be made every 2 to 4 weeks to 60, 90, and 180 mg/day until goals are achieved. Serum calcium and phosphorus should be measured within 1 week and at frequent intervals during dose titration to monitor for hypocalcemia. Intact PTH can be measured 1 to 4 weeks after initiation of therapy or a change in dose.[23]

Surgical Management
• Finally, surgical parathyroidectomy may become necessary in those with severe sHPT.
• The indications for parathyroidectomy are
  ○ Failure of maximal medical management with hypercalcemia, hypercalcuria, PTH >800 pg/mL, hyperphosphatemia (with calcium-phosphorus product > 70 mg^2/dL^2), osteoporosis, and symptoms: pruritis, pathologic bone fracture, ectopic soft tissue calcifications, severe vascular calcification, calcific uremia arteriolopathy (a.k.a. calciphylaxis), or bone pain
  ○ Medical observation not possible
  ○ Patient preference

Tertiary Hyperparathyroidism

In patients with tertiary hyperparathyroidism, medical treatment is not curative. The mainstay of treatment for tertiary hyperparathyroidism is surgery.[24]

Surgical Management
Evidence-based recommendation is still lacking. However, some experts agree the indications for parathyroidectomy in patients with tertiary hyperparathyroidism include the following:
• Severe hypercalcemia (serum calcium >12 mg/dL)
• Symptomatic hyperparathyroidism: fatigue, pruritis, bone pain or pathologic bone fracture, peptic ulcer disease, mental status changes, history of renal calculi
• Osteoporosis or high risk for osteoporotic fracture

Hypocalcemia

23

Prajesh M. Joshi and Michael P. Whyte

GENERAL PRINCIPLES

- Hypocalcemia is a common problem with multiple etiologies.
- Calcium homeostasis is essential for normal cell function, neural transmission, membrane stability, bone structure, blood coagulation, and intracellular signaling. Unrecognized or poorly treated hypocalcemic emergencies can lead to significant morbidity or mortality.

Definition

- Hypocalcemia is defined as serum ionized calcium <4.5 mg/dL or serum total calcium <8.6 mg/dL with a normal serum albumin.
- Normal reference range for serum total calcium is between 8.6 and 10.3 mg/dL (2.15 to 2.58 mmol/L) and that for ionized calcium is 4.5 to 5.1 mg/dL (1.13 to 1.28 mmol/L).
- Hypocalcemia can be classified into acute and chronic.

Epidemiology

Hypocalcemia is estimated to occur in up to 88% of patients in an intensive care unit (ICU) and 26% of those admitted to a non-ICU facility.

Etiology

Causes for hypocalcemia can be broadly classified (see Table 23-1) into:
- Inadequate parathyroid hormone (PTH) production (Hypoparathyroidism)
- PTH resistance
- Inadequate vitamin D
- Resistance to vitamin D
- Miscellaneous causes

Pathophysiology

- Approximately 99% of body calcium is found in bone. Of the 1% that is found in extracellular fluid, 50% is in the free (biologically active) ionized form, 40% is bound to protein (predominantly albumin), and 10% is complexed with anions (e.g., citrate or PO_4).[1]
- Variations in serum calcium levels depend upon serum pH, protein and anion levels, and calcium-regulating hormone function.
- Approximately 500 mg of calcium are removed from healthy bones daily and replaced by an equal amount. Calcium absorbed by the intestines is matched by urinary calcium excretion. Despite these large fluxes of calcium, serum levels of ionized calcium remain stable because of the rigid control by PTH and vitamin D levels and the vital role of the calcium-sensing receptor (CaSR).

TABLE 23-1 CAUSES OF HYPOCALCEMIA

Inadequate PTH production (Hypoparathyoidism)	• Surgical/postoperative • Autoimmune destruction • Genetic (DiGeorge's syndrome) • Postradiation therapy, infiltrative processes • CaSR receptor defect • Idiopathic
PTH resistance	• Pseudohypoparathyroidism • Magnesium deficiency
Inadequate vitamin D	• Nutritional deficiency • Lack of sunlight exposure • Malabsorption syndrome • End-stage liver disease and cirrhosis • Chronic kidney disease
Resistance to vitamin D	• Pseudovitamin D deficiency rickets (vitamin D–dependent rickets type 1) • Vitamin D–resistant rickets (vitamin D–dependent rickets type 2)
Miscellaneous	• Hyperphosphatemia • Drugs (e.g., foscarnet, IV bisphosphonate therapy in patients with vitamin D deficiency) • Rapid transfusion with citrate-containing blood • "Hungry bone syndrome" or recalcification tetany • Postthyroidectomy for Graves' disease • Postparathyroidectomy • Acute pancreatitis • Rhabdomyolysis or Tumor lysis syndrome • Acute critical illness

Calcium-sensing Receptor
• Changes in extracellular calcium levels are detected by a large extracellular amino-terminal region of the CaSR, a 7-transmembrane receptor found upon the cell membrane of parathyroid and kidney cells.
• Binding of calcium to the CaSR induces activation of phospholipase C through the G-protein signaling pathway. This leads to increases in free intracellular calcium concentration and, in turn, reduces transcription of the PTH gene. Conversely, a decrease in extracellular calcium increases PTH secretion.
• CaSR also regulates calcium excretion by the kidneys.

Parathyroid Hormone
• PTH is secreted by chief cells in the parathyroid gland in response to decreases in ionized calcium.
• It acts to maintain calcium levels by direct action on bone to promote resorption and on the kidney to conserve calcium and excrete phosphate. It also indirectly

enhances intestinal calcium absorption by mediating renal production of the active vitamin D metabolite, 1,25-dihydroxyvitamin D ($1,25(OH)_2D$, also referred to as calcitriol).

Vitamin D

- Vitamin D is derived from dietary sources or from conversion of cholesterol precursors in the dermis by exposure to UV light.
- Vitamin D is converted to more potent 25-hydroxyvitamin D (25(OH)D) by the liver and then to the active form $1,25(OH)_2D$ by PTH-regulated 1α-hydroxylase in the proximal renal tubular cells.
- Active vitamin D (calcitriol) stimulates intestinal absorption of calcium and regulates PTH release.
- To form vitamin D_3 (cholecalciferol), lightly pigmented individuals require at least 10 minutes of sun exposure daily, whereas individuals with darker skin may require longer exposure.

DIAGNOSIS

Clinical Presentation

- Ionized calcium levels, rather than serum total calcium primarily determine symptoms due to hypocalcemia.[1]
- Low extracellular fluid ionized calcium enhances neuromuscular excitability, an effect accentuated by hyperkalemia or hypomagnesemia.[1]
- Symptoms of hypocalcemia are more prominent and life-threatening when the presentation is acute; chronic hypocalcemia may cause few, if any, symptoms.[1]

History

- Patients with moderate to severe hypocalcemia often present with **symptoms of tetany** that include circumoral paresthesias, distal extremity numbness and tingling, and carpopedal spasm—the classic example of which is the main d'accoucheur (midwife) posture. This involves adduction of the thumb, flexion of the metacarpal joints, and flexion of the wrist.
- Patients may also develop potentially life-threatening **laryngeal stridor** due to laryngeal spasm.
- **CNS manifestations** like seizures, irritability, confusion, and delirium can occur. Children with chronic hypocalcemia may have mental retardation, and adults may develop worsening dementia. Mental retardation is typically irreversible, but dementia in adults can improve in 50% of cases with correction of hypocalcemia. Calcification of the basal ganglia may result in movement disorders.[2]
- **Cardiac manifestations** including syncope, congestive heart failure, and angina occur in the acute setting.
- **Gastrointestinal symptoms** include biliary colic, intestinal colic, and dysphagia from smooth muscle contractions. Diarrhea and/or gluten intolerance may be seen in cases of hypocalcemia that are due to malabsorption (e.g., from celiac sprue).
- **Chronic manifestations** include cataracts, dry skin, coarse hair, brittle nails, psoriasis, chronic pruritus, and poor dentition.
- **Related medical history** may include pancreatitis, renal or liver failure, gastrointestinal disorders, and hyperthyroidism or hyperparathyroidism.
- **Pertinent surgical history** includes thyroid, parathyroid, or bowel surgeries or recent neck trauma.

- Inquiry should be made about administration of radiocontrast media, estrogen, loop diuretics, bisphosphonates, denosumab, calcium supplements, antibiotics, and anti-epileptics to exclude secondary hypocalcemia.
- Family history of hypocalcemia may aid in the diagnosis of inherited conditions.

Physical Examination
- The two classic physical examination findings include Chvostek's sign and Trousseau's sign.
- **Chvostek's sign** is elicited by tapping the facial nerve 2 cm in front of the tragus and observing for ipsilateral contraction of facial muscles. The sign is neither sensitive nor specific and may be seen in normocalcemic individuals. If patients are undergoing parathyroidectomy, a Chvostek's sign should be elicited prior to surgery to determine the reliability of this sign.
- Trousseau's sign is elicited by inflating a blood pressure cuff to 20 mm Hg **above** the systolic blood pressure for 3 minutes and observing for main d'accoucheur posturing of the hand. It is reported to have a better sensitivity and lower false-positive rate compared to Chvostek's sign.
- Cardiopulmonary examination: S3 gallop and rales on auscultation suggests heart failure. Wheezing and stridor might result from bronchospasm and laryngospasm.
- Skin examination: impetigo herpetiformis, a form of acute pustular psoriasis, is associated with hypocalcemia in pregnancy.
- Features of Albright's hereditary osteodystrophy (AHO) may be seen (please see below for details).

Differential Diagnosis

Inadequate PTH Production (Hypoparathyroidism)
- Hypoparathyroidism is defined as an **inappropriately low secretion of PTH for given ionized calcium.** Characteristic laboratory findings of hypoparathyroidism are **hypocalcemia and hyperphosphatemia with normal renal function.** Twenty-four-hour urinary excretion of calcium is low, as is the blood $1,25(OH)_2D$ level.
- Hypoparathyroidism may have a surgical, autoimmune, familial (genetic), or idiopathic origin. All varieties share the same symptoms, although hereditary hypoparathyroidism tends to have a gradual presentation.
- **Postoperative hypoparathyroidism**
  - Postoperative hypoparathyroidism occurs on postoperative days 1 to 2 as a complication of parathyroid and thyroid surgery, although may occur years after the procedure. Patients undergoing thyroidectomy for Graves' disease are more likely to experience postoperative hypocalcemia than for other etiologies.[3] The incidence of hypoparathyroidism has been related more to the experience of the surgeon than to the exact procedure performed.
  - In the setting of parathyroidectomy, use of the intraoperative PTH values has been useful in predicting risk for developing postoperative hypocalcemia.[4] A combination of an early postoperative intact PTH (60 minutes postsurgery) <14 ng/mL and a serum calcium <8 mg/mL at 6 hours postoperative had 88% specificity in predicting hypocalcemia in a retrospective study.[5]
  - Postoperative hypocalcemia may occur after multiple blood transfusions due to calcium chelation by citrate preservative in the blood.
  - Postoperative hypocalcemia also results from "hungry bone syndrome" after surgery for either primary or secondary hyperparathyroidism. It is caused by rapid formation of calcium-containing hydroxyapatite crystals in the "hungry bone" when PTH

action suddenly stops. This can also be seen in the setting of total thyroidectomy in patients with hyperthyroidism, or in treatment of long-standing metabolic acidosis.
○ Hungry bone syndrome can be distinguished from hypoparathyroidism by measuring phosphorous and PTH levels. Phosphorus is low and the PTH appropriately elevated in hungry bone syndrome.
- **Hypoparathyroidism associated with autoimmune destruction**
  ○ The PTH gland destruction occurs either in isolation or as part of type 1 autoimmune polyglandular syndrome (APS1) (see Chapter 36).
  ○ APS1 can be sporadic or autosomal recessive, caused by mutations in the autoimmune regulator (AIRE) gene located on chromosome 21q22.3.
  ○ The destruction consists of the classic triad of *hypoparathyroidism*, *adrenal insufficiency*, and *mucocutaneous candidiasis*, two of which (diagnostic dyad) are required for diagnosis. The typical presentation is childhood candidiasis, followed by hypoparathyroidism, and then adrenal insufficiency during late childhood. The disease may also be associated with hypgonadism, hepatitis, pernicious anemia, type 1 diabetes mellitus, autoimmune thyroid disease, alopecia, and vitiligo.[6]
  ○ Antibodies against a parathyroid autoantigen, NACHT leucine-rich-repeat protein 5 (NALP5), which is predominantly expressed in the cytoplasm of parathyroid chief cells, has been identified in 49% of APS1 with hypoparathyroidism.[7] Patients with APS1 and isolated autoimmune hypoparathyroidism often have antibodies to CaSR. Although its role in the pathogenesis of the disease is unclear, stimulation of CaSR has been suggested.[8]
- **Hypoparathyroidism secondary to developmental disorders**
  ○ This hypoparathyroidism results from agenesis or dysgenesis of the parathyroid glands. This is often associated with the DiGeorge's syndrome, in which malformation of the third and fourth branchial pouches causes absence of the thymus and parathyroids. The DiGeorge syndrome presents with CATCH-22 (cardiac anomalies, abnormal facies, thymic aplasia, cleft palate, and hypocalcemia seen with a deletion in chromosome 22).
  ○ An autosomal dominant syndrome with hypoparathyroidism, deafness, and renal dysplasia (HDR) has been reported with presence of asymptomatic hypocalcemia with undetectable or normal PTH.[9] This has been shown to be caused by mutations in the transcription factor GATA3.[10]
- **Radiation therapy and infiltration**
  ○ Rarely, hypoparathyroidism has been described due to direct destruction of the parathyroid glands in patients who are transfusion-dependent through iron deposition, copper deposition in Wilson's disease, and aluminum deposition in dialysis patients. Infiltration of the gland by metastatic carcinoma, granulomatous disease, or amyloidosis can also cause hypoparathyroidism, as can extensive radiation to the neck and mediastinum.
- **Defect in CaSR receptor**
  ○ Autosomal dominant hypocalcemic hypercalciuria occurs as a result of gain of function mutation of gene encoding the CaSR leading to decrease in secretion of PTH.[11]
  ○ Activating antibodies to the CaSR has been suggested as a pathogenesis in autoimmune hypoparathyroidism.[8]
  ○ Similar effects are seen with use of calcimimetic agents, such as cinacalcet. These agents bind to the CaSR and lower the threshold for its activation by extracellular calcium. As a result, PTH release from parathyroid cells decreases. Hypocalcemia has been described in up to 5% of these patients.

- **Idiopathic hypoparathyroidism**
  - ○ Rare cases of autosomal dominant familial isolated hypoparathyroidism have been reported in association with mutation of preproparathyroid hormone gene.[12] Glial cells missing homolog B (GCMB), a transcription factor, is essential for development of the parathyroid gland. Autosomal recessive mutation in the gene encoding this molecule are uncommon cause of hypoparathyroidism.[13]

PTH Resistance
- **Pseudohypoparathyroidism**
  - ○ This cluster of inherited disorders is caused by decreased end-organ responses to PTH. The biochemical abnormalities mimic those of hypoparathyroidism (i.e., low serum calcium, high phosphorus); however, the PTH level is elevated.
  - ○ There are multiple possible defects in the PTH–receptor complex; therefore, there are several phenotypic presentations.
  - ○ Pseudohypoparathyroidism is classified into types 1 and 2. Type 1 is further subdivided into types 1a, 1b, and 1c.
    - Pseudohypoparathyroidism type 1 is caused by deficiency of α subunit of Gs, the signaling protein that couples PTH-receptor/adenylate cyclase complex and yields cyclic adenosine monophosphate (cAMP) as a secondary messenger in the cell. Patients with pseudohypoparathyroidism type 1 do not have a physiologic increase in cAMP in the urine after intravenous infusion of PTH. The defect of the Gs-alpha protein is not confined to the effects of PTH, but also affects other hormonal systems (e.g., resistance to glucagon, thyroid-stimulating hormone, gonadotropins) that use cAMP as a second messenger.
      - □ Pseudohypoparathyroidism type 1a, the most common variant, presents with the physical features of AHO, which include short metatarsals and metacarpals, short stature, rounded facies, obesity, mental retardation, and heterotopic ossification. The defect is due to mutation of the GNAS gene, which encodes the Gs-alpha protein and is located on chromosome 20. Inheritance of the disease is autosomal dominant, and the expression of the gene is tissue specific and imprinted, with the maternal allele being expressed in the kidney. Therefore, if one inherits the defective allele from the mother, hypocalcemia is present. If the allele is inherited from the father, there is the physical appearance of AHO, but serum calcium homeostasis is maintained. This latter disorder is termed pseudopseudohypoparathyroidism.
      - □ Pseudohypoparathyroidism type 1b is characterized by a defective kidney response to PTH. The patients do not have AHO; instead, they often have skeletal findings consistent with hyperparathyroidism. These patients have normal Gs-alpha protein, with hormonal resistance to PTH—an impaired cAMP response to PTH, suggesting that the defect resides within the receptor. The level at which the receptor is affected is not yet clear.
      - □ Pseudohypoparathyroidism type 1c presents with resistance to PTH along with multiple other hormones with physical features of AHO. A normal Gs-alpha protein expression distinguishes this condition from pseudohypoparathyroidism type 1a. Molecular studies suggest that these patients have GNAS mutations that result in functional defects of Gs-alpha protein that are not apparent in conventional in-vitro assays.[14]
    - Pseudohypoparathyroidism type 2 patients respond to PTH administration with an appropriate increase in urinary cAMP, but fail to increase urinary phosphate, suggesting that the defect is located downstream to the generation of cAMP. If the

patient presents with hypocalcemia, hypophosphaturia, and elevated immunoreactive parathyroid hormone (iPTH) levels, first rule out vitamin D deficiency, which has a similar presentation. In patients with a vitamin D deficiency, all parameters return to normal after vitamin D administration. Pseudohypoparathyroidism type 2 is quite rare, with <50 cases having been described.[15]

- **Magnesium deficiency**
  - Magnesium deficiency impairs PTH secretion from parathyroid glands or stops PTH biosynthesis. PTH resistance occurs when serum magnesium concentrations fall below 0.8 mEq/L (1 mg/dL or 0.4 mmol/L). Decreased PTH secretion occurs in patients with more severe hypomagnesemia. Malabsorption, diuretics, parenteral fluid administration, chronic alcoholism, and cisplatin therapy are the most common causes of hypomagnesemia.
  - Hyypocalcemia secondary to hypomagnesemia is resistant to administration of calcium and vitamin D.
  - Restoration of the calcium levels can occur only after the magnesium deficiency is corrected. Levels of phosphorus are not elevated in patients with hypomagnesemia (as found in hypoparathyroidism), which probably is related to associated nutritional deficiencies.
  - These patients present with low or inappropriately normal PTH levels in the presence of hypocalcemia.

Vitamin D Deficiency

- Vitamin D deficiency is the most common cause of hypocalcemia, which is caused by several mechanisms: (a) decreased absorption of dietary calcium; (b) decreased renal reabsorption of calcium; and (c) resistance to the osteoclastic effects of PTH on bone.
- In vitamin D deficiency and hypocalcemia, the compensatory increase in PTH results in mild increases in serum calcium. However, this comes at the expense of serum phosphate, since PTH increases phosphaturia. These combined effects lead to a loss of bone mineralization and, if uncorrected, cause syndromes of rickets and osteomalacia.
  - Rickets occurs in growing bone, typically in children, and results from diminished calcification of cartilage at the physis. The typical presentation involves bowing of the limbs and cupping of the costochondral junctions (the rachitic rosary).
  - Osteomalacia occurs after growth plates close and has a clinical appearance that may be difficult to distinguish from osteoporosis. Patients frequently have hypophosphatemia.
- Vitamin D deficiency may occur with inadequate exposure to sun, inadequate dietary supply of vitamin D, or intestinal malabsorption of fatty acids.
- Patients of darker skin pigmentation have decreased conversion of vitamin D_2 to calcidiol for a given amount of sunlight.
- Dietary insufficiency may occur in those who live in areas where vitamin D supplementation of dairy products is not standard practice. In addition, an inadequate dietary intake may occur in the elderly or in breastfed infants of vegetarian mothers.
- Malabsorption may occur in patients with gastrojejunostomy, gastric resection, or celiac disease causing deficiency. Liver disease with decreased synthetic function can cause vitamin D deficiency from several sources: impaired 25-hydroxylation of vitamin D, decreased bile salts with malabsorption of vitamin D, decreased synthesis of vitamin D-binding protein, or other factors. Patients with chronic pancreatitis, pancreatic insufficiency, and steatorrhea have malabsorption of calcium and vitamin D.

Vitamin D Resistance

- Patients with vitamin D–dependent rickets type 1, also known as pseudovitamin D deficiency, have a genetic deficiency of 1α-hydroxylase. This condition is rare and

is inherited in an autosomal recessive fashion typically manifesting prior to 2 years of age. These patients have normal or elevated levels of 25(OH)D, and calcitriol administration can correct the defect.

- Vitamin D–dependent rickets type 2, also known as hereditary calcitriol resistant rickets, involves typical symptoms of rickets as well as alopecia. It is inherited as an autosomal recessive disease and is the result of a mutation in the vitamin D receptor gene. These patients have high serum levels of $1,25(OH)_2D$ and can be treated with high doses of calcium as well as calcitriol. Calcium infusions are required if the resistance is complete.

Miscellaneous Causes of Acute Hypocalcemia

- **Acute hyperphosphatemia** can acutely lower calcium level, which is typically seen in rhabdomyolysis or tumor lysis syndrome. Rapid release of phosphorous from injured muscle cells or dying tumor cells can quickly complex calcium. This can be compounded by the acute renal failure often associated with these conditions.

- In addition, **malignancy** can cause hypocalcemia as a result of osteoblast activation in patients with blastic metastases from breast or prostate cancer via deposition of calcium in the lesions.

- **Chelation of calcium** by citrate (anticoagulant in banked blood or plasma), lactate, gadolinium-based contrast material used in magnetic resonance imaging (MRI, gadodiamide and gadoversetamide), and ethylenediaminetetraacetic acid (EDTA) reduce serum ionized calcium concentrations, but not serum total calcium concentrations. Calcium is also chelated in acute pancreatitis, most likely due to the release of free fatty acids. The degree of hypocalcemia seen with pancreatitis can be a prognosticator, with lower levels predicting a worse prognosis.

- Most patients in the ICU do not have an identifiable cause of hypocalcemia. Sepsis, especially if caused by gram-negative microorganisms, is associated with hypocalcemia, via endotoxins. Mortality rates increase among patients with sepsis and hypocalcemia.

- Multiple **medications** cause hypocalcemia. Those that inhibit bone resorption include calcitonin, plicamycin, gallium nitrate, and estrogens. Cimetidine decreases gastric pH, slowing fat breakdown, which is necessary to complex calcium for gut absorption. Anticonvulsants may stimulate microsomal enzymes with resultant abnormal metabolism of vitamin D. Reports also show that phenytoin interferes with the intestinal absorption of vitamin D. Patients on anticonvulsant therapy may present with hypocalcemia, normal calcitriol levels, and increased PTH levels.

- An increasing number of cancer patients are being treated with intravenous bisphosphonates for hypercalcemia or metastatic bone disease. In the setting of severe vitamin D deficiency, these patients can develop symptomatic hypocalcemia. This is most frequently reported with use of zoledronic acid, likely due to both its potency and frequency of use. Use of intravenous bisphosphonates is contraindicated in the setting of vitamin D deficiency; therefore, prior to use, serum 25(OH)D level should be obtained.

Diagnostic Testing

Laboratory Evaluation

- A patient with hypocalcemia should have his/her serum albumin quantified.
- To correct the total serum calcium in the setting of hypoalbuminemia, use the following equation:

$$\text{Corrected Ca}^{2+} = [4 - \text{serum albumin (g/dL)}] \times 0.8 + \text{serum Ca}^{2+} \text{ (mg/dL)}$$

- Alternatively, one can measure **serum ionized calcium** directly. However, this test is less reliable with a single measurement. It can be falsely elevated with prolonged ischemia of the arm during acquisition of the serum sample.
- Other tests should include measurement of **serum phosphorus, intact PTH, magnesium, creatinine,** and **vitamin D metabolites**.
- A low 25(OH)D level suggests vitamin D deficiency from poor nutritional intake, lack of sunlight, or malabsorption. Low levels of $1,25(OH)_2D$ in association with high PTH suggest PTH resistance or failure to induce the 1 α-hydroxylase, as observed in patients with chronic renal failure, vitamin D–dependent rickets type 1, and pseudohypoparathyroidism.
- Urinary cAMP may help to differentiate hypoparathyroidism from pseudohypoparathyroidism types 1 and 2.

Electrocardiography
The ECG finding of hypocalcemia includes prolongation of the QTc interval and shortening of RR interval, all proportional to the degree of hypocalcemia.[16,17]

Imaging
Skeletal x-rays show rickets or osteomalacia with pathognomonic "Looser zones" best observed in the pubic ramus, the upper femur, and the ribs.

TREATMENT

- Treatment depends on the severity and rapidity of development of hypocalcemia.
- Goals of treatment include alleviation of symptoms, correction of serum calcium to acceptable level, and avoidance of hypercalciuria or hypercalcemia.
- The indications for emergent correction of hypocalcemia include severe symptomatic tetany, stridor due to laryngospasm and bronchospasm, or seizures.

Medications
Acute Hypocalcemia
- This emergent condition is **treated by replacing calcium intravenously with either calcium gluconate or calcium chloride**. A 10 mL solution of 10% calcium gluconate (1 ampule) can be given over 10 minutes (rule of 10s) and can be repeated once or twice; calcium chloride, if used, is equally effective. Patients should be monitored using telemetry to detect cardiac arrthymias. The effect of this bolus is transient, and prolonged intravenous therapy should follow.
- For urgent, but non-emergent hypocalcemia, replacement with 1 mg/kg/hour of elemental calcium as an intravenous piggyback can be administered over several hours (10 mL of 10% calcium gluconate or 1 ampule = 93 mg elemental calcium). As such, if 6 ampules of calcium gluconate are mixed in 500 mL of D_5W, a drip rate of 0.92 mL/kg/hour will provide 1 mg/kg/hour of elemental calcium.
- Bicarbonate and phosphate solutions cause calcium to precipitate and should not be run simultaneously. **Serum calcium should be measured every 4 to 6 hours during intravenous infusion** and the rate adjusted to maintain a serum calcium level of 8 to 9 mg/dL.

Chronic Hypocalcemia
- Chronic management of hypocalcemia is accomplished using oral calcium salts, vitamin D metabolites and less commonly thiazide diuretics. Magnesium supplementation is needed for magnesium depletion.

- **The goal of chronic calcium replacement therapy is to keep the calcium in the low range of normal, especially in hypoparathyroid states to avoid hypercalciuria.** Approximately 1.5 to 3 g of elemental calcium should be given as a dietary supplement to ensure adequate intake. Supplementation should be given with meals to increase absorption and prevent hyperphosphatemia. There are multiple different preparations of oral calcium; in general, calcium carbonate is the cheapest, although absorption may be less than with other products.
- Vitamin D supplementation is typically given as ergocalciferol (vitamin D_2). This preparation is the least expensive and has the longest biological half-life. The typical dose range for patients with hypoparathyroidism is on the order of 50,000 to 100,000 IU orally daily (1.25 to 2.5 mg/day). Serum 25(OH)D levels can be measured along with serum calcium levels to assess for adequacy of treatment. Vitamin D is extremely lipophilic and may require several weeks to reach a steady state with a new dose. Calcitriol (1,25(OH)$_2$D), which has rapid onset of action and a shorter half-life (8 hours), may also be given with a typical starting dose of 0.25 to 0.5 mcg orally daily.

Hypocalcemia Secondary to Hypoparathyroidism and Pseudohypoparathyroidism

- Initial management is done with oral administration of calcium supplements, however, in patients with severe hypoparathyroidism, treatment with calcitriol is required due to lack of PTH-mediated conversion of inactive vitamin D (25(OH)D) to active vitamin D (1,25(OH)$_2$D).
- The aim in these patients is to maintain serum calcium at the lower end of the normal range to avoid development of hypercalciuria with a risk of nephrocalcinosis/nephrolithiasis due to loss of the renal calcium-conserving effect of PTH in hypoparathyroidism.
- Teriparatide has been shown to be effective in treatment of long-term hypoparathyroidism, but concerns about safety with long-term treatment have prevented its chronic use.[5] However, in the postparathyroidectomy setting, it could be used to decrease hospitalization and expedite achievement of normocalcemia.

Other Nonpharmacologic Therapies

In patients with a higher risk of developing permanent hypoparathyroidism, parathyroid tissue may be autotransplanted into the brachioradialis or sternocleidomastooid muscle at the time of parathyroidectomy.

COMPLICATIONS

- The goal of treatment of chronic hypocalcemia is a low-normal serum calcium level (8 to 8.5 mg/dL). If the calcium is kept below this level, the patient remains at risk for symptoms of hypocalcemia or cataracts. A higher calcium level may predispose patients to nephrolithiasis.
- In chronic hypocalcemia, the **calcium-phosphate product** (calculated by multiplying the calcium by the phosphate level) should be monitored. The goal is a product <60 to avoid calciphylaxis. In addition, **24-hour urine calcium-to-creatinine ratio** should be periodically checked for hypercalciuria. The ratio is determined by dividing urine calcium by urine creatinine. The ratio should be lower than 0.2; if it is higher, there is an increased risk of development of renal stones, particularly calcium phosphate stones.
- If hypercalcemia develops, vitamin D and calcium supplementation should be withheld until levels return to normal. The doses should be decreased. The effects of calcitriol typically last one week, but ergocalciferol can last more than 1 month.

• Patients treated with teriparatide for long duration have a potential risk for development of osteosarcoma.

PROGNOSIS

The prognosis for correcting hypocalcemia is good but is dependent upon the etiology. Most symptoms can be alleviated. However, cataract or mental retardation from long-standing hypocalcemia cannot be reversed.

REFERENCES

1. Favus MJ, Goltzman David. *Primer on the Metabolic Bone Diseases and Disorders of Mineral Metabolism,* 7th ed. Washington, DC: American Society for Bone and Mineral Research; 2009:104–108.
2. Fonseca OA, Cleverly JR. Neurological manifestations of hypoparathyroidism. *Arch Intern Med* 1967;120:202–206.
3. Pesce CE, Shiue Z, Tsai HL, et al. Postoperative hypocalcemia after thyroidectomy for Graves' disease. *Thyroid* 2010;20:1279–1283.
4. Mcleod Ik, Arciero C, Noordzij JP, et al. The use of rapid parathyroid hormone assay in predicting postoperative hypocalcemia after total or completion thyroidectomy. *Thyroid* 2006;16:259–265.
5. Graff AT, Miller FR, Roehm CE, et al. Predicting hypocalcemia after total thyroidectomy: Parathyroid hormone level vs. serial calcium levels. *Ear Nose Throat J* 2010;89:462–465.
6. Perheentupa J. Autoimmune polyendocrinopathy-candidiasis-ectodermal dystrophy. *J Clin Endocrinol Metab* 2006;91:2843–2850.
7. Alimohammadi M, Bjorklund P, Hallgren A, et al. Autoimmune polyendocrine syndrome type 1 and NALP5, a parathyroid autoantigen. *New Engl J Med* 2008;358:1018–1028.
8. Kifor O, McElduff A, LeBoff MS, et al. Activating antibodies to the calcium-sensing receptor in two patients with autoimmune hypoparathyroidism. *J Clin Endocrinol Metab* 2009;89:548–556.
9. Bilous RW, Murty G, Parkinson DB, et al. Autosomal dominant familial hypoparathyroidism, sensineural deafness and renal dysplasia. *N Engl J Med* 1992;327:1069–1084.
10. Adachi M, Tachibana K, Asakura Y, et al. A novel mutation in the GATA3 gene in a family with HDR syndrome (hypoparathyroidism, sensorineural deafness and renal anomaly syndrome). *J Pediatr Endocrinol Metab* 2006;19(1):87–92.
11. Pearce SH, Williamson C, Kifor O, et al. A familial syndrome of hypocalcemia with hypercalciuria due to mutations in the calcium-sensing receptor. *N Eng J Med* 1996;335:1115–1122
12. Arnold A, Horst SA, Gardella TJ, et al. Mutation of the signal peptide-encoding region of the preproparathyroid hormone gene in familial isolated hypoparathyroidism. *J Clin Invest* 1990;86:1084–1087.
13. Ding C, Buckingham B, Levine MA. Familial isolated hypoparathyroidism caused by a mutation in the gene for the transcription factor GCMB. *J Clin Invest* 2001;108:1215–1220.
14. Farfel Z, Brothers V, Brickman A, et al. Pseudohypoparathyroidism: Inheritance of deficient receptor-cyclase coupling activity. *Proc Nat Acad Sci* 1981;78:3098–3102.
15. Rao DS, Parfitt, AM, Kleerekoper M, et al. Dissociation between the effects of endogenous parathyroid hormone on adenosine 3-prime, 5-prime-monophosphate generation and phosphate reabsorption in hypocalcemia due to vitamin D depletion: An acquired disorder resembling pseudohypoparathyroidism type II. *J. Clin Endocrinol Metab* 1985;61:285–290.
16. Bechtel JT, White JE, Estes EH. The electrocardiographic effects of hypocalcemia induced in normal subjects with edathamil disodium. *Circulation* 1956;13:837–842.
17. Vanderark CR. Electrolytes and the electrocardiogram. *Cardiovasc Clin* 1973;5:269–294.

Vitamin D Deficiency

24

Amy E. Riek, Ana Maria Arbelaez, and Carlos Bernal-Mizrachi

GENERAL PRINCIPLES

Physiology

- Vitamin D is a nutrient and a pro-hormone largely regulated by environmental factors, including diet and exposure to the sun.[1,2]
- There are several nutritional forms of vitamin D: D_3 (cholecalciferol), which is generated in the skin of animals, and D_2 (ergocalciferol), which is derived from plants. In this chapter, any mention of vitamin D implies vitamin D_2 or vitamin D_3.
- D_2 and D_3 are biologically inert. To become physiologically active, vitamin D requires a first hydroxylation in the liver to 25-hydroxyvitamin D, or 25(OH)D, and then a second hydroxylation in the kidney to its active hormonal form 1α, 25-dihydroxyvitamin D, or $1,25(OH)_2D$.
- The main role of vitamin D in the body is calcium and phosphorous homeostasis, and deficiency of vitamin D is associated with negative balance of these minerals and osteomalacia. However, more extensive roles for vitamin D are suggested by the discovery of the vitamin D receptor (VDR) and the extrarenal production of active vitamin D in almost all tissues in the body. These observations have opened a new area of study in the physiologic and pharmacologic actions of vitamin D.

Synthesis of Vitamin D

- The skin is the main organ responsible for vitamin D production. Sunlight exposure, especially ultraviolet B (UVB) photons between 290 and 315 nm, causes photolysis of 7-dehydrocholesterol (7-DHC or provitamin D_3) in skin to form previtamin D_3, which isomerizes into vitamin D_3 proportionally to the number of UVB photons that penetrate the epidermis.
- Lengthy sun exposure does not produce toxic levels of vitamin D_3 because sunlight itself induces photodegradation of previtamin D_3 and vitamin D_3, thereby regulating the total output in the circulation and preventing intoxication.
- Vitamin D_3 then binds to the vitamin D binding protein (DBP) and is transported in the circulation.

Dietary Intake of Vitamin D

- Vitamin D is fat soluble and principally absorbed in the proximal small intestine. Absorption of dietary vitamin D requires bile salts and an intact absorptive surface.
- Enterocytes absorb vitamin D by passive diffusion and secrete it into the lymphatics in the form of chylomicrons. Endothelial lipoprotein lipase hydrolyzes triglycerides from chylomicrons, producing chylomicron remnants that are rapidly cleared via the liver. Most vitamin D is metabolized in this fashion.

Metabolism of Vitamin D

- Once vitamin D enters the circulation from the skin or from the lymph via the thoracic duct, it is rapidly stored in fat or metabolized in the liver. Fat stores of vitamin D are used during the winter; however, obese individuals are only able to increase their blood levels of vitamin D by half when compared with individuals of normal weight.

- The **first step** in the metabolic activation of vitamin D is hydroxylation of carbon 25, which occurs primarily in the **liver.** Several hepatic cytochrome P-450s have been shown to 25-hydroxylate vitamin D compounds. CYP2R1, present in the liver and in testis, appears to be the critical 25-hydroxylase involved in both vitamin D_3 and vitamin D_2 metabolism. Mutations in the *CYP2R1* gene have been identified in patients with low 25(OH)D levels and rickets.

- **25(OH)D is the major circulating form** of vitamin D and has a half-life in human circulation of 10 days to 3 weeks. Hepatic 25-hydroxylation is poorly regulated. **Serum levels of 25(OH)D increase in proportion to cutaneous synthesis and dietary intake of vitamin D, and thus represent the best indicator of vitamin D status** (Figure 24-1).

- The **second step** in vitamin D activation is the formation of $1,25(OH)_2D$ by 1α-hydroxylase, mainly in the **kidney.** The half-life of $1,25(OH)_2D$ in circulation of humans is approximately 4 to 6 hours. A congenital defect in renal tubular 1α-hydroxylase enzyme expression results in vitamin D–dependent rickets type I.

- Numerous cells and tissues including prostate, breast, colon, lung, placenta, pancreatic beta-cells, bone cells, activated immune cells, vascular wall and parathyroid cells express 1α-hydroxylase and are able to transform 25(OH)D to its active hormonal form. This increased local production of active vitamin D serves as an autocrine–paracrine factor, which is fundamental for cell-specific functions. The contribution of these extrarenal sources to circulating $1,25(OH)_2D$ levels is minimal and only occurs during pregnancy, chronic renal failure, sarcoidosis, tuberculosis, granulomatous disorders, and rheumatoid arthritis.

- Renal 1α-hydroxylase activity is highly regulated and functions to maintain serum calcium at normal levels. Low plasma calcium stimulates this enzyme by inducing parathyroid hormone (PTH) expression. Increased serum PTH enhances renal production of $1,25(OH)_2D$ directly by induction of 1α-hydroxylase expression and indirectly by the hypophosphatemia resulting from PTH-induced renal phosphate wasting. This compensatory event keeps the $1,25(OH)_2D$ hormone concentration nearly constant despite low levels of 25(OH)D. **Elevated $1,25(OH)_2D$ concentrations can mislead physicians into thinking that patients are vitamin D sufficient when they may be severely vitamin D deficient.**

- Vitamin D is excreted principally in the bile. Although some of it is reabsorbed in the small intestine, the enterohepatic circulation of vitamin D is not considered to be an important mechanism to sustain adequate levels. Vitamin D is also catabolized to more water-soluble compounds, which are transported by DBP and albumin and excreted by the kidney.

- Catabolism of both 25(OH)D and $1,25(OH)_2D$ is carried out by 24-hydroxylase, which catalyzes a series of oxidation steps resulting in side chain cleavage and inactivation. **The kidney is the major site of vitamin D catabolism.** $1,24,25(OH)D$ or $24,25(OH)D$ compounds are generated in the kidney under normal conditions; however, 24-hydroxylase is expressed throughout the body and attenuates the cellular responses induced by $1,25(OH)_2D$. $1,25(OH)_2D$ controls its own degradation directly by stimulating 24-hydroxylase activity or indirectly by reducing PTH levels.

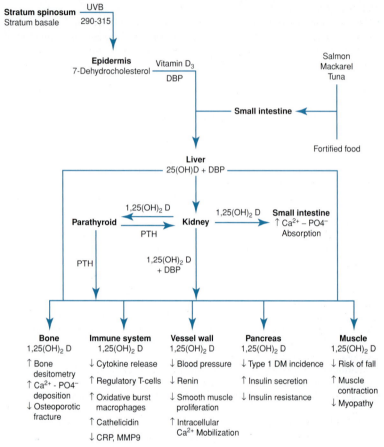

FIGURE 24-1 Synthesis and effects of vitamin D.

In the plasma, vitamin D is transported bound to plasma proteins. More than 99% of circulating vitamin D metabolites are protein-bound, mostly to DBP, and minimally to albumin and lipoproteins. DBPs have the highest affinity for 25(OH)D and 24,25(OH)$_2$D and less affinity for 1,25(OH)$_2$D. The levels of 1,25(OH)$_2$D are normally 1000 times lower than those of 25(OH)D. DBP may be reduced by liver disease, nephrotic syndrome, or malnutrition. DBP may be increased during pregnancy and estrogen therapy. Despite changes in DBP, the circulating concentration of free vitamin D active hormone remains constant. Therefore, DBP works as a buffer, preventing deficiency and/or intoxication of the active compound. DBP also facilitates 25(OH)D entry into the proximal tubule cells by a receptor-mediated uptake of DBP in the brush border. Megalin facilitates the endocytosis of the DBP and 25(OH)D complex. Once inside, 25(OH)D is released and is converted into 1,25(OH)$_2$D in the mitochondria by 1α-hydroxylase.

Molecular Actions of Vitamin D

- The VDR is expressed in almost all human tissues. $1,25(OH)_2D$ binds to the VDR, which acts as a ligand-activated transcription factor to regulate the expression of vitamin D–responsive genes. The VDR has a 100-fold affinity for $1,25(OH)_2D$ compared to $25(OH)D$ or other dihydroxy metabolites of vitamin D. Upon binding to VDR, vitamin D forms a heterodimeric complex with the retinoic acid X receptor, and the complex interacts with vitamin D–responsive elements on DNA and promotes transcription of vitamin D–regulated genes.
- Specific mutations in the VDR gene cause vitamin D–dependent rickets type II due to $1,25(OH)_2D$ resistance. Some VDR genetic variants are associated with changes in mineral homeostasis, skeletal remodeling, and modulation of cell proliferation.

Classification

Vitamin D status is usually estimated by measuring plasma $25(OH)D$ levels. Evidence that healthy outdoor workers, farmers, and lifeguards have $25(OH)D$ concentrations of 44 to 70 ng/mL suggest that an optimal healthy level may be higher than the accepted levels reported to prevent rickets and osteomalacia, though the majority of evidence to support this has been observational rather than interventional. Newer biomarkers such as intestinal calcium absorption and maximal PTH suppression have suggested that higher levels of $25(OH)D$ may be beneficial, but the specific levels reported by various studies have not been consistent, and the correlation of these levels in all age groups and races has not been tested. Therefore, based upon the best available evidence regarding clinical outcomes, primarily regarding bone mineral density (BMD) and fracture risk, the Institute of Medicine recently recommended the following classification for vitamin D status.[3] **An important concept is that most patients with suboptimal vitamin D levels are not hypocalcemic.**

- **Vitamin D Deficiency**—$25(OH)D$ levels <12 ng/mL.
- **Vitamin D Insufficiency**—$25(OH)D$ levels 12 to 20 ng/mL.
- **Vitamin D Adequacy**—$25(OH)D$ levels 20 to 50 ng/mL.
- **Vitamin D Toxicity**—$25(OH)D$ levels >150 ng/mL and hypercalcemia.[4,5]

Epidemiology

The prevalence of vitamin D deficiency is dependent upon the definition of deficiency, but appears to be widespread in all age groups. Latitude, time of day, season of the year, and race have a dramatic influence on the cutaneous production of vitamin D_3 (see Section Etiology). Data from The National Health Nutrition and Examination Survey (NHANES) 2003–2006 demonstrated $25(OH)D$ levels under 16 ng/mL (the median level of insufficiency) in 18.8% of those sampled: 10.6% of non-Hispanic whites, 53.6% of non-Hispanic blacks, and 27.2% of Mexican Americans.[6] The group at greatest risk includes African American men and women who live in the northern latitudes throughout the year. A study in noninstitutionalized elderly men and women in Boston (latitude 42°) during the winter showed vitamin D deficiency [$25(OH)D$ level <20 ng/dL] in 73% of blacks and 35% of whites, with severe vitamin D deficiency [$25(OH)D$ level <10 ng/dL] in 21% of African American and 11% of white subjects.[7]

Etiology

- **Decreased bioavailability**
  - Decreased fat absorption (malabsorption) resulting from cystic fibrosis, celiac disease, Whipple's disease, Crohn's disease, gastric bypass surgery, or medications that reduce cholesterol absorption.[8]

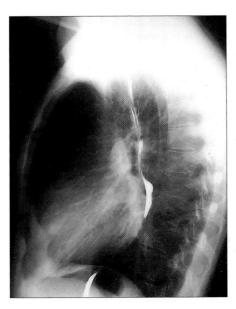

38
This patient presented with
dyspnoea and indigestion-like
pain.
i. What does the test show?
ii. What is the cause of the
dyspnoea?

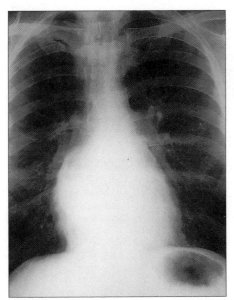

39
Describe the abnormalities on
the chest X-ray.

17

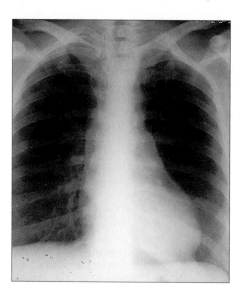

◄ 40

This chest X-ray is of a 29-year-old man with a history of dyspnoea. He underwent an interventional procedure in relation to his dyspnoea.

i. What is the underlying condition?

ii. What procedure was undertaken?

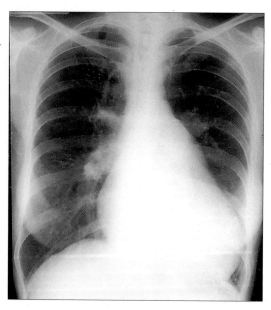

◄ 41

This chest X-ray is of a 30-year-old woman with a history of dyspnoea over a few years. She was found to have mild clubbing and cyanosis.

i. What are the abnormalities shown on the x-ray?

ii. What is the likely diagnosis?

iii. What non-invasive test would confirm the diagnosis?

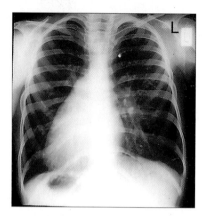

◄ 42

This chest X-ray is of a 25-year-old man who was found to have a soft systolic murmur and an early to mid-diastolic murmur. There was wide and fixed splitting of the second heart sound.

i. Describe the findings on the X-ray.

ii. What is the likely diagnosis?

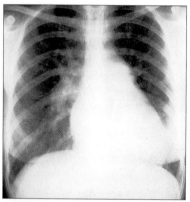

◄ 43

This chest X-ray is from a 35-year-old woman who presented with progressive dyspnoea and one episode of haemoptysis.

i. Describe the abnormalities.

ii. What is the most likely diagnosis?

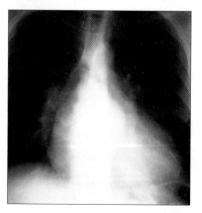

◄ 44

This chest X-ray is from a 60-year-old man who had a myocardial infarction nine years earlier.

i. What are the cardiological abnormalities seen?

ii. What is the commonest type of myocardial infarction to cause this abnormality?

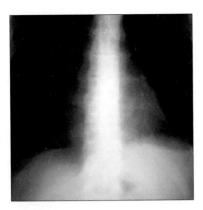

◀ **45**
What type of prosthetic valve does this patient have and in what position is it?

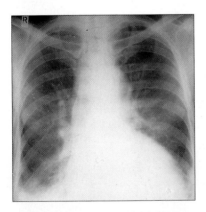

◀ **46**
This chest X-ray is of a 75-year-old man who presented with acute breathlessness.
i. Describe the radiological abnormalities.
ii. What is the likely diagnosis?

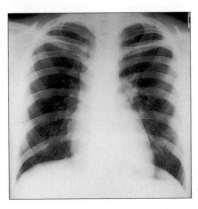

◀ **47**
This chest X-ray was performed for a routine health screen.
i. Describe the abnormality.
ii. What is its significance?

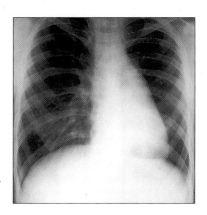

◄ 48

This chest X-ray is of a 30-year-old man who was referred by his doctor for investigation of breathlessness and a heart murmur. He had been healthy apart from a chest infection when aged seven years.

i. What abnormalities are seen?
ii. What are the likely diagnoses?

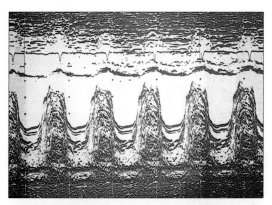

◄ 49

This echocardiogram is from a 40-year-old woman with a history of breathlessness, weight loss, pyrexia and episodes of dizziness.

i. Describe the findings on the echocardiogram.
ii. What is the likely diagnosis?

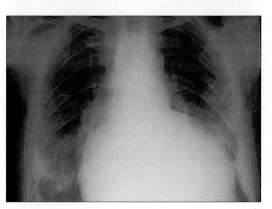

◄ 50

i. Describe the findings on the X-ray.
ii. What is the likely cause of the cardiological abnormality?

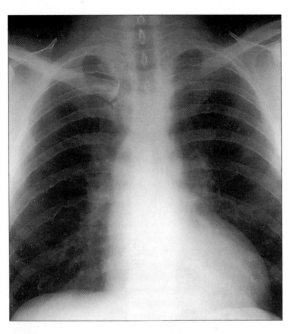

◄ **51**
This 25 year-old man was found to have raised blood pressure.
i. What is the abnormality on the X-ray?
ii. What other tests would confirm the diagnosis?

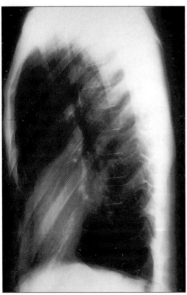

◄ **52**
i. Describe the abnormality of the X-ray.
ii. What is its cardiological significance?

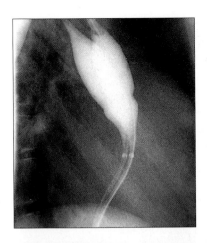

◄ 53

i. What procedure is being carried out?

ii. What are the complications associated with it?

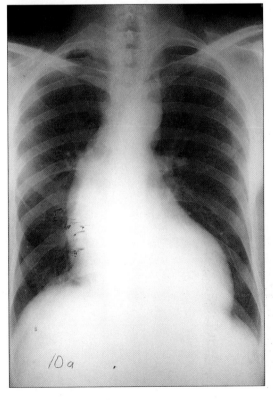

◄ 54

i. What is the main abnormality?

ii. What is the likely diagnosis?

iii. What test should be carried out?

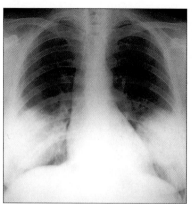

This chest X-ray is from a patient with vague chest pain. What abnormalities are seen on the X-ray?

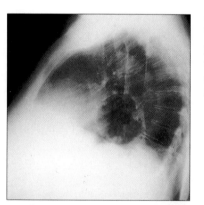

This X-ray is from a patient who presented with central chest pain which occurred both during exertion and at rest. What is the abnormality seen on the X-ray?

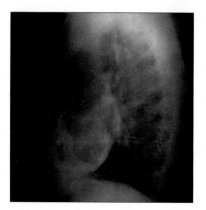

57

What are the cardiological abnormalities seen on this X-ray?

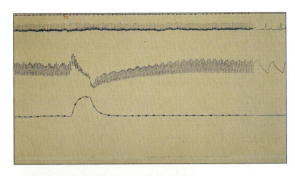

◀ 58
i. What is this test?
ii. What does it show?

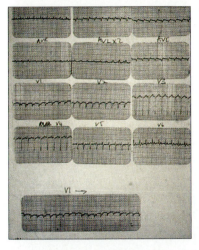

◀ 59
i. Describe the ECG.
ii. What rhythm is the patient's heart in?

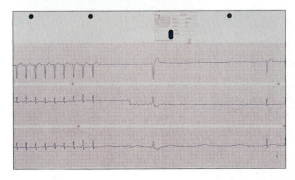

◀ 60
This rhythm strip was recorded from a patient with palpitations.
i. What is the rhythm?
ii. What was used to terminate it?

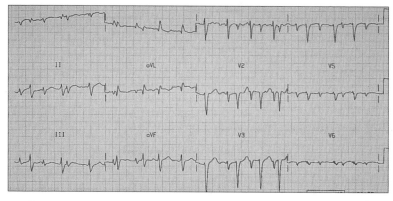

▲ 61

i.   Describe the findings on this ECG.
ii. What is the underlying condition that gives rise to this ECG?

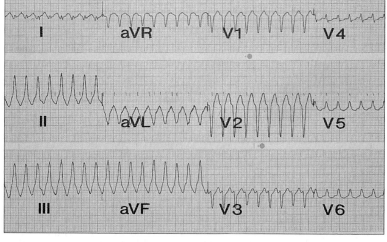

▲ 62

This ECG is from a 60-year-old man who presented with palpitations associated with chest pain and breathlessness.

i.   What are its characteristic features?
ii. What is the rhythm?

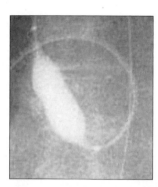

◄ 63
i. What procedure is being carried out?
ii. What are the indications for such a procedure?

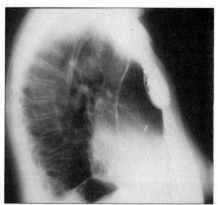

◄ 64
This patient had a dual chamber pacemaker implanted for complete heart block. Twenty four hours later he complained of an episode of dizziness. What is the abnormality that may be responsible for his dizziness?

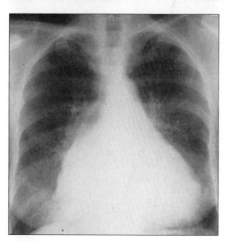

◄ 65
This X-ray is from a 57-year-old woman with a one year history of increasing breathlessness.
i. Describe the abnormalities.
ii. What are the possible diagnoses?

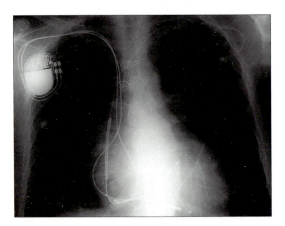

◄ 66
This X-ray is from a 62-year-old man with a history of palpitations and one episode of syncope. Describe the findings on the X-ray.

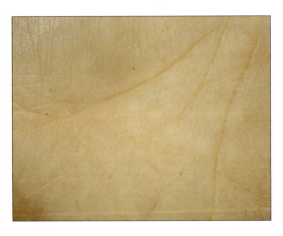

◄ 67
i. What is the abnormality in this patient's hand?
ii. What is the underlying condition and what is its significance?

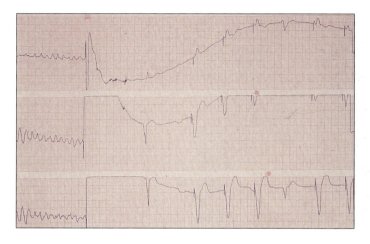

▲ 68
i. What is the cause of the events in the rhythm seen in this ECG?
ii. Describe their sequence.

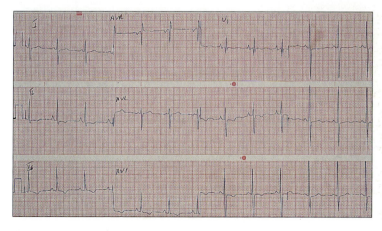

▲ 69
Describe the findings on this ECG.

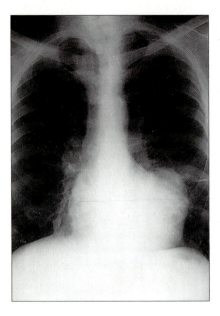

◄ **70**

This patient had a myocardial infarction eight months earlier.

i. Describe the main abnormality on the X-ray.

ii. In what type of myocardial infarction is this abnormality more common?

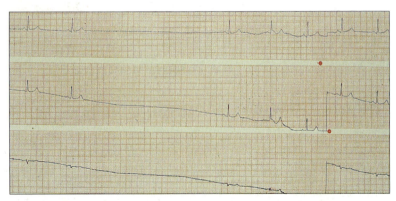

▲ **71**

This ECG rhythm strip is from a patient who has dizziness and near fainting attacks, particularly when shaving.

i. What is the abnormality?

ii. How could his symptoms be controlled?

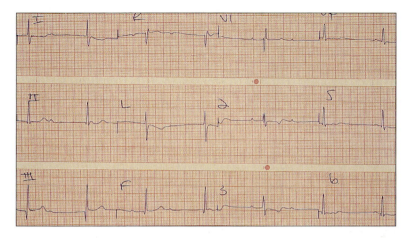

▲ 72

This ECG is from an 80-year-old man who presented with a syncopal attack.
Describe the ECG findings.

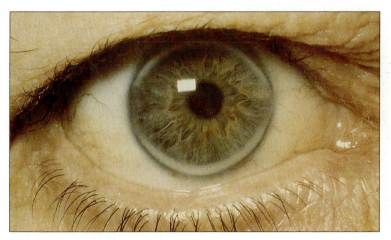

▲ 73

i. What abnormality is seen in this patient's eye?

ii. What is its significance?

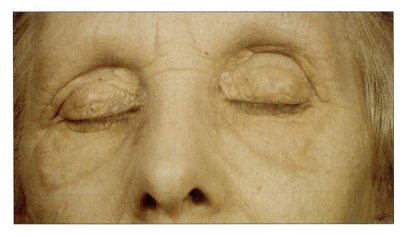

▲ 74
i. What are the lesions showing?
ii. In what conditions do they occur?

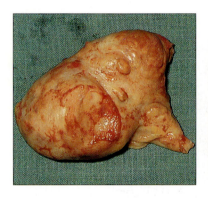

▲ 75
This mass was removed from a
patient who had a history of
dyspnoea, orthopnoea and weight
loss. The first two symptoms were
intermittent.
i. What is this mass?
ii. What other tests should be used
to diagnose this condition?

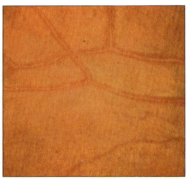

▲ 76
This patient was admitted with
acute abdominal pain.
i. What is the abnormality shown?
ii. With what conditions is it
associated?

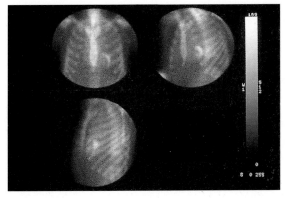

▲ 77

This patient had a severe episode of chest pain 12 months earlier. He has since had more frequent chest pain.

i. What test was carried out?

ii. What does it show?

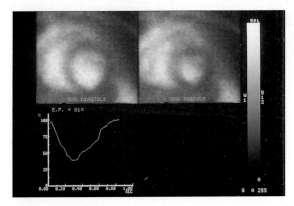

▲ 78

This patient had a history of ischaemic heart disease and breathlessness.

i. What is this test?

ii. What does it show?

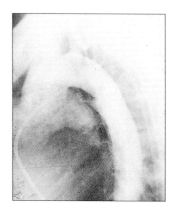

◄ 79
This procedure was
performed on a 30-year-old
woman with a heart
murmur and dyspnoea.
i. What is the procedure?
ii. What abnormality can be
   seen?

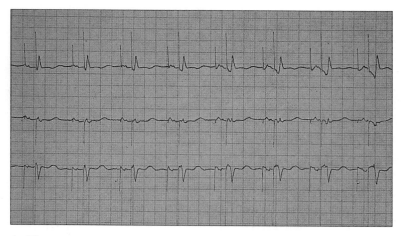

▲ 80
This is a paced rhythm strip.
i. What mode is the pacemaker in?
ii. What are the advantages and disadvantages of the possible modes?

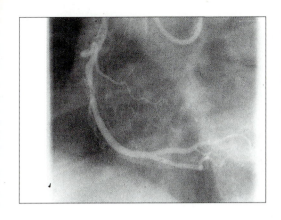

◄ 81

This 62-year-old woman presented with unstable angina.

i. Which coronary artery is shown?

ii. What is the treatment of choice?

iii. What is the incidence of recurrence?

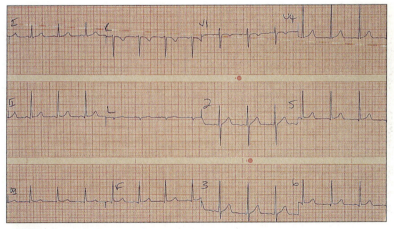

▲ 82

This ECG is from a 21-year-old man who had episodes of palpitations.

i. Describe the ECG.

ii. What is the likely diagnosis?

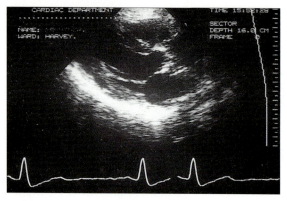

▲ 83

This echocardiogram is from a 70-year-old man with breathlessness, chest pain and a heart murmur.

i. Describe the findings on the echocardiogram.

ii What other investigations should be performed to confirm the diagnosis?

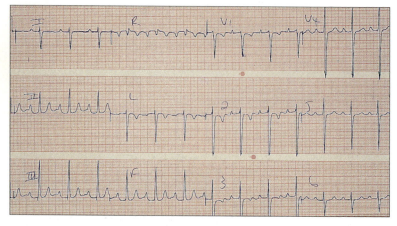

▲ 84

This ECG is from a 40-year-old man with breathlessness. He was noted to have had a heart murmur as a child.

i. Describe the ECG.

ii. Name two conditions that may cause these changes.

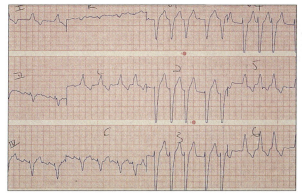

◀ 85
i. Describe the electro-cardiogram findings.
ii. What is the likely underlying condition?

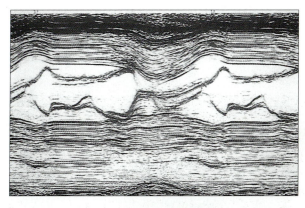

◀ 86
i. Describe the findings on this echo-cardiogram.
ii. What is the diagnosis?

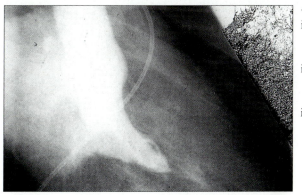

◀ 87
i. What procedure is this?
ii. What abnormalities are shown?
iii. What is the likely diagnosis?

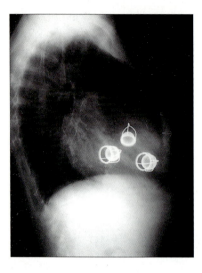

◄ 88
i. What prosthetic valves are these?
ii. In what positions are they sited?

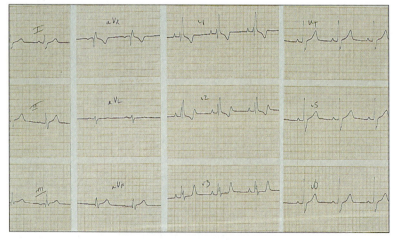

▲ 89
This is an ECG from a 19-year-old woman who was noted to have a heart murmur.
i. Describe the ECG findings.
ii. What is the likely diagnosis?

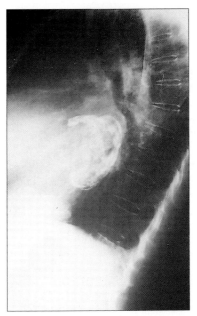

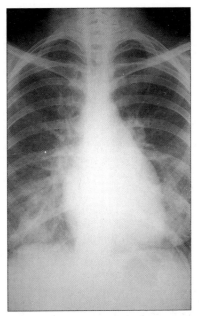

▲ 90

The chest X-ray is from a 62-year-old woman with increasing breathlessness.

i. Describe the radiological findings.
ii. What is the likely diagnosis?

▲ 91

This chest X-ray is from a 50-year-old woman who was admitted with acute breathlessness.

i. Describe the radiological abnormalities.
ii. What is the likely diagnosis?

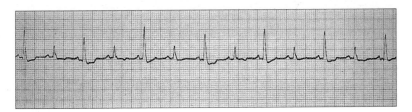

92 ▲

i. What is the abnormality on the ECG?
ii. What is its significance?

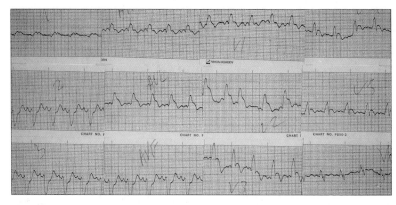

▲ 93
i. Describe the findings on the ECG.
ii. Name five conditions in which these findings may be present.
iii. What is the likely explanation in this case?

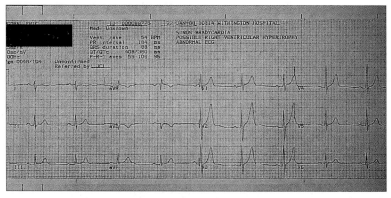

▲ 94
This ECG is from a patient who has angina. Describe the ECG findings.

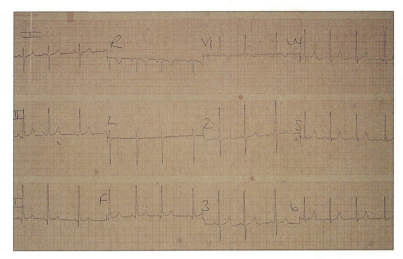

▲ 95
Describe the findings on this ECG.

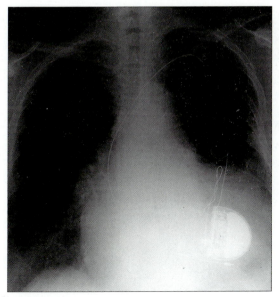

◄ 96
This patient presented with episodes of dizziness five years after a ventricular demand inhibited (VVI) pacemaker was implanted. Describe the findings related to the pacemaker which may have caused her symptoms.

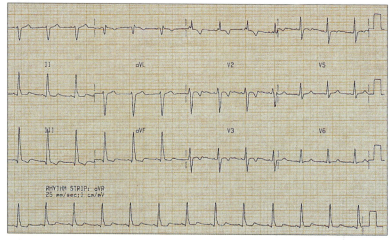

▲ 97
i. Describe the findings on this ECG.
ii. Name four conditions that may produce these changes.

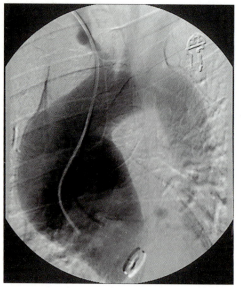

◄ 98
i   What is this investigation?
ii. What abnormalities can be seen?

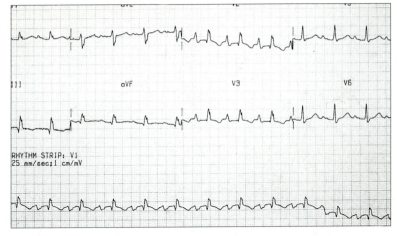

▲ 99

i. Describe the abnormalities on this ECG.

ii. Name two likely diagnoses.

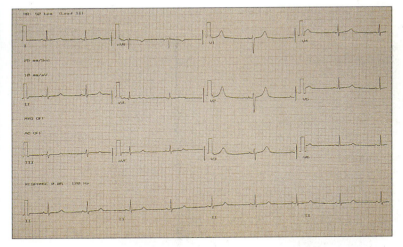

▲ 100

This ECG is from a 16-year-old female patient with deafness and a family history of sudden cardiac death.

i. What is the abnormality?

ii. Name the disorder.

iii. What is its mode of inheritance?

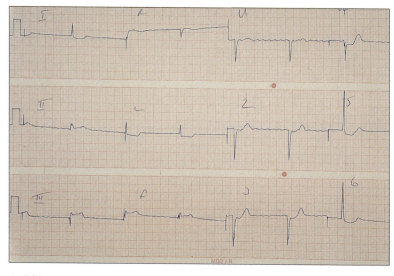

▲ **101**

This ECG is from a 70-year-old man who presented with chest pain and near fainting. Describe the findings on the ECG.

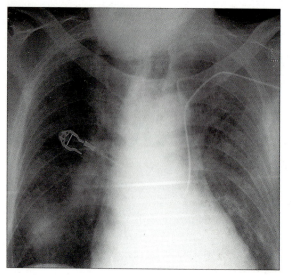

◄ **102**

i. Describe the abnormalities on this X-ray.

ii. What is the significance of the anatomical anomaly?

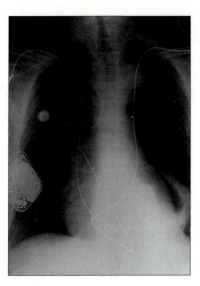

i. Describe the anatomical anomaly on this X-ray.
ii. What is its significance?

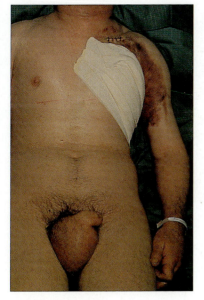

◀ 104

This patient had a permanent pacemaker implanted an hour earlier.

i. What complication has developed?
ii. Name three other complications relative to the implantation procedure.

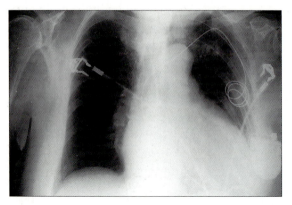

▲ **105**

This X-ray is from a 78-year-old woman who had a pacemaker implant nine years earlier. She presented on this occasion with dizzy spells. Her ECG showed atrial fibrillation without any signs of pacemaker activity. Describe the abnormality which resulted in pacemaker failure.

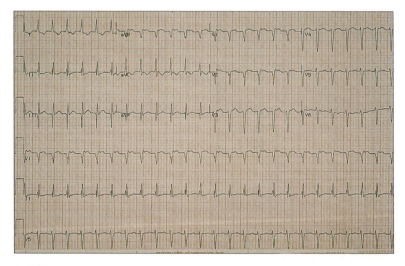

▲ **106**

i. What is the rhythm on this ECG?

ii. What are its characteristics?

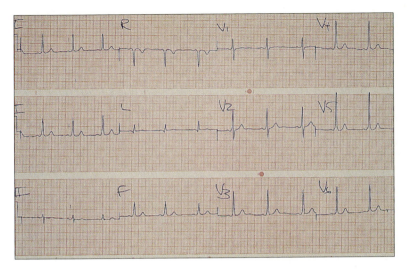

▲ 107
This ECG is from a 26-year-old man with a history of palpitations.
Describe the findings.

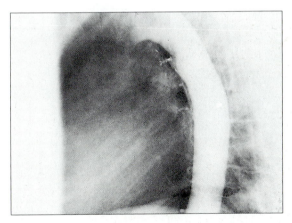

▲ 108
This procedure was carried out on a 30-year-old woman who had been
complaining of breathlessness.
i. What is the procedure?
ii. In what other circumstances could this procedure be carried out?

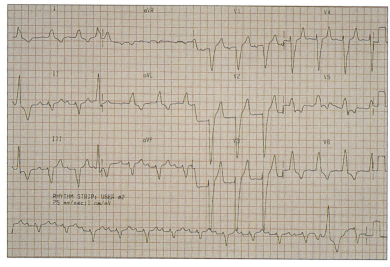

▲ 109

This ECG is from a 60-year-old man with a two-year history of exercise-induced chest pain.

i. What are the findings on the ECG?

ii. How would you investigate his chest pain?

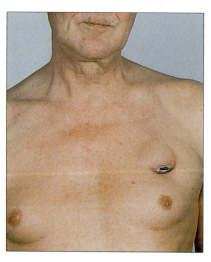

◀ 110

This patient had a pacemaker implanted six years earlier.

i. What has happened to the pacemaker?

ii. How would you remedy the situation?

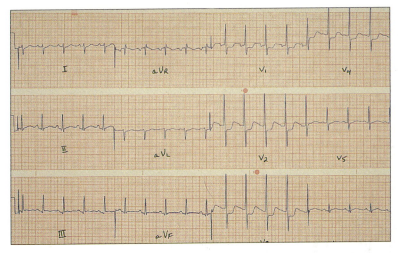

▲ 111

This ECG is from a 57-year-old man who presented with sudden tightness across his chest.

i. What are the abnormalities?

ii. What is the diagnosis?

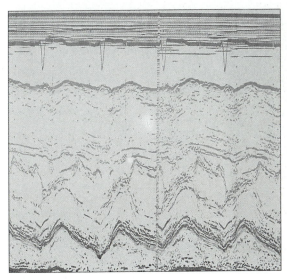

◄ 112

This echocardiogram is from a 32-year-old man with a family history of sudden cardiac death.

i. Describe the findings.

ii What is the most likely diagnosis?

49

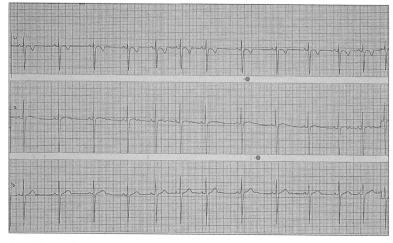

▲ 113

This is a rhythm strip from leads $V_1 - V_3$ in a 19-year-old healthy male.

i. Describe the abnormality.

ii. What is its significance?

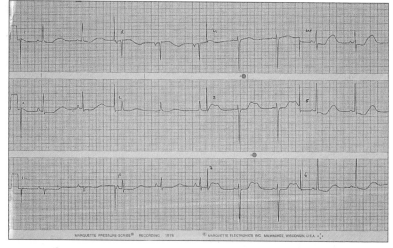

▲ 114

i. Describe the abnormalities on this ECG.

ii. What is the most likely cause?

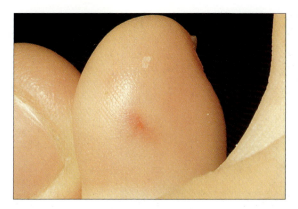

▲ 115

This patient has a prosthetic mitral valve. He presented
with a one week history of malaise, night sweats and
weight loss.

i.   What is the lesion?
ii. What is the underlying diagnosis?
ii. What imaging studies should be carried out?

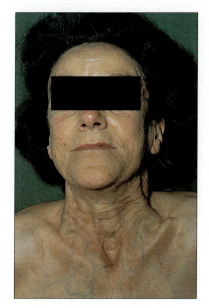

◄ 116

This 55-year-old woman was found
to have a high-pitched pansystolic
murmur, heard best in the fourth
intercostal space and subxiphoid
area. She had been relatively well.

i.   Describe the physical signs.
ii. What is the likely diagnosis?

51

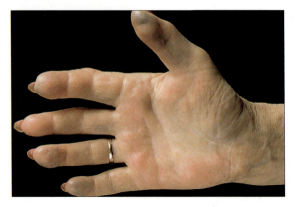

▲ 117

This patient presented with congestive heart failure.

i. What are the lesions in the hand?

ii. What are the cardiological manifestations of this condition?

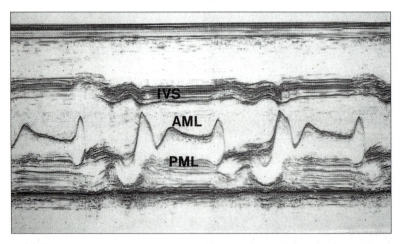

▲ 118

This echocardiogram is from a 28-year-old woman with a history of palpitations.

i. What does it show?

ii. What is the natural history of this condition?

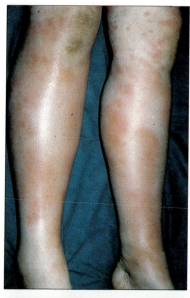

This patient presented with
lymphadenopathy and palpitations.
i. What are these lesions?
ii. What is the likely diagnosis?

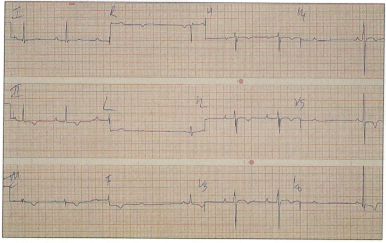

▲ 120
This ECG is from a 40-year-old man with a history of blackout and dizziness
since childhood.
i. Describe the ECG.
ii. What is the likely cause of the abnormality?

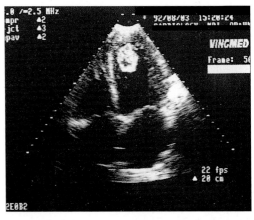

◀ 121
121
This echocardiogram is from a patient who had a myocardial infarction three years earlier. He now presents with episodes suggestive of transient cerebral ischaemic attacks.
i. What does the echocardiogram show?
ii. What is the likely cause of his symptoms?

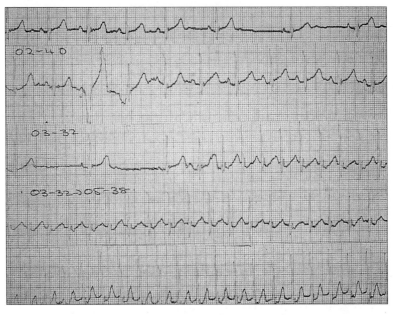

▲ 122
This continuous, ambulatory ECG monitoring trace is from a 50-year-old man who had a blackout during strenuous physical training.
i. What does it show?
ii. How can such an attack be prevented in future?

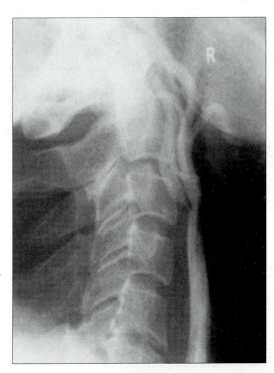

i. What artery is seen on this image and what abnormality can be seen?
ii. What diagnostic pulse wave can be seen in this artery in patients with aortic regurgitation and hypertrophic cardiomyopathy?

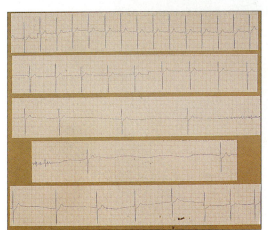

124

This ECG trace was recorded from a 60-year-old man whilst in a head-up position for the investigation of syncope.
i   What does the trace show?
ii. What is he suffering from?

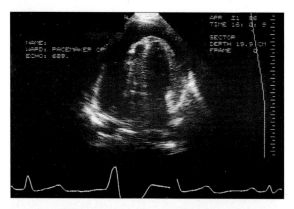

◄125
This echo-
cardiogram is from
a patient who had
a procedure
performed a short
time after a
collapse.
i. What does the
   echocardiogram
   show?
ii. What is the
    likely cause?

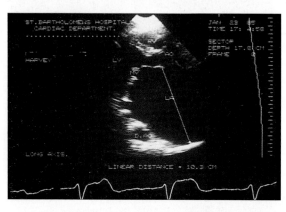

◄126
This transthoracic
echocardiogram is
from a 55-year-old
woman with a
history of effort-
related dyspnoea.
i Describe the
   findings.
ii. What is the
    likely diagnosis?

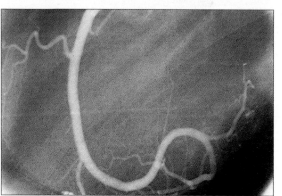

◄ 127
Which coronary
artery is this and
what course does it
take?

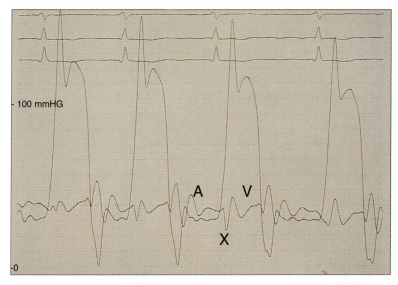

▲ **128**

These pressure tracings are taken from the LV and right atrium.

i. What haemodynamic abnormalities are shown?

ii. What is the most likely underlying condition giving rise to such pressures?

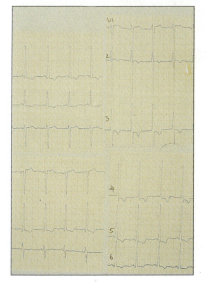

◄ **129**

This ECG is from a 40-year-old woman who presented to her doctor for a routine medical check up.

i. Describe the findings.

ii. What is the likely underlying condition?

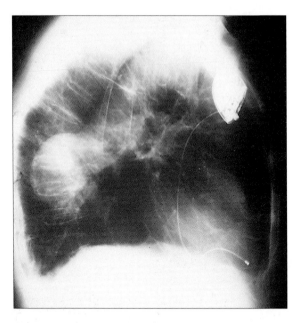

◄ 130
This lateral chest X-ray was taken routinely after the implantation of a permanent pacemaker.
i. What abnormality is seen?
ii. What is its significance?

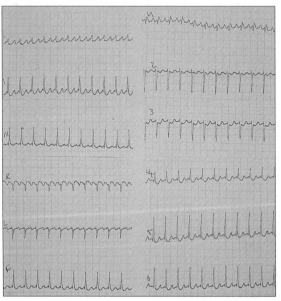

◄131
This ECG is from a 70-year-old man with a history of palpitations.
i. Describe the ECG.
ii. What would be the effect of digoxin, beta-blockers and verapamil on the rhythm?

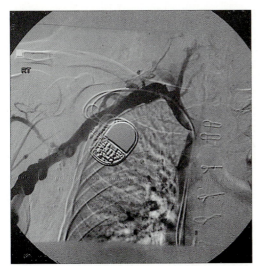

This patient presented with a few days' history of a slightly swollen right arm and right side of the neck. What does this image show?

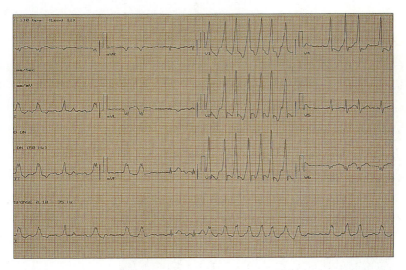

▲ 133

This patient has an accessory pathway which is responsible for this pre-excited atrial fibrillation. From the ECG, locate the site of the accessory pathway.

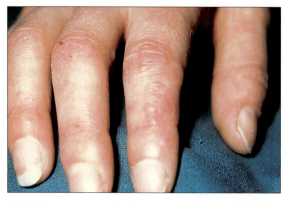

▲ 134

This patient had a syncopal episode. She had previously been healthy.

i. What are these lesions?

ii. What is the likely cause of her syncope?

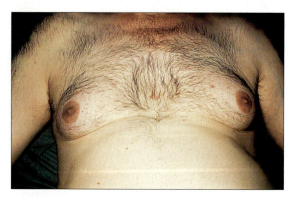

▲ 135

What cardiovascular drugs are responsible for this patient's abnormality?

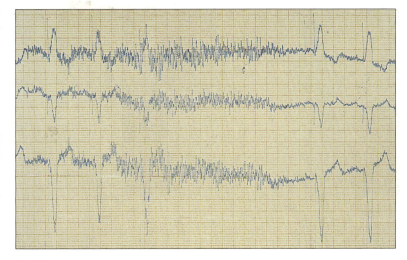

▲ 136

This patient is pacemaker-dependent. He has complained of dizziness whenever he tried to push-start his car. What is the cause of his dizziness?

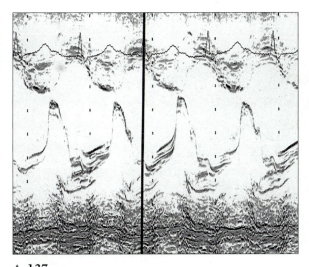

▲ 137

This echocardiogram is from a patient with a history of breathlessness. What abnormalities does the echocardiogram show?

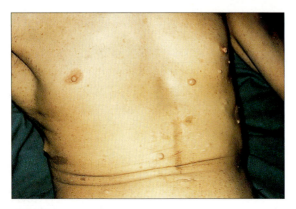

▲ **138**
This patient presented with a history of headaches, palpitations and sweating.

   What lesions are shown and what is the likely cause of the patient's symptoms?

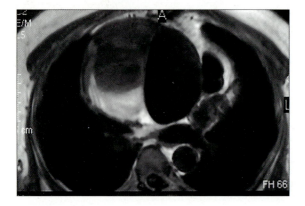

▲ **139**
This CT scan image was taken from a patient who had been complaining of chest pain. What abnormalities does it show?

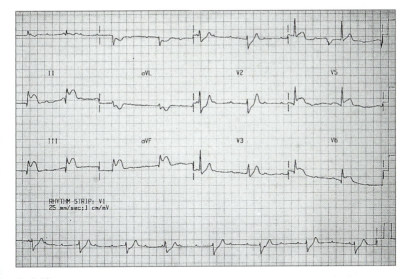

▲ 140

This ECG is from a 70-year-old man who was admitted with chest pain. Describe the ECG findings.

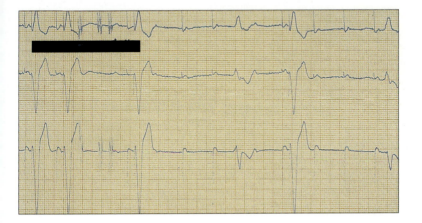

▲ 141

i. Describe the findings on this rhythm strip.
ii. What are the abnormalities due to?

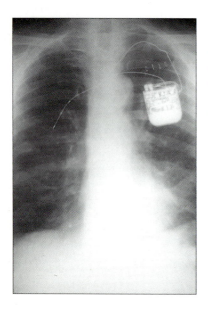

This chest X-ray is from a patient who had a permanent pacemaker implant.
i. What type of pacemaker was implanted?
ii. Where is the lead across the chest positioned?

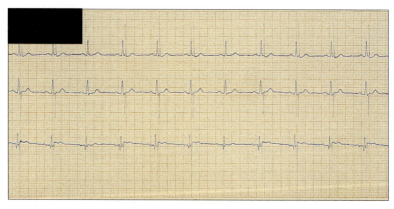

▲ 143
This rhythm strip is from a patient who had a pacemaker implanted a few days earlier.
i. What is the underlying rhythm?
ii. What is the abnormality?

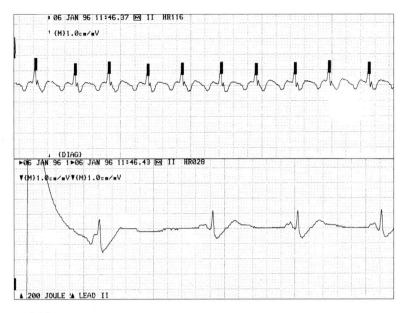

▲ 144

i. What does this rhythm strip show?

ii. What are the management options of this abnormal rhythm?

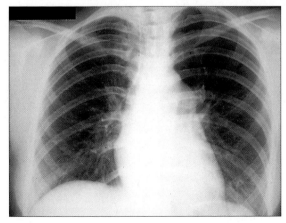

◀ 145

This chest X-ray is from a 40-year-old patient. The X-ray was performed for a routine medical examination.

i. What abnormality is seen?

ii. What is its significance?

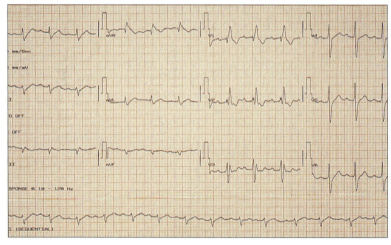

▲ 146

This ECG is from a 62-year-old man with one episode of syncope.

i. Describe the ECG findings.

ii. What is the appropriate course of action?

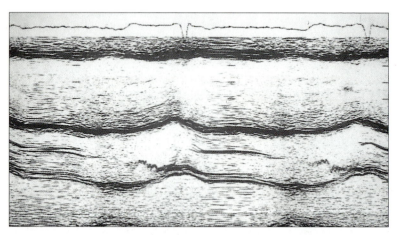

▲ 147

This echocardiogram is from a 30-year-old man with a history of breathlessness and one syncopal attack.

i. Describe the findings.

ii. What is the likely underlying condition?

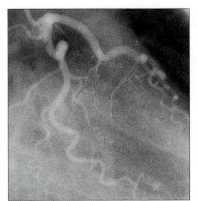

▲ **148**

i. Name these two coronary arteries?

ii. What course do they each take?

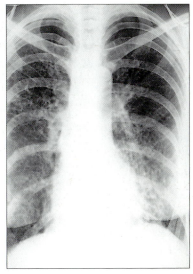

▲ **149**

This chest X-ray is from a 59-year-old woman who was admitted as an emergency with dyspnoea.

i. What are the findings on the X-ray?

ii. What is the likely diagnosis?

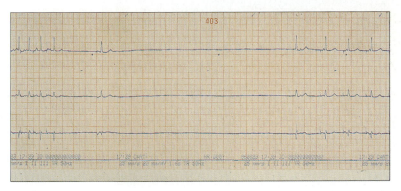

▲ **150**

i. What investigative procedure is used here?

ii. What mechanism is responsible for the asystole?

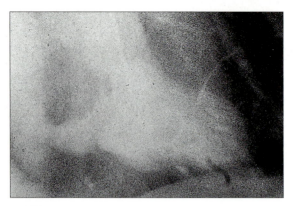

▲ 151

This left ventricular angiogram is from a 28-year-old woman with a history of dyspnoea, orthopnoea, haemoptysis and weight loss.

i.   Describe the abnormalities.
ii. What is the likely diagnosis?
iii. What other investigations should be carried out?

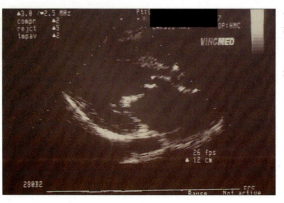

◄ 152

i. Describe the findings on this echocardiogram.
ii. What is the significance of the abnormal findings?

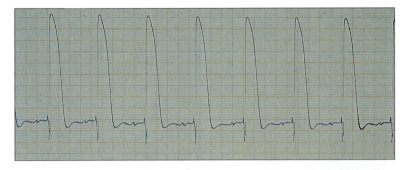

▲ 153
i. What does this ECG trace show?
ii. What is its significance?

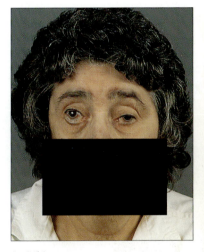

▲ 154
This 50-year-old woman presented with a history of breathlessness and a blackout.
i. What abnormalities can be seen?
ii. What is the diagnosis?
iii. What cardiac manifestations may be expected?

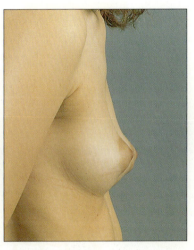

▲ 155
This patient presented for a routine medical examination for a health insurance. Her mother had emergency open heart surgery following an episode of chest pain at the age of 30.
i. What abnormality is seen?
ii. What is the diagnosis and what other physical signs support it?

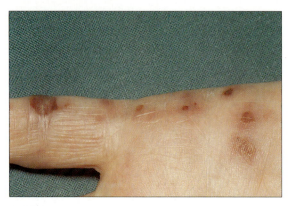

▲ 156

This 27-year-old man was admitted with a stroke affecting the left side of his body. He had recently been to his dentist for scaling. He was noted to have an early diastolic murmur.

i.   What are these lesions?
ii. What is the likely diagnosis?
iii. What other physical signs may be found?

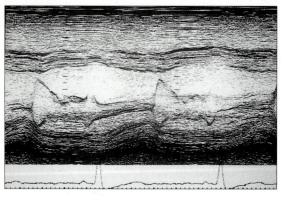

▲ 157

i. What does this M-mode echocardiogram show?
ii. What are the likely causes of the abnormality?

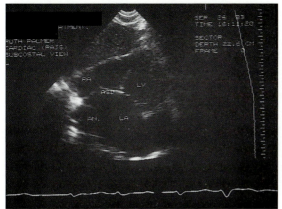

◀ **158**
This is from a 35-year-old man who was referred for echocardiographic study for a transient cerebral ischaemic attack.
i. Describe the findings.
ii. What is the significance of the abnormal findings?

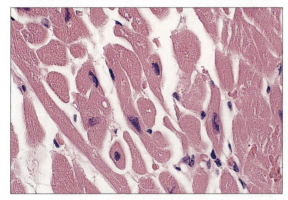

◀ **159**
This myocardial biopsy was taken from a 40-year-old man with a history of dyspnoea and palpitations.
i. Describe the findings.
ii. What is the diagnosis?

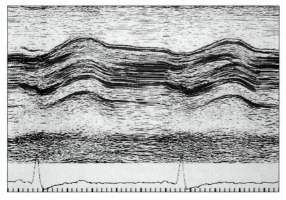

◀ **160**
This echocardiogram is from a 70-year-old woman with a history of chest pain, breathlessness and two blackouts.
i. What does the echocardiogram show?
ii. What other investigations should be carried out?

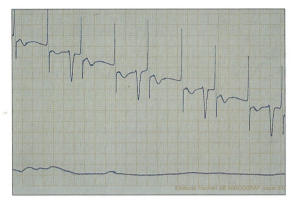

◀161
This ECG trace was recorded during a permanent pacemaker implantation. What does it show and what is its significance?

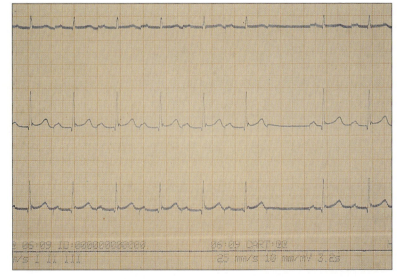

▲162
Describe the findings on this rhythm strip. What abnormality is seen and what is the likely cause?

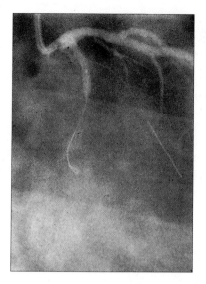

i. What procedure is being carried out?
ii. What are the recognised complications of such a procedure?

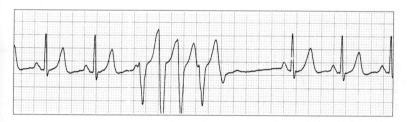

▲ 164

This rhythm strip was recorded five minutes after successful angioplasty to an acutely occluded left anterior descending coronary artery in a 42-year-old man.

i. What does the rhythm strip show?
ii. What is the mechanism and significance of the abnormality?

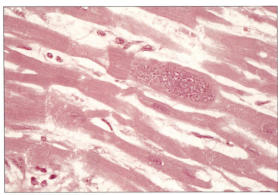

◄165

This myocardial biopsy was taken from a transplanted heart. The procedure was a routine follow-up.

i. What abnormality is seen?

ii. What are the most likely cardiac manifestations?

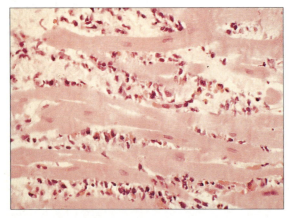

◄166

This myocardial biopsy was taken from a patient who had a heart transplant two months earlier.

i. What changes are seen?

ii. What other investigations are used in detecting this condition?

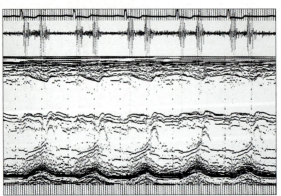

◄167

This echocardiogram is from a 49-year-old woman with a history of progressive breathlessness. She has had a murmur since childhood.

i. What does the study show?

ii. What is the differential diagnosis?

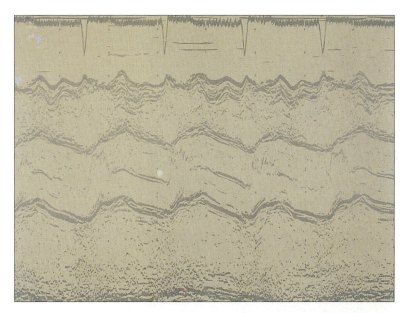

▲ 168
This echocardiogram is from a young man with a family history of sudden death.
i. Describe the findings.
ii. What is the diagnosis?
iii. What is the cause of sudden death in this condition?
iv. Name the risks of sudden death in this condition.

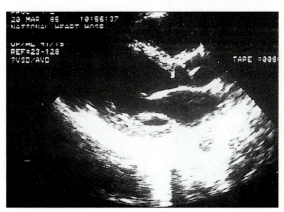

◀ 169
This echocardiogram is from a 16-year-old man who is asymptomatic but has had a systolic murmur since infancy.
i. What abnormality is seen?
ii. What auscultatory features may be present?

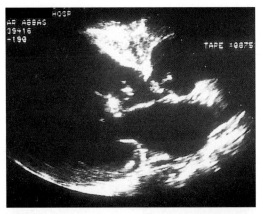

◀ 170

This echocardiogram is from a patient who presented with a left-sided hemiplegia. He was noted to have a mid-diastolic murmur in the apex and an enlarged spleen .

i. What does the echo-cardiogram show?
ii. What is the prognosis in this condition?

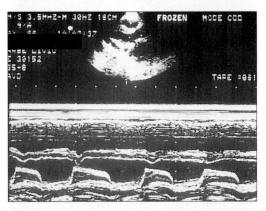

◀ 171

This echocardiogram is from a patient who had a rheumatic fever as a child.

i. Describe the findings.
ii. How would the severity of the condition be quantified on echocardiography?

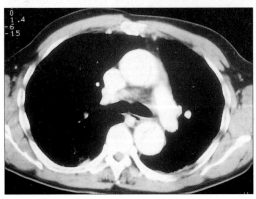

◀ 172

This CT scan is from a woman who presented with chest pain radiating through to the back.

i. What abnormality is seen?
ii. What is the prognosis for this condition?

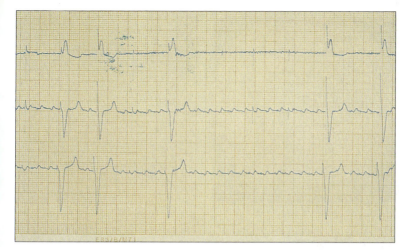

▲ 173

This rhythm strip is from a 70-year-old patient who had a pacemaker implanted 12 years earlier. He now presents with episodes of loss of consciousness.

i. Describe the findings.

ii. What are the possible causes for the abnormality?

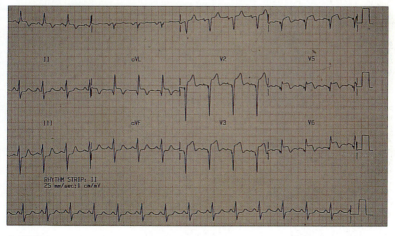

▲ 174

This ECG was performed, during a routine clinic visit, on a patient who had a myocardial infarction 12 months earlier.

i. Describe the morphological changes.

ii. What is the significance of these changes?

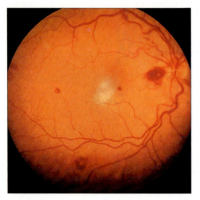

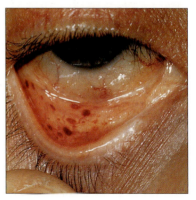

▲ 175

This patient had a prosthetic mitral valve replacement two years earlier. He presented with a four-week history of breathlessness and rigors.
i. What lesions are seen?
ii. What is the diagnosis?
iii. In what other conditions may this lesion be seen?

▲ 176

This patient presented with pyrexia and raised ESRs. A soft systolic murmur was found on examination.
i. What are these lesions?
ii. What is the differential diagnosis?

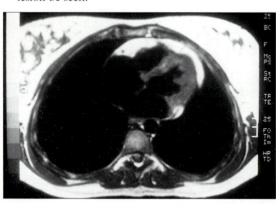

▲ 177

This nuclear magnetic resonance imaging (MRI) scan is from a patient with chest pain. His blood pressure was 130/80 mmHg.
i. What abnormalities can be seen?
ii. What is the likely diagnosis?
iii. What is the mechanism of pain in this condition?

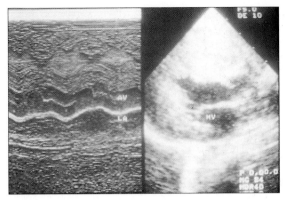

▲ 178
This echocardiogram is from a one-year-old boy who
was small for his age, lethargic and had a weak cry. He
had been breathless for a few weeks. His ECG showed
a short P-R interval.
i. Describe the findings.
ii. What is the likely diagnosis?

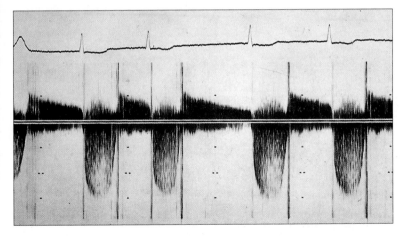

▲ 179
i. Describe the findings on this Doppler echocardiogram.
ii. What is the diagnosis?

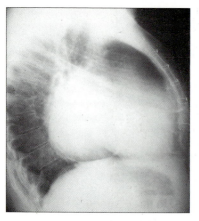

▲ 180

This chest X-ray is from a patient who had cardiac surgery in the past.

i. Describe the findings.

ii. What are the advantages and disadvantages of the prosthetic valve seen on the X-ray?

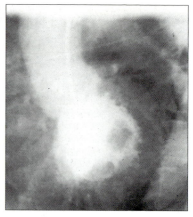

▲ 181

This patient had an anterior myocardial infarction six months earlier. He presented with chest pain and a transient cerebral ischaemic attack.

i. What does this radiological image show?

ii. What is the significance of the abnormality?

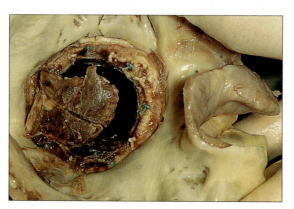

◄ 182

i. What does this specimen show?

ii. What are the causes of failure of the prosthetic valves?

80

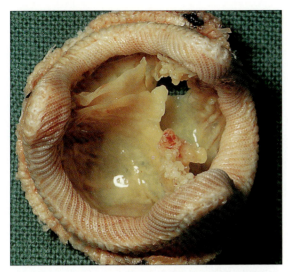

i. What type of
   prosthetic valve
   is this?
ii. What are the
    complications of
    such valves?

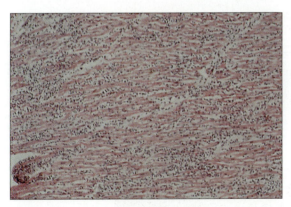

▲ 184
This myocardial biopsy is from a 19-year-old woman
who had a flu-like illness, associated with marked
dyspnoea. She had a sinus tachycardia with a third
heart sound on auscultation.
i. What does the biopsy show?
ii. What is the diagnosis?

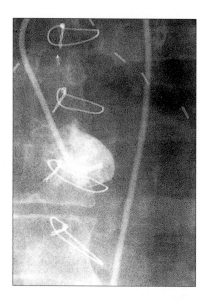

This angiogram is from a patient who had coronary artery bypass grafting to the left anterior descending, intermediate and circumflex coronary arteries.

i. What does this image show?

ii. How did this finding occur?

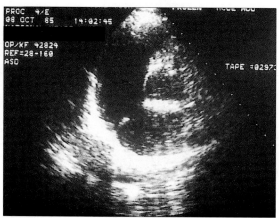

▲ 186

This echocardiogram is from a 35-year-old woman with a history of breathlessness. She has had a heart murmur since childhood.

i. What does the echocardiogram show?

ii. What are the electrocardiographic changes in this condition?

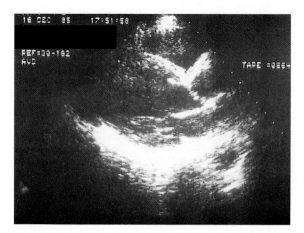

▲ 187
This echocardiogram is from a 25-year-old man who had been well. He was referred to this study because of the presence of a heart murmur.
i. What are the abnormal findings?
ii. What is the likely association?

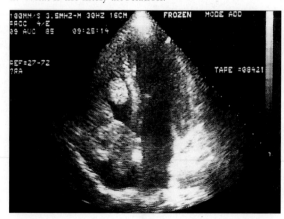

▲ 188
This echocardiogram is from a patient who presented with breathlessness, marked oedema from the waist down and haematuria.
i. What abnormalities are seen?
ii. What is the differential diagnosis?

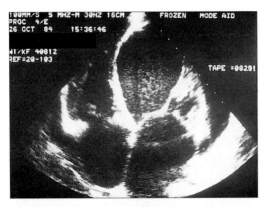

◄ 189

This echocardiogram is from a patient who presented with a few days' history of breathlessness following a sore throat.

i. Describe the findings.

ii. What factors are associated with a reduced survival rate?

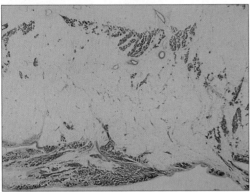

◄ 190

This myocardial biopsy is from a 40-year-old man who has had frequent palpitations and one episode of transient loss of consciousness.

i. What does the biopsy show?

ii. What is the diagnosis?

iii. What is the cause of the loss of consciousness?

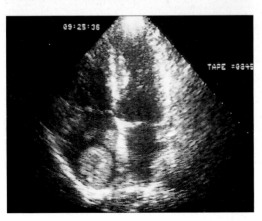

◄ 191

This patient had been in intensive care for several days. He had a Swan-Ganz catheter inserted on admission. He subsequently developed a sudden, severe pleuritic chest pain.

i. What abnormality is seen?

ii. What are the risks this patient is exposed to?

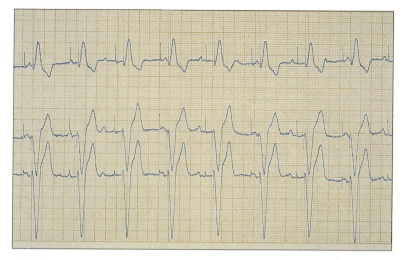

▲ 192

This rhythm strip is from a patient with a permanent pacemaker implant.
He complained of intermittent breathlessness.

i. What abnormalities can be seen?

ii. What are the possible causes?

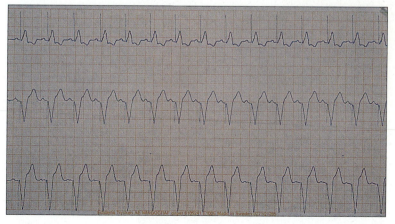

▲ 193

i. Describe the findings on this rhythm strip.

ii. What are the advantages and disadvantages of this pacing mode?

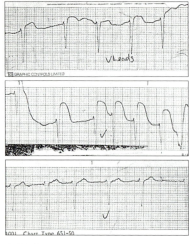

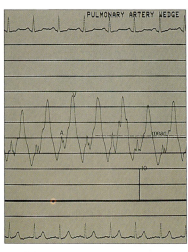

▲ 194

This rhythm strip was recorded from a patient while he was having a procedure. He had presented with raised jugular venous pressure, hypotension and cold clammy skin.

i. What procedure was carried out?

ii. What are its complications?

▲ 195

This is a pulmonary artery wedge pressure trace.

i. What does it show?

ii. What conditions cause raised pressure?

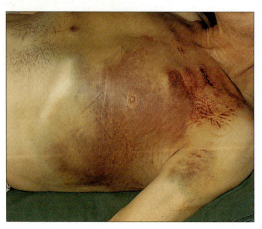

◄ 196

This patient had a temporary pacemaker lead inserted via the left subclavian vein two hours after an acute anterior myocardial infarction.

i. What is the likely cause of the bruising on his body?

ii. Discuss the common complications seen following pacemaker insertions.

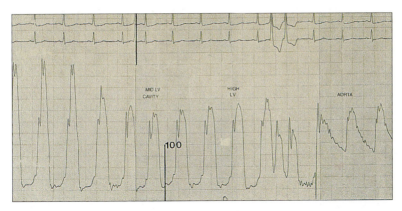

▲ 197
i. What do these pressure tracings indicate?

ii. What is the diagnosis?

iii. What is the aetiology of this condition?

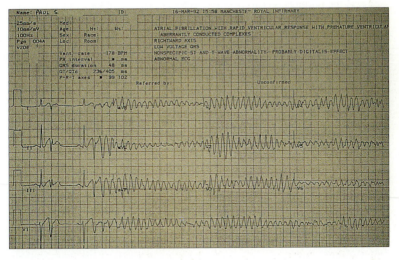

▲ 198
This ECG is from a 60-year-old man who was admitted with severe chest pain eight hours earlier.

i. Describe the appearances on the ECG.

ii. What are the relationships of this arrhythmia to the location and timing of antecedent infarction?

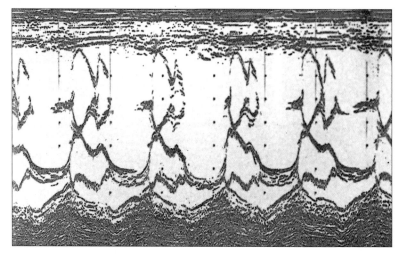

▲ 199

Describe the findings on this M-mode echocardiogram. What are the clinical manifestations of the condition?

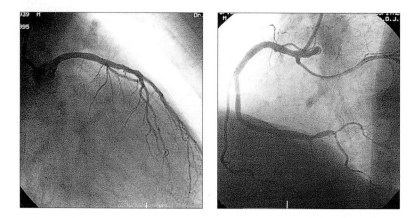

▲ 200

Describe the abnormality in these coronary angiographic images. What is its significance?

201 A 60-year-old man developed acute breathlessness three days after an anterior myocardial infarction. He was found clinically to have pulmonary oedema, a raised jugular venous pressure and hypotension. A systolic murmur was heard for the first time.
i. What is the differential diagnosis?
ii. What investigations should be carried out to confirm the diagnosis?

202 A 23-year-old woman presented with a ten-day history of progressive breathlessness preceded by a flu-like illness. Examination showed her to be breathless with a raised jugular venous pressure. She had a tachycardia with an S3 gallop.
i. What investigations should be carried out?
ii. What is the likely diagnosis and what is the prognosis?

203 A 27-year-old woman was referred by her doctor for investigation of breathlessness, fatigue and a syncopal attack. Her older sister had died suddenly aged 30 years. Auscultation of the heart revealed a loud second pulmonary sound.
i. What is the likely diagnosis?
ii .What are the haemodynamic features of this condition?

204 A 60-year-old man presented to the accident and emergency department with palpitations. He was mildly breathless. He was found to be in atrial fibrillation. His ventricular rate had been adequate five years earlier and no treatment was given. An ECG showed atrial fibrillation with a ventricular rate of 140 per minute. How would you manage this patient?

205 A 45-year-old man was admitted with central chest tightness. There were minor ST segment and T wave changes on his ECG. There was a minor rise in cardiac enzymes. Twenty-four hours after admission he developed recurrent ventricular tachycardia/fibrillation. How would you manage this patient?

206 A 47-year-old woman was admitted with severe central chest pain radiating through to the back. Blood pressure was 130/80 mmHg in the right arm and 100/70 mmHg in the left arm. There is no previous medical history of relevance.
i. What investigations should be carried out?
ii. What is the likely diagnosis and how should the patient be treated?

207 A 32-year-old woman with known mitral stenosis presented to the maternity unit in labour. How would you manage this patient?

208 A 50 year old man who had undergone coronary artery bypass surgery two years earlier was found to have cholesterol and triglyceride levels of 7.4 mmol/l and 3.7 mmol/l respectively. How would you manage his lipid levels?

209 A 58-year-old woman had an uneventful percutaneous transluminal coronary angioplasty to the left anterior descending artery. Six hours later she complained of central chest pain. An ECG showed raised ST-segment in the anterior precordial leads.
i. What has happened?
ii. How would you manage the patient?

210 A 51-year-old man with disabling angina and previous coronary artery bypass surgery was referred for consideration of a heart transplant. What are the criteria for considering such a patient for a heart transplant?

211 A 36-year-old man who had a heart transplant four months earlier presented with fever, lethargy and tachycardia. The only physical sign on examination was a soft systolic murmur.
i. What investigations should be carried out?
ii. What is the likely cause of the patient's symptoms?

212 A 19-year-old woman was referred for the investigation of breathlessness and a systolic murmur. The following pressures were obtained during cardiac catheterisation:

	Pressure (mmHg)
Right atrium	4
Right ventricle	21/5
Pulmonary artery	22/8
Pulmonary capillary wedge	7
High left ventricle (outflow tract)	130/10
Cavity of left ventricle	165/10

What is the likely diagnosis?

213 A 70-year-old man who had undergone coronary artery bypass surgery six hours earlier suffered a sudden haemodynamic deterioration with hypotension and raised systemic venous pressure.
i. What is the diagnosis?
ii. What is the treatment?

214 A 75-year-old man had a permanent pacemaker implanted through the right subclavian approach having previously had a system removed from the left infraclavicular position. He presented with a swollen right arm. The pacemaker site was slightly swollen but no external signs of infection were present. What has gone wrong and what needs to be done?

215 A 70-year-old woman who had a permanent pacemaker implanted through the left subclavian vein 12 years earlier presented with a twitch over the left pectoral muscles.
i.   What is the cause of the muscle twitch?
ii. What is the treatment?

216 A 50-year-old man who had a prosthetic valve fitted in the aortic position two years earlier was referred by his doctor with malaise, rigors and breathlessness.
i.   What investigations should be carried out?
ii. What is the likely diagnosis?
iii. What complications are likely?

217 A 22-year-old woman has a history of palpitations which are associated with vague discomfort in the chest and near fainting. She has a normal ECG. What investigations should be undertaken to reach a diagnosis?

218 A 29 year old woman was referred for the investigation of breathlessness. The following data were obtained during cardiac catheterisation:

	Pressure (mmHg)
Right atrium	5
Right ventricle	20/5
Pulmonary artery	30/10
Pulmonary capillary wedge	28
Left ventricle	130/10

i.   What is the diagnosis?
ii. How would you treat this patient?

219 A 78-year-old man with a permanent pacemaker presented to the accident and emergency department with acute breathlessness and palpitations. An electrocardiogram showed a paced rate of 210 per minute.
i.   What is the diagnosis?
ii. What is the treatment of the condition?

220 A 29-year-old woman was referred for investigation of breathlessness and cyanosis. The following data was obtained at cardiac catheterisation.

	Oxygen saturation (%)
Right atrium	68
Right ventricle	70
Pulmonary artery	70
Capillary wedge	95
Left ventricle (cavity)	80
Left ventricle (inflow tract)	95
Superior vena cava	65
Inferior vena cava	69
Aorta	95

What does this signify?

1 i. The patient had a heterotopic cardiac transplant 'piggyback' in which the donor heart is anastomosed in parallel with the retained recipient heart. The donor heart is in the right hemithorax.

 ii. Both hearts had retained their own sinus automaticity. The activities of the two hearts were synchronised by the pacemaker.

 iii. Four indications for this type of transplant procedure are:
 • permanently elevated pulmonary vascular resistance;
 • patient with a small donor heart;
 • donor heart with a long ischaemic time and anticipated poor early function;
 • patient with a reversible type of heart disease in which the graft may be removed when the native heart recovers.

2 This is a biplane trans-oesophageal echocardiogram showing a horizontal, four-chamber view. There is moderate mitral regurgitation. The jet is coming from the medial commissure.

 i. This patient had a percutaneous mitral commissurotomy using an Inoue balloon.

 ii. The following are complications related to percutaneous mitral commissurotomy:
 • systemic embolisation;
 • mitral regurgitation;
 • cardiac tamponade due to transseptal procedure;
 • small left-to-right shunt.

3 i. This patient had undergone cardiac catheterisation. The picture shows left ventricular angiography. The catheter had perforated the myocardium and contrast medium was injected into the pericardial cavity.

 ii. Immediately alert the cardiac surgeons to the possible need to intervene. Make haemodynamic observations with regular echocardiography to check that bleeding in the pericardial cavity does not progress to tamponade. If the latter occurs, surgical intervention may be necessary.

4 This is bluish-grey discoloration of the skin due to amiodarone. Amiodarone causes photosensitivity dermatitis in 20% of patients, with only 1–2% developing bluish-grey discoloration.

5 This is a longitudinal view from a biplane trans-oesophageal echocardiogram showing a paracommissural tear in the anterior mitral leaflet. This is a recognised complication following percutaneous balloon mitral commissurotomy.

6 i. Prolapse of the posterior leaflet of the mitral valve.

 ii. This condition is associated with:
 • primary mitral valve prolapse;
 • Marfan's syndrome;
 • coronary artery disease;
 • rheumatic endocarditis.

iii. Atrial and ventricular ectopic beats are common. Paroxysmal supraventricular tachycardia is the most common sustained arrhythmia associated with mitral valve prolapse. The mechanism of arrhythmia is not clear but primary mitral valve prolapse is sometimes associated with atrioventricular bypass tracts.

7   These are long fingers of Marfan's syndrome. Cardiological abnormalities associated with this include:
- mitral valve prolapse;
- arrhythmias;
- tricuspid valve prolapse;
- mitral regurgitation;
- aortic regurgitation;
- dilatation of the aortic root;
- aortic dissection.

The latter two are the most specific. The last is a common cause of death in this condition.

8   This is a four-chamber view showing a thickened and severely stenotic mitral valve. There is left and right atrial dilatation with a large mass in the left atrium. The differential diagnosis of this mass is thrombus, myxoma or a vegetation. A thrombus is most likely in this situation.

9   i. The main abnormality is prolonged Q-T interval (520 ms). The Q-T interval is heart rate dependent.
   ii. a. Prolonged Q-T interval can be congenital or due to ischaemic heart disease, cardiomyopathy and electrolyte changes.
      b. Amongst the drugs that commonly cause this condition are:
- sotalol;
- amiodarone;
- phenothiazine;
- quinidine.

10   The ECG shows a ventricular demand inhibited (VVI) paced rhythm. There is a right bundle branch block pattern of the QRS. A ventricular lead positioned in the right ventricle (RV) produces a left bundle branch block pattern. Here the ventricular lead was positioned in the left ventricle (LV) giving a right bundle branch block pattern.

11   i. This is a percutaneous balloon mitral commissurotomy using an Inoue balloon.
   ii. Recognised complications include:
- systemic embolisation;
- mitral regurgitation;
- cardiac tamponade due to transseptal procedure;
- small left-to-right shunt.

12 i.   These pressures represent the pulmonary wedge and left ventricular pressures. They were recorded during cardiac catheterisation. They show a gradient of around 25 mmHg across the mitral valve.
    ii. This indicates severe mitral stenosis.
    iii. The treatment requires intervention by mitral valvotomy, mitral valvuloplasty or mitral valve replacement, depending on the clinical situation, the condition of the valve and the available expertise.

13 i.   There is a moderate pericardial effusion.
    ii. The commonest causes are:
         • infection;
         • malignancy;
         • trauma;
         • connective tissue disease.

14 There is widening of the mediastinum with a rounded shadow projecting to the right from the mediastinum. A lateral view would be helpful in differentiating between an aortic aneurysm and a bronchial mass. An aortic aneurysm would be seen as a forward projection of the aortic arch. The history in this patient is suggestive of aortic dissection. The diagnosis can be confirmed by transthoracic or trans-oesophageal echocardiography, computerised tomography (CT) scan or magnetic resonance imaging.

15 i.   The main abnormality is a grossly dilated LV measuring 8 cm at end diastole. Septal contraction looks dyskinetic.
    ii. Ischaemic heart disease, dilated and alcoholic cardiomyopathy can cause left ventricular dilatation.

16 i.   Infected pacemaker site.
    ii. If not managed adequately thrombosis of the subclavian vein and superior vena cava could be a serious complication.
    iii. The whole pacemaker system, including the leads, must be extracted and a new system implanted after the infection is treated with antibiotics. If the patient is pacemaker dependent then a temporary pacemaker lead should be inserted.

17 There is bowing of the right femur due to Paget's disease of bone. The patient has high output heart failure giving breathlessness. Thyrotoxicosis, pregnancy and anaemia are other causes of high output heart failure.

18 i.   There is enlargement of the hilar and mediastinal lymph nodes.
    ii. The patient has sarcoidosis causing complete heart block. This occurs as a result of granulomatous involvement of the conducting tissue.
    iii. Other manifestations of cardiac involvement include arrhythmias (mostly ventricular), congestive heart failure, mitral incompetence and sudden death, the latter probably due to ventricular tachycardia.

19   i.   A shadow in the right cardiophrenic angle.

      ii.   This is due to a prominent fat pad which is an incidental finding and is of no significance. A shadow is more common in the left cardiophrenic angle when it sometimes gives the impression of cardiomegaly.

20   i.   This is a lateral chest X-ray showing pericardial calcification.

      ii.   Causes include:
- tuberculosis;
- connective tissue disease;
- trauma;
- irradiation;
- previous viral pericarditis.

21   i.   There are calcified pleural plaques. These are the consequence of previous exposure to asbestos.

      ii.   There is no direct cardiac involvement and the breathlessness is pulmonary in origin.

22   i.   This radiographic image was taken during electrophysiological studies.

      ii.   There are two major groups of complications:
      a. one related to intravascular catheterisation such as bleeding, thrombosis and myocardial perforation;
      b. the second related to the electrophysiological procedure such as adverse haemodynamic disturbances from rapid arrhythmias or bradycardias.

23   i.   There is both clubbing and cyanosis. The discoloration in the nail of the left index finger is due to trauma.

      ii.   This patient has cyanotic congenital heart disease.

24   This is a ^{201}Thallium chloride myocardial perfusion. There is reduced uptake of Thallium in the anterior wall of the LV and part of the septum during exercise. There is improvement of uptake following exercise, indicating the presence of exercise-induced ischaemia.

25   i.   The ECG shows an irregular, broad, complex tachycardia with right bundle branch block pattern. The QRS axis is −165. A delta wave can be seen in the lateral chest leads (V_4, V_5). This is atrial fibrillation with ventricular pre-excitation.

      ii.   The patient has Wolff-Parkinson-White syndrome.

26   At first sight the rhythm appears to be sinus. The QRS voltages in V_4–V_6 are low (consistent either with previous anterolateral infarction or with obesity). Examination of the rhythm strip indicates that the rhythm is unusual. It is sino-atrial Wenckebach block with the conduction delay at the delay junction of the sinus node and atrial myocardium. The P-R interval remains normal. The R-R and P-P intervals become progressively shorter and then suddenly lengthen. The

progressive shortening of the P-P interval before its sudden lengthening is equivalent to the progressive shortening of the R-R interval before its sudden lengthening seen in the typical atrioventricular-ventricular Wenckebach phenomenon.

27 i.   These are eruptive xanthomas. They are seen in diabetic patients with gross hypertriglyceridaemia.
   ii.   Diabetic patients and particularly those with hyperlipidaemia suffer from accelerated atherogenesis leading to premature and advanced coronary artery disease. There is also an increased risk of microangiopathy in the heart leading to left ventricular failure in the absence of coronary artery disease.

28 i.   These lesions are subperiosteal xanthomas. Xanthomatous deposits in the ascending aorta can cause supravalvar aortic stenosis. Involvement of the coronary ostia is frequently seen.
   ii.   This patient has familial hypercholesterolaemia. The condition is inherited as an autosomal dominant.

29 i.   This patient has café-au-lait spots. These are associated with neurofibromatosis.
   ii.   The likely diagnosis is phaeochromocytoma.

30 i.   The hands show sclerodactyly.
   ii.   This patient had systemic sclerosis, which involves the heart, leading to congestive heart failure.
   iii. This can cause cor pulmonale, conduction tissue abnormalities and pulmonary hypertension.

31 i.   There is ST elevation in most leads. The ST-segment is concave upwards, showing the typical changes of acute pericarditis. The ST depression in the cavity lead (in this case aV_R) is to be expected. The ST-segment is isoelectric in leads at right angles to the QRS (leads aV_L and aV_F). This is also to be expected.
   ii.   An echocardiogram should be performed to look for a pericardial effusion.

32 i.   There are tall peaked T waves.
   ii.   These changes are due to hyperkalaemia. Similar tall T waves may be found in true posterior ischaemia and, occasionally, as a normal variant in black people.
   iii. Hyperkalaemia is associated with depression of ventricular conduction, leading to ventricular ectopics, terminating in ventricular fibrillation.

33 i.   The P-R interval is short at 90 ms. The QRS duration is about 120 ms. There is initial slurring of the QRS complex representing a delta wave. The major part of the QRS complex is negative in V_1 and V_2.
   ii.   These changes represent a type B Wolff-Parkinson-White syndrome.
   iii. The cause of the palpitations would be paroxysmal tachycardia involving an accessory pathway, i.e. atrioventricular reentrant tachycardia.

34 i.   There is moderate cardiomegaly. The left ventricular contour is rounded, which is consistent with concentric left ventricular hypertrophy. There is dilatation of the ascending aorta suggesting aortic valvular disease. There is calcification in the aortic knuckle.

ii. This patient has hypertrophic cardiomyopathy, probably with outflow obstruction.

iii. Echocardiography will confirm the diagnosis and coronary angiography may be necessary to exclude coronary artery disease.

35 i.   There is a rounded, smooth shadow in the left hilar region.

ii. This is an aneurysm of the descending aorta. The cough may be due to bronchiolar compression or just an incidental occurrence.

iii. Aortography has been the diagnostic test. However, non-invasive imaging techniques, such as CT and nuclear magnetic resonance, are becoming the standard procedures.

36 i.   The heart size is normal. The left hilum is prominent due to pulmonary dilatation. There is also calcification in the pulmonary artery.

ii. This patient has a patent ductus arteriosus. This accounts for the continuous murmur. The mid-diastolic murmur is due to increased mitral flow as a result of the significant left-to-right shunt.

37 i.   There is cardiac enlargement. There is enlargement of the left atrium and enlargement of the pulmonary artery conus with pulmonary venous congestion.

ii. The pulmonary vascular changes indicate the presence of pulmonary hypertension. The left atrial enlargement shows that the underlying cause is restriction of the mitral valve. In this case, it is due to severe mitral stenosis.

38 i.   This is a barium swallow. The barium-filled oesophagus is displaced backwards towards the spine by an enlarged left atrium.

ii. The dyspnoea is probably related to mitral valve disease and the indigestion-like pain, to peptic ulceration. Detection of left atrial enlargement now is done easily (and non-invasively) by echocardiography.

39   The abnormalities on the X-ray are:
        • fullness of the left cardiac border;
        • possible double contour at the right cardiac border;
        • upper lobe blood diversion.
        These changes indicate left atrial enlargement with a degree of pulmonary congestion and are suggestive of mitral valve disease.

40 i.   This patient had a patent ductus arteriosus.

ii. He underwent percutaneous transvenous closure of the patent duct. The umbrella device is delivered transvenously and through the duct, to be sited on the aortic side of the duct. The catheter-based system can also be used to occlude atrial and ventricular septal defects.

41 i.   The heart is enlarged, with a Cardiothoracic Ratio (CTR) of 15.5/24.5. The pulmonary outflow tract is large with calcification in the main pulmonary artery. The large central pulmonary arteries suggest the presence of pulmonary arterial hypertension. The RV is also enlarged.

   ii.   This patient has cyanotic heart disease. The findings suggest a ventricular septal defect with a right-to-left shunt (Eisenmenger's syndrome).

   iii. An echocardiogram would confirm the diagnosis.

42 i.   There is complete situs inversus. The stomach gas shadow is located on the right. There is prominence of the 'left' mid-cardiac border with lifting of the apex, suggestive of enlargement of the RV and outflow tract.

   ii.   These findings, along with the physical signs, indicate the presence of an atrial septal defect.

43 i.   There is cardiomegaly with prominence of the main pulmonary conus and increased pulmonary blood flow. There is calcification in the right hilar region which may be due to old tuberculosis.

   ii.   Atrial or ventricular septal defects are the most likely causes for these changes. In view of the absence of strikingly increased pulmonary vascularity, a ventricular septal defect is more likely.

44 i.   There is significant enlargement of the heart. More importantly, there is bulging of the LV with a band of calcification. This is calcification in a ventricular aneurysm.

   ii.   About 85% of left ventricular aneurysms occur in the antero-apical area and 15% in the inferior surface of the heart.

45   This is a Björk-Shiley valve placed in the aortic position. Usually, it is seen better in a lateral chest X-ray, since in the postero-anterior view it overlies the spine. A mitral valve prosthesis would be clearly visible usually just to the left of the spine and slightly lower than the position of the prosthetic aortic valve.

46 i.   The heart is enlarged with diffuse haziness extending from both hila. There is a small effusion in the right side. These changes are due to early pulmonary oedema. The aortic root is dilated with linear calcification in the aortic wall of the ascending aorta.

   ii.   This is typical of syphilitic aortitis. The cardiomegaly and congestive changes may be due to valvular heart disease, particularly syphilitic valvular disease, cardiomyopathy or ischaemic heart disease.

47 i.   The aortic knuckle is situated on the right, indicating the presence of a right-sided aortic arch.

    ii. This is a normal variant of no clinical significance.

48 i. There is increased transradiancy of the right lung (compared with the left). Peripheral vascular shadows in the right lung are reduced. The mediastinum is central. The aortic knuckle is inconspicuous and the main pulmonary conus is dilated, indicating the presence of a left-to-right shunt.

    ii. In this case, the patient has an atrial septal defect. There are several causes for the lung abnormality including poorly centred film, scoliosis, congenital absence or embolic occlusion of a pulmonary artery, compensatory over-inflation and Macleod's (Swyer-James) syndrome.

49 i. This is an M-mode echocardiogram at the level of the mitral valve. A dense mass of echoes is seen behind the anterior mitral leaflet. During systole, the mitral valve is closed and looks normal. The dense echo during diastole is due to a mass extending into the atrioventricular canal.

    ii. This is likely to be a myxoma. During systole the mass is confined to the left atrium and, therefore, the dense echo is no longer seen.

50 i. The heart is grossly enlarged and is globular in shape. There are shadows in both lung fields. However, there are no signs of pulmonary congestion.

    ii. The cardiac abnormalities are typical of a large pericardial effusion. Sometimes, the right cardiophrenic angle is acute. The lung lesions are metastases which indicate that the aetiology of the pericardial effusion is likely to be malignant.

51 i. There is prominence of the LV. There are irregularities, or notching, of the inferior margins of the ribs posteriorly, more marked on the right side. These are due to collateral flow through the dilated, and pulsatile, intercostal arteries.

    ii. It is possible to see discrete coarctation of the aorta on two-dimensional echocardiography. Cardiac catheterisation would not only confirm the diagnosis, but would also assess the severity of the lesion. MRI scanning would reveal the anatomy of the lesion.

52 i. This patient has pectus excavatum. Note the reduction in the space between the sternum and spine.

    ii. On a postero-anterior view, the heart may be displaced to the left and may sometimes give the impression that it is enlarged.

53 i. This patient is having pulmonary valvuloplasty, using two balloons. Two balloons, rather than one, are used if the patient's pulmonary valve annulus exceeds 18–19 mm, as measured from right ventricular angiography.

    ii. Pulmonary valvuloplasty in older children and adults is safe. Ventricular ectopics and right bundle branch block are common and are due to catheter manipulation in the RV. Transient hypotension, femoral vein trauma and mild pulmonary regurgitation are seen occasionally.

54 i. The main finding is widening of the mediastinum. There is a prominent shadow to the right of the mediastinum. (This is lower than the usual position of a dilated ascending aorta seen in aortic valve disease.) This appearance is typical of gross dilatation of the aortic root.

   ii. This patient has Marfan's syndrome. In this condition, dilatation is confined usually to the first part of the aorta.

  iii. Echocardiography and/or magnetic resonance imaging will exclude or confirm aortic dissection.

55   There are well-defined, round, radio-opaque shadows at the lower zone of each lung. These represent bilateral mammary prostheses. They may obscure the borders of the heart, making its size difficult to assess.

56   This is a lateral chest X-ray. There is a large, air-filled structure just behind the heart. Its shape and size, as well as position, make it likely that it is a hiatus hernia. Hiatus hernia can produce pain similar in character to cardiac ischaemic pain. Sometimes it is difficult to determine the cause of the chest pain in patients known to have both coronary artery disease and hiatus hernia.

57   There is extensive calcification of the pericardium. Sometimes confusion may arise in distinguishing myocardial from pericardial calcification. Usually the distribution is different. Pericardial calcification is most abundant along the right atrial and ventricular borders and in the area of the atrioventricular groove. Pericardium adjacent to the LV is usually spared or less severely affected. Calcification rarely occurs along the left atrial border because of the absence of pericardium behind the left atrium.

58 i. These are ECG, aortic and mean right atrial pressure tracings during a Valsalva manoeuvre.

   ii. This is an abnormal trace. Normally, during the Valsalva manoeuvre, intrathoracic pressure rises, venous return to the heart diminishes, stroke volume falls and venous pressure rises. There is an initial rise in arterial pressure. With continuation of strain, the heart rate increases as a result of the reduction of venous return as well as the reduction in systolic, diastolic and pulse pressures. When the strain is released, a sudden drop in arterial pressure occurs equivalent to the fall in intrathoracic pressure. The sudden rush of blood into the heart results in an overshoot of arterial pressure and bradycardia. The changes in the intrathoracic and venous pressures are well shown on the right atrial pressure trace (bottom line). The abnormalities here are due to the absence of an overshoot in arterial pressure (middle line) when the raised intrathoracic pressure suddenly falls and there is a consequent absence of reflex bradycardia.

59 i. This is a narrow, complex tachycardia with a QRS rate of approximately 220/min. There is a P wave preceding each QRS complex (best seen in V_5, V_6).

    ii. These suggest a tachycardia, more likely to be atrial tachycardia, with 1:1 conduction.

60   i. The beginning of the rhythm shows a narrow complex tachycardia with a QRS rate of 120/min. The P waves are abnormal in morphology and appear to be inscribed at a regular rate, with one P wave to each QRS complex. This looks likely to be atrial tachycardia.

    ii. Carotid sinus massage or, as in this case, intravenous adenosine may terminate the tachycardia. Adenosine is more likely to cause such a prolonged sinus arrest.

61   i. This is a complex ECG. There are two different QRS complexes, each occurring at a different rate. The rhythm of the smaller complex in V_2 and V_3 appears to be regular with, possibly, a P wave with each complex (i.e. sinus rhythm). The rhythm of the other QRS complex appears to be irregular. There are no clear-cut P waves with these complexes.

    ii. Sometimes the two QRS complexes coincide, producing a summation of the voltage (first complex in aV_R, aV_L and aV_F) which is not fusion since the depolarisation pathways of the two different sets of ventricular myocardium are totally discrete. The ECG is from a patient with a heterotopic heart transplantation. The two types of QRS complex are therefore entirely separate and cannot influence one another in any way.

62   i. The QRS rate is about 200/min and is regular. There are minor differences in the configuration of the QRS complexes on a beat-to-beat basis. The QRS axis is –90 . The QRS duration is wide (120 ms). The minor difference in the QRS configuration is due to a superimposed P wave (best seen in V_5 and V_6) consistently related in time to the QRS complex. These findings suggest that the rhythm is ventricular.

    ii. This is ventricular tachycardia.

63   i. This patient is undergoing aortic valvuloplasty.

    ii. This procedure is indicated for patients:

      a. who are not suitable for surgery, but are incapacitated by symptoms of aortic stenosis (e.g. frail and/or senile patients);

      b. with calcific aortic stenosis who require urgent, non-cardiological surgery;

      c. who are in severe heart failure or cardiogenic shock due to aortic stenosis.

    The symptomatic and haemodynamic improvement after valvuloplasty in patients with degenerative aortic calcific stenosis is short-lived.

64   This is a lateral chest X-ray. The atrial lead is in a good position but the ventricular lead is not pointing anteriorly towards the apex of the RV. This makes it unstable, particularly as it is not an active fixation lead. As the patient is in complete heart block, the atrial impulses from the atrial lead will not produce adequate cardiac output to relieve his symptoms.

ANSWERS

65 i. There is marked dilatation of the heart. The left atrium is enlarged. The main
        pulmonary artery shadows are prominent. There is upper lobe blood diversion
        with early signs of congestion. The right heart border is prominent. The cardiac
        changes are likely to be associated with right ventricular enlargement.
    ii. Mitral valve disease is the likely underlying condition with predominance of (if
        not only due to) mitral regurgitation. Significant mitral stenosis would have
        resulted in a more significant left atrial enlargement. The changes in the heart
        indicate a severe degree of mitral valve disease with probable tricuspid
        regurgitation.

66   There are sternal wires indicating previous cardiac surgery. There are three leads
        positioned in the heart (two in the RV, one in the right atrium). This patient
        had a dual-chamber pacemaker and an automatic, implantable cardioverter-
        defibrillator. The defibrillator is sited in the anterior abdominal wall. Newer
        generations of defibrillators have pacing facilities and a separate pacemaker would
        not be necessary, although this is often used to save drain on the ICD battery
        by simple pacing function.

67 i. This patient has striate palmar xanthoma.
    ii. It occurs in remnant hyperlipidaemia (apolipoprotein E-II homozygosity).
    iii. It is associated with premature atherosclerosis leading to peripheral vascular,
        cerebral vascular and coronary artery disease.

68 i. This patient has an automatic, implantable cardioverter-defibrillator and also has
        had a permanent pacemaker. The defibrillator is being tested.
    ii. Ventricular fibrillation was induced under general anaesthetic. The device
        detected the abnormal rhythm and delivered a predetermined shock, to revert
        the rhythm to the patient's underlying paced rhythm.

69   In this ECG:
        • rhythm is sinus and the rate is 80/min;
        • frontal plane QRS axis is +105;
        • P wave amplitude in lead II is 3 mm with a P wave axis of +60;
        • P-R interval is normal;
        • QRS duration is approximately 80 ms;
        • dominant R wave is noted in V_1;
        • ST/T wave abnormalities are noted in leads V_1–V_4 with deep S waves in V_5
          and V_6;
        • QRS complex in V_1 is RSR, but the duration is only approximately 90 ms;
        • clockwise cardiac rotation is noted.
        These changes indicate the presence of right atrial hypertrophy, right ventricular
        hypertrophy and incomplete right bundle branch block. The presence of incom-
        plete right bundle branch block makes the underlying cause likely to be atrial
        septal defect.

70 i. There is a bulge on the left heart border. Its density appears to be the same as that of the heart. This is a moderately sized aneurysm of the LV.

ii. Aneurysms of the LV are more common after anterior myocardial infarction. Left ventricular aneurysms usually develop between five days and three months after infarction.

71 i. This patient has hypersensitive carotid sinus syndrome. Carotid sinus massage resulted in sinus arrest.

ii. Symptomatic patients with this condition require the implantation of a pacemaker. A dual-chamber pacing is preferred, as atrioventricular block may occur during periods of hypersensitive carotid reflex.

72 The ECG shows:
  • sinus rate is approximately 60/min with a ventricular rate of 40/min;
  • frontal plane QRS axis is +60;
  • no consistent relationship exists between the atrial and ventricular activity;
  • QRS rate is constant;
  • complete heart block.

73 i. The patient has arcus senilis.

ii. When occurring in men under age 40 this may indicate premature atherosclerosis.

74 i. These are eyelid xanthelasmata.

ii. They can be seen in familial hypercholesterolaemia, combined familial hyperlipidaemia and also in normocholesterolaemic subjects. The first two conditions are associated with premature atherosclerosis.

75 i. This is a myxoma. It was removed from the left atrium. A stalk is seen on the right of the mass which is the attachment, usually in the area of the fossa ovalis.

ii. Echocardiography, particularly trans-oesophageal, is very reliable in visualising atrial tumours. Nuclear magnetic resonance imaging is also of considerable value in detecting and delineating cardiac tumours.

76 i. This is lipaemia retinalis.

ii. It is seen in familial hypertriglyceridaemia and lipoprotein lipase deficiency. (The second condition is very rare.) Familial hypertriglyeridaemia is associated with pancreatitis, which is the cause of this patient's abdominal pain. Such patients are not particularly at risk of premature atherosclerosis.

77 i. This is a technetium ^{99m}Tc stannous pyrophosphate imaging scan. This test is used for hot-spot scanning of myocardial infarction. This tracer is not a specific marker of necrosis, but is a marker of both irreversible damage (necrosis) and of severe but reversible injury. The scan is unlikely to be positive in the first 12 hours.

ii. The hot-spot is seen as a half doughnut-shaped shadow.

78 i.   This is a gated cardiac blood pool imaging, also known as multigated acquisition (MUGA) imaging. It depends on the complete mixing of the marker (^{99m}Tc-labelled red blood cells) throughout the circulating volume. The marker should remain intravascular.

ii. This scan is used to determine the ejection fraction of the LV. In this case there is uniform contraction of the myocardium (left ventricular dimension in systole (top right) is uniformly less than that in diastole (top left)). The ejection fraction is 70%. (Bottom graph shows counts during cardiac cycle.)

79 i.   This is an aortogram. There is a catheter in the pulmonary artery. Contrast medium is clearly seen to be passing from the aorta into the pulmonary artery.

ii. This is due to the presence of a patent ductus arteriosis.

80 i.   Both chambers (atrium and ventricle) are being paced. The 'mode' is therefore either DDD or DVI (or theoretically DOO, although this is not a realistic option).

ii. If this were a DVI pacemaker, since the atrium is not being sensed, the pacemaker unit could compete with spontaneous atrial activity. In this trace, no competition is seen. DDD pacing is better (atrial activity is sensed) and is optimal if the sinus node behaves normally. If there is underlying sinus node disease, or failure of chronotropic response, a DDDR (rate responsive) unit would be preferable.

81 i.   This is the right coronary artery, which has a haemodynamically significant stenosis.

ii. In the absence of critical stenosing atheroma in the left coronary artery system, the management of choice is coronary angioplasty.

iii. The rate of restenosis is 40% in the first six months.

82 i.   The rhythm is sinus. The P-R interval is 100 ms, which is short. The QRS axis is normal at +75° and there are no abnormalities with the QRS, ST-segment or T waves.

ii. The ECG could be within normal limits but the short P-R interval suggests the possibility of Lown-Ganong-Levine syndrome.

83 i.   The main abnormality is heavy calcification of the aortic valve. This is typical of aortic stenosis. Considering the patient's symptoms, the degree of stenosis is probably severe.

ii. Echocardiography is accurate in measuring the gradient across the aortic valve. If surgery is contemplated, coronary angiography should be performed to determine the presence or absence of coronary artery disease.

84 i.   The ECG shows:
• rhythm is sinus;

ANSWERS

- P-R interval is 280 ms;
- right axis deviation with a QRS axis of +120 exists;
- T wave is inverted in aV_L and $V_1 - V_3$;
- P wave is prominent in leads II, III and aV_F (5 mm in amplitude);
- right atrial hypertrophy indicated by these findings;

ii. A left-to-right shunt and recurrent pulmonary embolism would result in pulmonary hypertension and right atrial hypertrophy. There is pronounced clockwise cardiac rotation but no definite QRS evidence of right ventricular enlargement. Severe right ventricular systolic overload (e.g. pulmonary hypertension or pulmonary stenosis) is unlikely in the absence of QRS changes of right ventricular hypertrophy.

85 i. The ECG shows:
- rhythm is irregular with a ventricular rate of 80–90/min;
- QRS duration is 150 ms;
- QRS axis is –60;
- Q waves are absent in V_5 and V_6;
- There is no rSr` in V_1 to indicate right bundle branch block. Therefore there is left bundle branch block and atrial fibrillation.

ii. The most likely underlying cause is either ischaemic heart disease or fibrosis in the conducting system.

86 i. The interventricular septum is disproportionately thicker than the posterior left ventricular wall. The left ventricular dimensions are small (especially at end systole). It is clear, from the visibility of both mitral leaflets, that the recording is taken from the left ventricular inflow area, where the cavity dimension would be expected to be greater.

ii. This is characteristic of hypertrophic cardiomyopathy. Another characteristic feature, not seen in this echocardiogram, is systolic anterior motion of the mitral valve.

87 i. This is a left ventricular angiogram.
ii. It shows thickened myocardium with almost total obliteration of the left ventricular cavity during systole. (Mitral incompetence is shown by opacification of dilated left atrium. This can occur in hypertrophic cardiomyopathy.)
iii. These findings are usually associated with hypertrophic cardiomyopathy, although systemic hypertension may produce a similar picture. An echocardiogram would differentiate between the two.

88 i. These are ball and cage valves (Starr-Edwards).
ii. The top one is in the aortic position, the left one in the mitral position and the right one in the tricuspid position.

89 i. The ECG shows:
- rhythm is sinus;

- frontal plane QRS axis is +90;
- QRS duration is 160 ms;
- secondary R wave exists in V_1;
- these changes represent right bundle branch block, which may occur congenitally in normal hearts.

   ii. With this patient's age and the murmur, the most likely cause is atrial septal defect.

90   i. This is a lateral chest X-ray. There is left atrial enlargement, clearly demonstrated by the air-filled oesophagus being pushed backwards. There is extensive calcification in the left atrium. Most likely, this is calcification in a mural thrombus.

   ii. These findings are generally associated with rheumatic mitral valve disease.

91   i. The heart size is normal but there is evidence of left atrial enlargement. There is marked pulmonary venous congestion with soft shadowing around both hila, representing early pulmonary oedema.

   ii. The combination of severe pulmonary venous congestion and dilated left atrium, with normal sized LV, implies mitral valve restriction. Most commonly, this is due to mitral stenosis or left atrial myxoma. Sometimes severe mitral stenosis may not be accompanied by detectable left atrial enlargement.

92   i. There is a difference in the amplitude of alternating QRS complexes. This is called electrical alternans.

   ii. Electrical alternans is seen, not uncommonly, in paroxysmal tachycardia (not relevant here). The finding of alternans in the absence of appreciable tachycardia (and with the virtually constant P-R interval and sinus rate) indicates alternating intraventricular conduction. This may be at His-Purkinje system, or bundle branch level. Sometimes it can occur in the presence of an accessory pathway. There is no evidence of ventricular excitation in this record.

93   i. This ECG shows:
- rhythm is sinus;
- right bundle branch block exists;
- frontal plane QRS axis is –90 indicating left axis deviation;
- initial R wave exist in leads II, III and aV_F.

These changes indicate right bundle branch block with left anterior hemiblock. There is ST-elevation in leads I and aVL which may be attributed to acute ischaemia.

   ii. Right bundle branch block is found most commonly in:
- elderly people without evidence of heart disease, (fibrous degeneration of the anterior division of the left and right bundle branches);
- chronic ischaemic heart disease;
- acute myocardial infarction;
- calcific aortic stenosis and hypertrophic cardiomyopathy.

iii. The most likely explanation is acute anterior infarction in a patient with right bundle branch block and left anterior hemiblock.

94   The most significant abnormality is the presence of prominent R waves in V_1 and V_2. (An R wave is abnormal when it equals or exceeds the S wave of the following lead.) There are also tall T waves in $V_1 - V_3$. Although these could be normal variants, the tall R waves indicate that the patient has had a posterior infarction in the past. Tall T waves are generally attributed to true posterior ischaemia. True posterior infarction is usually associated with inferior infarction (not seen here).

95   This ECG shows:
      • rhythm is sinus;
      • frontal plane QRS axis is +105;
      • dominant R wave exists in V_1 with an Rs QRS pattern;
      • QRS duration is about 60 ms.
      These changes are typical of right ventricular hypertrophy. In this case a left-to-right shunt, in a patient with ventricular septal defect, is a possible cause. Clear evidence of right ventricular hypertrophy points to the additional presence of pulmonary hypertension or pulmonary stenosis.

96   The pacemaker lead is twisted around itself. This is usually caused by the patient turning the pacemaker around in its pocket. This is known as 'twiddling'. This may result in the insulation or conductor in the lead breaking, thus interfering with its function.

97 i. This ECG shows:
      • rhythm is sinus;
      • frontal plane QRS axis is +105;
      • a defect exists in the right bundle branch system. There are no changes (such as those of right ventricular hypertrophy or clockwise cardiac rotation) to account for the right axis deviation.
      • QRS duration is about 100 ms;
    ii. These changes are seen in:
      • left posterior hemiblock;
      • vertical hearts in tall thin subjects;
      • emphysema;
      • atrial septal defect.
      It is not possible to confidently diagnose left posterior hemiblock with a 12-lead ECG.

98 i. This is an aortogram in a patient with a Björk-Shiley aortic prosthesis.
    ii. There is gross dilatation of the aortic root. This dilatation is not uncommon in aortic valve disease. There is no dissection.

99   i.   The ECG:
- rhythm is sinus;
- P-R interval is prolonged (310 ms);
- right bundle branch block pattern;
- marked right atrial enlargement;
- R wave in V_1 and V_2 is prominent with anterior ST/T wave changes.

These indicate right ventricular hypertrophy with systolic overload pattern.

     ii. These changes can be seen in pulmonary stenosis and atrial septal defect.

100 i.   The Q-T interval is prolonged (490 ms).

     ii. Prolonged Q-T interval in a young female with deafness is seen in Jervell and Lange-Nielsen syndrome. The risk of sudden cardiac death is higher in females than in males with this condition.

     iii. The inheritance is autosomal recessive.

101   In this ECG:
- R-R interval is regular;
- no P waves exist;
- baseline is irregular, indicating numerous localised depolarisation circuits in the atrial myocardia;
- QRS rate is 40/min;
- slight ST elevation exists in leads II, III and aV_F with q waves in lead $V_1 - V_4$;
- ST/T wave changes exist in leads I, aV_L and $V_4 - V_6$.

These changes show complete heart block with atrial fibrillation, evidence of an acute inferior myocardial infarction and, possibly, an old anterior infarction.

102 i.   There is cardiomegaly with signs of pulmonary congestion. The mediastinum is wide but this is an antero-posterior view with the patient sitting up and the chest rotated. A pacing lead appears to be running from the left subclavian vein into a left superior vena cava. A left superior vena cava is more commonly seen in situs inversus, but an isolated left superior vena cava is seen in the absence of any other congenital abnormalities.

     ii. It is of no great significance other than it may make manipulation of the pacing lead difficult.

103 i.   This patient has a left and right superior vena cava.

     ii. Anomalies of systemic venous drainage are commonly associated with atrial isomerism. Left atrial isomerism is characteristically associated with interruption of the inferior vena cava, with azygos continuation.

104 i.   This patient had a pneumothorax following a subclavian vein puncture for implantation of a permanent pacemaker. As a result marked subcutaneous emphysema developed. A pneumothorax is a recognised complication when the subclavian vein is used in this procedure.

ANSWERS

ii. Bleeding into the pocket, with the development of haematoma, air embolism and myocardial perforation are other complications encountered.

105 The tip of the pacemaker lead is in a satisfactory position. However, there is a break in the conductor of the lead, just below the left clavicle. This has resulted in loss of pacemaker activity. A conductor break in the distal part of the lead may produce pacemaker spikes on the ECG, whereas a more proximal break – as in this case – would not.

106 i. This is atrioventricular nodal re-entrant tachycardia.
ii. This ECG shows:
- narrow complex tachycardia with a regular rhythm. (QRS duration is 100 ms);
- rate is 160 beats per min;
- frontal plain QRS axis is 0°;
- P waves either occur immediately after, or are superimposed on, the QRS complex. This is best seen in leads $V_1 - V_3$. (It is difficult to decide whether the P waves are upright or inverted. They are probably inverted.)

107 In this ECG:
- rhythm is sinus;
- ventricular rate is around 64/min;
- P-R interval is about 90 ms;
- QRS is about 130 ms in duration;
- initial slurring of the QRS complex exists, connoting a delta wave. The delta wave represents the abnormal site of initiation of ventricular depolarisation.

This patient has Wolff-Parkinson-White (WPW) syndrome. As the major part of the QRS complex is positive in leads V_1 and V_2. This indicates a type A WPW.

108 i. This is an aortogram showing an embolisation device just distal to the aortic arch. This device was used to occlude a patent ductus arteriosus. It is a catheter-based system and the procedure is carried out percutaneously, under local anaesthesia.
ii. It could also be used to close small atrial and ventricular septal defects.

109 i. The abnormalities on this ECG include:
- prolongation of the P-R interval (280 ms);
- QRS duration of 160 ms;
- no septal Q wave in V_5 and V_6;
- frontal plane QRS axis of –60;
- no rSr` in V_1 to indicate that the intraventricular conduction disturbance is right bundle branch block.

These findings indicate the presence of first degree block, left bundle branch block and left axis deviation.
ii. The most likely aetiology is ischaemic heart disease. A treadmill exercise test would not be helpful as it would be difficult to interpret any ST-segment

changes. A Thallium exercise test would be preferable, though proceeding directly to coronary angiography may be more appropriate.

110 i. The pacemaker has eroded the skin and subcutaneous tissue and is now protruding through to the surface. This is due to chronic low grade infection.

ii. The whole system should be removed and, if the patient is not pacemaker-dependent, a new system implanted after a minimum 7-day course of antibiotics has been completed. If the patient is pacemaker-dependent, then a temporary epicardial system should be implanted to leave the right infraclavicular area clean for the new system.

111 i. Prominent R wave in V_1 and V_2 with ST-segment depression in leads $V_1 - V_4$.

ii. These changes are consistent with an acute posterior infarction.

112 i. This is an M-mode echocardiogram at the level of the left ventricular inflow tract. The interventricular septum is hypertrophied. Both mitral valve leaflets are visualised. There is abnormal motion of the mitral valve leaflets during systole.

ii. This is called systolic anterior motion of the mitral valve (SAM). SAM is commonly seen in hypertrophic cardiomyopathy. Mild SAM usually originates from chordal anterior motion, while severe SAM involves the body of the anterior mitral leaflet. SAM may be seen:
• in normal young subjects who are in hypovolaemic states;
• during inotropic stimulation;
• in hypertensive patients;
• in amyloid heart disease.

113 i. There is variation in the length of the P-P interval. This is sinus arrhythmia, better described as irregular sinus rhythm.

ii. The variation in cycle length is related to respiration. There is an increase in cycle length during expiration. This is commonly seen in athletes and children.

114 i. Abnormalities on this ECG are:
• slight ST-segment depression in most leads;
• increase in the amplitude of the T waves, seen best in leads $V_2 - V_5$;
• prominent U wave is present, seen best in V_2 and V_3.

ii. These changes occur due to hypokalaemia. Sometimes the duration of the QRS is prolonged.

115 i. This is a digital petechia.

ii. It may be seen in bacterial endocarditis. The lesion is not, however, specific for bacterial endocarditis, as it may develop in patients with haematological disorders, vasculitis and renal insufficiency.

iii. Two-dimensional echocardiography is important in demonstrating the presence of vegetations in 80% of patients with native valve endocarditis. It is of less value in demonstrating vegetations on non-tissue prosthetic valves. Cineradiography of the prosthetic valve would show abnormal motion in the presence of valve dehiscence.

116 i. There is marked jugular venous distention. There are also prominent temporal veins.

   ii. In the absence of significant symptoms such as breathlessness, the mostly likely diagnosis is tricuspid regurgitation. Examination of the jugular venous pulse shows absence of the normal 'x' and 'y' descents. (In fact, 'x' descents are unlikely to be relevant, since patients with severe tricuspid regurgitation are likely to have atrial fibrillation.) A prominent systolic wave (C-V wave) becomes apparent. The y descent is sharp, becoming the most prominent event in the venous pulse. If there is coexisting tricuspid stenosis, the y descent is slow.

117 i. These are amyloid deposits in the subcutaneous tissues of the hand.

   ii. Involvement of the heart commonly causes a restrictive cardiomyopathy. Other cardiac manifestations include arrhythmias, conduction defects and angina pectoris.

118 i. This is an M-mode echocardiogram at the level of the mitral valve. It shows mid-systolic bowing of the mitral valve leaflets as a result of mid-systolic mitral valve prolapse (MVP).

   ii. A large majority of children with MVP remain asymptomatic for many years. About 15% of patients develop progressive mitral regurgitation (MR) over a 10–15 year period. Men over the age of 50 years are more likely to develop severe MR. Patients with MVP are prone to infective endocarditis.

119 i. These are tender red swellings occurring mostly over the shin.

   ii. This is erythema nodosum. The likely diagnosis is sarcoidosis with cardiac involvement causing arrhythmia.

120 i. In this ECG:
   • QRS morphology is normal, but the rhythm is irregular;
   • QRS complexes not consistently preceded by a P wave; P waves not followed by a QRS complex;
   • P-R interval (taken from a PQRST complex) is variable. It is within normal limits at 160 ms in $V_4 - V_6$ and 320 ms in $V_1 - V_3$;
   • T wave abnormalities exist in leads II, III, aV_F and $V_2 - V_6$.
   This ECG shows a rhythm varying between first and second degree heart block.

   ii. The history going back to childhood suggests that the cause of the heart block is likely to be congenital. The T wave abnormalities may represent coincidental ischaemia.

121 i. This is a four-chamber view of a transthoracic echocardiogram. The main finding is a heavily calcified mass, in the apex of the LV. This most likely represents an old, calcified thrombus.

   ii. It is possible that the patient's symptoms are due to thrombo-embolic events from the LV, but this calcified thrombus is unlikely to be responsible. Another cause for the patient's symptoms, such as carotid artery disease, should be excluded.

122 i. The top two recordings show sinus rhythm but with variable rate. The P-R interval is constant. There is one premature ventricular beat. The bottom two and the right half of the middle recordings show a narrow complex tachycardia which, judging from the morphology of the QRS complexes, is supraventricular. This rhythm change is seen in bradycardia-tachycardia syndrome (sick sinus syndrome). The blackout occurred because excessive exercise heightens the vagal tone leading to profound bradycardia or even atrioventricular conduction abnormalities.

   ii. Symptoms are abolished by the implantation of a permanent pacemaker.

123 i. There is a tight lesion at the origin of the internal carotid artery (nearly 90%).

   ii. It is important that the internal and not the external carotid artery is palpated during physical examination. The internal carotid artery is usually lateral and easily palpated above the carotid bulb. In aortic stenosis, the carotid arterial pulse is small, slow-rising and showing prolonged duration. In aortic regurgitation, there is a rapid rise with a bifid peak, prolonged duration and a reduced dicrotic notch. In hypertrophic cardiomyopathy the rise is rapid but with an early abrupt peak and a plateau or a gentle second hump (known as bisferiens pulse).

124 i. This patient is having an upright tilt test, which shows progressive bradycardia leading to asystole. Upright posture is associated with pooling of blood in the lower extremities. This results in the fall of central venous pressure, stroke volume, and blood pressure. In normal individuals, head uptilting causes activation of arterial and cardiopulmonary baroreceptor reflexes (and activation of the renin-angiotensin system, as well as the release of vasopressin) which results in arterial and venous vasoconstriction, and an increase in the heart rate, preventing hypotension.

   ii. This patient is, however, suffering from vasovagal syncope (sometimes called neurally mediated syncope). The mechanism is not fully understood, but the hypotension is mainly due to vasodilatation in skeletal muscle vessels. The bradycardia is due to inappropriate vagal action and it aggravates the hypotension.

125 i. This is a four-chamber view from a transthoracic echocardiogram. It shows a large pericardial effusion. There is an echodense, long shadow in the RV.

   ii. The patient had a temporary pacing lead placed in the RV. This perforated the right ventricular wall causing an effusion. Perforation of the myocardium with a pacemaker lead is uncommon but is more likely in association with freshly infarcted myocardium.

126 i.   This is a long axis view. The mitral valve looks thickened and stenotic. The left atrium is grossly dilated. The aortic valve is also thickened but appears to open well.

   ii.   Mitral stenosis.

127   This is the right coronary artery. It arises from the right sinus of Valsalva and runs down the right atrioventricular groove to reach the inferior surface of the heart.

128 i.   These are superimposed left ventricular and right atrial pressure tracings. The pressures in these chambers in diastole are a) increased, and b) virtually identical. There is also a 'dip and plateau' configuration in the left ventricular trace. The x and y descents are both prominent in the right atrial pressure tracing. However, the x descent is dominant.

   ii.   These findings are strongly suggestive of constrictive pericarditis. In this condition the diastolic pressures in the left and right ventricles and the mean pressures in the left and right atria all tend to be about the same.

129 i.   On this ECG:
- rhythm is sinus;
- frontal plane QRS axis is 0;
- morphological changes of left ventricular hypertrophy exist;
- R waves in V_4 and V_5 exceed 27 mm;
- sum of the tallest R wave in the left precordial leads and the deepest S wave in the right precordial leads exceeds 40 mm;
- ST-segment depression and T wave inversion exist in the left precordial leads.

   ii.   These changes are seen in hypertension and aortic stenosis.

130 i.   The thoracic aorta is dilated and tortuous due to marked unfolding. This may occur in the elderly and is seen as widening of the aorta on a postero-anterior chest X-ray.

   ii.   With these findings, imaging should be considered to exclude a localised aneurysm.

131 i.   In this ECG:
- trace shows a narrow complex tachycardia with a QRS rate of around 160/min;
- flutter waves are clearly seen (best in leads I, aV_L and V_1);
- atrial rate is around 320/min;

A 2:1 atrioventricular block is confirmed showing that the estimated atrioventricular refractory period is longer than one, but shorter than two, atrial cycle lengths.

   ii.   Drugs such as digoxin, beta-blockers and verapamil, that affect the atrioventricular node, will tend to increase the degree of atrioventricular block to 3:1 or 4:1.

132   This is a digital subtraction venogram, showing the right subclavian vein. There is a stenosis just before the innominate vein. There is also a thrombus in the subclavian vein prior to it entering the superior vena cava. Contrast medium is seen in the superior vena cava. The thrombus is the likely cause of the patient's swollen arm and neck.

133   The delta wave is positive in the anterior precordial leads as well as in leads II, III and aV_F. It is isoelectric in V_5 and negative in V_6. These findings indicate that the accessory pathway is in the left lateral atrial wall.

134 i.   There are several nodules on all fingers, particularly the index finger. These lesions are due to sarcoidosis and represent accumulations of epithelioid granulomas in the dermis. These are more common in blacks than whites, and in women rather than men.

    ii.   The cause of the syncope is likely to be an ectopic arrhythmia, eg. ventricular tachycardia or a conduction disturbance (heart block).

135   This patient has gynaecomastia. Spironolactone and digitalis are commonly associated with this abnormality.

136   There is failure of pacemaker output. This occurs during contraction of muscles around the pacemaker. Muscle potentials may cause inhibition, or false driving, of a unipolar system. This is seldom of clinical relevance or dangerous for the patient.

137   This is an M-mode echocardiogram of the LV at mitral valve level. The mitral valve leaflets (MVL) are thickened, with the anterior leaflet moving slightly anteriorly at the onset of diastole. There is posterior excursion of the ventricular septum in early diastole. (This is best seen as a bump in the third, early diastolic event.) These findings indicate the presence of mitral stenosis and aortic regurgitation.

138   This patient has neurofibromatosis (von Recklinghausen's disease). This condition occurs in 5% of patients with phaechromocytoma which may be responsible for the patient's symptoms. On the other hand phaechromocytoma is found in only 1% of patients with neurofibromatosis.

139   This is a thoracic scan showing a grossly dilated ascending aorta. There is a flap separating the true lumen (on the right of the scan) from the false lumen (on the left). Static blood (in the false lumen) results in a dense shadow compared with that of moving blood. This patient had a chronic aortic dissection.

ANSWERS

140   In this ECG:
- rate is 60/min;
- ST-segment elevation exists in leads II, III, aV_F, V_5 and V_6;
- atrioventricular dissociation exists.

These represent an acute inferolateral myocardial infarction and complete heart block.

141 i. The first, second, fourth and eighth complexes are sequentially paced. There are several sensed P waves which are not followed by ventricular pacing.

     ii. This is due to electrical cross-talk. Cross-talk is the sensing of the output of one pacemaker channel in the other. In this rhythm strip, the atrial stimulus (spike followed by P wave) is sensed in the ventricular channel, resulting in inhibition of ventricular stimulus and ventricular output. Cross-talk causing ventricular inhibition is prevented by programming a blanking period, which begins simultaneously in the ventricular channel with the atrial stimulus. Depending on the pulse generator, this period is usually 12–50 ms in duration.

142 i. This is an old generation, rate-responsive pacemaker.

     ii. The system is a ventricular demand inhibited (VVI), with a respiratory rate sensor tunnelled in the subcutaneous tissue, transversely across the thorax. More recent rate-responsive pacemakers use other physiological parameters such as temperature, pressure, electrochemical and electrogram sensing.

143 i. All QRS complexes, except the third and seventh, are followed by a spike. If the pacemaker was recognising the intrinsic complexes, the spike should precede the QRS complexes. This rhythm strip shows ventricular undersensing.

     ii. This occurs because of:
- low-amplitude electrograms (the commonest cause);
- lead dislodgement;
- myocardial infarction;
- low-amplitude signal from premature ventricular complexes;
- failure of a component of the pulse generator.

144 i. The top half of the recording shows atrial flutter with 2:1 conduction. Sinus rhythm was restored by DC (direct current) cardioversion. The heavy markings on the QRS complexes in the left half of the recording indicate synchronisation – of the triggering circuit for the shock – to the QRS complexes.

     ii. When atrial fibrillation or flutter uccur, patients with underlying cardiac conditions such as mitral or aortic valve disease, hypertrophic cardiomyopathy, or those who have undergone Fontan procedure are usually acutely dyspnoeic, with signs of haemodynamic compromise. Treatment may be urgent and is preferred by DC cardioversion. DC cardioversion should always be undertaken under full anticoagulation cover. If time permits, warfarin should be given for 4–6 weeks. Otherwise, full intravenous heparinisation is indicated. Ideally the patient should remain anticoagulated for 4–6 weeks after cardioversion – with warfarin alone if this was used initially – or with intravenous heparin followed by warfarin if initial anticoagulation was with heparin. If atrial fibrillation recurs or if the patient is not haemodynamically compromised, digoxin should be given to control the ventricular rate. A beta-blocker or a calcium-channel blocker that acts on the A-V node (verapamil, diltiazem) may be added. Intravenous, verapamil or beta-blockers should not be used in patients with acute myocardial infarction as these drugs have a negative inotropic effect. Use of beta-blockers and diltiazem or verapamil together should be avoided because of the increased risk of complete heart block and heart failure.

145 i. The heart size is normal. The main pulmonary conus is enlarged, though the pulmonary vascularity is normal.
   ii. These appearances are typical of idiopathic dilatation of the pulmonary artery. Patients with the condition are asymptomatic. Physical signs, such as a late pulmonary ejection sound or 'click' preceding a soft murmur, may sometimes be found. The condition is compatible with a normal life span.

146 i. In this ECG:
   • rhythm is regular;
   • QRS morphology shows a right bundle branch block pattern;
   • P-R interval is prolonged (280 ms);
   • frontal plane QRS axis is –90 indicating left axis deviation;
   • an initial R wave exists in the inferior limb leads;
   • left axis deviation (more negative than –30) is present;
   • an initial R wave exists in the inferior leads, suggesting left anterior hemiblock.
   The overall ECG appearances indicate the presence of a conduction problem at these sites (right bundle branch, anterior division of left bundle branch). This is often inappropriately called 'trifascicular block.' The third fascicle (the posterior division of the left bundle branch) is not demonstrably affected. True trifascicular block would give complete heart block.
   ii. The combination of these types of block carries a high risk of sudden death. Therefore symptomatic patients with trifascicular block should be paced.

147 i. This is an M-mode echocardiogram at the level of the aortic valve. There is premature or mid-systolic closure of the aortic valve. Both the right and non-coronary cusps move briskly to the closed position.
   ii. This finding is seen in patients with hypertrophic obstructive cardiomyopathy. Such premature closure of the aortic valve is due to the Venturi effect of blood being ejected at high velocity, so that most of the stroke volume is evacuated within the first third of systole.

148 i. These are the two branches of the main left coronary artery.
   ii. The left anterior descending artery (on the right of the picture) lies to the left of the pulmonary conus before entering the anterior interventricular groove between the two ventricles. It runs the length of the interventricular groove to

reach the cardiac apex where it turns round, terminating in two small branches. The circumflex (on the left of the picture) runs posteriorly in the atrioventricular groove towards the crux of the heart.

149 i. The heart size is normal. There is widespread reticular shadowing involving both lungs. These are typical appearances of pulmonary fibrosis.

ii. These changes, and a normal sized heart, make the cause of the patient's dyspnoea most likely to be pulmonary rather than cardiac. However, such patients are likely to develop cor pulmonale in advanced stages.

150 i. Atrial overdrive pacing.

ii. This technique is used to measure the degree of suppression of sinus node automaticity following a period of rapid atrial overdrive pacing. The interval measured is that between the last paced atrial beat and the first spontaneous atrial beat. This is called the sinus node recovery time (SNRT). The degree of suppression depends on the inherent automaticity of the sinus node and the number of paced beats. Patients with sick sinus syndrome have a longer SNRT. No normal P waves are seen for nearly eight seconds following the end of overdrive pacing. This indicates severe depression of sinus node activity. The fact that there is no nodal escape beat for nearly eight seconds also indicates depression of A–V nodal activity.

151 i. The left atrium is filled with contrast medium, indicating the presence of mitral regurgitation which appears to be moderately severe. There is a filling defect within the left atrium.

ii. The differential diagnosis is between a myxoma and a large thrombus. The presence of weight loss makes it more likely to be a myxoma.

iii. Echocardiography is important to exclude the presence of mitral valve disease. A myxoma is more likely to be associated with a normal mitral valve.

152 i. This is a long axis view from a transthoracic echocardiogram. The aortic valve looks normal. The mitral valve is abnormal. The leaflets appear to be multicuspid in morphology. The left atrium is dilated.

ii. The mitral leaflet abnormality is the result of what is known as mitral cleft. This abnormality is congenital and is seen in isolated ostium primum defect. The morphology of the mitral valve in this case is pentacuspid. It causes significant mitral regurgitation, which would explain the dilated left atrium.

153 i. This is a trace from an intracardiac electrogram recorded during insertion of a ventricular pacing lead. Contact of the lead tip with the endocardium causes ST-segment elevation with an injury current (intracardiac signal).

ii. The intracardiac signal must be determined in order to ensure adequate and reliable post-implant sensing. It is usually not difficult to achieve a good R wave, in view of the large ventricular musculature. An R wave of at least 4 mV should be obtained; one of more than 8 mV is desirable.

154 i. There is persistent ptosis of the left eye while the patient is looking up.
  ii. This patient has Kearns-Sayre syndrome. This is a mitochondrial myopathy, characterised by progressive external ophthalmoplegia, pigmentary retinopathy and cardiac involvement.
  iii. Conduction defects are the commonest cardiac manifestation of the syndrome. Patients are usually at risk of having complete heart block. Other cardiac manifestations include dilated cardiomyopathy and heart failure.

155 i. She looks thin and has pectus excavatum.
  ii. With lateral thinking, the combination of these signs, and her mother's emergency surgery at a young age for chest pain (probably as a result of aortic dissection) suggests the possibility of Marfan's syndrome. The other common manifestations of Marfan's syndrome include tall stature, joint hypermobility, ectopia lentis, dilatation of the aortic root, and aortic dissection.

156 i. These are septic emboli.
  ii. The clinical situation is suggestive of endocarditis affecting the aortic valve (early diastolic murmur).
  iii. Other physical signs that may be present include splenomegaly, petechiae, splinter haemorrhages, Osler's nodes and Roth spots, which are retinal haemorrhages with a clear centre.

157 i. This M-mode echocardiogram shows the mitral valve. There is fluttering or vibration of the anterior mitral leaflet.
  ii. This effect is seen in aortic regurgitation and is due to the aortic regurgitant jet striking the anterior mitral leaflet. This effect, however, is not specific to aortic regurgitation – even if the chordae are intact.

158 i. This is a subcostal view. There is an aneurysm of the left atrium (to the left of the picture). There is also an atrial septal defect.
  ii. Aneurysms of the left atrium are usually congenital and clinically asymptomatic until the second to fourth decade. They are confined more frequently to the left atrial appendage though may occur in the atrial wall. They are usually associated with systemic embolisation and/or recurrent supraventricular arrhythmias. The atrial septal defect is usually asymptomatic early in life, although there are reports of infants and children developing congestive heart failure and recurrent pneumonia.

159 i. The cardiac muscle fibres show hypertrophy. There are areas in which cells are arranged in whorls rather than parallel. There is some interstitial fibrosis.
  ii. These findings are seen in hypertrophic cardiomyopathy. It should be noted, however, that disarray in the arrangement of muscle cells is not specific for hypertrophic cardiomyopathy. The diagnosis should not be made, or excluded, on the basis of a small biopsy specimen.

ANSWERS

160 i. This shows severe calcification of the aortic valve leaflets. Linear echoes are filling the aortic root and without clearly defined leaflet separation. This patient has severe aortic stenosis. Clearly the aortic valve needs replacing.

 ii. Cardiac catheterisation should be carried out to assess left ventricular function (though often the valve could not be crossed easily, in which case assessment by echocardiography would be sufficient). Coronary angiography should be performed to determine the necessity for coronary artery bypass surgery.

161 This is an intracardiac recording from the atrium during placement of the atrial lead in the right atrial appendage (atrial signal). This measures the P wave, which is important in ensuring reliable post-operative sensing; the larger the P wave, the better. A P wave of more than 4 mV is acceptable while a P wave equal to, or less than, 2 mV is not.

162 This is a paced rhythm strip. There is only one spike preceding each P wave, apart from the sixth wave. This indicates that the pacing mode is AAI, i.e. a single lead in the atrium. The sixth P wave is the patient's own and, therefore, is not preceded by a pacing spike. However, there is a pacing spike which is not followed by a P wave. This is due to exit block, in which a pacing spike is not followed by atrial depolarisation (and/or ventricular depolarisation, depending on the pacing mode). Exit block can be either permanent or intermittent. The problem in exit block usually lies at the interface between the electrode and the myocardium.

163 i. Percutaneous transluminal coronary angioplasty (PTCA) is being carried out. The dilating balloon is inflated in the circumflex coronary artery. A guide wire is positioned in the first marginal artery, to protect it from occlusion as its origin is in contact with the inflated balloon.

 ii. Complications include those common to any cardiac catheterisation procedure, such as arrhythmias, arterial embolisation and vascular injury at the site of catheter entry. Those related to lesion dilatation include dissection and occlusion of the coronary artery. Abrupt closure occurs in about 4% of patients, particularly those with long, eccentric or curved lesions. The mortality rate from PTCA in experienced hands is around 1%.

164 i. The first two complexes are sinus followed by a short run of non-sustained ventricular tachycardia.

 ii. Arrhythmias following opening of an acutely occluded coronary artery are well recognised (reperfusion arrhythmias). Reperfusion arrhythmias (ventricular tachycardia) differ from arrhythmias that occur early after occlusion of a coronary artery. There are two forms of reperfusion arrhythmia. One occurs within a few seconds after opening an acutely occluded artery. This is associated with fragmented and delayed activation of the ischaemic myocardium. Ventricular fibrillation is often an outcome. The second form appears within two to five minutes after reperfusion (by angioplasty or thrombolysis). This ventricular arrhythmia is slow and benign and rarely progresses to fibrillation. It is postulated that the washout of electrolytes and metabolites in the ischaemic myocardium cause electrical and chemical gradients which result in these arrhythmias. It is also believed that a transient increase in ventricular automaticity may be responsible for the slower ventricular arrhythmia.

165 i. The main abnormality is a toxoplasma cyst (in the centre of the picture). Bradyzoites of *Toxoplasma gondii* are packed tightly within the cyst.

ii. Most non-immunosuppressed adult cases are asymptomatic. However, severe, fatal myocarditis may occur. Other manifestations include arrhythmias, both atrial and ventricular, pericarditis, atrioventricular block and heart failure. Immunosuppressed patients, such as those with heart transplants, are most likely to develop symptoms.

166 i. There is widespread and diffuse interstitial infiltration by neutrophils, eosinophils and lymphocytes. There are also areas of myocardial necrosis. These changes indicate a severe degree of rejection.

ii. Endomyocardial biopsy is the most reliable tool for the detection and treatment of rejection. There are other investigations such as the detection of activated circulating lymphoblasts, echocardiography, nuclear magnetic resonance and a decrease in the summed QRS voltages. However, these are not totally reliable and, moreover, they do not detect early signs of rejection.

167 i. This is an M-mode echocardiogram, showing the RV at the top and LV at the bottom, separated by the interventricular septum. The RV is dilated (nearly 5 cm at end diastole). Septal contraction is paradoxical.

ii. Right ventricular dilatation can be seen in pulmonary hypertension, atrial septal defect and right ventricular infarction.

168 i. This scan is at the level of the outflow tract, showing the aortic valve. There is marked thickening of the septum and left ventricular wall.

ii. These changes are seen typically in hypertrophic cardiomyopathy.

iii. The cause of sudden death is presumed, though not definitely established, to be due to ventricular arrhythmias.

iv. Patients at high risk of sudden death include those who are less than 30 years of age at diagnosis, or have a family history of hypertrophic cardiomyopathy with sudden death. Those with a history of syncope as children, and who are offspring of patients with hypertrophic cardiomyopathy, are at high risk of sudden death. Symptoms, and the presence or severity of outflow tract obstruction, do not correlate with the risk of sudden death.

169 i. This is a long axis view of a transthoracic echocardiogram. There is a bright echo protruding from the proximal septum below the aortic valve. This is due to a discrete shelf which is causing subvalvular aortic stenosis. It is difficult clinically to differentiate this from valvular stenosis.

ii. However, the absence of an early systolic click, and the presence of auscultatory findings of aortic regurgitation, would favour subvalvular aortic stenosis. Aortic regurgitation is present in 50–75% of cases with subvalvular stenosis.

170 i. This is a parasternal long axis view from a transthoracic echocardiogram. There is an irregular echogenic mass attached to the anterior mitral leaflet. In the context of the clinical findings this mass is most likely a vegetation.

ii. The overall five-year survival in endocarditis ranges from 47%–90%; around 15%–25% of survivors remain incapacitated by heart failure through the embolic complications. The mortality rate varies with different causative organisms, being highest with staphylococci (40%) and lowest with streptococci (2%).

171 i. The findings of this echocardiogram include:
  • dense, heavy echoes arising from the anterior mitral leaflet, representing fibrosis and calcification;
  • immobile posterior leaflet;
  • flat E to F slope;
  • no A point as the patient is in atrial fibrillation.
  These findings indicate severe mitral stenosis.

ii. The severity of stenosis can be quantified by measuring the mitral valve orifice. The pressure gradient across the valve can be calculated through Doppler ultrasonography and from the Bernoulli equation:

$$P_1 - P_2 = 4 \ (Vmax)^2$$

where P_1 = pressure in left atrium during diastole
P_2 = diastolic pressure in LV
Vmax = maximum flow velocity across the mitral valve.

172 i. This is a thoracic CT scan with contrast enhancement. A flap can be seen clearly in the lumen of the ascending and descending aorta. This indicates aortic dissection (type 1).

ii. The mortality rate in untreated patients is 70% in the first two weeks after onset. Of those who survive, 50% or more will die within the first year. Younger patients, those without hypertension or other cardiovascular disease and patients without a primary tear in the descending aorta have a better prognosis.

173 i. There are five paced complexes in a ventricular demand inhibited (VVI) (single-chamber) pacing mode. There are several pacing spikes which are not followed by paced complexes. There is independent atrial activity. These are the typical appearances of failure to capture, i.e. loss of ventricular stimulation. It is intermittent, indicating that there is a problem in the electrode-tissue interface.

ii. Causes include displacement or unstable position of the pacing lead, lead fracture, insulation break and inappropriate programming of output parameters.

174 i. There are abnormal Q waves from $V_1 - V_6$, indicative of extensive anterior infarction. There is ST-elevation in leads V_2–V_6. This is probably related to the old infarction rather than being due to an acute anterior infarction.

  ii. Persistent ST elevation has always been thought to indicate the presence of a ventricular aneurysm in relation to a previous acute infarction. However, only two-thirds of patients with definite ventricular aneurysms have persistent ST-segment elevation, and probably less than two-thirds of patients with persistent ST-segment elevation have ventricular aneurysms at angiography.

175 i. There are small haemorrhages, each with a pale centre.

  ii. These are Roth spots in a patient who probably has bacterial endocarditis. Roth spots occur in less than 5% of patients with endocarditis.

  iii. They can also be seen in patients with connective tissue disease and haematological disorders.

176 i. There are conjunctival petechiae. They may be embolic or vasculitic.

  ii. They may occur in several conditions such as bacterial endocarditis, renal impairment, vasculitis, haematological disorders, scurvy and as a result of cholesterol or fat emboli.

177 i. This is a transverse magnetic resonance imaging (MRI) scan through the mid position of the LV. There is hypertrophy of the left ventricular wall with asymmetrical hypertrophy of the interventricular septum (ASH). There is no evidence of left ventricular outflow tract obstruction.

  ii. This patient has hypertrophic cardiomyopathy (HCM). (It must be noted that ASH is not specific for HCM. Of patients with idiopathic, chronic systemic and renovascular hypertension, 10–15% may have ASH.)

  iii. Cardiac ischaemic pain occurs as a consequence of increased muscle mass, raised diastolic filling pressure, abnormal intramural coronary arteries, systolic compression of arteries and increased myocardial oxygen demand.

178 i. There is marked left ventricular, as well as interventricular, septal hypertrophy. The mitral and aortic valves appear to be normal.

  ii. The clinical presentation, with these findings (and the fact that the P-R interval on the ECG was short), suggests a diagnosis of type II glycogen storage disease (Pompe's disease). The short P-R interval is thought to be due to facilitated atrioventricular conduction, owing to myocardial glycogen deposition.

179 i. This is a continuous-wave Doppler echocardiogram signal across the mitral valve. There is atrial fibrillation. The peak velocity across the valve is increased (2m/s) giving a gradient of about 16 mmHg in early diastole.

  ii. This indicates severe mitral stenosis. There is also a regurgitant flow. The intensity of the signal is strong, indicating severe mitral regurgitation.

180 i. This is a lateral chest X-ray showing an enlarged heart. The left atrium is grossly enlarged and is seen as a backward projection, close to the spine.

ii. There is a caged-ball prosthetic valve in both the aortic and mitral positions. Its durability and performance are well-known in comparison to other artificial valves. Its major disadvantage is that it is bulky and therefore not suitable in patients with a small left ventricular cavity or a small aortic arch composite graft. It tends to induce haemolysis in a small number of patients. When placed in the tricuspid position, it carries a lower risk of thrombosis than tilting-disc valves.

181 i. This is a left ventricular angiogram in the left anterior oblique position. The image is taken during systole. There are two filling defects. These represent two mural thrombi.

ii. These are common in patients dying from acute myocardial infarction (AMI). In one report, 44% of 924 patients who died from AMI were found at post mortem to have mural thrombi attached to the endocardium overlying the infarct. Mural thrombi are more common in large infarcts and in non-survivors than survivors. The vast majority occur in anterior myocardial infarction. The risk of embolism varies between 0–25%.

182 i. This shows a St. Jude prosthetic valve in the mitral position. A large thrombus has formed in, and caused obstruction of, the valve – in this case with fatal consequences.

ii. Around 60% of patients receiving prosthetic valves have a serious prosthesis-related problem within 10 years post-operatively. The most frequent complications leading to valve failure include:
  • thrombosis;
  • anticoagulant-related haemorrhage;
  • prosthetic valve endocarditis;
  • structural deterioration;
  • non-structural dysfunction such as pannus, suture and tissue entrapment and paravalvular leak.

183 i. This is a porcine heterograft valve. These are tissue valves which are treated with glutaraldehyde and mounted either on a Dacron-cloth-covered, flexible poly-propylene strut or on a Teflon-covered Eljiloy strut.

ii. They have limited durability. At least 20% require replacement within 10 years post-operatively as a result of cuspal tears, degeneration, fibrin deposition, perforation, fibrosis and calcification.

184 i. There is extensive infiltration by mononuclear cells, predominantly lymphocytes. There is focal necrosis to myocytes adjacent to the inflammatory cells.

ii. The absence of suppurative reaction and specific parasite reactions suggests that this is a myocarditis due to a viral infection.

185 i. This is a postero-anterior view showing contrast medium being injected into a stump. The fact that a left Judkins catheter is being used indicates that the stump is most likely that of the left coronary artery. As the patient had grafts to the

three main branches of the left main stem, this indicates that all three branches are occluded proximal to the graft anastomoses.

ii. Occlusion of a coronary artery proximal to a graft anastomosis may occur due to competitive blood flow, i.e. flow in the native artery is slower than that in the graft because of the presence of severe proximal disease.

186 i. This is a subcostal four-chamber view. The right atrium is enlarged (dark shadow to left of picture). The left atrium is not dilated (dark shadow at bottom of picture). There is an atrial septal defect, clearly seen between the right and left atrium.

ii. The ECG changes consist of a right axis deviation, right ventricular hypertrophy and rSR` or rsR` pattern. The left axis deviation and superior orientation, and counterclockwise rotation of the QRS loop in the frontal plane, suggests the presence of either an ostium primum defect or a secundum defect in association with mitral valve prolapse.

187 i. This is a parasternal long axis view. The important finding is prolapse of the right coronary cusp during diastole.

ii. Prolapse of the aortic valve cusps and sometimes the whole sinus of Valsalva is seen most frequently in association with a ventricular septal defect (not seen on this study). Prolapse of the cusp causes a decrease in the size of the defect, as well as creating aortic regurgitation.

188 i. This is an apical four-chamber view. There is a lobulated mass occupying most of the right side of the heart.

ii. The differential diagnosis would be between a thrombus, a primary cardiac tumour or an extension of a primary non-cardiac tumour. Lobulated primary cardiac tumours are uncommon, particularly in older people. In the context of the clinical picture, this most likely represents an extension from a primary tumour in the abdomen, upwards via the inferior vena cava. Leiomyomata from uterine neoplasms and renal cell carcinomata are known to invade the right side of the heart. In this patient, the primary tumour originated in the kidney.

189 i. This is an apical four-chamber view showing a dilated LV. The left atrium is possibly slightly dilated. There is a pericardial effusion. This patient has a dilated cardiomyopathy.

ii. A patient may have a dilated LV but remain asymptomatic for months or years. Reduced survival is associated with:
   • raised filling pressure;
   • the presence of a third heart sound;
   • left ventricular conduction problems;
   • cardiac enlargement;
   • age greater than 55;
   • reduced ejection fraction;
   • ventricular arrhythmias.

190 i.   The muscle fibres have been replaced by fibrous and fatty tissue.
   ii. These changes are seen in right ventricular dysplasia. In this condition the RV is enlarged and is paper-thin.
   iii. Such patients have recurrent ventricular tachycardia, especially with left bundle branch block pattern on the ECG.

191 i.   This is an apical four-chamber view. There is a large mass in the right atrium which appears to be attached to the atrial wall, rather than the septum, which makes it likely to be a thrombus (atrial myomata are usually attached to the septum).
   ii. It is unusual for a thrombus to develop following Swan-Ganz catheterisation. (There have, however been a few reported cases.) The patient had already had a small pulmonary embolus. There is a risk that a larger embolus may dislodge and embolise to the pulmonary arteries, with possible fatal consequences.

192 i.   This patient has a dual-chamber pacemaker. The first, fourth, sixth and eighth complexes are sequentially paced, i.e. the atrial impulse was sensed by the pacemaker. In the other complexes, the pacemaker spike occurred on or after the P wave, having failed to sense atrial activity.
   ii. This failure to sense atrial activity, known as undersensing, can usually be corrected by programming. Undersensing may also occur with component failure of the generator, inappropriate programming of sensitivity or refractory period and an abnormal (jammed) magnetic reed switch, which fails to restore sensing when the magnet is removed.

193 i.   This shows atrial synchronous pacing from a VAT mode pacemaker (also known as an atrial synchronous ventricular pacemaker). VAT pacing consists of a single, atrial sensing circuit that detects depolarisation and triggers ventricular stimulation after a pre-set, fixed interval that mimics the normal atrioventricular interval. DDD pacemakers can function in VAT mode since they have a ventricular pacing and atrial sensing mechanism. They do (normally) function in VAT mode when the spontaneous atrial (sinus) rate is such that the P wave is seen before completion of the atrial pacing escape interval.
   ii. Ventricular activity is not sensed, leading to possible competitive ventricular pacing and ventricular tachycardia. The disadvantage applies only to a VAT pacemaker and not to a DDD unit functioning in VAT mode. The advantage is the inherent ability to increase cardiac output during exercise, secondary to the associated increase in sinus rate.

194 i.   This patient is having pericardiocentesis. The ECG strip recording is directly from the aspiration needle. It shows the typical ST-segment elevation, due to myocardial injury, when the needle reaches the epicardium.
   ii. The risk of a life threatening complication is 0–5%. Haemopericardium secondary to laceration or puncture of the heart, leaking left ventricular or aortic aneurysm,

may occur. A rare complication is the development of ventricular dilatation and acute pulmonary oedema following the relief of cardiac tamponade.

195 i. The V wave is large (about 35 mmHg). The mean pressure is raised to about 20 mmHg. (Normally it is 1–10 mmHg.)

   ii. A large V wave may be seen in patients with mitral regurgitation. Pulmonary artery wedge pressure will be raised in mitral stenosis, reflecting raised left atrial pressure.

196 i. Thrombolysis.

   ii. The commonest complication of thrombolysis is bleeding which may occur cerebrally, intraperitoneally and pericardially. Therefore, if a patient requires the insertion of a temporary pacemaker or a central line, the subclavian vein route should be avoided because of the risk of increased bleeding from the vein or occidental arterial puncture. The internal jugular vein is a safer route. Reperfusion arrhythmias, both tachyarrhythmias and transient bradycardias may occur. Anaphylaxis or allergic reactions have been reported in 2–5% of patients. Anaphylactic shock occurs in up to 0.1% of patients.

197 i. There is a pressure gradient between the apex and the outflow tract of the LV, as well as between the apex of the LV and the aorta.

   ii. This is seen in hypertrophic cardiomyopathy (HCM).

   iii. Several factors have been postulated as possible causes for HCM. Asymmetrical septal hypertrophy has been used as a marker in demonstrating a familial component. Some studies have shown that this occurs on an autosomal dominant basis. Human leucocyte antigen HLA DRWH has been found to be associated with hypertrophic cardiomyopathy in several studies, indicating a genetic link. Some have postulated that HCM develops as a response to increased catecholamine stimulation. However, the true cause remains unknown.

198 i. This is a 12-lead ECG and a rhythm strip. The first and third complexes are sinus. The second is a premature ventricular beat (PVB) occurring on top of the T wave. The fourth, fifth and sixth are also PVBs, with the fourth occurring on top of the T wave. The second and fourth complexes represent the typical R on T appearance, which in this case has led to ventricular fibrillation (VF).

   ii. Ventricular fibrillation occurs with equal incidence in patients with anterior and inferior transmural infarctions. It is rare in patients with non-Q wave infarctions. About 60% of VF arrhythmia occurs in the first four hours and 80% within 12 hours from the onset of chest pain. This is called primary VF. Secondary VF occurs at an end stage of a progressive downhill course of left ventricular failure and cardiogenic shock. Those patients with anterior infarction and intraventricular conduction defects and those with atrial fibrillation, flutter or persistent sinus tachycardia are at a higher risk of developing VF late in their inpatient stay. (Note the ECG machine computer analysis of the ECG.)

199   Both atrioventricular valves (mitral and tricuspid) are recorded without interposing septal echoes. This echocardiographic image is seen in single ventricle hearts (which are also known as common ventricle or univentricle hearts). The clinical manifestations depend on the presence or absence of significant pulmonary stenosis or atresia. Common presenting features are cyanosis and congestive heart failure. The findings on palpatation and ascultation of the heart are not specific for a single ventricle but mimic those of a large ventricular septal defect, tetralogy of Fallot or transposition of the great vessels.

200   The circumflex coronary artery arises from the proximal segment of the right coronary artery. This occurs in less than 0.5% of the population. The circumflex coronary artery may arise from the right aortic sinus. In the absence of atherosclerosis in the coronary arteries, this anomaly has no great clinical significance.

201 i. Several complications after acute myocardial infarction are associated with a new systolic murmur and haemodynamic deterioration. These include rupture of the interventricular septum, papillary muscle disfunction or rupture, massive pulmonary embolism with right hear failure and tricuspid regurgitation, and right ventricular failure with tricuspid regurgitation.
    ii. An ECG may show conduction disturbances, including complete heart block which occurs in septal rupture. ST-segment elevation may be seen. Echocardiography is important in differentiating between septal rupture and acute mitral regurgitation. Right heart catheterisation offers a definitive diagnosis of a left-to-right shunt at ventricular level by documenting a 'step-up' in oxygen saturation in the right ventricle or main pulmonary artery. Left ventricular and coronary angiography are essential in defining the extent of coronary artery disease and locating the septal defect.

202   The patient probably has viral myocarditis which has progressed to heart failure. Electrocardiography will show a tachycardia and non-specific ST-segment and T wave changes. Echocardiography is important in detecting dilatation of the LV and diminished cardiac function. Serological tests are necessary to find the infectious agent. The results of these tests take time and therefore treatment should not be delayed.

203   Age, symptoms, family history and the absence of significant auscultatory findings (apart from the loud pulmonary sound) strongly suggest pulmonary hypertension. The sudden death in the family points towards primary pulmonary hypertension. Haemodynamic studies would reveal markedly raised pulmonary artery pressure and resistance with diminished cardiac output. Systemic arterial oxygen saturation may be reduced in some patients.

204   He appears to be tolerating the arrhythmia well. It is unlikely that DC cardioversion would be successful in restoring sinus rhythm as he must have been

in atrial fibrillation for the previous five years. Intravenous procainamide may be used to restore sinus rhythm but again the chronicity of the arrhythmia would make it unlikely. In this case the important thing is to control the ventricular rate by digoxin. A small dose of a beta-blocker may be added if there are no contraindications. Anticoagulants should be administered. If drugs fail to control the ventricular rate, ablation of the atrioventricular node and implantation of a permanent pacemaker should be considered.

205   This patient probably has significant coronary artery disease and will need urgent coronary angiography. His arrhythmia should be controlled until angiography is performed. If anti-arrhythmic agents fail, pacing the ventricle at a rate faster than the patient's own sinus rate may be successful. If the patient has no significant coronary artery disease, or the arrhythmia recurs despite anti-arrhythmic drugs, an implantable cardioverter/defibrillator should be considered.

206   The likely diagnosis is acute aortic dissection. However, a myocardial infarction should be excluded. Echocardiography (particularly trans-oesophageal) may confirm the diagnosis. Magnetic resonance imaging (MRI) or computed tomography (CT) are also diagnostic. Treatment depends on the type of dissection. Results from surgery are better than drug therapy in types I and II dissection. Urgent surgery is recommended in these patients. In patients with type III (distal) dissection, drug therapy is instituted. Surgery is performed if pain persists and the dissection is not stabilised.

207   Cardiac workload may double during the active stage of labour and women with even relatively mild cardiac disease may experience decompensation at this stage. The important objective is to reduce stress on the heart. Relief of pain, which causes less anxiety and reduces the swings in cardiac work, can be achieved by epidural anaesthesia. The second stage of labour should be shortened as much as possible, delivering by forceps if necessary. Caesarean section in women with functional classes I and II cardiac disease is indicated along the same lines as in healthy mothers; those with functional classes III and IV are at very high risk of maternal death. Caesarean section is indicated as the maternal mortality from vaginal delivery is more than 50%.

208   Hyperlipidaemia contributes to the development of coronary artery disease. Vein grafts tend to suffer from accelerated atherogenesis particularly in the presence of hyperlipidaemia. Dietary control is important and although the levels of cholesterol and triglycerides are not excessively high, lipid lowering agents should be introduced. As the triglycerides also are raised, fibrates rather than statins should be used in the first instance. The aim should be to achieve a total cholesterol level of less than 5.0 mmol/l.

ANSWERS

209   The left anterior descending coronary artery has occluded. Total arterial occlusion is the most common serious complication. It is usually due to a thrombus rather than arterial dissection and occurs within the first six hours post-operatively. Adequate anticoagulation with intravenous heparin and the administration of aspirin may prevent this complication. The patient should be re-studied and the artery re-opened. If attempts to open the artery fail, emergency coronary artery bypass surgery should be considered. The patient should be restudied by angiography.

210   Patients should be symptomatic either with intractable angina or refractory heart failure (ejection fraction of less than 20%). The gradient between the mean pulmonary artery and mean left atrial pressures should be less than 15 mmHg. The patient should be psychologically stable and motivated. There should be no sepsis or malignancy. Generalised atheroma, active peptic ulceration and recent pulmonary embolisation are exclusion criteria. The age cut-off varies from one centre to another. However, most centres have a cut-off at 55 years for ischaemic heart disease and 60 years for non-ischaemic cardiomyopathy.

211   The patient is still in the vulnerable period both for acute rejection and infection as a consequence of immunosuppression. A myocardial biopsy should be performed to exclude rejection. In the absence of rejection an infection screen is carried out. C-reactive protein, ESR, full blood picture, chest X-ray and blood culture are necessary. Viral, protozoal and fungal screens should be done. The lungs are the commonest site of infection, usually with *Nocardia spp.* Cytomegalovirus, *Toxoplasma* and *Aspergillus* organisms are common causes of infection in immunosuppressed patients.

212   The only abnormal finding is the systolic pressure gradient (35 mmHg) between the cavity of the left ventricle and the outflow tract. This indicates the presence of a narrowing in the left ventricular outflow tract. This could be due to subvalvar aortic stenosis or hypertrophic obstructive cardiomyopathy.

213   Pericardial effusion with tamponade is the likely diagnosis. An echocardiogram would confirm this. Urgent re-opening of the chest and drainage of the effusion is essential.

214   The most likely cause is right subclavian vein obstruction secondary to chronic low grade infection. Bilateral upper limb venogram should be done. It is likely that both subclavian veins are stenosed or occluded. If this is the case, the entire pacemaker system should be removed to prevent recurrence of infection in the new system. A new epicardial system should be implanted after a course of antibiotics (if both subclavian veins are occluded). If the patient is pacemaker-dependent, a temporary epicardial pacing system should be used.

215   This is most likely due to a break in the insulation along the pacing lead. As a result the conductor is in direct contact with the pectoral muscle, causing it to twitch at the same rate as that of the pacemaker. If the muscle twitch is occurring at low output, the pacing system should either be repaired or extracted and a new one implanted.

216   This patient is likely to have prosthetic valve endocarditis. Urea, creatinine, electrolytes, full blood picture, ESR and CRP should be done. The patient should be transferred to the cardio-surgical unit immediately. A further replacement of the valve is likely to be necessary. Blood cultures are important and several sets should be taken within 48 hours. A baseline chest X-ray is necessary to determine the presence of pulmonary congestion. Echocardiography is of value in looking for vegetations both on the prosthetic valve and other valves in the heart, assessing valve damage and monitoring left ventricular failure. Infective endocarditis causing severe congestive heart failure is associated with a 40-93% mortality. Other complications include myocardial infarction, conduction defects, emboli, metastatic infection, renal failure and central nervous system abnormalities.

217   Heightened awareness of the normal heart beat is the most common explanation for palpitations. However, an adequate history should distinguish this from palpitations due to tachyarrhythmia. Hyperthyroidism should be excluded. The presence of cardiac abnormalities that may cause arrhythmias, such as mitral valve prolapse and cardiomyopathy, can be excluded by echocardiography. Ambulatory ECG monitoring is a vital test in documenting any arrhythmias. However, the patient may not experience palpitations while wearing the recorder. In this case the patient is supplied with a cardiomemo to record the heart rate and rhythm whenever an attack occurs; he or she relays the recording to the hospital by telephone. Whether an arrhythmia is documented or not, electro-physiological studies should be undertaken because the palpitations were associated with near syncope. This is done not only to induce any arrhythmia but also to document the presence or absence of an accessory pathway and assess the option of management.

218   These show a gradient of 18 mmHg across the mitral valve, indicating significant mitral stenosis. In such a young patient it is unlikely that the valve would be calcified, and therefore percutaneous balloon mitral commissurotomy would be the treatment of choice. However, a trans-oesophageal echocardiogram should be carried out to exclude the presence of calcification and ensure there are no significant anatomical abnormalities.

219   This is probably called a runaway pacemaker and it constitutes a life-threatening condition. It is due to a technical fault with the pacemaker causing it to pace at a fixed fast rate. The treatment is the emergency exploration of the pacemaker. If the patient is pacemaker-dependent, a temporary pacing lead should be

inserted. However, if the pacing system is in a DDD mode, the patient may be having a supraventricular tachycardia which is tracking into the ventricular component of the pacing system, thus pacing the ventricle at the same rate as that of the atrium. This is unlikely to happen in a rate-responsive pacing mode as the upper rate limit is usually set at much lower than 210/minute.

220   The oxygen saturation in the left ventricle cavity is low with normal saturations in the other chambers. This suggests a right-to-left shunt across the two ventricles through a ventricular septal defect.

INDEX

Numbers refer to Question and Answer numbers.